THE ANATOMY OF THE EYE AND ORBIT

First Edition	.	.	.	.	.	1933
Reprinted .	.	.	.	.	.	1936
Reprinted .	.	.	.	.	.	1938
Reprinted .	.	.	.	.	.	1939
Second Edition	.	.	.	.	.	1940
Reprinted .	.	.	.	.	.	1942
Reprinted .	.	.	.	.	.	1945
Third Edition	.	.	.	.	.	1948
Reprinted .	.	.	.	.	.	1949
Reprinted .	.	.	.	.	.	1951
Fourth Edition	.	.	.	.	.	1954
Reprinted .	.	.	.	.	.	1958
Fifth Edition	.	.	.	.	.	1961
Reprinted .	.	.	.	.	.	1964
Reprinted .	.	.	.	.	.	1966
Sixth Edition	.	.	.	.	.	1968
Reprinted .	.	.	.	.	.	1969
Reprinted .	.	.	.	.	.	1970
Reprinted .	.	.	.	.	.	1972
Reprinted .	.	.	.	.	.	1973
Reprinted .	.	.	.	.	.	1975
Seventh Edition .	.	.	.	.	.	1976

EUGENE WOLFF'S

ANATOMY OF THE EYE AND ORBIT

Including the central connexions, development, and comparative anatomy of the visual apparatus

SEVENTH EDITION

Revised by

ROGER WARWICK

B.Sc., Ph.D., M.D. (GOLD MEDAL).

PROFESSOR OF ANATOMY, UNIVERSITY OF LONDON,
DEPARTMENT OF ANATOMY, GUY'S HOSPITAL MEDICAL SCHOOL,
EXAMINER IN THE UNIVERSITIES OF
LONDON, MANCHESTER, OXFORD, LIVERPOOL, BELFAST, HONG KONG,
SINGAPORE, ROYAL COLLEGE OF SURGEONS OF ENGLAND
SOCIETY OF APOTHECARIES OF LONDON

WITH 467 ILLUSTRATIONS, INCLUDING
56 IN COLOUR

W. B. SAUNDERS COMPANY
Philadelphia and Toronto

Library of Congress Catalog Card Number 76-17429

ISBN 0 7216 9124 2

PRINTED IN GREAT BRITAIN

PREFACE TO THE SEVENTH EDITION

EUGENE WOLFF'S book has now passed through six editions and ten reprints in less than forty years, growing in pages from 309 to 553 and in illustrations from 173 (initially none in colour) to 467 (56 in colour). Both text and illustrations contain much that is of historical interest, and—like my predecessor—I have wished to avoid tampering unnecessarily with the author's creation. However, very considerable changes have been necessary which have entailed a rewriting of about a quarter of the text. Only the chapters on the osseous orbit and comparative anatomy have required less extensive deletions and replacement by new writing. In all sections many old citations (limited in interest and often undocumented) have been omitted; and yet the Bibliography has almost doubled in length, a measure of the injection of new contributions. The accumulations of knowledge, particularly in such fields as the ultrastructural detail of ocular tissues, analysis of ocular movements, and organization in the visual pathways, have demanded particular attention; and it is to these that revision has been deliberately directed. These and other fields of study have evoked many highly specialized monographs and a countless legion of original papers, many of which can only be quoted briefly. But it is my belief that readers of such a generalized textbook as this will thus find useful signposts by which to look elsewhere for further detail.

There are 75 new illustrations in this edition, the majority being replacements. In this regard I am much indebted to my friend, Mr. Richard E. M. Moore, D.F.A. (London), M.M.A.A., F.R.S.A., who works in my own department; he has contributed 28 new illustrations and diagrams. I am also most grateful to Dr. John Marshall and his assistant, Mr. P. L. Ansell (both of the Institute of Ophthalmology, University of London), who have provided much improved substitutes for 40 electron- and photo-micrographs. I must also thank Dr. N. A. Locket (of the same Institute) for the loan of preparations for photomicrography. My colleagues, Mr. Kevin Fitzpatrick and Mr. Joe Curtis, have also helped in the replacement of several illustrations. Dr. Gordon Ruskell (The City University, London) has helped with much useful criticism. From the publishing staff, and particularly Mr. John Goodhall, I have received most efficient and patient support. Despite all this help I am solely responsible for any inaccuracies and omissions in this text. While hoping that readers will find it improved in its usefulness, I hope equally that they will volunteer their criticisms and suggestions.

ROGER WARWICK

GUY'S HOSPITAL MEDICAL SCHOOL,
UNIVERSITY OF LONDON, S.E.1.

February 1976

EXTRACTS FROM
PREFACE TO THE FIRST EDITION

THIS *Anatomy of the Eye and Orbit* is based mainly on lectures and demonstrations which I have had the honour to give during ten years as Demonstrator of Anatomy at University College, and for the last three years as Pathologist and Lecturer in Anatomy to the Royal Westminster Ophthalmic Hospital.

It is an attempt to present to the Student and Ophthalmic Surgeon the essentials of the structure, development, and comparative anatomy of the visual apparatus in conjunction with some of their clinical applications. The motor nerves to the eye muscles have received special attention, as have also the illustrations, many of which are from my own preparations.

EUGENE WOLFF.

HARLEY STREET,
    LONDON, W.1.
  1933

CONTENTS

ANATOMY OF THE EYE AND ORBIT

CHAPTER I

THE BONY ORBIT AND PARANASAL SINUSES

THE BONY ORBIT

THE two orbital cavities are placed on either side of the sagittal plane of the skull between the cranium and the skeleton of the face. Thus situated they encroach about equally on these two regions (Winckler, 1927).

Above each orbit is the anterior cranial fossa, medially are the nasal cavity and ethmoidal air sinuses, below is the maxillary sinus (antrum), while laterally from behind forwards are the middle cranial and the temporal fossæ.

The orbit is essentially intended as a socket for the eyeball and also contains the muscles, nerves and vessels, which are essential for its proper functioning. Moreover, it serves to transmit certain vessels and nerves destined to supply the areas of the face around the orbital aperture. Seven bones take part in the formation of the orbit, namely: the maxilla and palatine, the frontal, the sphenoid and zygomatic bone, the ethmoid and the lacrimal bone.

The orbit has *roughly* the shape of a quadrilateral pyramid whose base, directed forwards, laterally and slightly downwards, corresponds to the orbital margin, and whose apex is the optic foramen or, as some hold, the medial end of the superior orbital fissure; or the bar of bone between these two apertures (Whitnall, 1911).

As stated above, the comparison with a quadrilateral pyramid is a rough one only, for since the floor (which is the shortest orbital wall) does not reach the apex, the cavity is triangular on section in this region.

Also, since the orbit is developed around the eye, and is bulged out by the lacrimal gland, it has a tendency towards being spheroidal in form, and its widest part is not at the orbital margin but about 1·5 cm behind this. Moreover, this results in the fact that its four walls are for the most part separated from each other by ill-defined rounded borders, so that Whitnall compares the shape of the orbit to a pear whose stalk is the optic canal. It is important to note that the medial walls of the orbits are almost parallel, whereas the lateral walls make an angle of about 90° with each other. The direction of each orbit is given by its axis which runs from behind forwards, laterally and slightly downwards.

The roof or vault of the orbit is triangular in shape. It is formed in great part by the triangular orbital plate of the frontal bone and behind this by the lesser

1

wing of the sphenoid. It does not look directly downwards but slightly forwards as well. It is markedly concave anteriorly and more or less flat posteriorly. The anterior concavity is greatest about 1·5 cm from the orbital margin and corresponds to the equator of the globe.

It presents:

(a) *The fossa* for the lacrimal gland. This lies behind the zygomatic process of the frontal bone. It is simply a slight increase in the general concavity of the anterior and lateral part of the roof, and is better appreciated by touch than by sight. It contains not only the lacrimal gland but also some orbital fat found principally at its posterior part (accessory fossa of Rochon-Duvigneaud). It is bounded below by the ridge corresponding to the zygomaticofrontal suture, at the junction of roof and lateral wall of the orbit. It is usually quite smooth, but may be pitted by the attachment of the suspensory ligament of the lacrimal gland when this is well developed.

(b) *The fovea* for the *trochlea* of the superior oblique is a small depression situated close to the frontolacrimal suture some 4 mm from the orbital margin (Figs. 1 and 2). Sometimes (10 per cent) the ligaments which attach the U-shaped cartilage of the pulley to it are ossified. Then the fovea is surmounted most often posteriorly by a spicule of bone (the *Spina trochlearis*). Extremely rarely a ring of bone, representing the trochlea completely ossified, may be seen (Winckler). Above the fovea the frontal sinus separates the two plates of the frontal bone; the cavity extends lateral and posterior from the fovea to a very variable extent.

(c) *The frontosphenoidal suture*, which is usually obliterated in the adult, lies here between the orbital plate of the frontal bone and the lesser wing of the sphenoid.

The roof of the orbit is separated from the medial wall by fine sutures between the frontal bone above and the ethmoid, lacrimal and frontal process, and those of the maxilla below. In or just above the frontoethmoidal suture are the anterior and posterior ethmoidal canals (Figs. 1 and 2). The roof is separated from the lateral wall posteriorly by the superior orbital fissure, anteriorly by the slight ridge that marks the frontozygomatic suture. The orbital aspect of the roof is usually quite smooth, but may be marked by certain small apertures and depressions. The apertures known as the *Cribra orbitalia* are most commonly apparent to the medial side of the anterior portion of the lacrimal fossa. They are not always present and are best marked in the fetus and infant (Winckler). They give the bone a porous appearance, and, according to Toldt, are for veins which pass from the diploë to the orbit.

In the posterior part of the orbit, in or around the lateral part of the lesser wing of the sphenoid, small orifices may also be found which serve as communications between the orbit and the cranial dura mater and contain vessels during life.

Numerous small grooves may be seen in the roof of the orbit. These lead to the above orifices and are made by vessels or nerves.

THE BONY ORBIT AND PARANASAL SINUSES

Very rarely one may find an anteroposterior fissure up to 14 mm long with periorbita and dura mater.

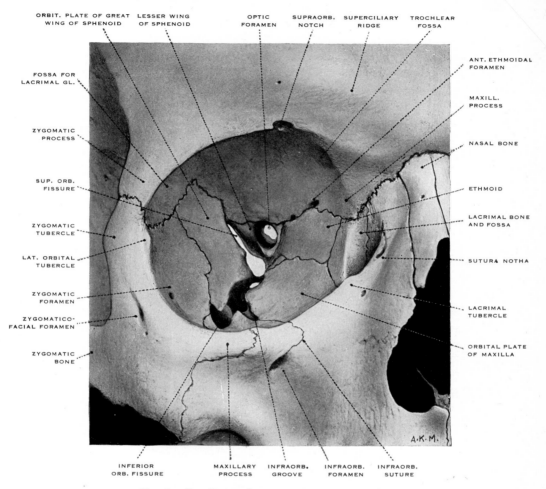

FIG. 1.—THE RIGHT ORBIT VIEWED ALONG ITS AXIS.

Structure.—The roof of the orbit is very thin, translucent and fragile except where it is formed by the lesser wing of the sphenoid, which is 3 mm thick. If the bone be held up to the light, one can make out the ridges and depressions on the cranial aspect formed by the sulci and gyri of the frontal lobe of the brain. This is especially true of the posterior two-thirds. The translucency of the anterior third enables the outline of the orbital extension of the frontal sinus to be seen.

Occasionally in old age portions of the bone may be absorbed, and then the periorbita is in direct contact with the dura mater of the anterior cranial fossa.

It is quite easy, in the disarticulated skull, to break the roof of the orbit by slight pressure with the finger.

Penetrating wounds through the lids are sometimes inflicted with the points of umbrellas or walking-sticks, and the roof of the orbit may easily be fractured by direct violence, leading to frontal lobe injury.

The roof of the orbit is invaded to a varying extent by the frontal sinus and sometimes by the ethmoidal sinuses. The frontal sinus may extend laterally to the zygomatic process and backwards close to the optic foramen. The sphenoidal or the posterior ethmoidal sinuses not infrequently invade the lesser wing of the sphenoid and the former may surround, more or less completely, the optic canal.

Relations.—The frontal nerve lies in direct contact with the periorbita for the whole extent of the roof (Figs. 278 and 279). The supraorbital artery accompanies it only in the anterior half. Beneath the nerve is the levator palpebræ, and deep to this again is the superior rectus.

The trochlear nerve lies medially, in contact with the periorbita, on its way to the superior oblique muscle.

The lacrimal gland adjoins the lacrimal fossa, and the superior oblique lies at the junction of the roof and the medial walls.

Invading the roof to a variable extent, as seen above, are the frontal and the ethmoidal sinuses; the former usually extends to about its midpoint. Above the roof are the meninges covering the frontal lobe of the brain (Fig. 282).

The medial wall of the orbit (Fig. 2) is the only wall which is not obviously triangular. It is roughly oblong, either quite flat or slightly convex towards the orbital cavity. It runs parallel with the sagittal plane, and consists from before backwards of four bones united by vertical sutures.

(*a*) The frontal process of the maxilla.

(*b*) The lacrimal bone.

(*c*) The orbital plate of the ethmoid.

(*d*) A small part of the body of the sphenoid.

Of these the orbital plate of the ethmoid takes by far the largest portion. It often shows a characteristic mosaic of light and dark areas. The dark areas correspond to the ethmoidal sinuses, while the light lines between them correspond to the partitions between the cells (Fig. 19).

In the anterior part of this wall is the *lacrimal fossa*, formed by the frontal process of the maxilla and the lacrimal bone. It is bounded in front and behind by the *anterior* and *posterior lacrimal crests*. Above there is no definite boundary, while below the fossa is continuous with the bony nasolacrimal canal. At their point of junction the hamulus of the lacrimal bone curves round from the posterior to the anterior lacrimal crest and bounds the fossa to the lateral side (Fig. 2). At this point the fossa is some 5 mm deep, while it gradually gets shallower as we trace it upwards. It is about 14 mm in height. The lacrimal bone and frontal process of the maxilla take varying parts in the formation of the fossa; and so the position of the vertical suture between them varies also.

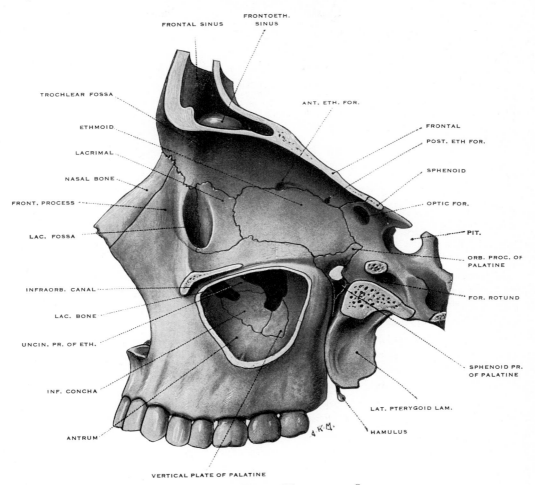

FIG. 2.—THE MEDIAL WALL OF THE ORBIT.

The anterior lacrimal crest on the frontal process of the maxilla is ill-defined above but well marked below, where it becomes continuous with the lower orbital margin and here often presents a *lacrimal tubercle* (Fig. 1).

The lacrimal bone separates the upper half of the fossa from the anterior ethmoidal sinuses, and the lower part from the middle meatus of the nose (see also p. 229).

The Structure of the medial wall.—The medial is by far the thinnest orbital wall (0·2–0·4 mm). It is translucent, so that if held up to the light, the ethmoidal sinuses can be plainly seen, and they usually produce a mosaic pattern upon the wall.

The orbital plate of the ethmoid, as its former name (lamina papyracea) implies, is, in fact, as thin as paper, and infection from the ethmoidal sinuses can easily get into the orbit. *This is the reason why ethmoiditis is the commonest cause of orbital cellulitis.*

Despite its thinness, however, the orbital plate but rarely shows senile absorptive changes, whereas the thicker lacrimal bone, especially that portion which enters into the formation of the lacrimal fossa, is often absorbed.

VARIETIES.—The lacrimal bone may be divided by accessory sutures into several parts (Schwegel, Henle, Hyrtl).

A sutural bone may be developed in its upper and fore part.

An accessory lacrimal bone, such as is found in many lower animals, may be split off the front of the ethmoid.

The hamulus may be absent, may exist as a separate bone, or may be double.

Relations.—Through the medial wall lie, from before backwards (Fig. 3), the lateral wall of the nose, the infundibulum and ethmoidal sinuses, and the sphenoidal air sinus. The optic foramen lies at the posterior end of the medial wall (Fig. 2).

The superior oblique occupies the angle between the roof and medial wall, and the medial rectus runs along this wall, while between the two muscles are the anterior and posterior ethmoidal and the infratrochlear nerves and the termination of the ophthalmic artery (Fig. 279).

Anteriorly the lacrimal sac lies in its fossa, surrounded by the lacrimal fascia, while just behind it is the attachment of the lacrimal fibres of orbicularis oculi (Horner's muscle), the septum orbitale, and the check ligament of the medial rectus (Figs. 222 and 223).

The floor of the orbit is roughly triangular, corresponding to the shape of the roof. It is not quite horizontal, but slopes slightly downwards from the medial to the lateral side. The lowest part of the floor of the orbit is found in a concavity some 3 mm deep at the lateral and anterior part. The floor (47·6 mm long), the shortest of the orbital boundaries, is formed by three bones:

(1) The orbital plate of the *maxilla*.

(2) The orbital surface of the *zygomatic*.

(3) The orbital process of the *palatine bone*.

Of these the *maxilla* takes by far the largest portion. The *zygomatic* forms the anterolateral part, while the *palatine bone* occupies a small area behind the maxilla.

The floor of the orbit is traversed by the *infraorbital sulcus*, which runs almost straight forwards from the inferior orbital (sphenomaxillary) fissure. At a variable distance (usually about half-way) it is converted into a *canal* by a plate of bone which grows over it from its *lateral* side to meet the medial in a suture (the infraorbital suture), which is but rarely obliterated (Fig. 3). This suture can be traced over the lower orbital margin to the medial side of, and into, the infraorbital foramen (Fig. 1). It sometimes cuts across the zygomaticomaxillary suture.

The infraorbital canal, formed as described above, sinks anteriorly into the orbital floor and opens at the infraorbital foramen some 4 mm from the orbital

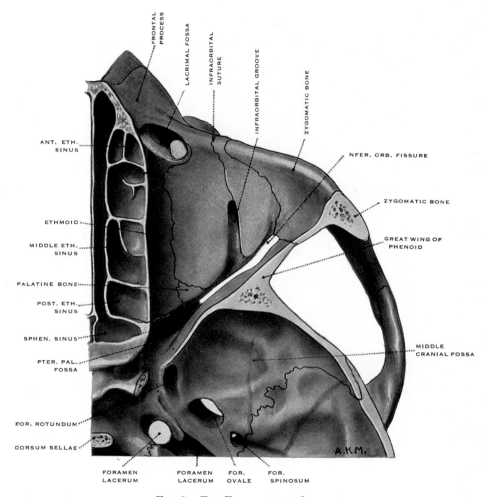

FIG. 3.—THE FLOOR OF THE ORBIT.

margin. It transmits the infraorbital vessels and nerve. Along its course it gives off the *middle* and *anterior superior alveolar (dental) canals* for the corresponding nerves and vessels.

Lateral to the opening of the nasolacrimal canal a small pit or roughness marking the origin of the inferior oblique muscle may (rarely) be found.

The floor of the orbit is separated from the medial wall only by a fine suture; the lateral wall is separated from it posteriorly by the inferior orbital (spheno-maxillary) fissure, while anteriorly it is continuous with it (Fig. 3).

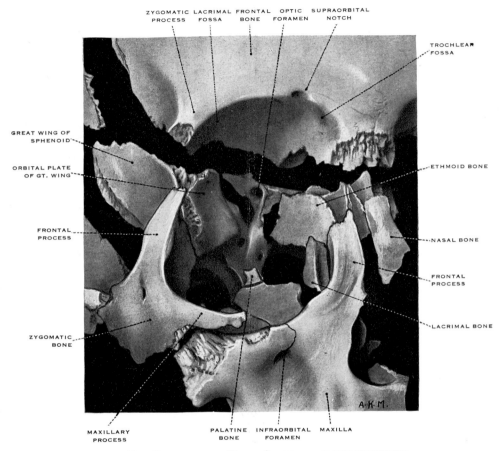

FIG 4.—THE BONES OF THE RIGHT ORBIT *IN SITU* BUT SEPARATED.

VARIETIES.—Not infrequently the roof of the infraorbital canal and sometimes its floor may be incomplete, but otherwise only very rarely does the floor of the orbit show holes, the result of senile absorption. Langer has seen three cases where the infraorbital canal ran in the suture between the maxilla and the zygomatic bone.

Relations and Structure.—*Below* the floor of the orbit for nearly its whole extent is the maxillary sinus, a most important practical relation. *For as the bone between them is only 0·5–1 mm thick, tumours of the sinus can easily invade the orbit, causing proptosis.* It is in fact thinnest at the inferior orbital groove and canal (Fig. 14).

More posteriorly is a small sinus in the orbital process of the palatine bone and sometimes extensions from the ethmoidal sinuses may invade the floor.

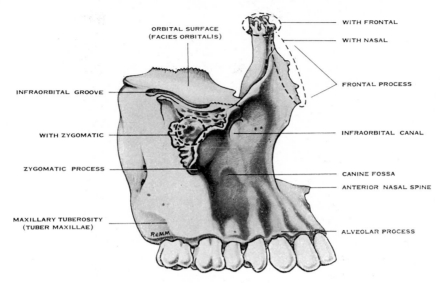

FIG. 5.—RIGHT MAXILLA (LATERAL ASPECT).

The inferior rectus is in contact with the floor near the apex of the orbit, but anteriorly it is some distance away, being separated from it by the inferior oblique muscle and some fat. Lateral to the inferior rectus and lying on its lateral edge or between it and the lateral rectus is the nerve to the inferior oblique (Fig. 283).

The inferior oblique arises just lateral to the opening of the nasolacrimal canal and passes backwards, laterally and upwards for the most part near the floor (Fig. 277).

The infraorbital vessels and nerve lie in the infraorbital sulcus and canal.

The lateral wall of the orbit is triangular in shape, the base being anterior. It makes an angle of 45° with the median sagittal plane and faces medially, forwards and slightly upwards in its lower part. It is slightly convex posteriorly, flat at its centre, while anteriorly the orbital surface of the zygomatic bone 1 cm behind the orbital margin is concave.

The lateral wall of the orbit is formed by two bones:

(*a*) Posteriorly by the orbital surface of the greater wing of the sphenoid.

(*b*) Anteriorly by the orbital surface of the zygomatic (malar) bone.

The sphenoidal portion is sharply separated from the roof and floor by the superior and inferior orbital fissures respectively.

The zygomatic portion passes imperceptibly into the floor, and is separated from the roof by the frontozygomatic suture, which is roughly horizontal and

A.E.—2

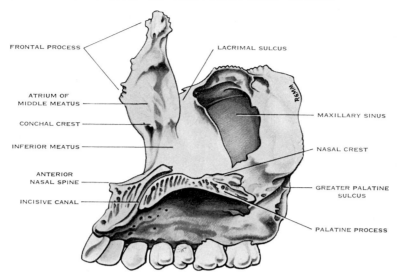

FIG. 6.—RIGHT MAXILLA (MEDIAL ASPECT).

often marked by a slight ridge. The suture between the two portions of the lateral wall is vertical (Fig. 1).

The lateral wall presents:

(1) *The Spina recti lateralis.*—This is a small bony projection situated on the inferior margin of the superior orbital fissure at the junction of its wide and narrow portions. It may be pointed, rounded or grooved, and gives origin to a part of the lateral rectus muscle, but it is produced mainly by a groove which lodges the superior ophthalmic vein. This groove is prolonged upwards, then runs anterior to the spine. Not infrequently the spine is duplicated.

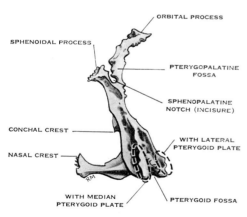

FIG. 7—RIGHT PALATINE BONE (POSTERIOR ASPECT).

(2) *The Zygomatic Groove and Foramen.*—The groove which lodges the nerve and vessels of the same name runs from the anterior end of the inferior orbital fissure to a foramen in the zygomatic bone. This leads into a canal which divides into two, one branch opening on the cheek, the other in the temporal fossa. Thus the branches of the zygomatic nerve reach their destination. If the nerve divides before entering its canal, there may be two or even three grooves and foramina in the orbit.

(3) *The Lateral Orbital Tubercle* (Whitnall).—This is a small elevation on the orbital surface of the zygomatic bone just within the lateral orbital margin and about 11 mm below the frontozygomatic suture. It gives attachment to:

(*a*) The check ligament of the lateral rectus muscle.

(*b*) The suspensory ligament of the eyeball.

(*c*) The aponeurosis of the levator palpebræ superioris (Fig. 277).

(4) Not infrequently there is a foramen in or near the suture between the greater wing of the sphenoid with the frontal, near the lateral end of the superior orbital fissure. This leads from the orbit to the middle cranial fossa, and transmits a branch of the meningeal artery and a small vein.

Structure.—Being the one most exposed to stress, the lateral is the thickest of the orbital walls, and is especially strong at the orbital margin. Behind this is a relatively weaker part, then comes a thicker portion, and the most posterior portion, walling in the middle cranial fossa, is thinner again (Fig. 3). The most posterior is, in fact, the feeblest portion. Here on either side of the sphenozygomatic suture it is only 1 mm thick and its lamellar structure makes it translucent. In 30 per cent of cases, according to Nippert, there exist in this area supplementary fissures which represent the extensive primitive communication between the orbit and the temporal fossa.

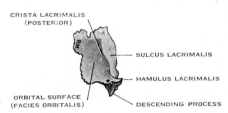

FIG. 8—RIGHT LACRIMAL BONE
(LATERAL ASPECT)

Relations.—The lateral wall separates the orbit *anteriorly* from the temporal fossa containing the temporal muscle; posteriorly from the middle cranial fossa and the temporal lobe of the brain (Figs. 3 and 284).

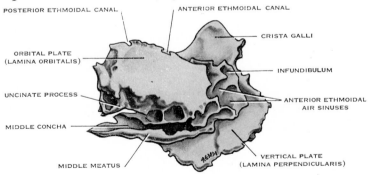

FIG. 9.—THE ETHMOID BONE (RIGHT LATERAL ASPECT).

Inside the orbit the lateral rectus muscle is in contact with the whole of this wall. Above it are the lacrimal nerve and artery.

The spina recti lateralis and the *orbital tubercle* with their attachments have already been described, as has the zygomatic canal and its contents.

The lacrimal gland reaches down on to the lateral wall, and the *lacrimal nerve* receives a parasympathetic branch from the zygomatic (Fig. 283).

The following **fissures** and **canals** lie between the various orbital walls:

The superior orbital (sphenoidal) fissure.

The inferior orbital (sphenomaxillary) fissure.

The anterior and posterior ethmoidal canals.

The superior orbital (sphenoidal) fissure lies between the roof and lateral wall of the orbit. It is the gap between the lesser and greater wings of the sphenoid, and is closed laterally by the frontal bone.

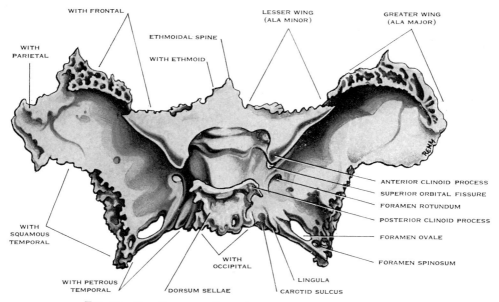

FIG. 10.—THE SPHENOID BONE (SUPERIOR, ENDOCRANIAL ASPECT).

It is wider at the medial end, where it lies below the optic foramen, and is often described as comma- or retort-shaped. Sometimes there is gradual reduction in size towards the lateral extremity, but usually it is composed of two limbs, a narrow *lateral* portion and a wider *medial* part. At the junction of the two limbs is the *spine* for the *rectus lateralis* (Fig. 1).

The superior orbital fissure is some 22 mm long, and is the largest communication between the orbit and the middle cranial fossa. Its tip is 30 to 40 mm from the frontozygomatic suture. Its medial end is separated from the optic foramen by the posterior root of the lesser wing of the sphenoid on which is found the infraoptic tubercle. This lies below and lateral to the optic foramen on the middle of the vertical part of the medial border of the wide part of the superior orbital fissure (Fig. 1).

The common tendinous ring (*anulus tendineus communis*) spans the superior orbital fissure between the wide medial and narrow lateral parts. The lateral rectus arises here, from both margins of the fissure.

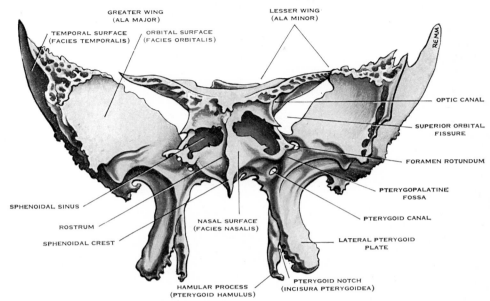

FIG. 11.—THE SPHENOID BONE (ANTERIOR ASPECT).

One or more frontosphenoidal foramina may be present in the frontosphenoidal suture and transmit an anastomosis between the middle meningeal and the lacrimal arteries.

According to Hovelacque *the lateral limb is closed by dura mater and nothing passes through it.* This is not the usual teaching, but it is borne out by my own (Eugene Wolff) dissections (Figs. 261 and 262). Passing above the anulus are the trochlear, frontal, and lacrimal nerves, superior ophthalmic vein, and the recurrent lacrimal artery.

Passing within the anulus or between the two heads of the lateral rectus are

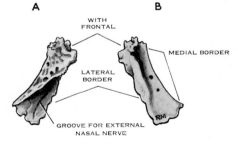

FIG. 12.—THE RIGHT NASAL BONE
(A, MEDIAL ASPECT; B, LATERAL ASPECT).

the superior division of the oculomotor nerve, the nasociliary and sympathetic root of the ciliary ganglion, the inferior division of the oculomotor nerve, then the abducent nerve (and then sometimes the ophthalmic vein or veins)—in that order from above downwards. The abducent nerve is actually passing from below the inferior division of the oculomotor nerve to lie lateral and between the two divisions (Fig. 263).

As a rule nothing passes below the anulus, rarely the inferior ophthalmic vein.

The inferior orbital (sphenomaxillary) fissure lies between the lateral wall and floor of the orbit. Through it the orbit communicates with the pterygopalatine and infratemporal fossæ. It commences below and lateral to the optic foramen, close to the medial end of the superior orbital fissure. It runs forwards and laterally for some 20 mm, its anterior extremity reaching to about 2 cm from the inferior orbital margin (Figs. 1 and 3).

The inferior orbital fissure is bounded anteriorly by the maxilla and the orbital process of the palatine bone; posteriorly by the whole of the lower margin of the orbital surface of the greater wing of the sphenoid. In the majority of cases it is closed anteriorly by the zygomatic (malar) bone.

The fissure is narrower at its centre than at its two extremities, the anterior end sometimes being markedly expanded.

The width of the inferior orbital fissure depends on the development of the maxillary sinus and thus is relatively wide in the fœtus and infant. The lateral border is sharp and may have grooves above and below it; it is higher than the medial border anteriorly, but lower posteriorly. It is closed in the living by periorbita and the muscle of Müller (p. 270).

The inferior orbital fissure is near the openings of the foramen rotundum and the sphenopalatine foramen (Figs. 1 and 2). It transmits the infraorbital nerve, the zygomatic nerve, branches to the orbital periosteum from the pterygopalatine ganglion, and a communication between the inferior ophthalmic vein and the pterygoid plexus (Fig. 282).

The ethmoidal foramina lie between the roof and medial wall of the orbit either in the frontoethmoidal suture *or actually in the frontal bone*. They are the openings of canals which are formed in greater part by the frontal but are completed by the ethmoidal (Figs. 1, 2, 9 and 19).

The anterior ethmoidal canal is inclined posterolaterally. Its posterior border is ill-defined and continuous with a groove on the orbital plate of the ethmoid. It opens in the anterior cranial fossa at the side of the cribriform plate of the ethmoid, and transmits the anterior ethmoidal nerve and artery.

The posterior ethmoidal canal transmits the posterior ethmoidal nerve and artery. Supplementary foramina are common.

The optic foramen, or rather the **optic canal**, leads from the middle cranial fossa to the apex of the orbit, and it is formed by the two roots of the lesser wing of the sphenoid. It is directed forwards, laterally, and somewhat downwards, its axis making an angle of about 36° with the median sagittal plane. If produced forwards, the axis passes approximately through the middle of the inferolateral quadrant of the orbital opening. Hence it is neither in the axis of the orbit nor in that of its lateral wall. If produced backwards it meets its fellow at the dorsum sellæ at an angle of 90°. The canal is funnel-shaped, the mouth of the funnel being the anterior opening. This is oval in shape, with the greatest diameter vertical. The cranial opening, on the other hand, is flattened from above down, while in its middle portion the canal is circular on section. With regard to the intra-cranial opening, the upper and lower borders are sharp, the medial and lateral rounded. The interoptic groove is thus continuous with the medial wall without line of demarcation (Fig. 10). Rarely, the optic foramen may be double (Warwick).

The lateral border of the orbital opening is more or less well defined. It is formed by the anterior border of the posterior root of the lesser wing of the sphenoid. The medial border is less well defined.

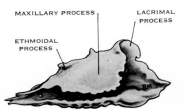

FIG. 13.—THE RIGHT INFERIOR CONCHA (LATERAL ASPECT).

The distance between the intracranial openings of the two canals is 25 mm. The distance between the orbital openings is 30 mm.

The roof of the canal reaches farther forwards than the floor, while posteriorly the floor projects beyond the roof. This gap in the roof is filled in by a fold of dura mater with a free posterior edge (the falciform fold) (Fig. 274).

The optic canal is close to the sphenoidal air sinus, sometimes to a posterior ethmoidal sinus. According to Fazakas (1933), the longer the optic canal, the thinner its medial wall and the more likely it is to encroach on a posterior ethmoidal sinus. Often only a very thin plate of bone separates the optic canal from these. At times the canal makes a ridge inside the sinus. Not infrequently the sinus or a posterior ethmoidal sinus may invade the lesser wing to a greater or smaller degree, and they have been known to surround the canal completely. Above the canal is the posterior part of the gyrus rectus and olfactory tract.

The optic canal is separated from the medial end of the superior orbital fissure by a bar of bone, on which there is a tubercle or roughness for the anulus tendineus (Fig. 1). It transmits the optic nerve and its coverings of dura, arachnoid, and pia (Figs. 293, 294) (p. 325); the ophthalmic artery which lies here below then lateral to the nerve and embedded in its dural sheath (Figs. 294, 295); and a few twigs from the sympathetic which accompany the artery. Separating artery and nerve is a layer of fibrous tissue which may (rarely) be ossified.

The average measurements of the optic canal are as follows:

The orbital opening is 6 to 6·5 mm by 4·5 to 5 mm.

In the middle portion it is 5 by 5 mm.

The canal is further narrowed by the periosteum.

The lateral wall is 5 to 7 mm long, which is the width of the posterior root of the lesser wing of the sphenoid. The roof, 10 to 12 mm in length, varies with the development of the lesser wing of the sphenoid between the anterior clinoid process and the body of the sphenoid. The upper and medial walls are longer than

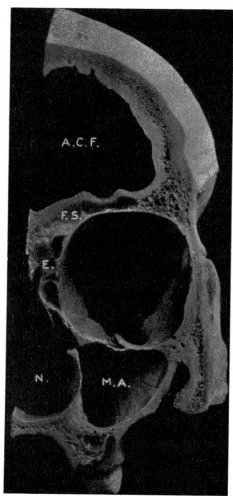

FIG. 14.—FRONTAL SECTION OF THE LEFT HALF OF SKULL JUST BEHIND ORBITAL MARGIN AND PASSING THROUGH LARGEST PART OF CAVITY (GREATEST ORBITAL HEIGHT = 37·5 MM); SEEN FROM IN FRONT. NATURAL SIZE.

The floor of the orbit is deeply grooved by the infraorbital sulcus.

A.C.F. = Anterior cranial fossa.
F.S.   = Frontal sinus.
E.   = Ethmoidal sinuses.
N.   = Nasal cavity.
M.A.   = Maxillary sinus (showing the ostium maxillare).
(From Whitnall, 1932.)

the others. The longer the optic canal, the narrower it is, and *vice versa* (Fazakas).

A thorough investigation of the optic canal shows that variations in contour, as seen radiologically, are produced by the development of the lower root of the lesser wing of the sphenoid (Kier, 1966).

The orbital margin is most commonly quadrilateral with rounded corners. The orbital margin usually has the form of a spiral; the inferior orbital margin is continuous with the anterior lacrimal crest, while the superior is continued down into the posterior lacrimal crest. The lacrimal fossa thus lies in the orbital margin (Poirier).

Each side measures some 40 mm, but usually the width is greater than the height; the relation between the two is given by the *orbital index*,[1] which varies in the different races of mankind. The opening is directed forwards and slightly laterally, and is tilted so that the upper and lower margins slope gently downwards from the medial to the lateral side.

The orbital margin is made up of three bonds, the frontal, zygomatic, and maxilla.

[1] The orbital index (of Broca)—
$$= \frac{\text{Height of Orbit} \times 100}{\text{Width of Orbit}}$$

Taking the orbital index as the standard, three classes of orbit are recognised:

1. *Megaseme (large).*—The orbital index is 89 or over. This type is characteristic of the yellow races, except the Esquimaux. The orbital opening is round.

2. *Mesoseme (intermediate).*—Orbital index between 89 and 83. This type is found in the white races (European 87, English 88·4, according to Flower).

3. *Microseme (small).*—Orbital index 83 or less. This type is characteristic of the black races. The orbital opening is rectangular.

The superior orbital margin is formed entirely of the frontal bone, i.e. by its orbital arch.

It is generally concave downwards, convex forwards, sharp in its lateral two-thirds, and rounded in the medial third. At the junction of the two portions, some 25 mm from the mid-line and situated at the highest part of the arch, is the *supraorbital notch*, whose lateral border is usually sharper than the medial. Not infrequently it is converted into a foramen by the ossification of the ligament which closes it below. The posterior opening then is 3 to 6 mm from the orbital margin. It transmits the supraorbital nerve and vessels. Notch and foramen are easily palpable in the living.

Sometimes medial to this a second notch (of Arnold) or foramen is found. This transmits the medial branches of the supraorbital nerves and vessels where these have divided inside the orbit.

Supraorbital grooves leading from these notches or foramina are sometimes seen.

A groove may also be present some 10 mm medial to the supraorbital notch for the supratrochlear nerve and artery.

A supraciliary canal (Ward, 1858) is found in about half the cases (Fig. 1). It is a small opening near the supraorbital notch, and transmits a nutrient artery and a branch of the supraorbital nerve to the frontal air sinus.

The lateral orbital margin, being the most exposed to stress, is the strongest portion of the orbital outlet. It is formed by the zygomatic process of the frontal and by the zygomatic bone. If looked at from the side it appears to be concave forwards and not to reach as far forward as the medial margin.

In the sphenozygomatic suture there are not infrequently ossicles resembling the Wormian bones of the cranium.

Another suture occurs in 21·1 per cent of Japanese skulls, in which the zygomatic bone may be in two parts (*Os Japonicum*).

The inferior orbital margin is raised slightly above the floor of the orbit. It is formed by the zygomatic bone and the maxilla, usually in equal portions.

The zygomatic portion forms a long thin spur (the maxillary or marginal process) which lies on the maxilla (Figs. 1 and 4).

The suture between the two, which is not infrequently marked by a tubercle, can be felt lying usually about half-way along the margin just above the infra-orbital foramen (Fig. 1).

Sometimes, however, the zygomatic (malar) may reach the anterior lacrimal crest, thus excluding the maxilla, or may take only a very small part itself in the formation of this margin.

The medial margin is formed by the anterior lacrimal crest on the frontal process of the maxilla and the posterior lacrimal crest on the lacrimal bone. These crests overlap; the medial margin is thus not a continuous ridge, but runs up from the anterior lacrimal crest across the frontal process of the maxilla to the superior margin (Fig. 1).

Age and Sex Changes

The changes in the orbit during the period of growth depend partly on the development of the cranium and skeleton of the face, between which the orbit is placed, and also on the growth of the neighbouring air sinuses.

The orbital margin is sharp and well ossified at birth. As Fisher (1904) points out: "The eyeball is therefore well protected from stress and injury during parturition. When we recollect the relatively large size and the advanced stage of development of the eye at birth, it is clearly specially desirable that such protection should be afforded; that it is efficacious, the rarity of birth injuries of the globe in cases of unassisted labour can testify."

The orbital margin is sharp at birth; at seven years, except at its upper part, it is less sharp, and as the superomedial and inferolateral angles are better marked than the others the orbital opening tends to be triangular.

The form of the orbit on coronal section behind the orbital margin is that of a quadrilateral with rounded corners. In the newborn it has the form of an ellipse higher on the lateral than on the medial side.

The infantile orbits look much more laterally than the adult, i.e. their axes, of the lines drawn from the middle of the orbital opening to the optic foramen, make an angle of 115°, and, if produced backwards, meet in the middle at the nasal septum. In the adult the axes make an angle of 40°–45° with each other, and, if produced backwards, meet at the upper part of the clivus of the sphenoid. These axes, too, lie in the horizontal plane in the infant, whereas in the adult they slope downwards from 15° to 20°.

The orbital fissures are relatively large in the child owing to the narrowness of the orbital surface of the greater wing of the sphenoid, and the wide and narrow portions are not well differentiated.

The orbital index is high in the child, the vertical diameter of the orbital opening being practically the same as the horizontal, but later the transverse increases more than the vertical (see table p. 19). The size of the orbits is relatively great; thus they do not grow much after seven years.

The interorbital distance is small. This is of some practical importance. *Children are not infrequently brought to the ophthalmic surgeon because they are thought to squint when the strabismus is apparent only. This appearance is due to the narrow interorbital distance, which makes the eyes look too close together. With the growth of the frontal and ethmoidal sinuses the interorbital distance increases, and so causes the "squint" to disappear.*

The infraorbital foramen is usually present at birth; but at times it may be represented by the terminal notch of an infraorbital groove whose roof has not grown over to convert it into a canal and which thus reaches to the orbital margin.

The orbital process of the zygomatic (malar) bone may almost reach the lacrimal fossa, and this condition may persist to ten years.

The roof of the orbit is relatively much larger than the floor at birth compared with the adult proportions. The fetal skull has a large cranium (orbital roof) and a small face (orbital floor). The fossa for the lacrimal gland is shallow, but the accessory fossa (p. 2) is well marked.

The optic canal has no length at birth, *so that it is actually a foramen*; at one year it measures 4 mm. The axis also changes with age; essentially while facing forwards and laterally it looks much more downwards at birth than in the adult.

The periosteum or periorbita is much thicker and stronger at birth than in the adult.

The following table gives a résumé of the changes in the orbital opening (Winckler).

	Form	Height	Width	Index
Fetus (8 months) . .	Oval	14 mm	18 mm	77·7
New-born (6 months) .	Rounded	27 mm	27 mm	100
Child (7 years) . .	Quadrilat.	28 mm	33 mm	84·8
Adult	Quadrilat.	35 mm	39 mm	89·7

Senile Changes.—Here the changes are those due to absorption of the bony walls. Thus in the skulls of old people holes are sometimes found in the *roof* of the orbit. In such cases the periorbita is in direct contact with the dura mater.

The medial wall, although normally very thin, rarely shows senile holes in its ethmoidal portion. Parts of the lacrimal bone are, however, commonly absorbed.

The lateral wall not uncommonly shows holes or such marked thinning that it becomes very fragile in these places.

As regards the *floor*, senile changes very rarely produce holes apart from those in the roof or floor of the infraorbital canal.

In old people, too, the orbital fissures, especially the inferior, become wilder owing to absorption of their margins.

In longheaded (dolichocephalic) skulls the orbits tend to look more laterally than in the shortheaded (brachycephalic) (Mannhardt, 1871).

Mensuration.—There is a great difference between the measurements given by different authorities. The following is a useful average:

Depth of orbit . . . . . . 40 mm
Height of orbital opening . . . . 35 mm
Width of orbital opening . . . . 40 mm
Interorbital distance . . . . . 25 mm
Volume . . . . 30 ml
Volume of orbit: Vol. of eye = 4·5 : 1 (Ovio)

Sex Differences.—Up to puberty there is little difference between the orbits and, in fact, the skulls of male and female.

After this the male skull takes on its secondary sexual characters, seen especially in the formation of the lower jaw and in the forehead region.

The female remains more infantile in form. The orbits tend to be rounder and the upper margin sharper than in the male. The glabella and superciliary ridges are less marked or almost absent. The forehead is more vertical and the frontal eminences more marked. The contours of the region are rounder and the bones smoother. The zygomatic process of the frontal bone is more slender and pointed.

The female orbit is more elongated and relatively larger than the male (Merkel).

The Periorbita (Figs. 15, 16, 278)

The periorbita or orbital periosteum lines the bones of the orbit. Generally it adheres but loosely to the bones which it covers, so that for the most part it may be lifted from them by blood or pus or during the course of certain operations.

At various points, however, it is firmly fixed:

(1) At the orbital margin, where it is thickened to form the arcus marginale and becomes continuous with the periosteum covering the bones of the face.

(2) At the sutures.

(3) At the various fissures and foramina; and

(4) At the lacrimal fossa.

Through the superior orbital fissure, the optic foramen, and anterior ethmoidal canal (Fig. 278) it becomes continuous with the periosteal layer of the dura mater.

In the superior orbital fissure it becomes a dense membrane, which just allows sufficient room for the various structures to pass through.

In the optic foramen the fibrous (dura mater) sheath of the optic nerve is closely adherent to the periosteum of the canal (p. 327).

At the optic foramen, also, the periorbita splits, a portion becoming continuous with the dural covering of the optic nerve; here also it gives origin to the muscles and sends processes which are continuous with the muscle sheaths. Fine lamellar processes also pass from the periorbita, divide which the fat into lobules and form coverings for the vessels and nerves.

Through the inferior orbital fissure it is continuous with the periosteum covering the bones of the infratemporal and pterygopalatine fossæ, through the temporal canal with that of the temporal fossa and via the zygomatic canal with that on the front of the zygomatic bone.

It is adherent to the posterior lacrimal crest, and here gives off a layer to enclose the lacrimal fossa, being separated from the sac by some loose areolar tissue, and then passes down the duct to become continuous with the periosteum of the inferior meatus.

These facts can be made out and should be remembered in doing an exenteration of the orbit. Having divided the periosteum at the orbital margin, one finds little

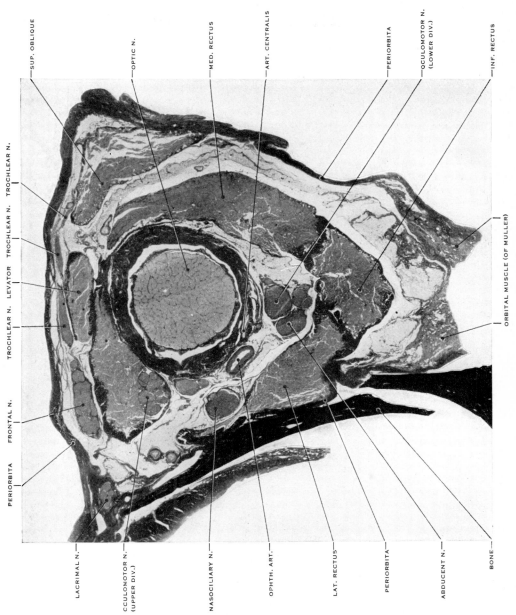

SUP. OBLIQUE

OPTIC N.

MED. RECTUS

ART. CENTRALIS

PERIORBITA

OCULOMOTOR N. (LOWER DIV.)

INF. RECTUS

TROCHLEAR N.

TROCHLEAR N.

TROCHLEAR N.

LEVATOR

TROCHLEAR N.

FRONTAL N.

PERIORBITA

LACRIMAL N.

OCULOMOTOR N. (UPPER DIV.)

NASOCILIARY N.

OPHTH. ART.

LAT. RECTUS

PERIORBITA

ABDUCENT N.

BONE

ORBITAL MUSCLE (OF MULLER)

FIG. 15.—CORONAL SECTION OF RIGHT ORBIT NEAR APEX.

21

difficulty in removing the periosteal cone except at the above places, where bands of varying strength have to be divided.

The periorbita consists of two layers. In the outer, next to bone, oblique fibres are well seen. These cannot be made out in the inner, which is much weaker than the outer. It is this inner layer which gives a covering to the frontal and lacrimal nerves and forms the space in which the lacrimal gland is lodged.

The periorbita is liable to become ossified, especially where it roofs over the infraorbital canal and where it is attached to the posterior lacrimal crest.

Orbital periosteum, like that elsewhere, is sensitive. It is supplied by those trigeminal nerve branches which lie in contact with it—frontal, lacrimal, zygomatic, infraorbital and ethmoidal.

The Muscle of Müller (*Musculus orbitalis*).—In the region of the inferior orbital (sphenomaxillary) fissure some plain muscle fibres are found with the periorbita, which give the latter in this region a rosy tint. This is the muscle of Müller. It is more extensive than one would imagine. It not only spans the inferior orbital fissure but extends backwards, deep to the anulus tendineus, to the front of the cavernous sinus, while anteriorly it gradually gets lost in the periorbita. It has a width of 12 mm. Its action in the human is very doubtful. In certain mammals, where there is no long lateral wall to separate the orbit from the temporal fossa, the muscle of Müller is large and takes the place of this wall (see also pp. 194, 270, 499).

Relations.—Above is orbital fat in which are the inferior ophthalmic vein and its tributaries. The inferior surface lies on the fatty tissue of the pterygopalatine fossa in which are found the infraorbital nerve, the pteryopalatine ganglion with the arteries and veins surrounding it. Through the muscle pass anastomotic branches between the ophthalmic vein and the pterygoid plexus.

Nerve supply.—Branch from the pterygopalatine ganglion (sympathetic) (Fig. 17).

Function.—The muscle was held by some to be the cause of the proptosis in exophthalmic goitre, either directly, or indirectly through pressure on the veins which pass through it. But while the muscle acts as a protruder in some of the lower animals, it does not act in this way in man, in whom it is vestigial. The free venous anastomosis, moreover, negatives any effect which a compression of the veins might have had. True proptosis in exophthalmic goitre is due to increased volume of the infraorbital fibro-fatty tissue produced by a myxomatous type of œdema. Apparent exophthalmos is a widening of the palpebral fissure due to overaction of the smooth muscle component of levator palpebræ superioris.

CERTAIN POINTS OF IMPORTANCE IN THE NEIGHBOURHOOD OF THE
ORBITAL MARGIN

The Superciliary Ridges are elevations above the orbital margins which meet in the mid-line in the *glabella* which forms the prominence above the nose. The

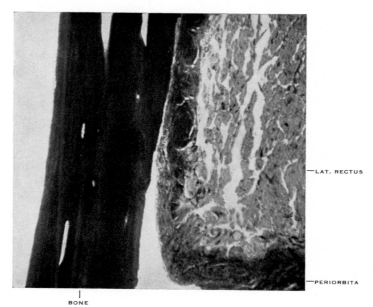

—LAT. RECTUS

—PERIORBITA

BONE

FIG. 16—DETAIL OF FIGURE 15.
Note how loosely attached periorbita is to the bone.

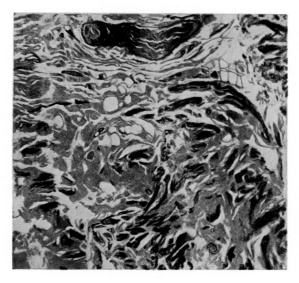

FIG. 17.—DETAIL OF FIGURE 15.
To show fibres of the orbital muscle of Müller.

prominence of the ridges and of the glabella has nothing to do with the size of the frontal sinuses. They are larger in the male than in the female and absent in the infant.

The Frontal Eminences are rounded elevations on the vertical plate of the frontal bone some 5 cm above the orbit; they are more prominent in the female and even more so in the infant.

The Infraorbital Foramen lies 4–5 mm below the tubercle on the lower orbital margin which marks the suture between the zygomatic bone and the maxilla. It is usually oval, and looks downwards as well as forwards. Its upper margin is sharp and crescentic, while the lower border is ill-defined. The foramen may be double—indeed, up to five have been described.

The supraorbital notch, the infraorbital foramen, and the mental foramen are on the same vertical line, which passes between the two bicuspid teeth.

The Temporal Crest runs from the zygomatic process of the frontal bone upwards and backwards to become continuous with the temporal lines on the parietal bones.

The Sutura Notha (Fig. 1) is a groove on the frontal process of the maxilla, and runs parallel with the anterior lacrimal crest. It lodges a branch of the infraorbital artery.

SURFACE ANATOMY

The Upper Orbital Margin forms a well-marked prominence, more so in the lateral sharp portion than in the medial more rounded part. Its form can be made out easily by touch.

It should be noted carefully that the eyebrow corresponds in position only in part to the upper orbital margin.

The head of the eyebrow lies for the most part *under* the medial part of the margin, to palpate which the finger must press *upwards*.

The body lies *along* the margin, while the tail runs well above the lateral part of the margin, which can be felt and usually seen below it.

The zygomatic process of the frontal bone often forms a marked prominence under the skin.

The Supraorbital Notch can be felt at the junction of the lateral two-thirds with the medial third, and not infrequently the supraorbital nerve can be rolled under the finger.

The Lateral Orbital Margin is only visible down to the level of the lateral canthus, but can easily be felt in its whole extent.

The Lower Orbital Margin, as opposed to the upper, forms no prominence, since the skin of the lower lid passes without sudden change of plane into that of the cheek. Just beyond it, especially in the old, lie the nasojugal and malar furrows.

It is easily palpable as a sharp ridge beyond which the finger can pass into the orbit. On the lower and lateral side the little finger can pass between the eye and the orbital margin for about 1·25 cm.

The **Lacrimal Tubercle** can be felt in the sharp anterior lacrimal crest, as can the **tubercle** at the middle of the lower margin which marks the suture between the zygomatic bone and maxilla.

The trochlea of the superior oblique is easily felt with the tip of the thumb, just within the superomedial angle of the orbital margin.

The **Lateral Orbital Tubercle** (Whitnall's) can be felt just within the lateral orbital margin at its middle by passing the finger into the orbit and rubbing it up and down against the margin.

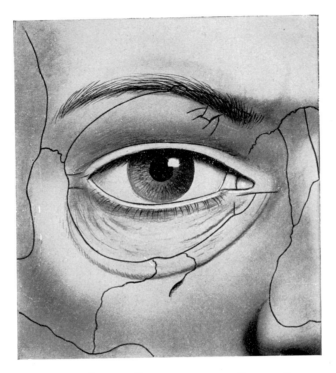

FIG. 18.—THE SURFACE PROJECTION OF THE ORBITAL OPENING.

The **Infraorbital Foramen**, or rather its sharp crescentic upper margin, can, not infrequently, be made out 4–5 mm below the tubercle on the lower orbital margin which marks the zygomaticomaxillary suture.

The **Zygomatic (Malar) Tubercle** can be felt below and behind the zygomatic process of the frontal bone, and between the two is a V-shaped interval, at the bottom of which is the frontozygomatic suture.

The **Anterior Lacrimal Crest** is easily defined. Behind it the finger passes into the lacrimal fossa, and behind this again the posterior lacrimal crest can be felt.

It should be noted carefully that the finger in the lacrimal fossa lies below the medial angle of the eye and not under the ridge made by the medial palpebral ligament.

The Temporal Crest can be felt arching backwards from the zygomatic process of the frontal bone.

The Nasal Bone, sitting on the frontal process of the maxilla, can be seen and palpated down to its lower end, where it joins the mobile cartilage of the nose.

The Paranasal Sinuses

The Maxillary Sinus.—The maxillary sinus (antrum of Highmore) is a pyramidal cavity situated in the maxilla (Figs. 2, 19).

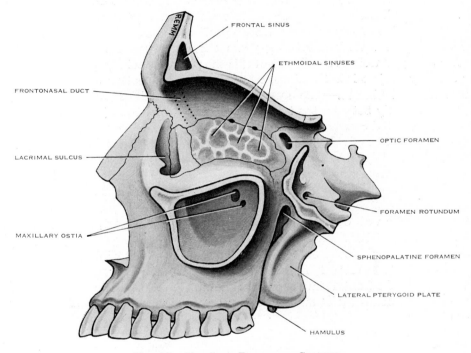

FRONTAL SINUS

ETHMOIDAL SINUSES

FRONTONASAL DUCT

OPTIC FORAMEN

LACRIMAL SULCUS

FORAMEN ROTUNDUM

MAXILLARY OSTIA

SPHENOPALATINE FORAMEN

LATERAL PTERYGOID PLATE

HAMULUS

Fig. 19.—The Left Paranasal Sinuses.

Its base forms part of the lateral wall of the nose; its apex lies under the zygomatic bone. In the disarticulated skull the base presents a large opening, which is, however, partly closed in the articulated skull by the uncinate process of the ethmoid above, the inferior concha below, the palatine behind, and the lacrimal in front (Fig. 2). The mucous membrane covers this in still further, so that finally there is only one small opening (sometimes two) situated near the roof of the antrum, and therefore bad for gravitational drainage if the antrum contains excess fluid. The ostium opens into the middle meatus of the nose in the hiatus semi-

A.E.—3

lunaris (Fig. 20). The nasolacrimal duct forms a ridge in the anterior part of this wall (Fig. 19).

The anterolateral wall looks on to the face, and may be reached by everting the upper lip. In it are the canals containing the anterior and middle superior alveolar (dental) nerves (Fig. 288).

The posterior wall faces the infratemporal fossa, of which it forms the anterior wall. In it are the canals for the posterior superior alveolar (dental) nerves.

The roof of the antrum is formed by the orbital plate of the maxilla, which constitutes the floor of the orbit. In it is the infraorbital canal containing the infraorbital nerve and vessels. The canal raises a ridge in the front part of the roof.

The floor is formed by the alveolar process, and is about 1·25 cm below the nose. The sinus lies above the posterior five teeth (i.e. the two premolars and the three molars). The roots of these teeth occasionally produce elevations on the floor of the sinus. With advancing years the floor descends by resorption of alveolar bone; sometimes as a result of this the roots, especially of the first molar, may actually project into the sinus, covered only by mucous membrane.

The Frontal Sinuses.—The frontal sinuses are cavities of variable extent situated anteriorly between the two plates of the frontal bone (Figs. 2, 278, 280). They are separated by a septum, which is often deviated to one or other side. In the peripheral parts of the sinus there are also small partitions forming loculi. In some cases a frontal sinus may extend laterally to the zygomatic process; in others, especially if the septum is much to one side, it may be reduced to a mere slit.

On an average (Logan Turner, 1901, 1908) the height is 3 cm, the breadth 2·5 cm, and depth 2 cm.

The posterior wall of the sinus is thin, contains little diploë, and separates it from the meninges and frontal convolutions.

The anterior wall looks on to the forehead. It contains diploë, hence osteomyelitis spreads more readily in this than in the posterior wall.

The floor of the frontal sinus separates it from the orbit and nose.

Behind and below the ethmoidal sinuses are only separated from the sinus by a thin plate of bone. Not infrequently a *frontoethmoidal* forms a prominence in the floor of the sinus (Fig. 2).

The frontal sinus opens into the nose by the infundibulum. This narrow canal passes between the anterior ethmoidal sinuses and opens into the hiatus semilunaris in the middle meatus, in front of the openings of the anterior ethmoidal and the maxillary sinuses (Fig. 20).

Hence infection in one sinus can and does easily spread to the others.

The Ethmoidal Sinuses.—The ethmoidal sinuses are situated for the most part in the lateral mass of the ethmoid, but are completed by the frontal, palatine, sphenoid, maxillary, and lacrimal bones.

Above them are the meninges and frontal convolutions in the anterior cranial fossa.

In front is the infundibulum of the frontal sinus, behind is the sphenoidal sinus. Below is the nose, laterally the orbit and lacrimal fossa (Figs. 3 and 278).

The sinuses are separated from these structures by very thin plates of bone, which are not good barriers to the spread of infection. Thus the orbital plate is not much thicker than paper: hence the reason why ethmoiditis is the commonest cause of orbital cellulitis.

The ethmoidal sinuses are divided by irregular septa into anterior, middle, and posterior groups (Fig. 19).

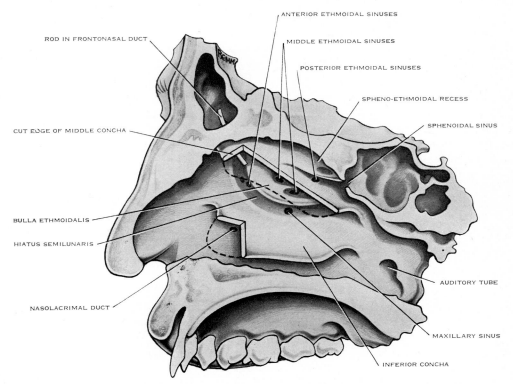

FIG. 20.—THE RIGHT LATERAL WALL OF THE NASAL CAVITY TO SHOW THE OPENINGS OF THE PARA-
NASAL SINUSES AND NASOLACRIMAL DUCT.

The anterior and middle open into the middle meatus of the nose; the anterior in the hiatus semilunaris, the middle on the bulla ethmoidalis (Fig. 20).

The posterior lie anteromedial to the optic canal and open into the superior meatus.

The Sphenoidal Air Sinuses.—The sphenoidal sinuses are in the body of the sphenoid bone (Figs. 20, 317, 368).

There is a vertical median septum often deviated to one or other side of the mid-line. A variable amount of a transverse septum is also usually present, and runs most often from above downwards and forwards. It is known as the "carotid buttress" (Cushing), because it is used as a landmark for protecting the internal carotid artery when approaching the pituitary body by the nasal route. According to Cope (1916–1917) it can be seen in 25 per cent of the X-rays of the region. The sphenoidal sinus lies in front of the pituitary fossa. The sinus gradually enlarges by resorption of bone. As age advances the sinus extends below the pituitary fossa and into the root of the lesser wing. It may excavate the basisphenoid and basi-occiput till close to the anterior margin of the foramen magnum.

Above the sphenoidal sinuses are the pituitary body and optic nerves, which often makes a ridge inside each sinus. It is this close relation which causes the optic nerve to be involved at times in sinusitis, giving rise to a sudden loss of vision (retrobulbar neuritis) (Fig. 294).

Below is the nose, and in the floor of the sinus is the pterygoid canal which may make a ridge in the sinus.

In front are the ethmoidal sinuses, the posterior of which often bulges into the sinus.

Laterally are the cavernous sinuses, containing the internal carotid artery and abducent nerve. In front of this the body of the sphenoid bone forms the medial wall of the orbit.

Each sphenoidal sinus opens into the highest meatus, or sphenoethmoidal recess.

When a sphenoidal sinus is very large it may send a prolongation between the foramen rotundum and the foramen ovale. Such an extension of the sinus may explain certain cases of involvement of the nerves in sinus disease.

NERVE SUPPLY

The *maxillary sinus* is supplied by multiple branches of the maxillary nerve. The infraorbital nerve supplies the roof by perforating branches. The superior alveolar nerves on their way to the teeth supply the posterior, lateral and anterior walls. The anterior superior alveolar nerve supplies the nasal wall alongside the nasolacrimal duct, and behind this the anterior (greater) palatine nerve supplies the nasal wall and ostium.

The *frontal sinus* is supplied by the supraorbital nerve. The *anterior* and *middle ethmoidal sinuses* are supplied by the anterior ethmoidal nerve, while the *posterior ethmoidal sinuses* and the *sphenoidal sinus* are supplied by the posterior ethmoidal nerve.

LYMPH DRAINAGE

The sphenoidal and posterior ethmoidal air sinuses drain back to retro-pharyngeal lymph glands. The remainder (i.e. middle and anterior ethmoidal, frontal and maxillary sinuses) drain to the submandibular lymph nodes.

DEVELOPMENT

The accessory sinuses of the nose all arise as out-buddings from the nasal mucosa. They are at the most rudimentary and largely absent at birth.

The bud which is to form each frontal sinus passes up from the ethmoid bone, and at one year is just present in the frontal bone. The stalk remains as the infundibulum. At 7 years it is about the size of a pea. Then it starts growing rapidly, but does not reach its full size till about 25 years.

Similarly, the ethmoidal sinuses are just present at birth as small depressions, and grow rapidly after 7 years.

At 2 years the sphenoid bone is still spongy, each sphenoidal sinus being represented by a slight depression at its future opening. It really only starts growing at 8 years.

The maxillary sinus is a groove in the lateral nasal wall at birth. At 1 year it has just reached the infraorbital canal. It grows rapidly with the second dentition, so that at 12 years it is nearly like the adult, whose form, however, it does not acquire till 18 years.

CHAPTER II

THE EYEBALL

ALTHOUGH we speak of the globe of the eye, it is not a true sphere, but consists of the segments of two somewhat modified spheres placed one in front of the other. The anterior of these two segments is the smaller, more curved than the posterior, and called the cornea. Their respective radii are about 12 and 8 mm.

It is for this reason that the anteroposterior diameter of the globe is greatest (24 mm). Also the eyeball is slightly flattened from the above down, hence the vertical diameter (23 mm) is slightly less than the horizontal (23·5 mm).

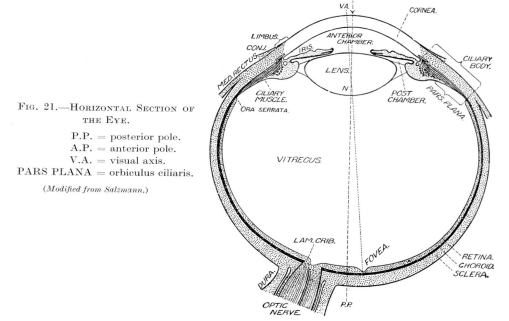

FIG. 21.—HORIZONTAL SECTION OF
THE EYE.

P.P. = posterior pole.
A.P. = anterior pole.
V.A. = visual axis.
PARS PLANA = orbiculus ciliaris.

(Modified from Salzmann.)

So constituted, the eyeball is placed in the anterior part of the orbit, nearer the roof than the floor, and slightly closer to the lateral than the medial wall.

As regards the depth that it normally occupies in its socket, a straight-edge placed against the superior and inferior orbital margins will just touch or just miss the front of the cornea. A line joining the medial and lateral margins will have nearly one-third of the globe in front of it. The eyeball is, in fact, least protected on

30

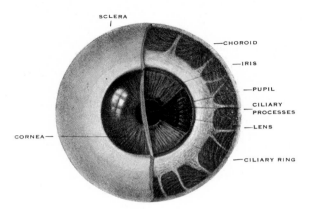

FIG. 22.—ANTERIOR ASPECT OF THE EYE.
Parts of the cornea, sclera, and iris have been removed to show internal structures.
(*From Hirschfeld and Leveillé, 1853.*)

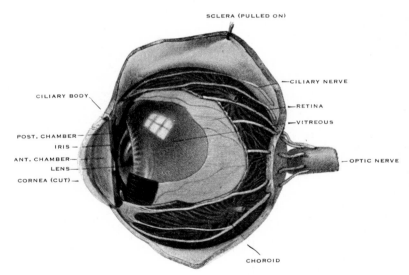

FIG. 23.—PREPARATION TO SHOW THE COATS AND CONTENTS OF THE EYE.
Parts of the sclera, cornea, choroid, ciliary body, iris, and retina have been removed.
(*From Hirschfeld and Leveillé, 1853.*)

the lateral side, and it is therefore from this side that the surgeon finds his easiest approach.

For this reason, too, rupture of the globe takes place most frequently up and medially from blows which come from the lower and lateral side.

The globe of the eye consists of three concentric coverings or tunics enclosing the various transparent media through which the light must pass before reaching the sensitive retina:

1. The outermost coat is fibrous, protective in function, and made up of a posterior five-sixths, which is white and opaque and called the *sclera*, and an anterior part which is transparent, the *cornea*.

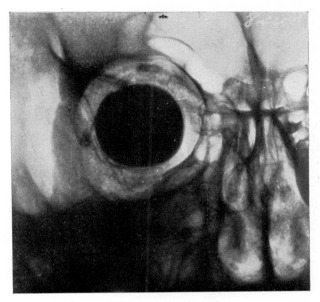

Fig. 24.—To show the Position of the Eye in the Orbit.
The eye was injected with a saturated solution of lead nitrate before the X-ray was taken.
The actual injection fluid was kindly suggested by the late Professor H. A. Harris.

2. The middle coat is mainly vascular and nutritive in its function. It is made up from behind forwards of choroid, ciliary body and iris.

3. The innermost tunic is the retina, consisting essentially of nerve elements and forming the true receptive portion for visual impressions.

The scleral tunic also provides a passive resistance to the intraocular pressure which maintains the choroidal and retinal layers against the sclera, preserving thus the optical dimensions of the eyeball. The choroidal circulation provides not only the source of the intraocular fluid but also maintains the more external, non-vascularized layers of the retina (p. 145). The retina also is not a simple array of

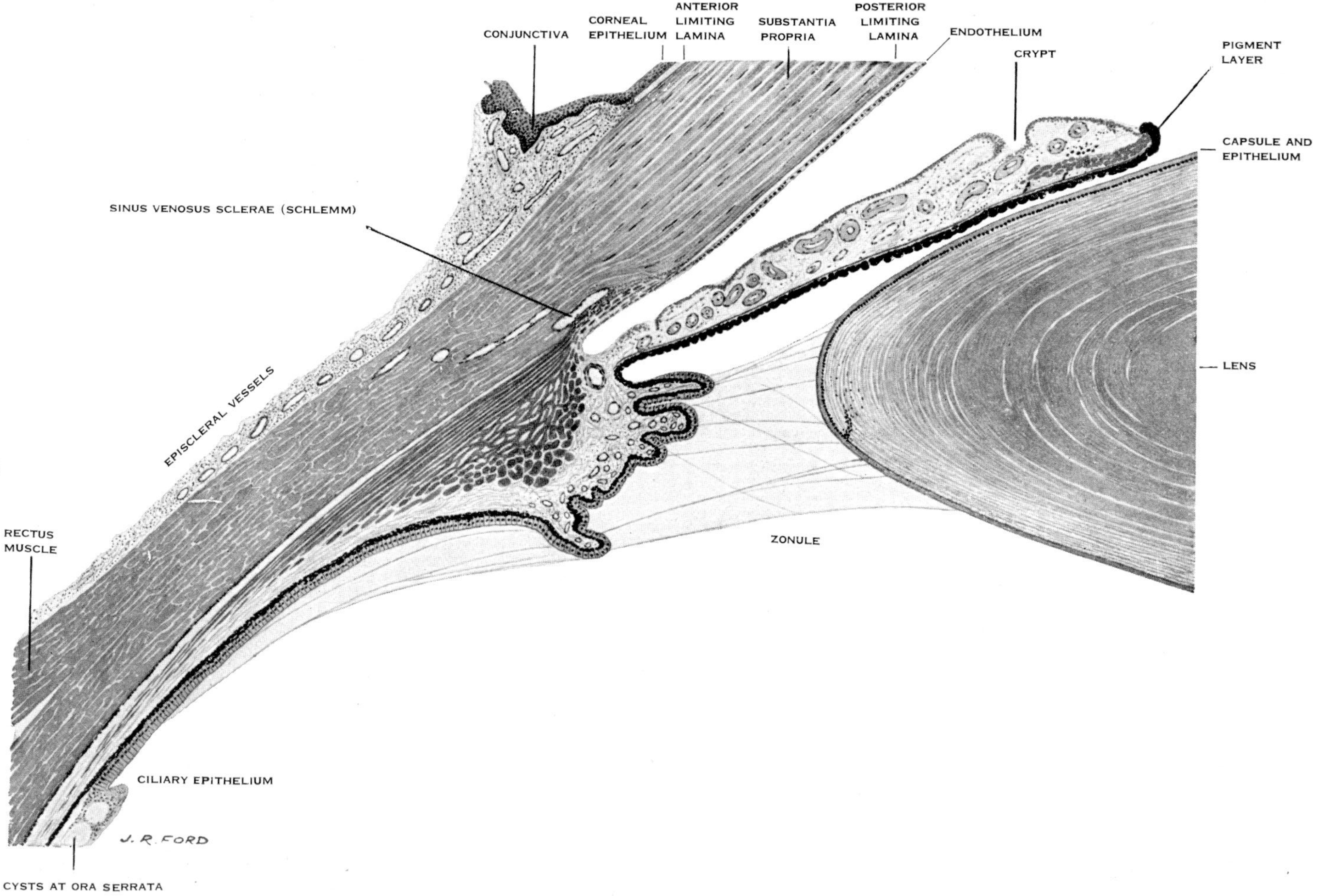

PIGMENT
LAYER

CAPSULE AND
EPITHELIUM

LENS

ENDOTHELIUM

CRYPT

POSTERIOR
LIMITING
LAMINA

SUBSTANTIA
PROPRIA

ANTERIOR
LIMITING
LAMINA

CORNEAL
EPITHELIUM

CONJUNCTIVA

ZONULE

SINUS VENOSUS SCLERAE (SCHLEMM)

EPISCLERAL VESSELS

CILIARY EPITHELIUM

J. R. FORD

CYSTS AT ORA SERRATA

RECTUS
MUSCLE

32

FIG. 25.—MERIDIONAL SECTION THROUGH THE LIMBIC REGION OF THE EYE.

photoreceptors and their neurons; considerable "processing" of visual information occurs in the retina itself (p. 121).

THE CORNEA

The cornea is transparent, and resembles a little watch-glass. Its curvature is somewhat greater than the rest of the globe, and so a slight furrow (the sulcus scleræ) separates it from the sclera.

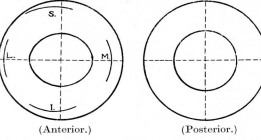

FIG. 26.—IN THE ANTERIOR ASPECT THE CORNEA IS TRANSVERSELY ELLIPSOID, WHEREAS ITS POSTERIOR ASPECT IS CIRCULAR. S, M, I AND L INDICATE THE POINTS OF ATTACHMENT OF THE RECTI.

(Anterior.)   (Posterior.)

This furrow is best demonstrated in the living by making the image reflected from a mirror pass from the cornea to the sclera. The image is first narrowed horizontally (Tscherning, 1898), then may divide into two.

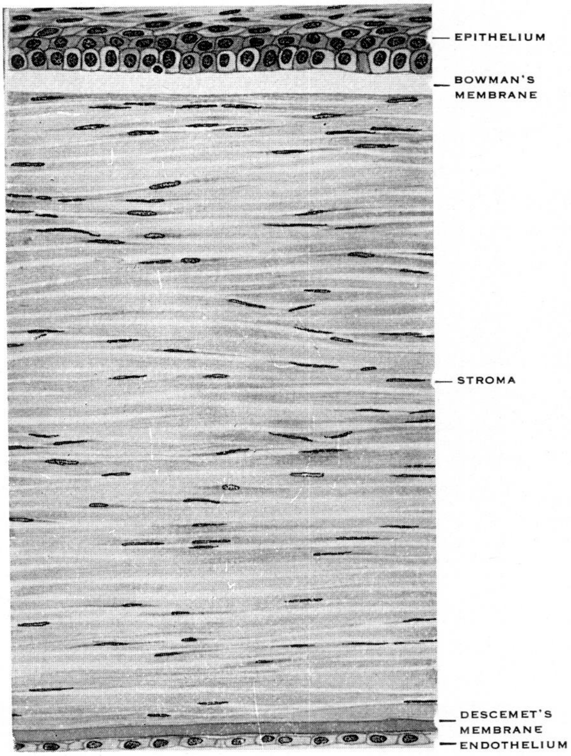

The cornea and sclera are structurally continuous, and even histologically it is very difficult to tell where one ends and the other begins. The line of junction between the two is best seen (with the naked eye) when an eye which has just been removed from the living is divided by a meridional section. Looked at from in front, the cornea is elliptical, being 12 mm in the horizontal meridian and 11 mm in the vertical.

From behind, the cornea appears circular, about 11·5 mm in diameter. This difference is due to the fact that the sclera and conjunctiva overlap the cornea anteriorly more above and below than laterally.

Ideally the cornea forms part of the surface of a sphere, but very often it is curved more in

EPITHELIUM

BOWMAN'S MEMBRANE

STROMA

DESCEMET'S MEMBRANE
ENDOTHELIUM

FIG. 27.—TRANSVERSE SECTION OF CORNEA.

one meridian than another, *giving rise to the condition of astigmatism*. Usually it is more curved in the vertical than in the horizontal meridian, i.e. astigmatism with the rule.

The radius of curvature of the anterior surface is about 7·8 mm, that of the posterior 6·5 mm, in adult males. These radii only hold good for the central third, or optical zone, the peripheral portions being more flattened. *Hence a higher convex glass is often necessary when looking at the periphery of the fundus with the ophthalmoscope.* The cornea is thicker at the periphery than at the centre, optical estimates being 0·67 and 0·52 mm (Maurice, 1969).

Contrary to popular opinion, most of the refraction of the eye takes place, not in the lens, but at the surface of the cornea. Maintenance of transparency is an obvious essential; this is a function mainly of the epithelial cells on its surfaces. The living cells are rich in glycogen, enzymes and acetylcholine; their activity regulates that of the corneal corpuscles and controls the transport of water and electrolytes through the lamellæ of the substantia propria (*The Cornea World Congress, London*, 1965). Consonant with its great optical importance, and its exposure to frequent minor injury, the corneal epithelium is replaced by growth from its basal cells with perhaps greater rapidity than any other stratified epithelium. According to Hanna (1961) it has a replacement period of seven days.

Structure.—Behind the precorneal film (p. 240) there are the following five layers:

1. *Layer of Stratified Squamous Epithelium.*—This may be regarded as the continuation of the conjunctival epithelium forwards. But unlike the limbal epithelium its two surfaces are, as near as matters, parallel to each other. This layer is approximately 50 μm thick and consists of five or six layers of cells. The deepest of these, the *basal* cells, stand in a palisade-like manner, in perfect alignment, on a basement membrane. These basal cells are columnar with rounded heads and flat bases, which often present processes which spread out on the basement membrane. Each has a slightly oval nucleus whose long axis is that of the cell and placed near the head of the cell. The cells are connected with the membrane by fine denticulations which are not very strong. They vary somewhat in dimensions, with a height of about 15 μm and a diameter of 10 μm; but the various types of "short", "dark", and dendritic basal cell described by some observers are not significantly established for human tissue. The basal cells are, of course, the germinal layer, and are continuous at the corneal periphery with the same layer in the conjunctiva.

The next layer (the *Wing* or umbrella cells) consists of polyhedral cells whose rounded heads are directed anteriorly and whose concave bases fit over the heads of the basal cells and send processes, the wings, between them. Each contains an oval nucleus whose long axis is parallel with the surface of the cornea (Fig. 30).

The next two or three layers are also polyhedral, and the most superficial are flattened but do not lose their nuclei, *nor do they normally show keratinization*. The

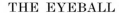

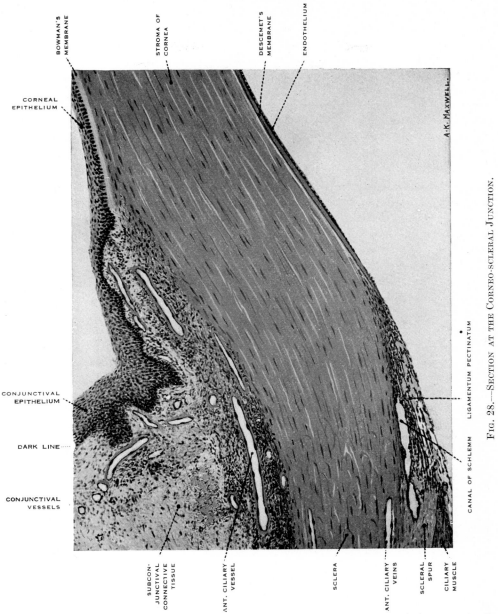

FIG. 28.—SECTION AT THE CORNEO-SCLERAL JUNCTION.

flattened nuclei of the surface cells project backwards leaving the surface perfectly smooth, which makes it the most brilliant in the body.

As in the epidermis, the various cells appear to be united by cell bridges forming prickle-cells. The spaces between the cells, which are difficult to make out in the normal eye, form a lymph space which can be injected, and *which may be greatly distended pathologically, for instance in glaucoma.* These spaces are best seen between the basal cells, and gradually disappear in the more superficial ones. A few leucocytes (wandering cells) may be found normally in the spaces between the basal cells just in front of Bowman's membrane (Fig. 27). Pathologically they may increase greatly in number. In spite of its avascularity the corneal epithelium possesses a very active power of regeneration after abrasion.

Electron microscopy of corneal epithelium. Ultrastructural studies have, as elsewhere, clarified the nature of the "prickles" or cell bridges. The adjoining surfaces of epithelial cells are intricately and reciprocally folded. Adhesion is maintained by numerous desmosomes. The basal cells are similarly adherent to an underlying basement membrane. The membrane is strongly osmiophilic, of even thickness and merges with the anterior limiting membrane (of Bowman). The most superficial cells display microvilli and microplicæ extending into the superjacent film of tear fluid. Zonulæ occludentes occur between these superficial cells.

2. *The Anterior Limiting Lamina* (*Bowman's Membrane*) or the anterior "elastic" lamina does not consist of elastic tissue. It is a thin homogeneous sheet about 8–14 μm thick between the basement membrane and the substantia propria. It is separated from the epithelium by a sharply defined border, *and under pathological conditions as well as after death the epithelium separates readily from the limiting layer.* The anterior surface of "Bowman's membrane" is absolutely parallel with the surface of the cornea. Hence the difficulty often of seeing abrasions which have removed the whole thickness of the epithelium. Posteriorly the line of demarcation from the stroma is ill-defined. In fact, it may be regarded as a modified portion of the stroma and hence the objection to regarding it as a "membrane" or as a "limiting" structure. Peripherally it ends abruptly in a rounded border (Figs. 25 and 28).

The anterior limiting lamina is not truly elastic, nor does it regenerate when once it has been destroyed. It, however, shows a good deal of resistance to injury or infection.

Electron microscopy of the anterior limiting lamina.—An acellular mass of collagen fibrils are disposed irregularly. They are much finer than the fibres of the underlying substantia propria (Figs. 29, 32) but lamellæ of the latter can be traced into

3. *The Substantia Propria* of the cornea is composed of a modified connective tissue of which the constituents have very nearly the same refractive index so that in the perfectly fresh condition it is difficult to make out any indications of structure. After death, and with the aid of certain reagents, the cornea may be ascertained to consist of alternating lamellæ of collagenous tissue (about 200–250 in number) the planes of which are parallel to the surfaces of the cornea. It is about 0·5 mm in thickness.

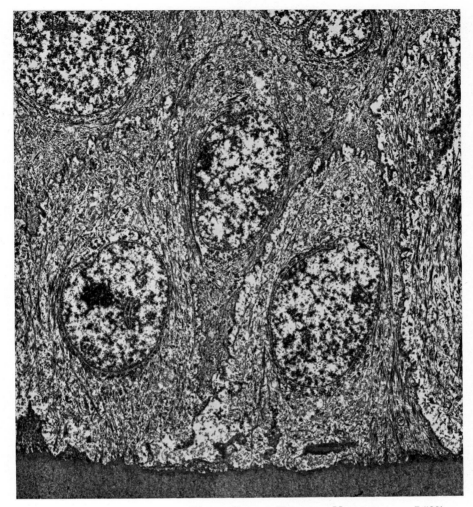

FIG. 29.—THE BASAL CELLS OF HUMAN CORNEA (ELECTRON MICROGRAPH, ×7,500).

The basal cells adjoin a basement membrane contiguous with the limiting layer of Bowman's membrane (below).

(By courtesy of Dr. John Marshall and Mr. P. L. Ansell, Institute of Ophthalmology, London.)

The lamellæ are multiple bands each composed of fine collagen fibrils, which can be identified clearly by electron microscopy (p. 40), but which are individually beyond the resolution of light microscopy. The lamellæ branch, and hence appear to be cut in different directions in any section. The union between neighbouring bands makes it impossible to separate the cornea into lamellæ or bands without much tearing taking place. The bands of each lamella are parallel to each other but

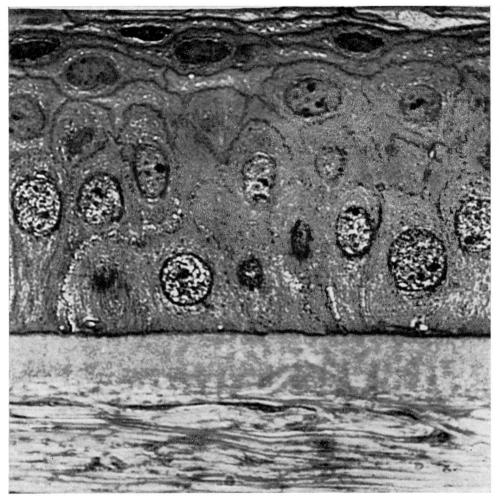

FIG. 30.—THE SURFACE CELLS OF HUMAN CORNEA (ELECTRON MICROGRAPH, ×3,750).

Blunt microvilli project from the flat surface cells. The wing cells fit over the rounded heads of the basal cells. Note also Bowman's membrane and part of the substantia propria below.

(Courtesy of Dr. John Marshall and Mr. P. L. Ansell, Institute of Ophthalmology, London.)

those of alternate layers make a right angle or near this with each other. Each lamella crosses the whole of the cornea, being about 2 μm thick and with a highly variable width of 10–25 μm.

While most corneal fibres are parallel to the surface some *oblique* ones are found, especially anteriorly. They probably run along the perforating corneal nerves.

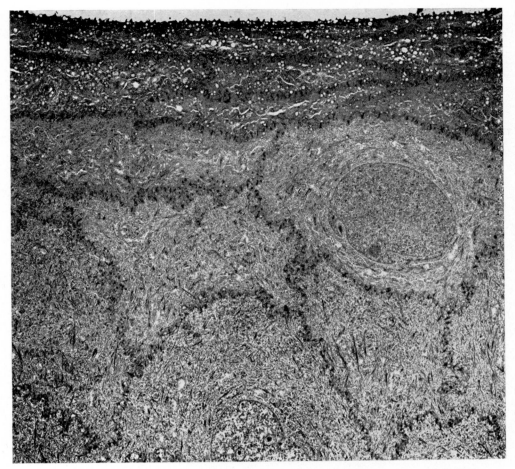

FIG. 31.—THE SURFACE CELLS OF HUMAN CORNEA (ELECTRON MICROGRAPH, × 69,000).

These flattened cells are vital and show no sign of keratinization. Microvilli project from the free surface. Note reciprocal folding of adjoining surfaces of the cells at all levels.

(*By courtesy of Dr. John Marshall and Mr. P. L. Ansell, Institute of Ophthalmology, London*).

Among the lamellæ of the corneal stroma are considerable numbers of "fixed" cells, the corneal fibroblasts, or keratocytes. They are flattened cells, with flattened nuclei and multiple cytoplasmic processes which form contacts with other cells in the same layer. They do not, however form a syncytium.

Wandering macrophages may also be seen, and occasional lymphocytes or polymorphonuclear leucocytes. They escape from the marginal loops of the corneal blood-vessels, are few in number normally, but play an important part in inflammation.

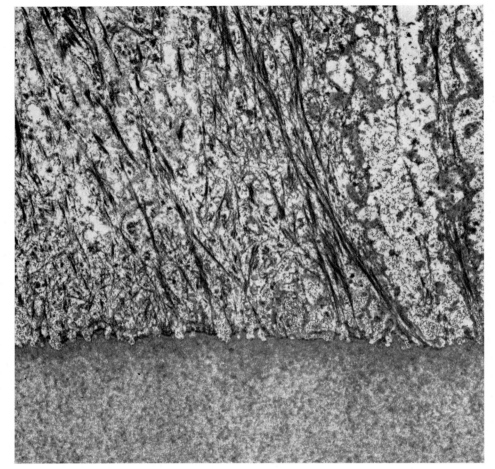

FIG. 32.—BOWMAN'S MEMBRANE

The irregular arrangement of an acellular feltwork of very fine fibrils is typical. Note the interlocking of the surfaces of the two basal cells shown. The cells of the basal layer of epithelium lie on a basement membrane (arrow). Human cornea (× 16,000.)

(By courtesy of Mr. P. V. Rycroft, F.R.C.S.)

Electron microscopy of substantia propria.—This confirms the alternating direction of the fibres; in each layer they are parallel, and in alternate layers they lie at right angles. The presence of elastic fibres has not been confirmed. In man the corneal corpuscles commonly lie *within*, and not between, the collagen lamellæ (Figs. 33, 34). For further details see Takus (1964) and Hogan, Alvarado and Weddell (1971).

4. *The Posterior Limiting Lamina* (Descemet's membrane, posterior elastic membrane) is a strong, homogeneous, and very resistant membrane. It is 10–12 μm

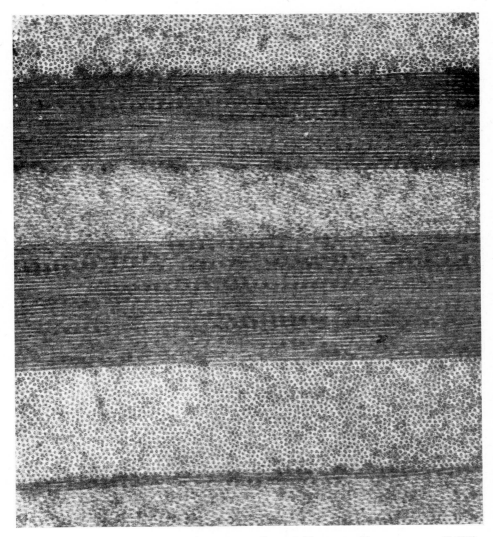

Fig. 33.—The Substantia Propria of Human Cornea (Electron Micrograph, ×48,000).

The layers of collagen fibres, lying alternately at approximately right angles, are well shown. Note slight degree of variation in the width of the lamellae.

(*By courtesy of Dr. John Marshall and Mr. P. L. Ansell, Institute of Ophthalmology, London.*)

A.E.—4

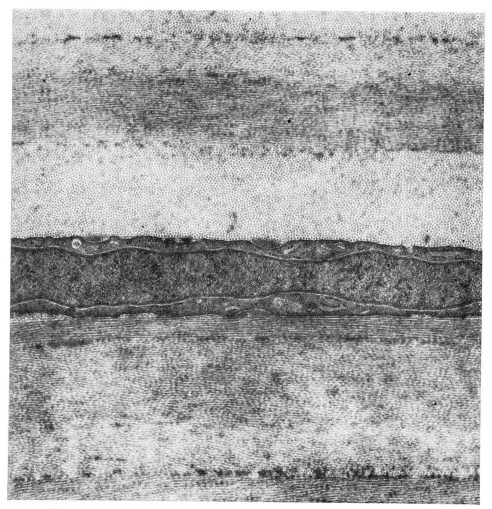

FIG. 34.—A HUMAN CORNEAL CORPUSCLE (ELECTRON MICROGRAPH, ×30,000).

A corneal corpuscle is visible in part, within a lamella of transversely divided fibres, but very close to a thin stratum of fibres divided longitudinally.

(By courtesy of Dr. John Marshall and Mr. P. L. Ansell, Institute of Ophthalmology, London. Preparation by Mrs. R. Tilly.)

thick. Unlike the anterior lamina it is sharply defined from the corneal stroma. There is in fact a plane of separation between them which is made use of in lamellar keratoplasty. It is very resistant to chemical reagents and likewise to pathological processes going on in the cornea. When the entire cornea has broken down into pus, we often see the thin Descemet's membrane offering resistance and remaining unimpaired for days (Fuchs).

The posterior lamina is normally in a state of tension: if torn it gapes slightly and tends to assume a curve which is the opposite of the normal, i.e. it tends to curl up into the anterior chamber. While showing this type of elasticity it does not stain with all elastic stains although it does with some and does not therefore consist of true elastic tissue. In fact, it agrees very much in its staining reactions with those of the capsule of the lens, being PAS-positive. Unlike the anterior lamina, which never regenerates, the posterior can be re-formed. The posterior lamina tapers at its edge, but although it appears to end here, at the Ligamentum pectinatum iridis (p. 60), some claim that it forms part of the corneoscleral trabecular tissue of the ligament, a view now substantiated by the most recent observations.

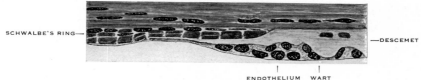

SCHWALBE'S RING —

— DESCEMET

ENDOTHELIUM   WART

FIG. 35.—THE EDGE OF DESCEMET'S MEMBRANE.

Note the oval nuclei (black) in single file in front of Schwalbe's ring.

At the periphery of the cornea the posterior surface of the membrane presents rounded wart-like elevations, the Hassal-Henle bodies, which tend to increase with age (p. 239, and Fig. 359).

Electron microscopy of the posterior limiting lamina (Descemet).—It is composed of very regular strata of fine collagenous fibres. In man they are disposed in two layers, an outer "banded" layer against the corneal substantia propria and an inner stroma against the endothelium (Figs. 36, 37). Although the posterior layer displays the physical property of elasticity there is no evidence that the fibres themselves are composed of elastin.

5. *The Endothelium* is the most posterior layer of the cornea, and consists of a single layer of flattened *epithelial-like* cells, continuous round the angle of the anterior chamber with any remnants of the fetal endothelium which may persist on the front of the iris (p. 81). The endothelium of the cornea can be seen by slit-lamp in the living eye—the only place in the body where this is possible (p. 238).

Electron microscopy of the endothelium.—There is no basement membrane. Adjacent cells interlock by reciprocal tortuous surfaces. Abundant cellular organelles (Fig. 38) indicate a high degree of metabolic activity. The posterior limiting lamina is sometimes considered to be the basement membrane, and specialized contacts can be seen between the two layers by electron microscopy.

Embryologically the cornea is the continuation forwards of three structures:

(a) The epithelium and Bowman's membrane of the conjunctiva.

(b) The substantia propria of the sclera.

(c) Elements of the uveal tract.

Pathologically, too, this is of importance, for the epithelium is liable to be affected in diseases of the conjunctiva, the stroma in diseases of the sclera and the posterior lamina and endothelium in diseases of the uveal tract.

THE LIMBUS

The limbus is the transition zone between the conjunctiva and sclera on the one hand and the cornea on the other. The transparent corneal tissue ends just behind a line which joins the peripheries of the limiting laminæ.

The Conjunctivocorneal Junction.—The conjunctiva is a thin and transparent skin; i.e. a fibrous membrane surfaced with epithelium. It is rather loosely attached to the sclera by a tenuous subconjunctival connective tissue. *The conjunctiva ends at the limbus, and only the epithelium passes centrally to surface the cornea* (Figs. 28, 47). The overlap of conjunctival and subconjunctival tissue forms a translucent membrane over the extreme margin of transparent cornea (Fig. 57). The width of this film when studied with the naked eye is seen to vary greatly. At times the white sclera ends sharply without any film.

The anterior lamina, usually ending suddenly in a rounded border but often bevelled, gives place to a thin layer of conjunctival fibrous tissue which is here closely adherent to the sclera.

The basal layer of the corneal epithelium, kept rigidly aligned by the anterior lamina, becomes wavy and may even become papillary as soon as it loses the support of this membrane. The five-layered corneal epithelium gives place to one of ten to twelve layers. The cells of the basal layer become smaller and poorer in protoplasm and the nuclei more densely staining. This causes the basal layer to appear under the low power of the microscope as a *dark line.*

The marginal vessels (superficial marginal plexus) occupy a triangular area whose apex lies where the lamina ends and whose base is formed by episcleral tissue and sclera.

The Sclerocorneal Junction.—If, in a preparation of the anterior segment of the eye which has been fixed in formalin or alcohol, we make two incisions through the centre of the cornea at right angles to each other, we obtain four segments. If now we pick up at the apex of one segment some corneal tissue with forceps, we can strip the laminæ quite easily till we come to the white sclera, where we are stopped abruptly. Under the microscope this point corresponds to the place where the regular corneal lamellæ give place to the oblique and circular fibres of the sclera which, as it were, form a frame to the cornea (Rochon-Duvigneaud). The regular corneal lamellæ continue a little beyond the line joining the limiting laminæ. The oblique fibres and star-shaped cells characteristic of the sclera commence a little sooner anteriorly than posteriorly; but the main overlap of the cornea is by conjunctiva and subconjunctival tissue rather than by sclera as usually stated (Rochon-Duvigneaud). Neither does the cornea fit into the groove in the sclera like a watch-glass, as generally described (and in previous editions of

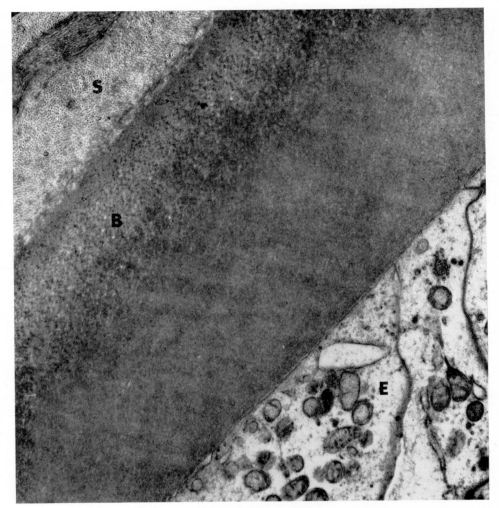

FIG. 36.—DESCEMET'S MEMBRANE (HUMAN, ELECTRON MICROGRAPH, ×13,500).

Lying against the substantia propria of the cornea (S) is the banded layer (B) of Descemet's membrane. Deep to this is the stroma of Descemet's membrane, lined by the endothelium (E).

(By courtesy of Dr. C. Pedler, Institute of Ophthalmology, London. Preparation by Mrs. R. Tilly.)

this anatomy). In fact, the fibres of the corneal lamellæ (transparent and regular) run directly into the fibres of the sclera (opaque and less regularly arranged).

THE VESSELS AND NERVES OF THE CORNEA

The cornea is avascular. It is generally stated, however, that small loops derived from the anterior ciliary vessels invade the periphery for about 1 mm. But

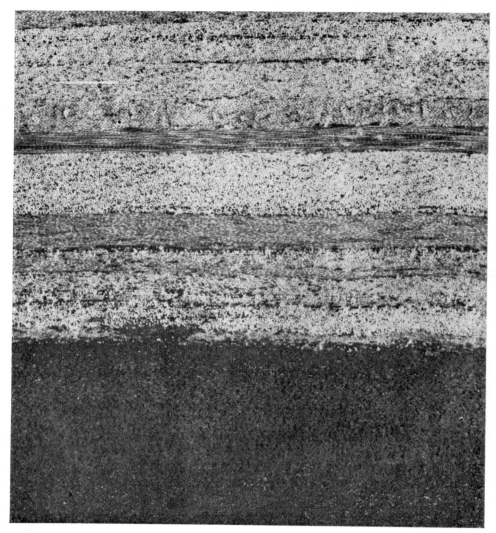

FIG. 37.—ANTERIOR LIMITING MEMBRANE (DESCEMET) (HUMAN, ELECTRON MICROGRAPH, × 19,000).

Compare with Fig. 36. Details of the junction between the membrane (below) and the substantia propria (above) are clearer at this higher magnification.

(*By courtesy of Dr. John Marshall and Mr. P. L. Ansell, Institute of Ophthalmology, London.*)

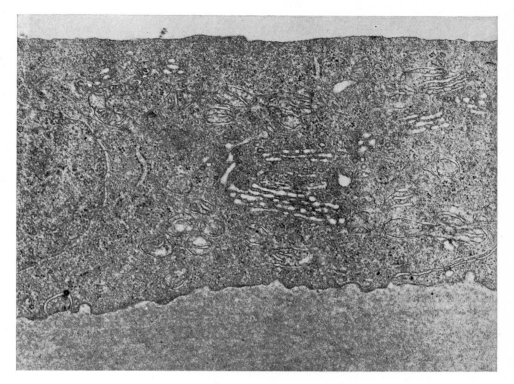

FIG. 38.—CORNEAL ENDOTHELIUM (HUMAN, ELECTRON MICROGRAPH, ×28,000).

Part of a cell only is shown (nuclear profile on left). The adjoining limiting membrane is below.

(*By courtesy of Dr. John Marshall and Mr. P. L. Ansell, Institute of Ophthalmology, London.*)

these vessels are not in the cornea. They are in the subconjunctival connective tissue which overlaps it. The termination of these vessels, visible in the living, is at the periphery of the anterior limiting lamina (Bowman). The nourishment is obtained by lymphatic permeation through the spaces between the lamellæ. No actual lymphatic vessels lined by endothelium are found.

Nerves.—The cornea is supplied by the ophthalmic division of the trigeminal nerve, via the ciliary nerves and those of the surrounding conjunctiva. *The first division of the trigeminal nerve, in fact, supplies almost the whole of the eye and its appendages, giving warning of injury, for instance, of a foreign body, and hence may well be called the sentinel of the eye.* The anterior ciliary nerves enter the sclera from the perichoroidal space a short distance behind the limbus. They connect with each other and with the conjunctival nerves, forming pericorneal plexuses at various levels. The nerves pass into the cornea as 60–80 myelinated trunks at its junction with the sclera. After having gone about 2–4 mm, they usually lose their myelin sheaths (Fig. 233) and divide into two groups—anterior and posterior. The anterior (40–50) pass through the substance of the cornea and then form a plexus subject to the anterior limiting membrane. Having traversed this, the fibres connect again to form a subepithelial plexus and lastly, actually in amongst the epithelial cells, an intraepithelial plexus is found. The posterior (40 or 50) pass to

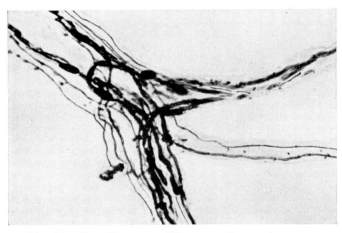

the posterior part of the cornea. This classical description of distinctly stratified corneal plexuses is less clear in human tissues than in the corneæ of the experimental animals originally studied. (Consult Zander and Weddell, 1951 and Toussaint for details.) However, it is certain that all levels, except the posterior limiting membrane (Descemet) are richly supplied.

FIG. 39.—FLAT SECTION OF NERVES AT LIMBUS (STAINED BIELCHOWSKY).

The sheaths of Schwann cells (lemmocytes) extend far into the corneal tissue, but probably not into the epithelium. According to Dogiel, the nerves in the stroma at the periphery of the cornea end in small plates with serrated edges. Krause's end-bulbs may occur beneath the epithelium at the limbus (Fig. 216), but no specialized nerve-endings have been identified in the cornea.

THE SCLERA (FROM σκληρός = HARD)

The sclera forms the posterior opaque five-sixths of the fibrous external tunic of the eye. Its anterior portion is visible, and constitutes the "white" of the eye.

In childhood (or pathologically) when the sclera is thin it appears bluish owing to the uvea showing through. In old age it may become yellowish owing to a deposition of fat. The internal surface of the sclera is brown owing to adherent choroidal pigment cells and is marked by grooves in which the ciliary nerves and vessels lie.

The sclera is thickest behind (about 1 mm), and gradually becomes thinner when traced forwards. It is very thin at the insertion of ocular muscles (0·3 mm), but the thickness of tendon and muscle = 0·6 mm (Fig. 25). At the site of attachment of the optic nerve 3 mm to the medial side of and just *above* the posterior pole of the eye, the sclera becomes a thin sieve-like membrane—the *lamina cribrosa*, through the holes of which the axons of the ganglion cells of the retina pass. It forms most of a sphere 22 mm in diameter.

The lamina cribrosa forms the weakest spot in the outer fibrous tunic of the eye. In glaucoma, therefore, it is here that the eye will give, and result in the cupped disc—characteristic of the *chronic* form of the disease when the intraocular pressure has been raised for some time. Moreover, as the fibres of the optic nerve pass through the lamina cribrosa they lie in canals whose walls are little distensible and hence are easily strangulated by inflammatory swelling.

The outer surface of the sclera is in contact with the fascia bulbi, to which it is connected by fine trabeculæ (see also p. 265).

The sclera is pierced by three sets of apertures—posterior, middle, and anterior.

The Posterior apertures are situated round the optic nerve, and through them pass the long and short ciliary vessels and nerves.

The Middle apertures, 4 mm behind the equator of the eye, give exit to the venæ vorticosæ, which come from the choroid, and some lymphatics.

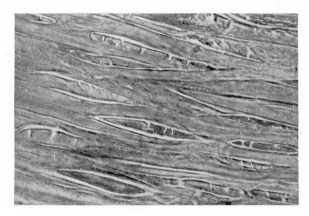

FIG. 40.—ANTEROPOSTERIOR SECTION OF SCLERA.

The Anterior apertures are for the anterior ciliary vessels (which come from the muscular branches to the recti), perivascular lymphatics, and sometimes nerves which may have ganglia on them (see also p. 51).

The sclera contains the sinus venosus scleræ (canal of Schlemm), which indents its deep surface at the corneoscleral junction. A circular flange of sclera thus lies deep to the outer circumference of the sinus venosus scleræ. Wedge-shaped in section, it is known as the *scleral spur* (Figs. 28, 42, 43, 46, 51, 58, 64).

Structure.—The sclera consists of dense bundles of collagen fibres some 10–16 μm in thickness and 100–140 μm in width. The bands are mostly parallel with the surface and cross each other in all directions. They may divide dichotomously and then reunite. The imbrication of the fibres is so dense, especially in its posterior part, that it is almost impossible to separate them by dissection. The deeper bands are stronger than those next the episclera. The tendons of insertion of the recti penetrate into the sclera as parallel fibres and then spread out in a fan-shaped manner to become lost among the meridional fibres of the sclera. The tendons of the oblique muscles behave similarly but here they lose themselves among the oblique or equatorial fibres of the sclera (Kokolt, 1934).

Just as the direction and strength of the trabeculæ of bone are determined by the stresses and strains to which they are subject, so the plan of the scleral fibres is determined by the intraocular tension and the pull of the various muscles. The adaptation of the sclera to these stresses and strains is effected by the disposition

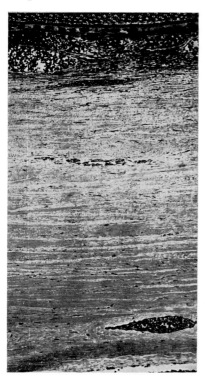

of the fibrous bands, by the wavy course of the connective tissue fibres, and by the great abundance of the elastic fibres (Redslob).

The different parts of the sclera have different functions to perform. This is recognized by the orientation of the fibres. In the posterior portion the external fibres are arranged like the net around a balloon, while the internal fibres spread out fanwise.

The sclera contains no true elastic fibres; collagen is relatively inelastic, but the fibres are not straight and a limited viscoelastic property has been demonstrated experimentally in strips of scleral tissue (Gloster *et al.*, 1957 ; St. Helen and McEwen, 1961). Although in certain pathological states the sclera may gradually yield to increased intraocular pressure, it provides, in normal circumstances, an opposing resistance to the internal pressure; and by this balance the retina and choroid are maintained in correct optical shape within the curve of the sclera.

The anterior portion has a further function. It forms a rigid skeleton for the insertion of the ocular muscles. This rigidity is brought about by the strictly circular direction of the scleral fibres. With age the connective tissue fibres tend to become sclerosed. This conden-

FIG. 41.—SECTION OF CHOROID (ABOVE) AND SCLERA (× 260). A long ciliary nerve appears between the two strata.

(*By courtesy of Dr. John Marshall, Institute of Ophthalmology, London.*)

sation is seen especially around the canals of the venæ vorticosæ.

The fibroblasts of the scleral tissue resemble those of the cornea, but the nuclei are more irregular, and the syncytium formed by the processes not so closed (Salzmann). Pigmented cells of various shapes are met with, especially in the deeper layers near the choroid, and on the vessels and nerves which pass through the sclera. Also at the points where the anterior ciliary vessels enter there is often a collection of pigment, especially in dark people.

These pigment cells have obviously migrated from the uvea, and point the way by which malignant disease of the interior of the eye often makes its way to the outside. In

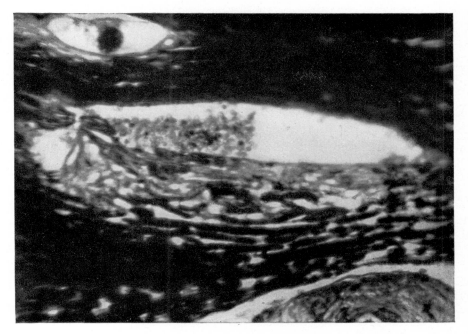

FIG. 42.—SECTION OF SINUS VENOSUS SCLERÆ (CANAL OF SCHLEMM).

Note multinuclear cap in projection of inner wall, and fine fibrils beneath endothelium.   The canal contains blood.

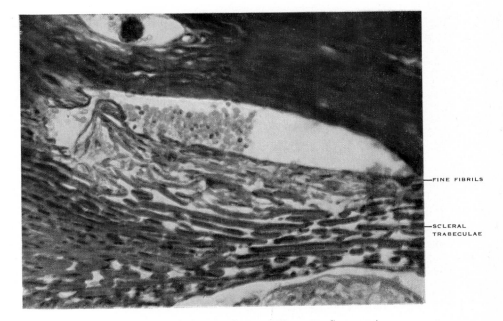

FINE FIBRILS

SCLERAL
TRABECULAE

FIG. 43.—SINUS VENOSUS SCLERÆ (CANAL OF SCHLEMM).

Inner wall juts into canal. Fine fibres beneath endothelium. In the trabeculæ a darker core is visible.

fact, the transition between the most internal scleral laminæ and the most external levels of the choroid is imperceptible (see Lamina fusca, p. 62).

If a section be taken passing through the cornea and sclera, no line of demarcation can be made out, the fibres of one being continuous with those of the other. At their junction, however, we find the sinus venosus scleræ (canal of Schlemm).

The sclera is almost avascular except for the vessels which pass through it to and from the interior of the eye.

Posteriorly around the optic nerve and in the substance of the sclera is the circulus vasculosus of the optic nerve (vascular circle of Zinn or Haller)—see p. 148.

The episcleral tissue is the loose connective and elastic tissue which covers the sclera and anteriorly connects the conjunctiva to it. It is for the most part continuous superficially with the loose tissue of Tenon's space, while its deeper layers become more and more dense and gradually give place to sclera proper. It differs both from the loose tissue of Tenon's space and the sclera, both of which are relatively avascular, by containing quite a fair number of vessels.

Behind the ocular attachments of the recti the episcleral tissue is thin and the vessels, two veins to each artery, form a wide-meshed net. The arteries here come from the posterior ciliaries. In front of the attachment of the muscles the episclera is much thicker and much richer in vessels. The meshes of the vascular net, too, are much smaller. A capillary net exists only in this anterior zone of the sclera. It is a marked filling of this net which is called "ciliary injection".

Nerves of the Sclera.—The ciliary nerves pierce the sclera around the optic nerve. The long ciliary nerves accompany the long posterior ciliary arteries and so reach the ciliary body. At the level of the orbiculis ciliaris the nerves divide into branches. Some go to the ciliary body, some accompanied by vessels penetrate the sclera, most commonly at the equator or some 2–4 mm from the limbus (Fig. 39). When they reach the surface, the branches connect, forming loops around the limbus, from the convexity of which branches pass into the cornea. Nerves also pass from the episcleral tissue inwards into the sclera.

Some scleral nerves have a curious course. They enter the sclera and may even reach its outer surface. They then bend round sharply and turn back to the point of entrance. The extremity of the loop sometimes presents a mushroom-like thickening. These scleral loops are found most commonly about 1·6 mm from the limbus. In their intrascleral course the nerves are often accompanied by pigment and appear under the conjunctiva as hyaline elevations surrounded by a ring of pigment, which are very sensitive (Redslob). Most of the "scleral" nerves are in transit to other tissues, but some afferent fibres, of uncertain function, appear to innervate the sclera itself.

SINUS VENOSUS SCLERÆ (THE CANAL OF SCHLEMM)

Position and Form.—The sinus venosus scleræ is a circular venous canal at the corneoscleral junction at the bottom of the so-called scleral furrow. For most of its course it is single (with perhaps a very small companion) but there may be two or more canals. It has been likened to a river which divides into branches and then unites again. According to Leber, there may be a plexiform arrangement of these branches, which may number up to seven, especially in the region where the canal is joined by branches from the ciliary muscle.

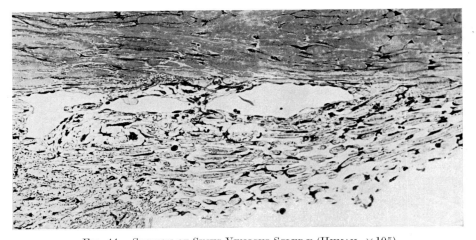

FIG. 44.—SECTION OF SINUS VENOSUS SCLERÆ (HUMAN, × 105).
Note the loosely arranged trabecular tissue between the sinus and anterior chamber (below).
(*By courtesy of Dr. John Marshall and Mr. P. L. Ansell, Institute of Ophthalmology, London.*)

The canal is flattened from without inwards and tends to be wider posteriorly. It may be oval or triangular with the apex nearest the cornea. It occupies approximately the posterior half of the distance between the scleral spur and the posterior limiting lamina, and thus is about 0·5 mm across. Its width is always less than that of the trabecular rete.

Structure and Relations.—The sinus venosus is lined by endothelium whose nuclei project in towards the lumen; it has a thin fibrous wall, but is otherwise closely surrounded by scleral tissue. The wall of the canal is a mere 10 μm in thickness on its external aspect, away from the trabecular tissue. The basement membrane of the endothelial cells is incomplete and much interrupted. The cells are joined side-to-side by zonulæ occludentes, but not by tight junctions. Many of the endothelial cells are prominently vacuolated and exhibit pinocytic activity, especially in the wall of the sinus adjoining the scleral trabeculæ.

Here and there partly and more rarely completely crossing the lumen of the canal are partitions of sclera resembling those of the dural venous sinuses. The

anterior ciliary veins have in general the same structure as the canal. The canal is
bounded posteriorly by the scleral spur which also overlaps it somewhat to the
inner side.

The inner wall of the sinus venosus scleræ, next to the scleral trabeculæ, is
usually flat but it projects in places like a villus (Figs. 41, 42, 43), and may indeed
reach the outer wall. The cells in these projections are loosely arranged, and here,

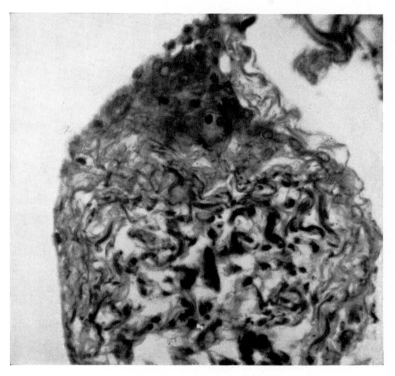

FIG. 45.—ARACHNOIDAL VILLUS.

Note multi-nuclear cap. Also fine fibrils below endothelium and coarse subarachnoid
trabeculæ forming core.

as elsewhere in the endothelium, vacuoles may sometimes provide temporary
intracellular canaliculi from the trabecular spaces to the venous sinus. (See
Ashton, 1969; Tripathi, 1971, 1972.) The inner wall of the sinus venosus scleræ is
sometimes described as being formed by the trabeculæ of the ligamentum pectinatum iridis and, although both Salzmann and Rochon-Duvigneaud have noted a
different type of tissue directly under the endothelium, their descriptions are no
doubt the result of noting the appearance seen when hæmatoxylin and eosin or
van Gieson has been used as the stain. For Salzmann says it resembles the tissue
under the endothelium of the outer wall of the canal, while Rochon-Duvigneaud

describes it as compact or dense. With Mallory's triple stain after Zenker fixation this tissue is seen to consist of a reticulum of very fine fibrils. This layer probably has the consistency of cotton wool and I (Eugene Wolff) would suggest is homologous with the tissue under the endothelium of an arachnoidal villus, that is with the protruded arachnoid (Fig. 44). Deep to this are some fibres which resemble those of the main mass of the ligamentum, but are frailer and contain no core of connective and elastic tissue. These no doubt represent the subarachnoid trabeculæ. Modern views emphasize that the tissue in this region is largely endothelial, and assert that connective tissue is minimal. It is, however, interesting to

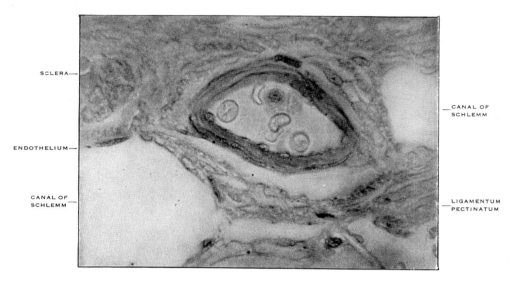

FIG. 46.—PORTION OF THE SINUS VENOSUS SCLERÆ (CANAL OF SCHLEMM) WITH AN ANTERIOR CILIARY ARTERY ACTUALLY IN THE CANAL.

note the similarity in the problems of return of aqueous fluid and cerebrospinal fluid to the venous system. (Consult Tripathi, 1973). It is also worth noting that direct canaliculi through the endothelium have been described in arachnoid granulations in some animals (Jayatilaka, 1965).

The Normal Content of the Canal.—It is generally stated that on section the canal usually contains no blood and that Schlemm (1830) found it full of blood because he examined the eye of a man who had been hanged and in whom therefore the veins of the head were engorged.

But Leber in sections of normal eyes (or eyes which were affected with cataract only) found blood in the canal of fifteen out of seventeen eyes. It is true in some there was very little blood, but this does not alter the argument. Also in favour of the canal normally containing some blood is the fact that Fuchs found that in individuals with a thin sclera a dark line concentric with the limbus can be made out by focal illumination. The evidence derived from gonioscopy is equivocal. With the gonioscope the canal may appear grey, that is without blood, or pink, that is with blood; the pink staining may affect a section only. It seems to depend largely on whether the gonio-glass presses on the limbus or the cornea (see Busacca, 1945).

A large volume of physiological experimentation, carried out to establish the mechanisms of return of aqueous fluid to the venous circulation by the inter-mediation of the scleral venous sinus, indicates that the latter usually, if not al-ways, contains no blood.

Communication with the Anterior Chamber.—The dispute started by such workers as Schwalbe (1887) and Leber (1903), and perpetuated by Sondermann (1953), François (1955), and others recently, as to whether direct endothelialized channels conduct aqueous from the scleral trabecular spaces to the scleral venous sinus has not been entirely resolved. There seems little doubt that such communi-cations exist. Equally, it is improbable that they are a major mechanism in the transport of aqueous.

Communicating and Neighbouring Vessels.—The intrascleral venous plexus receives junctional branches from the scleral sinus which form very characteristic collecting trunks. They run from the convex anterior aspect of the canal into a vein of the plexus, as a straight vessel or after having made a hook-shaped bend. They are minute, flattened, and have an oblique course. They may thus act as valves, the usual type of which are absent (Maggiore).

There are 25–35 collector channels leaving the scleral sinus at irregular intervals, but mostly near the horizontal meridian (Theobald). Some fourteen or more branches from the ciliary muscle also traverse the sclera to join the plexus of veins in the neighbourhood of the canal (Leber).

The arteries near the canal probably form a circular vessel which runs close to and parallel with the canal. It is so figured by Maggiore. Sometimes the artery may actually be found in the canal (Wolff) (Fig. 45). Also Friedenwald has de-scribed fine arterial branches actually opening into the canal. These he holds are important in explaining the draining of aqueous from the canal. This work, however, has not been confirmed.

According to Maggiore, the canal of Schlemm receives junctional branches from a vas-cular plexus situated in the depths of the limbus and composed of a reticulum mainly venous with which are constantly associated some fine arterial branches and capillary loops. The arterial branches which had not been described before are branches of the anterior ciliaries. These vessels, which are generally very fine, run into the deep layers of the sclera and, giving off successive anastomosing branches, form a net with large and irregular meshes which accompanies the venous plexus and is joined to this by means of fine loops of very characteristic aspect, which insinuate themselves radially into the peri-phery of the cornea and running up to the commencement of the canal of Schlemm not infrequently pass beyond it in a centripetal direction. This vascular plexus, unlike the episcleral, is hidden from clinical observation, but is responsible for the violet colouring which the limbus assumes in inflammation of the uveal tract.

Maggiore describes four plexuses in the region of the limbus:

1. Conjunctival (see p. 216).
2. The plexus of the fascia bulbi.
3. Episcleral plexus (see p. 217).
4. The intrascleral plexus.

Aqueous Veins.—The aqueous veins of Ascher (1942, 1949) vary in size from 0·01 to 0·1 mm in diameter. Thus while a slit-lamp is usually necessary to see

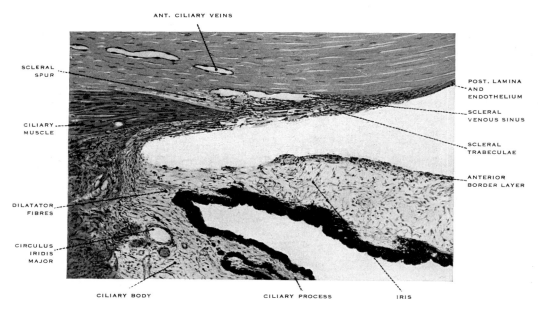

FIG. 47.—SECTION OF THE ANGLE OF THE ANTERIOR CHAMBER. (Same slide as Fig. 28.)

them, the largest can just be made out with a loupe. They are found near the limbus (about 2 mm from it), most often inferonasally and often commencing in a hook-shaped bend where they come out of the sclera. They contain a clear fluid or very diluted blood and run a short course from 10 mm to just over a centimetre. They join an episcleral vein, the blood of which may become more diluted, or clear fluid and blood may run side by side unmixed. Thus is formed a laminated vein of Goldmann (1946). Sometimes a clear central stream is flanked by a blood column on either side.

Aqueous veins are exit channels of the aqueous, hence the name. Indeed, Ashton (1952) has traced one of these vessels, seen during life, into the canal of Schlemm after the removal of the eye. An aqueous vein is therefore an efferent from the canal of Schlemm which remains separate or nearly so until it has passed through the sclera.

To summarize, the aqueous fluid, having reached the venous sinus of the sclera, passes first into the neighbouring deep scleral plexus of veins, and thence *via* the intrascleral plexus to the episcleral plexus and even the subjunctival plexus at the limbus. In addition, direct connections (aqueous veins) pass from the deep scleral to the episcleral plexus (Fig. 51).

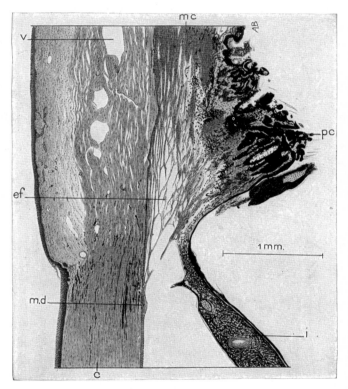

FIG. 48.—MERIDIONAL SECTION OF ANGLE OF ANTERIOR CHAMBER OF HYENA.

mc, the ciliary muscle of which the deep portion goes with the ciliary processes while the superficial portion is adherent to the sclera; pc, ciliary processes; i, iris and scleral trabeculæ; ef, the cilioscleral space or space of Fontana; c, cornea with an interstitial pigmentary zone; md, posterior limiting lamina; v, sinus venosus scleræ.

(*From Rochon-Duvigneaud.*)

COMPARATIVE ANATOMY OF THE ANGLE OF THE ANTERIOR CHAMBER (THE IRIDOSCLERAL OR CILIOSCLERAL ANGLE)

In the quadruped mammals (and also in birds and reptiles) the ciliary body of the adult is divided into two layers by a fissure (the intraciliary sinus or the cilioscleral space or space of Fontana) which passes more or less deeply from before backwards between the ciliary processes and the ciliary muscle always placed directly against the sclera.

In the primates the ciliary body is, on the contrary, compact and has no fissure or sinus, because the ciliary processes throughout their length are adherent by their line of insertion to the ciliary muscle. This is fundamentally the difference which exists between the angle of the anterior chamber of the primates and that of the other mammals (Rochon-Duvigneaud).

The intraciliary space or sinus of the latter is filled by the trabeculæ of the true pectinate

A.E.—5

ligament, of which the most superficial attach the ciliary processes and the root of the iris (which otherwise would hang loose) to the sclera from the region of the canal of Schlemm to the posterior limiting lamina (Descemet). Hence Hueck described the ligament as iridis, i.e. of the iris.

The obliteration of the ciliary sinus in the primates necessarily does away with the necessity of cilioscleral trabeculæ and further causes an attachment of the iris to the tendon of the ciliary muscle (Fig. 46), thus forming a cilioiridial arcade which makes the fibres of the true pectinate ligament unnecessary. These fibres present in the human fetus (see p. 442 and Fig. 400) have largely disappeared in the adult. Hence, in the human the cilioiridial arcade limits the anterior chamber while in quadrupeds this is prolonged through the meshes of the true pectinate ligament or space of Fontana to the bottom of the cilioscleral sinus, well beyond the scleral attachment of the tendon of the ciliary muscle.

The adherence of the ciliary processes to a strong ciliary muscle which is characteristic of the primates, assures the direct action of the muscle on the lens through the Zonule. It thus makes for an improved mechanism of accommodation. In other words, the necessity of a more extensive power of accommodation has brought about the adherence of the surface of origin of the zonular fibres, represented by the ciliary epithelium to the ciliary muscle. This adhesion makes for the obliteration of the ciliary sinus and the disappearance of the trabeculæ of the pectinate ligament, which partition its cavity. The more central fibres which form arcades and which attach the iris to the posterior limiting lamina (that is the true pectinate ligament) become unnecessary when the iris gains attachment to the tendon of the ciliary muscle (to form the cilioiridial arcade). Their almost complete disappearance in the primates and more especially in man practically clears the angle of all trabeculæ and hence the anterior chamber is limited by the cilioiridial arcade and the space of Fontana is obliterated (Rochon-Duvigneaud).

NORMAL APPEARANCES AS SEEN WITH THE GONIOSCOPE

The structures which may be made out with the gonioscope are:

(1) The root of the iris.

(2) A portion of the anterior surface of the ciliary body.

(3) The iris processes.

(4) The scleral trabeculæ (ligamentum pectinatum) with the scleral spur behind Schwalbe's ring in front, and the scleral venous sinus external.

(5) The posterior aspect of the cornea.

(1) The most prominent portion here is the last ridge.

(2) The anterior surface of the ciliary body which is responsible for the ciliary band forms a concave recess or sinus. It has the same colour as the iris, but is much darker (Troncoso, 1947).

(3) The iris processes, that is the remains of the fetal or true ligamentum pectinatum, bridge over the angle and are usually visible as thin yellowish semitransparent lines which run vertically from the edge of the iris upwards to disappear in the line formed by the scleral trabeculæ (Troncoso). The iris processes vary in number and so the amount that the angle is hidden varies also.

(4) The scleral trabeculæ (ligamentum pectinatum) forms a band which in young persons is bluish or grey, but in older people is yellowish, possibly with pigment deposits. Behind this the scleral spur forms a narrow whitish line (the

posterior annular line) while anterior to it Schwalbe's ring also forms a whitish line which may or may not project (the anterior annular line).

When the canal of Schlemm contains blood, it forms a narrow but well-marked reddish line just in front of the line formed by the scleral spur and taking in about

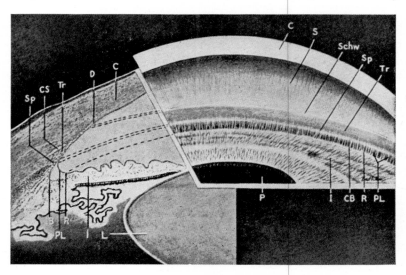

FIG. 49.—SECTION OF THE ANGLE OF THE ANTERIOR CHAMBER WITH THE CORRESPONDING PARTS AS SEEN BY THE GONIOSCOPE.

P, pupil; I, iris; R, ciliary border of iris; CB, ciliary body; Sp, scleral spur; PL, iris processes; Tr, corneoscleral trabeculæ covering canal of Schlemm, CS; Schw, Schwalbe's ring; S, dome of cornea with limbal vessels; D, termination of Descemet's membrane; C, cornea; L, lens.

(From François, 1948; after Troncoso.)

half the band formed by the ligamentum. When empty, the canal of course is invisible. Whether it contains blood or not appears to depend largely on the fit of the contact glass: where this presses on the limbus the canal appears empty; while opposite this point it tends to be full of blood (see Busacca, 1945).

THE LIGAMENTUM PECTINATUM IRIDIS.[1] (CORNEO-SCLERAL TRABECULAR SYSTEM OF ROCHON-DUVIGNEAUD) (CRIBRIFORM LIGAMENT OF HENDERSON.)

The so-called ligamentum pectinatum iridis—better called the scleral trabeculæ—is a circular zone consisting essentially of reticulated tissue between the

[1] The name ligamentum pectinatum iridis is misleading, for, as Fuchs points out, Hueck introduced it because he found that in ungulates, on stripping the iris from the sclera, the tissue that unites these parts projects in a series of ridges resembling the teeth of a comb (pecten). In mammals and birds the ridges are formed by large pigmented trabeculæ which cross the angle of the anterior chamber from the corneoscleral junction to the front of the iris (see Rochon-Duvigneaud). In man similar ridges occur up to the sixth month of fetal life, but after that largely disappear. They occur, however, in the adult human eye much more frequently than is commonly supposed

sinus venosus sclerae and the anterior chamber. It reaches from the scleral spur to the periphery of the posterior limiting membrane (about 1 mm). On examination after teasing of a stained preparation it may be shown that superficially (i.e. next the anterior chamber) near the scleral spur the meshes of the ligament are wide, irregular, and bounded by fine trabeculæ. Deeper, the trabeculæ are wider, flattened, and surround meshes which are much narrower. Posteriorly there are some twelve to fifteen planes. As we go anteriorly the planes tend to fuse, so that

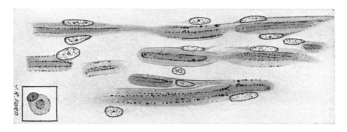

FIG. 50. — DETAIL OF LIGAMENTUM PECTINATUM (in Figs. 28, 47) UNDER HIGHER MAGNIFICATION (ABOUT 800) TO SHOW THE FOUR LAYERS OF WHICH EACH TRABECULA CONSISTS. (INSET, CROSS-SECTION.)

near the posterior lamina (Descemet) there are only three or fewer perforated plaques.

Microscopically. On meridional section the trabecular network is triangular. The apex of the triangle is attached to the posterior layers of the cornea (including the posterior lamina) at Schwalbe's "anterior limiting ring" (Fig. 47). The inner side of the triangle lies in the anterior chamber. The outer side is in contact anteriorly with the sclera; farther back for half to two-thirds of its length it is internal to the scleral venous sinus.

The base of the triangle is formed by the scleral spur and the ciliary muscle, while the posterocentral angle is, as it were, continued in front of the ciliary body into the iris. The triangle is filled with the segments of the trabeculæ which run in straight lines from the apex to the base, diverging slightly. They appear as a rule as little rods of different lengths with rounded and slightly tapering ends, placed end to end. Each represents a distinct plane. Sometimes a segment is oval or, where the section is perpendicular to its length, round.

According to Ranvier, each trabecula consists of a core and a peripheral portion, the whole being covered by endothelium. The endothelium consists of large flat cells whose nuclei usually lie at the bifurcation of a trabecula. These cells are obviously the continuation of Descemet's endothelium but are flatter and larger. The nuclei also instead of being round are slightly flattened.

The peripheral portion is hyaline and is the continuation of Descemet itself.

(Fig. 63). Thus Fritz showed that some can be seen in most eyes if the angle is opened up and examined with a binocular microscope. In eyes with dark irides they are pigmented and easily seen, while in blue eyes they are non-pigmented, very fine, and easily missed. With the introduction of the gonioscope, they can be found in most eyes (see iris processes, above). It must be added, too, that the region does not behave as a ligament.

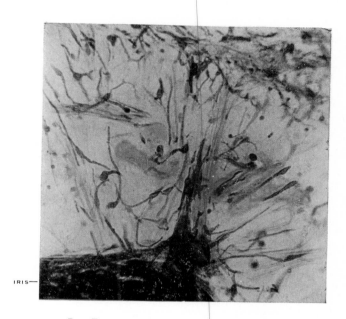

IRIS—

FIG. 51.—SECTION ALONG IRIS PROCESS SHOWING STRANDS OF LIGAMENTUM PECTINATUM IRIDIS.

A.E.—60]

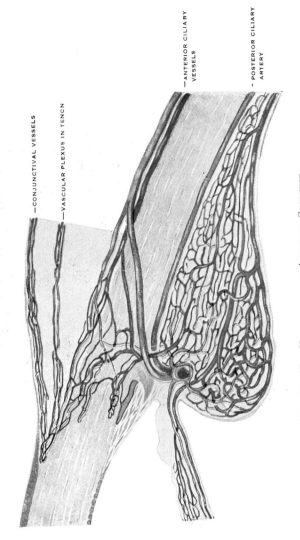

CONJUNCTIVAL VESSELS

VASCULAR PLEXUS IN TENCN

ANTERIOR CILIARY VESSELS

POSTERIOR CILIARY ARTERY

Fig. 52.—The Vessels of the Anterior Segment.

(From Lauber, after Maggiori.)

The core which takes in a little more than a third of the whole thickness consists of elastic and connective tissue. According to Salzmann (and Fig. 52), the elastic fibres lie on the connective tissue (Salzmann thus described four layers: endothelial, hyaline, elastic, and collagenous). At the apex of the triangle the nuclei of the ligamentum arrange themselves in single file in front of the anterior limiting ring or termination of Descemet (Fig. 35). The trabeculæ of that portion which lies next the anterior chamber and passes into the root of the iris (uveal part of lig. pect. iridis) are much finer than the remainder (scleral part of lig. pect. iridis), and in them the elastic fibres are absent.

Electron Microscopy on the whole confirms these appearances of the fibres and their endothelial covering (p. 43). The holes in the sponge are known as the spaces of Fontana, and on the outer side lie near the venous sinus and on the inner communicate with the anterior chamber.

The anterior limiting ring of Schwalbe (Fig. 35) is a bundle of connective tissue and elastic fibres anterior to or at the periphery of the posterior limiting lamina. Histologically it consists of the same tissue as the scleral trabecular network but the fibrils have a different direction: from being meridional they have become circular. The ring varies in position and size not only from eye to eye but in different portions of the same eye. It may form a projection into the anterior chamber (Fig. 49), in which case it can be seen with the gonioscope. It is probably only visible when this region is abnormally prominent.

The scleral furrow of Schwalbe. It should be carefully noted that this furrow is not present normally. It is only formed as an artefact after the inner wall of the venous sinus and scleral trabeculæ have been torn away. It is limited anteriorly by the anterior limiting ring and posteriorly by the scleral spur which is the *posterior limiting ring.*

THE VASCULAR TUNIC OR UVEAL TRACT

The vascular tunic consists from behind forwards of the choroid, ciliary body, and iris, all continuous with each other. This continuity can easily be made out if the cornea and sclera be carefully dissected off the underlying structures. Such a dissection would show a dark brown sphere attached to the optic nerve behind and having a central hole, the pupil, in front. On account of the similarity to a grape (uva) of the dark sphere hanging on the optic nerve as on a stalk, the middle coat of the eye has received the name of uvea or uveal tract (Fuchs).

THE CHOROID

The choroid is the most posterior part of the vascular coat of the eye. It is the homologue of the pia-arachnoid, and just as the latter vascularizes the brain, so does the choroid maintain the outer part of the retina. It is a thin membrane, extending from the optic nerve to the ora serrata, that is, the jagged line where the retina ends. It is very difficult to estimate the thickness of the choroid, for it consists largely of vessels—it has been compared to the corpus cavernosum—and hence diminishes in thickness on enucleation and as the result of fixation. But it is thicker posteriorly (about 0·22 mm) than anteriorly (about 0·1 mm), and is especially thick in the macular region (Fig. 150). Its inner surface, which can be examined by removing the vitreous and retina after opening the eye, is smooth and brown. On separating the choroid from the sclera, on the other hand, the outer surface of the former is found to be rough and shaggy.

The choroid is firmly attached to the margin of the optic nerve, and slightly at the points where vessels and nerves enter it. It is more firmly attached to the

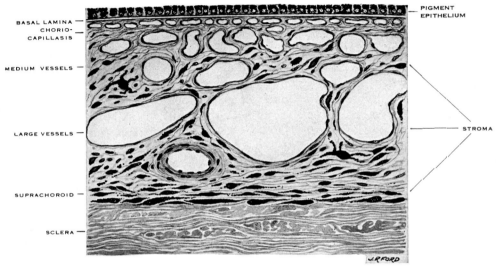

FIG. 53.—CHOROID, TRANSVERSE SECTION.

(After Fuchs and Wolff's preparation.)

sclera behind the coronal equator than in front of this (Moses). Moses (1965) has measured in the excised eye the strength of the suprachoroidal lamellæ and of their attachments to the sclera. A strip of this tissue, one centimetre in width, resists a tensile force of 6 g.

Structure.—The choroid consists mainly of blood-vessels, but on each side of these is a nonvascular layer. Externally, i.e. nearest the sclera, is the *lamina suprachoroidea*, and most internally the homogeneous *basal lamina* (*membrane of Bruch*). The vessels of the choroid are classically described as being arranged in three superimposed strata—the largest being nearest the sclera and the smallest, the capillaries, called the *chorio-capillaris*, towards the retina.

Thus we may divide the choroid into five layers, which from without inwards are as follows:

1. *The suprachoroid lamina* or lamina fusca is some 10–34 μm in thickness. It consists of flattened laminæ closely applied to each other which limit potential spaces. These become evident pathologically when the suprachoroid is distended with fluid. It is then seen that the laminæ join each other at acute angles at certain points and then separate again, giving the whole the appearance of a grill.

The laminæ consist of a delicate mesh of collagen fibres. They always run from the sclera anteriorly to the choroid and are shorter posteriorly. Schwalbe taught that these were covered by an endothelial layer limiting lymphatic spaces; but this view is now discredited. The laminæ contain numerous melanocytes and fibroblasts.

The laminæ are more adherent to each other posteriorly than anteriorly. Hence it is in the anterior portion that a detachment of the choroid usually takes place. The melanocytes here are more stunted, with shorter processes than those in the

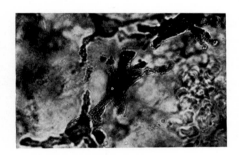

FIG. 54.—HUMAN CHOR-
OIDAL MELANOCYTES (× 675).
(*By courtesy of Dr. John Marshall and Mr. P. L. Ansell, Institute of Ophthalmology, London.*)

vessel layer. They are more pigmented posteriorly and may be poor in pigment anteriorly. The nucleus is always non-pigmented (Figs. 54, 55). The melanocytes spread out in the plane of the surface of the choroid and are thus seen properly only in a flat section (compare Figs. 53 and 54).

Unstriped muscle fibres are also found. These are more numerous in front of the equator, where they tend to form star-shaped figures or *muscle stars* (see p. 70). They have also been described around the optic nerve (Fuchs). On separating the choroid from the sclera this layer divides, part of its adhering to the former, part to the latter. It is this fact that gives the outer surface of the choroid its shaggy appearance.

The suprachoroidal space contains the long and short posterior ciliary arteries and nerves. The nerves break up into smaller and smaller branches, which eventually supply the choroid. At the points of division of the nerves are placed multipolar ganglia, which are probably vasomotor in function.

2 and 3. *The Layer of Vessels.*—Classically this layer is divided into two:

    (*a*) The layer of large vessels (Haller's layer).

    (*b*) The layer of medium-sized vessels (Sattler's layer).

But, while it is possible in places so to separate them, usually one cannot do so owing to the irregularity of their distribution, and the whole region is better described as the *stroma* of the choroid.

The larger vessels are external and tend to diminish in size as we go towards the choriocapillaris. The innermost of them are arterioles which join the capillaries by oblique branches and veins that receive oblique venules from them. As regards the large vessels, the arteries are deep posteriorly but more anteriorly they are superficial. In fact, in the greater part of the choroid only veins are found next to the suprachoroid lamina. The veins are largest posteriorly, especially in the macular region and where they join the venæ vorticosæ after undergoing an ampullary dilatation. No choroidal vein is supplied with valves.

By light and electron microscopy the vessels show no peculiarities. The ciliary arteries have the typical structure of smaller arteries. The second, external endothelial tube ascribed to the veins by Salzmann is a misinterpretation.

The Stroma consists of loose collagenous tissue with some elastin and reticulin fibres. The collagen fibres are arranged circularly as an adventitia to the vessels. The stroma is especially characterized by the presence of *pigment cells* or melanocytes. These are variable in number depending on the part of the choroid, the age of the individual, his race and general pigmentation. The region round the optic nerve is richest in these cells. The cells spread out for the most part in a plane parallel to the surface of the choroid and are, therefore, best seen in a flat section. Hence one only infrequently comes across a whole pigment cell in a vertical section. This is especially true of the suprachoroid; in the choroid itself the processes may be three-dimensional.

The cells usually anastomose with each other so as to form a syncytium but may be found isolated. The nuclei are most often round or oval, rarely kidney-shaped. They contain no pigment and their chromatin is evenly spread, there being no nucleolus. The size of the cells and their pigmentation varies; usually the more pigmented, the plumper they are. The pigment granules, *which are of the same size in any particular cell*, are very fine and evenly distributed in the cell body and processes. It is only in the embryo that the region round the nucleus is less or non-pigmented. The granules are light yellowish brown to dark brown; but never so dark as the retinal pigment. The size of the pigment granule is the same for the same individual, but differs from race to race; but always much smaller than those of the pigment epithelium. The cells are melanoblasts.

The connective tissue cells have a very fine and evenly granular cytoplasm which is difficult to make out with ordinary stains. The nucleus is usually oval, but may be round or kidney-shaped. The achromatic ground work is very fine. The chromatin is evenly divided and finely granular. Nucleoli are very rare.

Other cells present in the stroma are macrophages, lymphocytes, mast cells (mastocytes), and plasma cells.

4. *The Choriocapillaris* consists of capillaries of wide bore (Figs. 87, 90), packed closely together. *They nourish the outer part of the retina.* Unlike the other

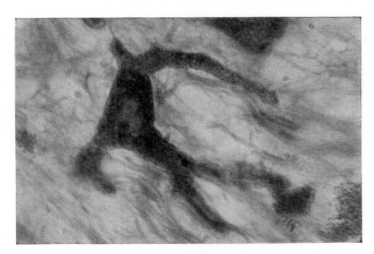

FIG. 55.—MELANOCYTE OF CHOROID (FLAT SECTION).
Nucleus visible (Mallory's triple stain).

vascular layers, the choriocapillaris contains no pigment. Indeed, it is obvious, on looking at any section of the normal choroid, *that it is more pigmented towards its external aspect.*

The choriocapillaris ends at the ora serrata, whereas the other layers continue on into the ciliary body.

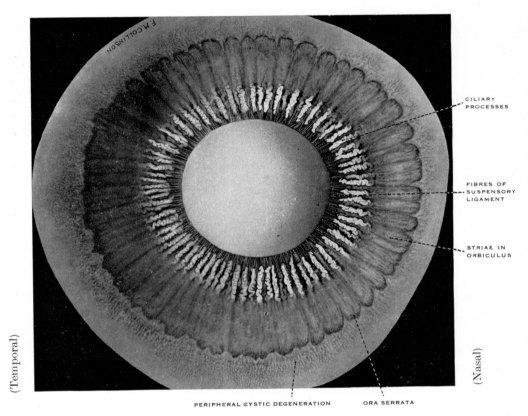

(Temporal)   (Nasal)

CILIARY PROCESSES

FIBRES OF SUSPENSORY LIGAMENT

STRIAE IN ORBICULUS

PERIPHERAL CYSTIC DEGENERATION   ORA SERRATA

FIG. 56.—CILIARY BODY, SUSPENSORY LIGAMENT, LENS, AND ORA SERRATA (SEEN FROM BEHIND).

Note that the serrations of the ora are less evident temporally, where cystic degeneration (shown by the mottled appearance) is most developed.

The capillaries of the choriocapillaris are much wider than elsewhere and show many sac-like dilatations. They form a net which is densest, i.e. with the smallest meshes, at the macula. Also here the capillaries have the widest bore and so ensure the richest blood-supply to the cones of the area centralis. Towards the periphery the meshes are larger and tend to be more and more elongated. The dimensions of the intercapillary spaces vary from 5×20 μm in the perimacular region to about 20×200 μm at the equator.

The capillaries vary in diameter from 18–50 μm, being about 20 μm at the macula. Ultrastructurally these vessels resemble those of many viscera in being fenestrated, but these openings have a diaphragm (Leeson, 1971). Around the capillaries are supporting collagen fibres, nerve fibres, and ganglion cells. The nerves are arranged as plexuses with amyelinate branches to the capillary wall.

5. *The Basal Lamina* (membrane of Bruch; lamina vitrea; hyaloid membrane) is a thin complex membrane about 2 μm in thickness, placed next the pigment layer of the retina, which indeed used to be regarded as belonging to the choroid, since it remains adherent to the membrane when the rest of the retina is removed or detached. It is normally smooth and regular in the visual region. The ease of separation of the retina from its own pigment epithelium, as in detachment of the retina (p. 102), is due to mode of development of the optic cup (p. 425). The outer layer of the basal lamina gives firm attachment to the fibres which bind together the whole thickness of the choroid. The inner layer of the lamina consists of a dense network of extremely delicate fibres. When the two portions separate, either pathologically or as an artefact, fine fibrils can be seen traversing the potential space between them. As will be seen later, the layers do separate at the ora serrata, and in the ciliary body a well-marked layer of connective tissue is interposed between them (Figs. 68, 69).

The earlier light microscopy of the basal lamina has been amplified by the use of more selective stains and electron microscopy. The simple division into a "cuticular" layer, adjacent to the retinal pigment cells and a connective tissue zone merging with the choriocapillaris is no longer adequate. The former layer, about 3 μm thick, is the basement membrane of the retinal pigmented epithelium, is PAS positive, and composed of fine fibres, with a space of about 100 nm between it and the epithelial cell walls. The rest of the lamina is a sandwich of elastic fibres between two layers of collagen fibres. (For details see Sumita, 1961; Hogan, 1961, 1971). Its choroidal aspect is an interrupted basement membrane derived from the endothelium of the capillaries. (The existence of two basement membranes in the layer renders the current official term, basal lamina, a little confusing).

Posteriorly the lamina reaches the edge of the optic papilla, where the elastic fibres assume a circumferential orientation, the collagen fibres merging with the connective tissue of the optic nerve.

THE CILIARY BODY

If the eyeball is bisected antero-posteriorly and the vitreous, lens and retina removed, we see the choroid, ciliary body and iris in continuity.

The choroid, as we have seen, extends up to the ora serrata—that is, the denticulated line where the retina has been torn away anteriorly. Beyond this the ciliary body starts, and can be easily recognized by the fact that it is black, whereas the choroid is brown. If we examine the inner surface of the ciliary body, we see that usually the part just beyond the ora serrata is smooth *to the naked eye* and hence is known as the *pars plana* (orbiculus ciliaris or ciliary ring).

Under low magnification, however, one sees the ciliary *striæ* (of Schultze) in the pars plana. These are slight dark ridges which converge anteriorly from the teeth of the ora serrata to the valleys between the ciliary processes (Fig. 56). Also there

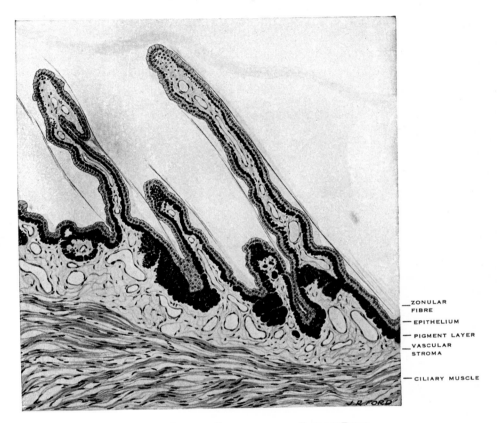

ZONULAR
FIBRE

EPITHELIUM

PIGMENT LAYER

VASCULAR
STROMA

CILIARY MUSCLE

FIG. 57.—OBLIQUE SECTION OF THE CILIARY BODY.

Note that the pigment does not reach the apex of the main ciliary processes. Hence they are white in the living. The ones in between, however, appear black, since pigment reaches to the apex.

(*Wolff's preparation.*)

is often a dark band just in front, and following the indentations of the ora serrata (Fig. 56). This marks the posterior attachment of the suspensory ligament of the lens. Further forward the inner surface presents about seventy radiating ridges of various sizes. These ridges are the *ciliary processes,* and are lighter in colour than the valleys between them. The region in which they occur is called the *pars plicata* (corona ciliaris) (Fig. 56). The whole ciliary body forms a ring whose width is 5·9 mm on the nasal side and 6·7 mm on the temporal: the pars plicata occupies about 2 mm of this.

On sagittal section (Fig. 25) the ciliary body is triangular in form, with its shortest side anterior. The anterior side of the triangle in its outer part usually enters into the formation of the angle of the anterior chamber, but may be covered by the mesh-work of the angle. From about its middle the iris extends, and makes, with the remaining part of the anterior surface, an angle, usually quite acute, which opens in the posterior chamber (Fig. 25). The outer side of the triangle corresponds to the ciliary muscle, and lies against the sclera, the suprachoroidal tissue, however, coming between them. The inner side corresponds to the ciliary processes,

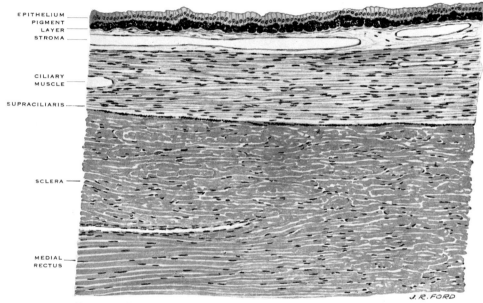

EPITHELIUM
PIGMENT
LAYER
STROMA

CILIARY
MUSCLE

SUPRACILIARIS

SCLERA

MEDIAL
RECTUS

J. R. FORD

FIG. 63.—CILIARY BODY (ORBICULUS). ANTERO-POSTERIOR SECTION.
(*Wolff's preparation.*)

and is in relation anteriorly with the fibres of the suspensory ligament which are bathed in aqueous, and posteriorly with the vitreous. The equator of the lens is about 0·5 mm from the ciliary processes.

Structure.—From without inwards we find the following layers: (1) Suprachoroidal lamina or "supraciliaris"; (2) ciliary muscle; (3) the ciliary processes, with: (4) the basal lamina and stroma; (5) the epithelium; and (6) the internal limiting membrane.

1. *The Suprachoroid Lamina* (more suitably named the "supraciliaris") resembles that of the choroid. It consists of strands of pigmented collagen fibres, partly derived from the suprachoroidea proper but also from the external, longi-

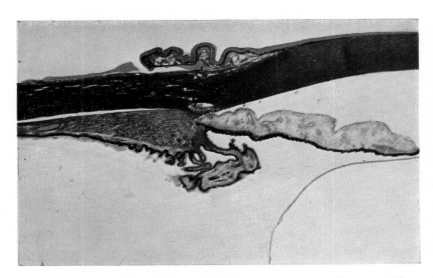

Fig. 58.—Meridional Section of Anterior Segment of Eye. (Zenker. Mallory's Triple Stain.)

This section is from an eye with a small malignant melanoma at the macula. The narrowness of the angle of the anterior chamber is an artefact.

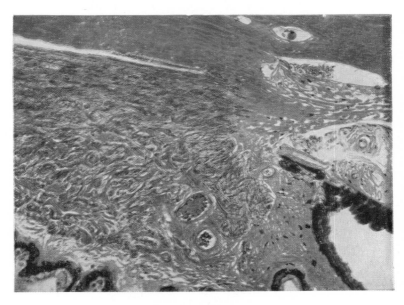

FIG. 59.—DETAIL OF FIGURE 58.
To show differential staining of muscle (red) and connective tissue (blue) in the ciliary body. The meridional fibres show little connective tissue. (Zenker. Mallory's triple stain.)

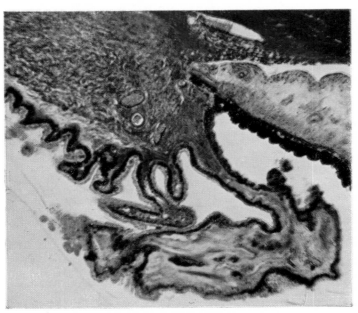

FIG. 60.—DETAIL OF FIGURE 58.
Note large anterior ciliary process.

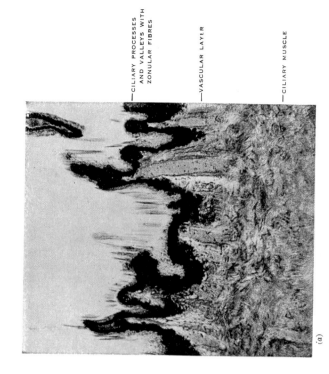

CILIARY PROCESSES
AND VALLEYS WITH
ZONULAR FIBRES

VASCULAR LAYER

CILIARY MUSCLE

(a)

Fig. 62.—Coronal Section of Posterior Portion of the Corona Ciliaris. (Zenker Fixation. Mallory's Triple Stain.)

(a) = Artery passing through ciliary muscle.

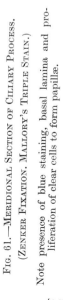

PIGMENT CELLS
SURFACE CELLS

Fig. 61.—Meridional Section of Ciliary Process. (Zenker Fixation. Mallory's Triple Stain.)

Note presence of blue staining, basal lamina and proliferation of clear cells to form papillæ.

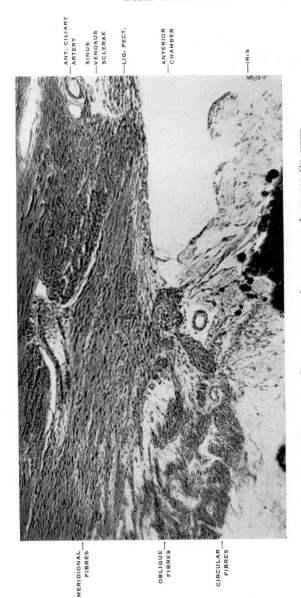

FIG. 64.—MERIDIONAL SECTION OF THE ANGLE OF THE ANTERIOR CHAMBER.

Note how the deepest fibres of the ligamentum pectinatum pass outwards to give attachment to circular fibres and also to some radial fibres of the ciliary muscle. Also anterior ciliary artery entering muscle. An iris process crosses the angle. (Zenker. Mallory's triple stain.)

tudinal layers of the ciliary muscle. There is no endothelium forming a true suprachoroidal space. Among the collagen fibres are melanocytes and fibroblasts. Fluid may accumulate between the collagenous lamellæ, forming large, pathological "spaces".

2. *The Ciliary Muscle* in a meridional section has the form of a right-angled

triangle, the right angle being internal and facing the ciliary processes. The posterior angle is acute and points to the choroid, the hypotenuse runs parallel with the sclera. The form of the whole ciliary body depends on that of the muscle, which consists of flat bundles of nonstriated fibres, the most external being longitudinal or meridional, the intermediate fibres oblique or radial, the most internal being circular or "sphincteric". There are other views on the "parts" of the ciliary muscle (see Rohen, 1964; Calasans, 1953).

The Longitudinal Fibres, also called Brücke's muscle, take origin largely by tendinous fibres from the scleral spur and adjacent trabeculæ (described collec-

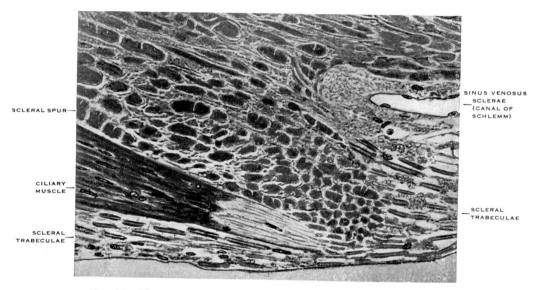

SCLERAL SPUR —

SINUS VENOSUS
SCLERAE
(CANAL OF
SCHLEMM)

CILIARY
MUSCLE

SCLERAL
TRABECULAE

SCLERAL
TRABECULAE

FIG. 65.—MERIDIONAL SECTION TO SHOW RELATIONS OF SCLERAL SPUR.
Note tendon of ciliary muscle and circular fibres of scleral spur.

tively by Calasans as the *ciliary tendon*). This attachment to the corneascleral limbus is the main union between the uveal tract and the fibrous coat of the eye. The origin from the scleral spur (Figs. 64, 65, 66) is by a narrow tendinous ring the fibres of which pass between the circularly running fibres of the spur and can be traced to the scleral trabecular network which bounds the chamber aspect of the canal, with which in fact they are developmentally continuous (see p. 448). The muscle fibres can be traced posteriorly into the suprachoroid lamina to the equator or even beyond. They end usually in branched stellate forms, the epichoroidal muscle starts with three to five primary processes and a variable number of dichotomous, terminal secondary processes.

The muscle stars are flattened in keeping with the lamellar structure of the suprachoroid lamina and, therefore, appear as very slender spindles in meridional

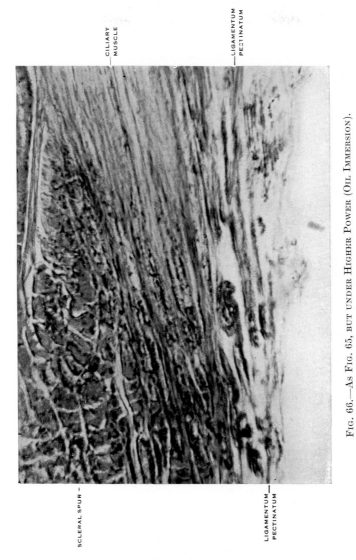

FIG. 66.—As FIG. 65, BUT UNDER HIGHER POWER (OIL IMMERSION).

The tendinous fibres of origin of the ciliary muscle are seen running into the scleral spur and the ligamentum pectinatum (scleral trabeculae). (Zenker. Weigert's elastic stain.)

sections (Salzmann). Their true form can best be studied in teased preparations. They occur on both surfaces of the suprachoroidal lamellæ and become continuous with or are inserted into fine radiating elastic fibres which run into the elastic plexus of neighbouring lamellæ (Salzmann).

The longitudinal fibres often exist as V-shaped bundles, and some are described as inclining obliquely towards the ocular interior to become continuous with the circular fibres, thus forming the oblique or radial layer.

A *radial* or oblique layer is, however, commonly described as a discrete entity (Figs. 25, 64), although many authorities regard all three layers as exchanging fibres.

The Circular Fibres (or Müller's muscle) occupy the anterior, most internal part of the ciliary body. They lie nearest to the lens, and run parallel with the margin of the cornea. The fibres are thus cut transversely in a meridional section (Fig. 64). In many cases those fibres of the scleral trabeculæ which lie next the inner border of the ciliary muscle pass outwards to give a tendinous attachment to some of the circular fibres and also often to some of the radial fibres of the muscle. As a whole these tendinous fibres of origin form a ring. Passing through the muscle are branches of the long posterior ciliary and the anterior ciliary arteries which supply it. The venous return is via the ciliary processes to the choroidal veins and

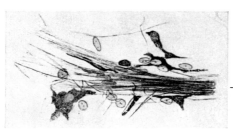

FIBRES OF
—CILIARY
MUSCLE

FIG. 67.—A SMALL BUNDLE OF SMOOTH MUSCLE FIBRES IN THE LAMINA SUPRA-CHOROIDEA (SURFACE VIEW.) TEASED PREPARATION; STAINING WITH MALLORY'S PHOSPHO-MOLYBDIC-ACID HÆMATOXYLIN. × 200.

(From Salzmann.)

partly via the anterior ciliary veins. *The circulus arteriosus iridis major* lies in the ciliary body in front of the circular portion of the muscle (Figs. 25, 47, 64).

The ultrastructural details of the ciliary muscle (Ishikawa, 1962) differ little from those of other nonstriated muscles. Basement membranes are occasionally interrupted by tight junctions between the cells, mitochondria are unusually numerous.

The Stroma of the Ciliary Muscle.—In the longitudinal portion the stroma forms thin longitudinal lamellæ which are continuous with those of the supra-choroidal lamina, from which pigment cells can often be traced into the muscle. In the radial portion the stroma has a reticular structure, and consists of dense connective tissue in which are found blood-vessels, nerves, and, in deeply pig-mented eyes, a few melanocytes. In the circular portion the stroma is looser, and resembles that of the root of the iris, with which it is continuous.

The differentiation between stroma and muscle fibres comes out very well with van Gieson's stain, the former being coloured pink, the latter yellowish green. With Mallory's triple stain muscle fibres are red and connective tissue blue (Fig. 59). The stroma is little apparent in the new-born and increases with age. In the old it tends to become sclerosed and may undergo a hyaline degeneration which indeed is the fate of all the connective tissue of the ciliary body.

The action of all parts of the ciliary muscle is to slacken the suspensory ligament of the lens. This results in decreased tension on the capsule of the lens, which therefore becomes more convex (see Fincham, *infra*)—as in looking at near objects. The circular fibres act directly as a sphincter diminishing the circumference of the ring formed by the ciliary body. This probably also applies to the radial portion of the muscle (Fincham). While all are agreed about the sphincteric action of the circular fibres and this probably also applies to the radial fibres, there is still a great deal of dispute as to how the longitudinal portion of the muscle slackens the suspensory ligament of the lens.

Most authors state that it acts by drawing the choroid forwards. When we remember, however, that the insertion of the muscle is into the very delicate tissue of the suprachoroid lamina which also lies to the outer side of the choroid proper, it becomes very difficult to see how it can draw forward the ciliary epithelium to which the suspensory ligament is attached. Even if this were possible it would entail the retina moving forward, which is hardly likely.

Also the posterior attachments of the ciliary muscle consisting largely of delicate elastic tissue seem to be admirably adapted to allow the posterior ends of the muscle to pass forwards during contraction and to guide them back to their original positions on relaxation. They appear, in fact, so constituted that the action of the ciliary muscle far from pulling the choroid forward shall disturb this structure as little as possible. It must be remembered that all fibres of the muscle, no matter of what part, will get thicker during contraction. The effect of this will be to increase the cross-sectional diameter of the whole muscle and make the inner border of the muscle move inwards towards the inner edge of the ciliary body. Thus the whole muscle, including the longitudinal fibres, will in effect act as a sphincter to the ciliary ring. In this connection it should be noted that the ciliary muscle is thickest approximately opposite the equator of the lens. It will therefore presumably bulge inwards most just where one would expect it to have the greatest slackening effect on the zonular fibres.

According to Fincham the general mechanism of accommodation is as follows:

When the eye is in its passive state with the ciliary muscle at rest, the lens capsule is held under tension by the elastic zonule and vitreous by which it is suspended from the wall of the eyeball, and the zonule is then stretched. Under these conditions the lens substance is in its normal undistorted form, the capsule exerting no influence upon it. When the muscle contracts the ciliary ring is reduced in diameter, thus reducing the tension of the lens suspensions. The zonule gives up some of its stretch and the elastic capsule, under the freedom now given to it, presses upon the soft lens substance and moulds it into the accommodated form by compressing it at the equator and in those regions where the capsule is thickest, allowing it to bulge in the thinner parts (see Fig. 175).

Thus, the normal state of the crystalline lens is the passive state: the accommodated form is impressed upon it by the capsule when it is freed to do so by the contraction of the ciliary muscle.

According to Thompson (1912) the longitudinal part of the muscle *takes origin* in the epichoroid, and is *inserted* into the scleral spur. He holds that it exerts a *pumping action* on the canal of Schlemm, which is responsible for the drainage of the aqueous from the anterior chamber. The pull of the muscle on the spur opens the canal and sucks in the aqueous, while the elastic tissue around will pull the spur to its normal position and thus tend to empty the canal.

But thousands of children every year have their ciliary muscles paralysed with atropine, often for long periods, without any increase of tension. This pumping action then, if it does exist, can be of no real importance.

According to Iwanoff the circular fibres of Müller are much better developed in the hypermetropic than in the myopic eye. This accords with the fact that the hypermetropic eye has to accommodate more than the myopic. He also pointed out that normal eyes may show great differences in the relative amounts of the two portions of the muscle.

But Heine showed that if the eye of a monkey, which had been atropized before death, be sectioned its ciliary muscle has the form of the hypermetropic type, whereas an eye similarly treated with eserine has a "myopic" ciliary muscle.

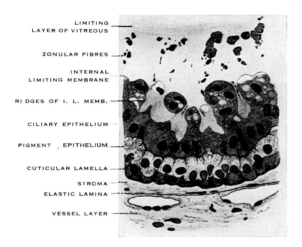

LIMITING LAYER OF VITREOUS

ZONULAR FIBRES

INTERNAL LIMITING MEMBRANE

RIDGES OF I. L. MEMB.

CILIARY EPITHELIUM

PIGMENT EPITHELIUM

CUTICULAR LAMELLA

STROMA

ELASTIC LAMINA

VESSEL LAYER

Fig. 68.—Bleached Transverse Section of the Orbiculus Ciliaris near the Corona Ciliaris ($\times 380$).

(*From Salzmann.*)

It is probable that the differences in form of the ciliary muscle (which are present at birth) depend simply on the length of the eye, e.g. the long myopic eye has a long ciliary muscle.

The Effect of the Sympathetic on Accommodation.—In the human, as is well known, atropine which acts on the postganglionic fibres of the oculomotor nerve produces a hypermetropia of 1 dioptre in the emmetrope. This is no doubt the result of abolishing the tone of the ciliary muscle, a state of slight contraction present in all muscles when at rest. Hence, presumably, the oculomotor nerve can not only bring the ciliary muscle to a state of rest when the lens is in focus for distance, but can actually make the eye hypermetropic. Hence there is no real need for help from the sympathetic. But that the sympathetic does help is suggested by the following.

(*a*) Cocaine, which stimulates the sympathetic while it does not paralyse the accommodation, does weaken it slightly (Fuchs).

(*b*) In Horner's syndrome it has been found that the near point is closer to the eye on the affected side.

(*c*) Graves showed that in a patient whose lens had been absorbed after an injury, looking in the distance make the capsule relatively taut and cocaine made it quite taut.

(d) In dogs and rabbits stimulation of the sympathetic has been shown by some observers (although not by all) to cause flattening of the lens.

This action of the sympathetic is probably brought about by inhibition of the same fibres as the oculomotor nerve stimulates and not by stimulation of the meridional fibres.

Accommodation for Distance.—Latterly the idea that there is an active accommodation for distance as well as for near has again been brought forward.

It is said that it is effected by the meridional fibres of the ciliary muscle which are held to be supplied by the sympathetic, thus bringing it (the ciliary muscle) into line with the reciprocal innervation of unstriped muscle elsewhere in the body.

In the human, however, atropine which paralyses the endings of the oculomotor nerve, causes a hypermetropia of 1 dioptre in an emmetrope. It would appear, then, that paralysis of the parasympathetic can not only bring the lens to a state where it focuses for distance, but can make the eye hypermetropic.

It is of course possible that stimulation of the sympathetic may diminish the blood supply to the ciliary body and thus reduce its size, which might cause a pull on the suspensory ligament. But, as stated above, it is quite unnecessary to invoke the aid of the sympathetic and, indeed, it is difficult to see how the meridional fibres could in any case affect the suspensory ligament in the manner suggested above.

Lyle, however, states that the radial fibres of the ciliary muscle are innervated by the sympathetic. Knowledge on this point remains incomplete. The evidence is largely pharmacological, and the presence of adrenergic fibres in the parasympathetic could explain the apparent double innervation of the ciliary muscle.

Despite the above prolonged, and somewhat speculative analysis, exact knowledge of the mode of action of the ciliary muscle is in many respects still unsolved, as is the precise role of its supposed sympathetic nerve supply.

Nerve Supply.—The ciliary muscle is innervated by fibres from the ciliary ganglion which reach the eyeball in the short ciliary nerves (p. 309). These form rich plexuses amongst the muscle cells. Several types of motor-ending have been described, but older accounts of proprioceptive and other sensory endings have not been substantiated. Anatomical evidence for sympathetic innervation of muscle cells in the ciliaris and blood-vessels of the region, derived from the superior cervical ganglion, is equivocal, in contrast to the pharmacological evidence (Alpern, 1969).

3. *The Ciliary Processes.*—Each ciliary process is a ridge some 2 mm long and 0·5 mm high, which becomes wider as we trace it anteriorly, where it ends in an expansion known as the head of the process. Its colour is almost white, which makes it stand out in strong contrast to the deep pigmentation of the valleys between the processes (see Fig. 71).

If we separate two ciliary processes, we see smaller dark ridges of various sizes between them.

The ciliary processes consist essentially of blood-vessels (for the most part veins), the continuation forwards of those of the choroid with the exception of the choriocapillaris. This is the most vascular region of the whole eye, and the ciliary muscle takes no part in its formation (Figs. 57, 61, 62).

In the pars plana of the ciliary body the vascular layer is much like that of the choroid, with which, indeed, it is directly continuous; but it is not so wide *and there is no choriocapillaris* (Figs. 63 and 68). Since also the arteries of supply to the whole region passes through the ciliary muscle, the vessels consist almost entirely of veins which run backwards parallel with each other. The ciliary processes are essentially a great thickening of the vascular layer.

4. *The Basal Lamina.*—To the inner side of these vessels is the forward continuation of the basal lamina of the choroid, which, however, has quite a different structure here. For as we trace the choroidal lamina towards the ora serrata we find that it splits into two laminæ, the outer elastic and inner "cuticular", and by the time we reach the ciliary body a layer of avascular connective tissue is found

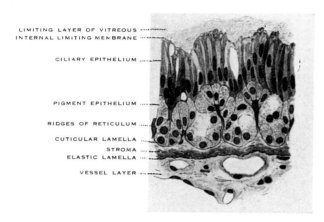

LIMITING LAYER OF VITREOUS

INTERNAL LIMITING MEMBRANE

CILIARY EPITHELIUM

PIGMENT EPITHELIUM

RIDGES OF RETICULUM

CUTICULAR LAMELLA

STROMA

ELASTIC LAMELLA

VESSEL LAYER

Fig. 69.—Bleached Transverse Section of the Orbiculus Ciliaris (pars plana) near the Ora Serrata (× 320).

(*From Salzmann.*)

between the two. The inner layer, which is the basement membrane of the retinal pigment epithelium, is continued into the ciliary region in the same relation to its deeper layer of pigmented epithelial cells (a prolongation of the external layer of the optic cup and hence a retinal homologue). (Figs. 68, 69 and 74.)

The Stroma of the vascular portion of the ciliary body resembles that of the choroid. But the melanocytes are not so plentiful, and indeed may disappear entirely in the anterior portion and in the ciliary processes; also the collagen tissue, in which are found some elastic fibres, is denser and shows up exceedingly well with van Gieson's stain. There is a considerable condensation of connective tissue between the ciliary muscle and epithelium in the pars plicata, especially along the summits of the ciliary processes. Most of the vessels in the stroma are capillaries and veins. Loose connective tissue separates the ciliary muscle from the anterior chamber. The major arterial circle of the iris is in fact in the ciliary stroma in this region, close to the anterior chamber and the circular fibres of the ciliary muscle (Figs. 64, 86).

5. *The Epithelium* (Pars ciliaris retinæ).—Lining the basal lamina are two layers of cells, the outer of which consists of pigment cells and represents the forward continuation of the pigment layer of the retina. But where the rods and cones cease the cells of the pigment epithelium diminish in height and lose their

pigment processes. The cells become much more pigmented so that the nucleus is usually entirely masked. It is continuous with the dilator cells of the iris anteriorly. The pigment consists of rounded granules, which are larger and darker than those of the choroid (and retina). Hence the ciliary body (except the corona ciliaris) is darker than the choroid.

The superficial layer of epithelial cells, derived from the internal layer of the optic cup and hence the equivalent of all retinal laminæ except the pigment layer, extends from the periphery of the iris over the whole of the ciliary region. It is a single layer of nonpigmented cells of low columnar or cubical form of an average dimension of 10–15 μm; but on the summits of the ciliary processes they are distinctly columnar and may reach 30 μm in height. The cells are adherent to the subjacent pigmented epithelium and are covered on their free (vitreous) aspect by the internal limiting membrane (*vide infra*).

Electron Microscopy. The ciliary stroma is dense and contains characteristically thin-walled, fenestrated capillaries (Fig. 72). The cells of both layers are united at their

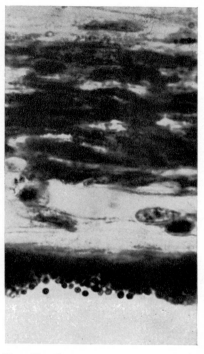

FIG. 70.—SECTION OF RETINA AND CHOROID NEAR ORA SERRATA.

Only rounded pigment granules are seen. But spindle forms also occur here.

adjoining apices by occluding type junctions, and in each layer adjacent cells show elaborate reciprocal foldings (see Bairati and Orzaleri, 1966). Both layers have a basement membrane, that of the pigmented epithelium tying the cells very firmly to the ciliary stroma, while that of the nonpigmented layer is part of the internal limiting membrane (*vide infra*). The junctional zone between the two epithelia may be opened up by pathological accumulations of fluid.

The cytoplasm of the ciliary epithelium has attracted much attention. Mawas (according to Redslob) has found in the cell refractile granules, mitochondrial formations most marked in the apical portions of the cell, vacuoles containing crystalloids and lipoid vesicles. He has seen changes in the position of the nucleus, changes in its form and chromatin content, all characteristics of secretory cells. After depigmentation he finds the same formations in the pigment epithelium. The mitochondria increase after puncture of the anterior chamber. Diamico has found iron-containing granules in the pigment epithelium, which makes the melanin here unique and probably points to a special function of the epithelium. Apart from the mitochondria, Schmeltzer has discovered, in the cytoplasm of the nonpigmented

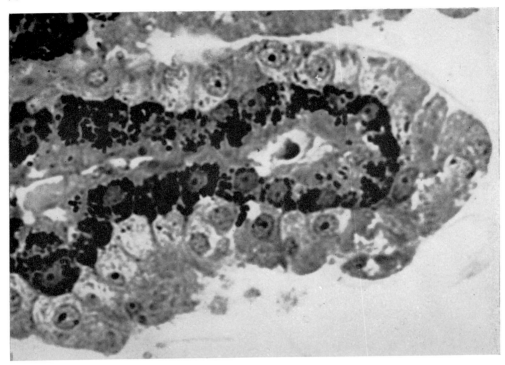

FIG. 71.—THE TWO LAYERS OF CILIARY EPITHELIUM FROM A RHESUS MACAQUE ($\times$ 1,500).

(By courtesy of Dr. C. Pedler, Institute of Ophthalmology, London. Preparation by Mrs. R. Tilly.)

cells, granules which stain blue with indo-phenol. All these facts appear to point to a secretory function of the ciliary epithelium. However this may be, the formation of the aqueous humour is still much disputed. It would seem that the tissue fluid of the ciliary processes, which comes from the capillaries, has the same composition as the tissue fluid elsewhere in the body. It is changed into aqueous in its passage through the ciliary epithelium which takes up certain of its constituents. Electron microscopic studies of the ciliary epithelium (Holmberg, 1959; Fine and Zimmerman, 1963; Hogan *et al.*, 1971) indicate intense secretory activity, particularly in the nonpigmented cells. Mitochondria are numerous, granular endoplastic reticulum well developed, with abundant cisternæ.

6. *The Internal Limiting Membrane* (Membrana limitans interna ciliaris).— On the inner side of the nonpigmented epithelium is the membrana limitans interna ciliaris, the continuation forwards of the internal limiting membrane of the retina (Figs. 61, 72, 143). It is a very thin membrane which is said to be absent over the posterior part of the orbiculus ciliaris. It is of even thickness in young eyes, but becomes thick and less regular with increasing age.

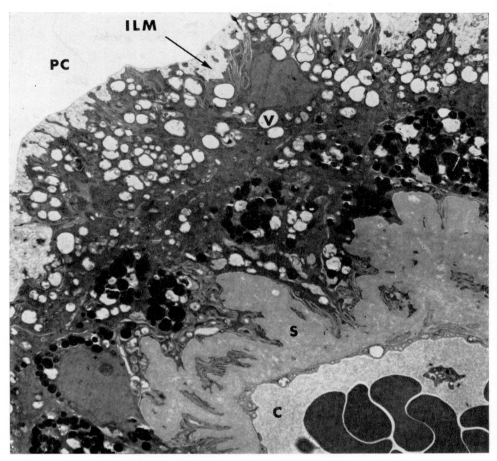

FIG. 72.—CILIARY PROCESS OF RHESUS MONKEY (ELECTRON MICROGRAPH FROM FIG. 71, GLUTARALDE-
HYDE AND OSMIUM TETROXIDE FIXATION, ×4,000).

The capillary (C), with its contained erythrocytes, has an extremely thin wall; this is characteristic of the ciliary body. Two layers of cells lie on the stroma (S). Pigment granules are seen in the
cells of the outer (i.e. the deeper) layer. The cells of the inner layer show great irregularity at adjacent
surfaces, with infolding (called β-cytomembranes) of the cell membrane; this is a characteristic feature
of cells engaged in water transport. The pale areas (V) are interpreted as vesicles or, perhaps, sheets
of tubules cut across; they *may* be secreting or transporting aqueous humour, but this is not certain.
Tormey (1966), believes they are osmium fixation artefacts. The pale surfaces of the cells of the inner
layer are a meshwork that forms the internal limiting membrane (ILM). The human membrane is
almost identical, but in many other animals it is quite different. PC—posterior chamber.

(By courtesy of Dr. C. Pedler, Institute of Ophthalmology, London. Preparation by Mrs. R. Tilly.)

THE IRIS

The iris is the most anterior portion of the vascular tunic of the eye. It differs from the choroid and ciliary body in being placed in a more or less frontal plane. It is a thin circular disc, corresponding to the diaphragm of a camera, and is perforated near its centre, usually slightly to the nasal side, by a circular aperture called the pupil. This varies greatly in size under different conditions, being, for instance, pinpoint in bright sunlight and widely dilated in the dark. It thus regulates the amount of light which reaches the retina. It contracts also to accommodation; this serves to sharpen the focus by diminishing spherical aberration. Its average diameter is 12 mm, with a thickness of about 0·5 mm, except at the collarette (*vide infra*).

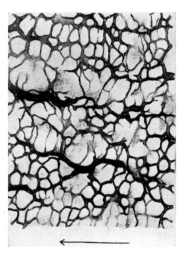

FIG. 73.—SURFACE VIEW OF THE RETICULUM OF H. MÜLLER IN THE ANTERIOR PART OF THE ORBICULUS CILIARIS STAINED BY MALLORY'S HÆMATOXYLIN (× 285). THE ARROW POINTS FORWARDS.
(*From Salzmann.*)

The iris is continuous at its periphery with the middle of the anterior aspect of the ciliary body. It will be noted that it does not arise from the corneo-scleral junction but farther back, and that, therefore, *not only does part of the sclera actually come into the anterior chamber of the eye* (p. 159) *but as a rule part of the ciliary body as well.*

Its so-called "root" is thin and it tears away easily from the ciliary body (irido-dialysis) as the result of contusion injuries. The pupillary margin is lightly in contact with the anterior surface of the lens, which projects farther anteriorly than the junction of the iridial perimeter with the ciliary body. The iris thus has the shape of a low cone with a truncated apex. (When the lens is removed the iris becomes flat and is often tremulous.) It divides the space between the cornea and lens into *anterior* and *posterior chambers*, and is bathed in the aqueous fluid on both aspects, the pupil permitting free flow of the fluid between the two parts of the aqueous cavity of the eyeball.

MACROSCOPIC APPEARANCE OF THE IRIS

The anterior surface of the iris. (Figs. 74, 89.)

The peripheral region (ciliary zone—*vide infra*) presents a series of radial streaks. These are straight when the pupil is small and wavy when it is dilated.

If the iris contains much pigment, as in the darker races of mankind, the anterior surface appears smooth, homogeneous, velvety, the structure being masked by the melanin.

Near to the pupillary margin is an incomplete circular series of ridges overlying an incomplete vascular circle (circulus vasculosus iridis minor—p. 94). The surface of the ridges is marked by a zigzag line which represents the attachment of the pupillary membrane. This line, called the collarette, divides the anterior surface of the iris into two zones—the outer, the *ciliary zone* and the inner, the *pupillary*

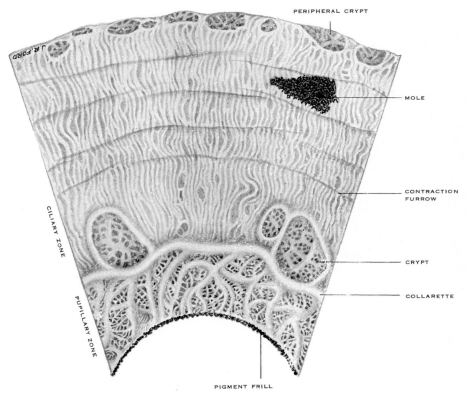

FIG. 74.—THE SURFACE ANATOMY OF THE FRONT OF THE IRIS.

zone, which often differ in colour (Fig. 89). At the collarette, which is about 1·6 mm from the pupillary margin, the iridial thickness is slightly increased.

In the region of the circulus minor are many pit-like depressions called the crypts of Fuchs. At these points, as will be seen later, the superficial tissue layers of the iris are deficient so that fluid can get quickly in and out of the iris—for instance, during contraction and dilatation of the pupil. Similar crypts occur near the margin of the iris, but are small and not easily seen in the living eye. This is due partly to their size and partly because they are concealed by the margin of the sclera, which projects in front of them. It is only in blue eyes, especially in children, that the peripheral perforated zone becomes apparent as a dark, almost black, circle, close to the root of the iris. In the new-born neither collarette nor crypts are present. They develop later.

At the pupillary margin there is a fringe of black pigment, better marked when the pupil is small or is thrown into relief by the white of an opaque lens. Under the magnification of a loupe it is seen to have a beaded appearance. It represents the

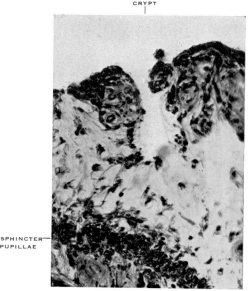

CRYPT

SPHINCTER—
PUPILLAE

FIG. 75.—MERIDIONAL SECTION OF CRYPT OF
FUCHS.

anterior edge of the optic cup (Figs. 74, 89) and is due to a slight extension of the posterior, pigmented epithelium of the iris round the edge of the pupil. Its crenated appearance (hence the term "ruff") is due to the radial folds in this epithelium.

At times when the pupillary zone has an especially delicate structure the sphincter pupillæ can be seen as a whitish band about 1 mm in width close to the pupillary border (p. 85).

The inner part of the ciliary zone is fairly smooth, but near the outer part one sees several concentric lines which become deeper as the pupil dilates. They are, in fact, *contraction furrows* corresponding to the folds in the palm of the hand. At the bottom of the furrow there is less pigment than elsewhere in the stroma, so that they are best seen in a dark iris with a contracted pupil (Fuchs).

The posterior surface of the iris is dark brown or black and smooth to the unaided eye. With low magnification the following fine radial and circular furrows can be made out:

Schwalbe's Contraction Folds are numerous little radial furrows which commence 1 mm from the pupillary border, wind round this, notching it, and giving it its crenated appearance (*vide supra*).

Schwalbe's Structural Furrows—so-called because they are present in the vessel layer as well—start about 1·5 mm from the pupillary margin and, narrow and deep at first, become broader and shallower as they approach the ciliary margin.

The Circular Furrows are finer than the radial. They cross the structural furrows at regular intervals, and are due to the difference in thickness of the pigment epithelium. They occur near the pupillary margin.

Structure.—The iris consists from before backwards of the following layers:

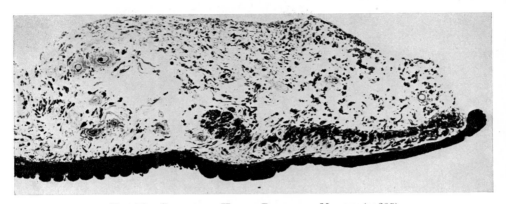

FIG. 76.—SECTION OF HUMAN PUPILLARY MARGIN (× 285).

(By courtesy of Dr. John Marshall and Mr. P. L. Ansell, Institute of Ophthalmology, London.)

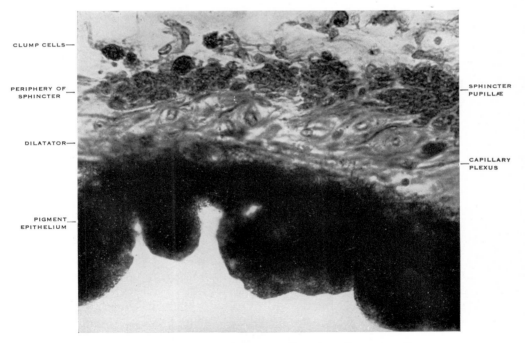

FIG. 77.—MERIDIONAL SECTION OF POSTERIOR LAYERS OF IRIS.

The so-called anterior endothelium.
1. The anterior limiting (border) layer.
2. The stroma.
3. The posterior membrane (anterior epithelium).
4. The posterior pigment epithelium.

While a complete epithelial covering on the anterior aspect may occur in some other mammals (Walls, 1963), the long dispute as to its occurrence in the human

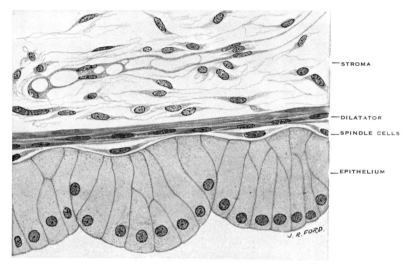

— STROMA

— DILATATOR
— SPINDLE CELLS

— EPITHELIUM

J. R. FORD.

FIG. 78.—BLEACHED SECTION OF IRIS.
(*Wolff's preparation.*)

eye has been resolved by electron microscopy (Vrabec, 1952; Tousimis and Fine, 1959). The anterior surface is in fact formed by elements of the stroma of the iris, but these form a distinctive layer.

1. *The Anterior Limiting Layer* (Figs. 25, 47) is really a condensation of the anterior part of the stroma. It consists of a dense matting produced by anastomosing and intertwining processes of connective tissue and pigment cells. In it are found *obliterated* blood-vessels and numerous nerve endings. The connective tissue cells are star-shaped, have the characteristics of primitive mesenchyme cells, and spread out mostly parallel to the surface. The anterior limiting layer is deficient at the crypts and much thinned at the contraction furrows. On it depends the definitive colour of the iris. In the blue iris the anterior limiting layer is thin, and has only a few pigment cells; in the brown iris it is thick and densely pigmented. Electron microscopy (Smelser and Ishikawa, 1966) shows two main types of cell—melanocytes and fibroblasts, the latter forming a fairly complete surface layer, but without intercellular junctions. A few of these cells may be ciliated on their free surface. They blend at the iridial periphery with similar cells in the

ciliary body and processes. The melanocytes are in many places more numerous. They are orientated in dense sheets subjacent to the fibroblasts, forming frequent contacts but no specialized junctional apparatus.

2. *The Stroma* consists of a loosely arranged collagenous network in which are embedded the following structures:

(*a*) The sphincter pupillæ muscle.
(*b*) The vessels and nerves of the iris.
(*c*) Pigment cells.

The wide spaces in the collagenous stroma contain a mucopolysaccharide ground substance and some fluid. There are no elastin fibres in the stroma proper. The stromal fibres are attached to the iridial muscles, the anterior border layer, and to the ciliary stroma. The collagen bundles are somewhat randomly arranged, with condensations around the vessels and an annular orientation near the pupil. This loose arrangement allows free permeation of fluid and of particles up to 200 μm.

(*a*) *The Sphincter pupillæ* consists of a flat bar of intertwining plain muscle fibres whose predominant direction is circular, separated by connective tissue containing vessels. It is 1 mm broad, forming a ring all round the pupillary margin near the posterior surface of the iris. It is derived from ectoderm, and its inner edge comes close to the pupillary zone of pigment cells which gave it origin. When it contracts it constricts the pupil, and tends to pull the edge of the pigment on to the anterior surface of the iris. It is supplied by the oculomotor nerve via the short ciliaries (p. 312).

The sphincter muscle does not lie loose in the stromal tissue. Each portion adheres firmly to surrounding structures by vessels and by radial bundles of connective tissue. Hence *after an iridectomy the portion of the sphincter remaining does not contract up and the pupil can still react to light.*

Electron microscopy shows that the muscle cells are grouped in small bundles, and that tight junctions exist between the cells. Nerve fibres end peripheral to these bundles. All the usual organelles occur. The muscle cells have a basement membrane.

(*b*) *The Vessels* form the bulk of the iris: they run radially for the most part, giving rise to the streaks which can be seen on the anterior surface. Their course is sinuous to allow for movements of the iris. They straighten out as the pupil constricts and become more wavy as it dilates. At the root of the iris and near the pupillary margin, however, there are circular anastomoses, known as the circulus vasculosus iridis major and minor. The former is arterial, and lies actually in the ciliary body in front of the circular portion of the ciliary muscle (Figs. 25 and 46). The latter is arterial and venous, hence the name circulus *arteriosus* is not correct. As regards the origin of these vessels, they are derived from the long and anterior ciliary arteries in the following way:

The long ciliary arteries—two in number—pierce the sclera on the lateral and medial sides of the optic nerve. They run in the suprachoroidal space between choroid and sclera, often grooving the latter. Just behind the attached margin of the iris each divides. The branches so formed anastomose with each other and the anterior ciliary arteries (which come from the muscular vessels and pierce the sclera) to form the circulus arteriosus iridis major (see also pp. 90, 91). From here radial branches run towards the pupil, but near its edge arterial and venous anastomoses take place to form the circulus *vasculosus* iridis minor.

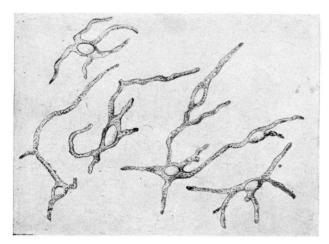

FIG. 79.—MELANOCYTES OF IRIS.
(*From Poirier.*)

The iridial arteries, like those of the major iridial circle, have a muscular layer but no internal elastic lamina. Most of the vessels in the iris have a particularly well developed adventitious tunic, and internal to this is a much less dense collagenous zone, sometimes regarded as a lymph space. The endothelium of the capillaries is not fenestrated. All these peculiarities (except the last) have been ascribed to adaptation of the vessels to the great mobility of the iris (p. 96).

The *nerves* are derived from the long and short ciliaries. These follow the course of the corresponding arteries, piercing the sclera around the optic nerve and running in the space between choroid and sclera. Some end in the vessels of the uveal tract, others supply the various intrinsic muscles of the eye. They are curious in having many gangliform enlargements. Most of the fibres are non-myelinated. (See Chap. VIII.)

(*c*) *The Pigment Cells* (melanocytes) are branching elements, with processes which may reach 100 μm or more; through these processes they form networks, especially around vessels (Fig. 79). Melanin granules in various stages of development can be seen. These cells have small, oval nuclei, devoid of pigment, of course. The average granule size is 0·5 μm. Granules extend into all the cell processes.

Apart from fibroblasts, certain other cells occur in the iris stroma, including lymphocytes, macrophages, mastocytes, and the so-called "clump" cells. These occur in the neighbourhood of the sphincter pupillæ and sometimes near the ciliary border (Figs. 25, 64, 80, 81). They may be up to 100 μm in diameter, and by electron microscopy their surfaces show villous processes. They are rounded pigment cells without processes. Their pigment consists of large, round, and very dark granules, which resemble those of the cells of the posterior surface of the iris, from which, in fact, they are derived (Elschnig, Lauber) (Figs. 25, 80). They often retain their pigment in blue and partially albinotic irides, and in these cases can be seen easily with the slit-lamp. When depigmented they are seen to be large rounded cells with slightly granular protoplasm and a relatively small nucleus like that of the pigment epithelium. On cursory examination they might easily be taken for ganglion cells.

3. The *Posterior Membrane*, better known as the anterior epithelium (a confusing term, considering its position), is also sometimes equated with the dilatator

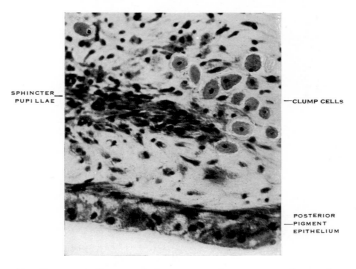

SPHINCTER PUPILLAE

—CLUMP CELLS

POSTERIOR —PIGMENT EPITHELIUM

FIG. 80.—BLEACHED SECTION OF PORTION OF IRIS TO SHOW CLUMP CELLS.
(*By courtesy of Dr. N. Ashton.*)

pupillæ and even regarded as the homologue of the membrane of Bruch (see p. 65). The latter concept is due to the derivation of the anterior epithelium from the outer layer of the optic cup, like certain elements of Bruch's membrane.

The anterior epithelium consists essentially of a layer of nonstriated muscle cells which, like those of the sphincter pupillæ, are derived from the external layer of the optic cup, and are hence ectodermal in origin (p. 444). The apices of these muscle cells contain their nuclei and form the actual epithelium; their basal parts are contractile elongated processes which form the thin sheet known as the sphincter pupillæ. Near to the pupil, where the sphincter closes and unites with the sphincter, the cells become cuboidal epithelial in shape.

Close to the edge of the pupil the dilatator fuses with the sphincter; also about midway along the length of the sphincter the dilatator sends a few junctional fibres accompanied by pigment (Fuchs' spur).

Von Michel's spur is a similar bundle of dilatator fibres, accompanied by pigment which is attached to the peripheral border of the sphincter. At the iris root a third spoke of dilatator fibres (Grünert's spur) runs into the iris stroma. The dilatator is continued into the ciliary body (Fig. 47), where it takes origin.

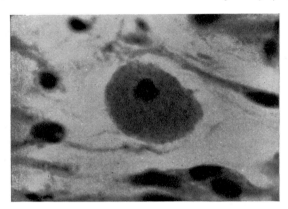

FIG. 81.—ENLARGED VIEW OF BLEACHED CLUMP CELL.

When it contracts it draws the pupillary margin towards its origin, and thus dilates the pupil. The dilatator is poorly developed in the new-born, in whom it is difficult to dilate the pupil fully with a mydriatic. It is supplied by the sympathetic via the long ciliary nerves.

It should be mentioned here that the presence of these dilatator fibres is denied by many. As Grynfelt and others have shown, they can only be demonstrated when the iris is bleached. These observations, together with the experiments of Langley and Anderson, put the existence of the dilatator beyond dispute, and the evidence of electron microscopy is unequivocal. This also demonstrates tight junctions between adjoining muscle processes. The latter contain large filaments and densities resembling the Z-discs of striated muscle.

4. *The Posterior Pigment Epithelium* is a layer of cells which is derived from the internal layer of the optic cup. Being highly pigmented, it is difficult to make out except in albinotic eyes, or in preparations which have been decolorized. The pigment cells form an approximately columnar epithelium, being however somewhat higher (about 40 μm) than wide (about 20 μm).

The pigment granules are dark brown, and for the most part round, but some are spindle-shaped (Fig. 82). Electron microscopy shows a basement membrane, and the adjoining cell walls are much infolded. The lateral walls of the cells are reciprocally serrated and display tight

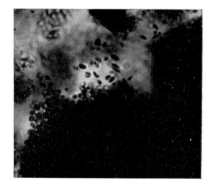

FIG. 82.—PIGMENT CRYSTALS OF POS-
TERIOR EPITHELIUM OF IRIS.
Spindles are still present.

junctions. The granules show average diameters of 0·8 μm and 2·5 μm.

After lining the back of the iris the pigment epithelium curls round the pupillary margin, where it gives rise to the black fringe which can be seen with the naked eye (Figs. 74 and 89).

Just as the pigment epithelium of the retina adheres firmly to the basal lamina of the choroid in a detachment of the retina, so, when the posterior of the two layers at the back of the iris remains adherent to the lens in the rupture of a posterior synechia, the anterior remains attached to the posterior membrane.

Thus it will be seen that the iris has fundamentally the same structure as the ciliary body. It consists of uveal and retinal elements. The uveal stratum is anterior. The retinal ratum is represented, as in the ciliary body, by two layers of cells, but here both are pigmented. Here also the ectodermal cells have become metamorphosed into muscle fibres.

The Colour of the Iris.— Most babies belonging to the white races of mankind

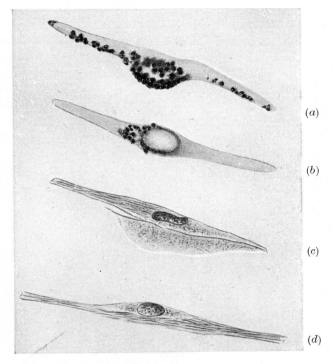

FIG. 83.—CELLS OF DILATATOR PUPILLÆ.
(*a*) and (*b*) after Heerfordt; (*c*) and (*d*) after Wolfrum; (*c*) is unipolar.

are born with blue irides. The reason for this is that the dark pigment on the posterior aspect of the iris seen through the translucent stroma (which as yet has no pigment of its own) appears blue, just as the veins (although the blood in them is of a port-wine colour) look blue through the skin. As time goes on, pigment is deposited in the anterior limiting layer and the stroma, and, varying with the amount so laid down, the colour changes. If little is deposited, the eye remains blue or grey—if there is much, the eye becomes brown. In darker races the iridial stroma contains pigmented melanocytes even at birth, and this pigmentation increases thereafter. Hence the iris in such individuals is not blue at birth.

THE CILIARY ARTERIES

The ciliary arteries comprise:
  (1) The short posterior ciliary arteries.
  (2) The long posterior ciliary arteries.
  (3) The anterior ciliary arteries.

These supply the whole of the uveal tract, the sclera and the edge of the cornea with its neighbouring conjunctiva.

(1) **The Short Posterior Ciliary Arteries.**—The posterior ciliary arteries usually come off the ophthalmic as two trunks while the artery is still below the optic

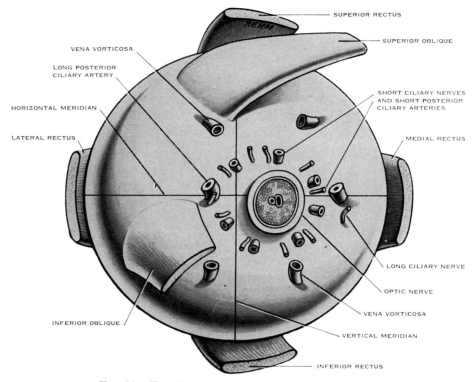

FIG. 84.—THE GLOBE OF THE LEFT EYE FROM BEHIND.

To show the attachment of the oblique muscles and optic nerve. Also the points of entry of the posterior ciliary arteries and nerves and exit of the venæ vorticosæ. Note that the inferior oblique is fleshy almost up to its insertion and that the venæ vorticosæ *appear* to converge towards a common trunk.

nerve. These divide into some 10–20 branches which, running forwards, surround the nerve and pierce the eyeball around it. The majority of these constitute the short posterior ciliary arteries, while the two which pierce the sclera to the medial and lateral side of the nerve respectively are called the *long ciliary arteries* (Fig. 84).

The majority and largest of the short posterior ciliaries, after giving branches to the sclera, pierce it (the sclera) in the region of the posterior pole of the eye (and macular region), i.e. lateral to the optic nerve (Fig. 84). A smaller number and of smaller size pierce the sclera all round but closer to the optic nerve. The canals in the sclera through which they pass are almost directly anteroposterior. The

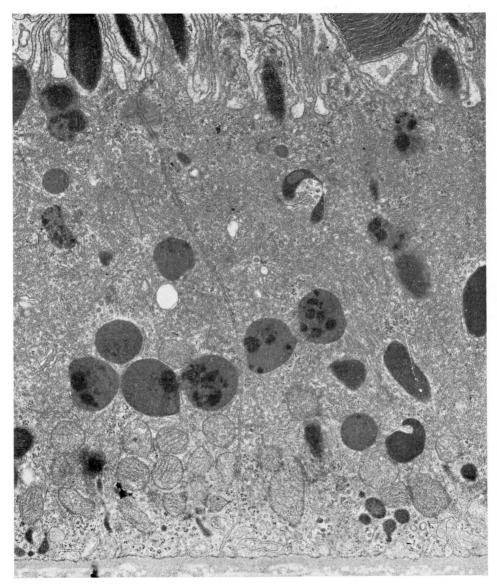

Fig. 102.—Junction between two Pigment Cells from a Monkey's Retina (× 22,000).
Parts of photoreceptor members appear above. The almost vertical line between the two cells
(only partially included) shows a variety of junctional complexes.

(*By courtesy of Dr. John Marshall and Mr. P. L. Ansell, Institute of Ophthalmology, London.*)

2. **The Visual Cells,** i.e. the rods and cones, form the receptive element, the *photoreceptors* of the retina, the remainder mediating transmission. Both rods and cones may be called "Neuro-epithelium", designating a specialized form of epithelium capable of transforming physical energy into nerve impulses, similar to the hair cells in the internal ear or the epithelial cells of taste buds. They transmit through synapses to the bipolar cells, in the external nuclear zone. The rods and cones are arranged like a palisade across the external limiting membrane, which gives this layer under the low power of the microscope a characteristic finely striated appearance at right angles to the choroid.

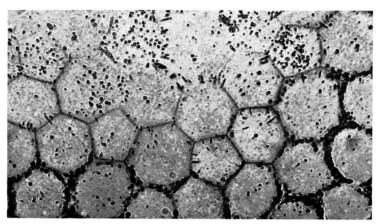

FIG. 103.—TANGENTIAL SECTION OF PIGMENT EPITHELIUM OF HUMAN RETINA ($\times 3{,}375$).

(By courtesy of Dr. John Marshall and Mr. P. L. Ansell, Institute of Ophthalmology London.)

Transformation of light energy into the (visual) nerve impulse depends on breakdown of "visual" pigments contained in the visual cells of the neuro-epithelium. The rod and cone processes of the photoreceptors both contain photo-sensitive substances or visual pigments, which have been much studied in other vertebrates but much less so in man. Human rod processes contain "visual purple", a rhodopsin, belonging to a group of substances containing Vitamin A. The existence of a similar pigment, sometimes called iodopsin, in human cone processes, has been detected. (Consult Rushton, 1962, Partmaller Lythgoe, 1965, Pirense, 1967, and Rodieck, 1973.)

The rod and cone pigments evince different absorption maxima, this duality being reflected in the different roles of these photoreceptors in "photopic" and "scotopic" vision. However, at least three kinds of cones appear to exist, perhaps corresponding to trichromatic colour vision theory.

Indeed, electron microscopy in its present state of progress suggests that "the concept of the 'rod' and 'cone' no longer fits the morphological facts well enough, and is due for replacement". In particular the one-to-one synapse between cones and bipolar cells while actual in places appears to be far from universal. The foveal cones of man may have rod-like form, but stain like cones; yet they have complex (i.e. multichannel) feet (Pedler, 1965).

It is important to note that while the processes (rods and cones) of the photoreceptor cells have attracted most notice, both in light and electron microscopy, they are parts of cells (Fig. 105). In the following account the older views of light microscopists have been preserved, and these are followed by the more recent observations of electron microscopy.

Each *rod*, whose length varies from 40 μm to 60 μm, consists of two segments, an outer and an inner. The outer is cylindrical, highly refractile, and transversely

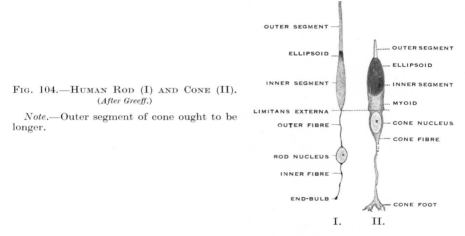

FIG. 104.—HUMAN ROD (I) AND CONE (II).
(*After Greeff.*)

Note.—Outer segment of cone ought to be longer.

OUTER SEGMENT

ELLIPSOID

INNER SEGMENT

LIMITANS EXTERNA

OUTER FIBRE

ROD NUCLEUS

INNER FIBRE

END-BULB

OUTER SEGMENT

ELLIPSOID

INNER SEGMENT

MYOID

CONE NUCLEUS

CONE FIBRE

CONE FOOT

I.   II.

striated, and contains the visual purple. It is surrounded by a very fine sheath of neurokeratin. The outer segment stains with osmic acid; the inner segment takes on nuclear stains. Apart from this, a longitudinal striation can also be made out. This, according to Schultze, is due to furrows, which lodge the processes of the pigment epithelium.

The inner segment is slightly thicker than the outer. In the fresh state its protoplasm is transparent and homogeneous, but soon after death becomes finely granular.

From the inner end of each rod runs a thin varicose *outer fibre* which passes through the external limiting membrane (Figs. 98, 104), swells out into its densely staining nucleus, the *rod granule*, in the outer nuclear layer, and then terminates as an *inner fibre* in the outer molecular layer, whose dendrites of the bipolar cells arborise round it.

According to Balbuena, the terminal *spherules* of the rods are in contact with the cone feet. In certain regions where the cones are surrounded by a palisade of rods, one sees a bunch of spherules enveloping the cone feet.

The Visual Purple is absent in the rods in a zone 3–4 mm wide at the ora serrata. It is also, of course, missing at the fovea centralis, where there are no rods. The whole of a retina which has just been removed from an eye kept in the dark will therefore appear purplish red except at these places, but visual purple bleaches so easily that it is difficult to demonstrate it in this manner.

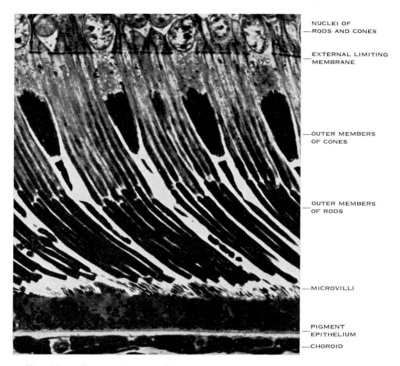

NUCLEI OF RODS AND CONES

EXTERNAL LIMITING MEMBRANE

OUTER MEMBERS OF CONES

OUTER MEMBERS OF RODS

MICROVILLI

PIGMENT EPITHELIUM

CHOROID

Fig. 105.—Photoreceptor Processes of Monkey Retina (× 3,375).
Note microvilli of pigment epithelial cells, some of which contain pigment granules.
(*By courtesy of Dr. John Marshall and Mr. P. L. Ansell, Institute of Ophthalmology, London.*)

Each *cone*, whose length varies from 85 μm at the fovea to 40 μm at the periphery, also consists of two segments. Classically the outer segment of the cone is described as conical in shape and much shorter than that of the rod (Fig. 113, A and B), but it has, however, been shown that the outer segment of the cone is much like that of the rod (Fig. 97), only it is very much more fragile. It does, in fact, reach to the pigment epithelium everywhere in the fundus and not only in the macular region. It contains no visual purple. But Eichner (1958) showed that *during dark adaptation* in man the outer segment of the cone is an expanded funnel lying in contact with the surface of a pigment cell and appearing to absorb pigment granules (Fig. 105). The lipoid from the granules lies in zones which

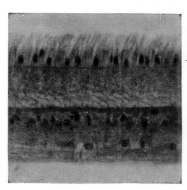

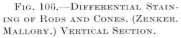

RODS AND
—CONES

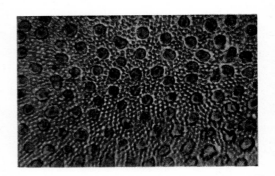

FIG. 106.—DIFFERENTIAL STAIN-
ING OF RODS AND CONES. (ZENKER.
MALLORY.) VERTICAL SECTION.

    Inner members of cones are red;
rods are blue.

FIG. 107.—DIFFERENTIAL STAINING OF RODS
AND CONES. (MALLORY'S TRIPLE STAIN.)
TANGENTIAL SECTION.

Cones larger and red; rods smaller and blue.

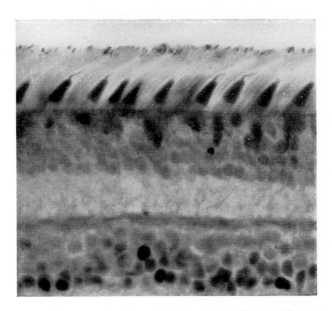

FIG. 108.—DIFFERENTIAL STAINING OF RODS AND CONES OF RHESUS MONKEY. (WEIGERT-PAL.)
Inner members of the cones are darkly stained.

Fig. 109   Fig. 110   *Trans. Section.*

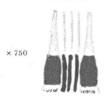
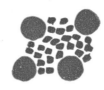

× 750   × 1500

DIFFERENTIAL STAINING OF RODS AND CONES. (ZENKER. MALLORY'S TRIPLE STAIN.)
Cones red; rods blue.

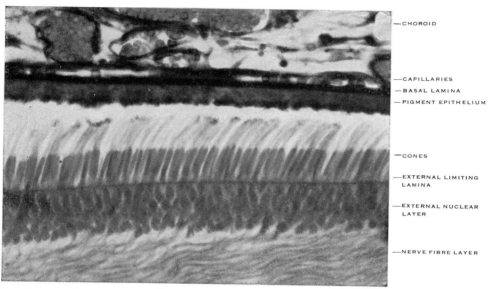

—CHOROID

—CAPILLARIES
—BASAL LAMINA
—PIGMENT EPITHELIUM

—CONES
—EXTERNAL LIMITING LAMINA
—EXTERNAL NUCLEAR LAYER
—NERVE FIBRE LAYER

FIG. 111.—VERTICAL SECTION OF THE EXTERNAL RETINAL LAYERS AND ADJOINING CHOROID AT THE
MACULA. (ZENKER. MALLORY'S TRIPLE STAIN.)

Note that the cones here look like rods but stain like cones. The space between the pigment
epithelium and the outer part of the cones is an artefact.

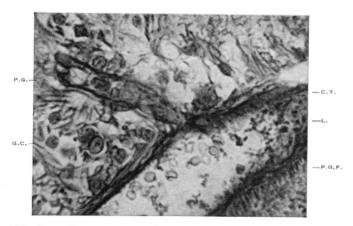

P.G.—

—C.T.

—L.

G.C.—

—P.G.F.

FIG. 112.—FLAT SECTION OF THE GANGLION LAYER OF THE RETINA. × 600.
(ZENKER. MALLORY'S TRIPLE STAIN.)

Perivascular glia is stained red. P.G. = perivascular glia; P.G.F. = perivascular glia and feet of
glial fibres; G.C. = ganglion cell; C.T. = connective tissue in wall of vessel (stained blue); L. =
lumen of vessel.

(Photomicrograph.)

produce the cross-striations seen in the outer segment. In its passage through the cones this altered pigment takes on a "visual-receptor" function, being presumably elaborated into the visual pigment (iodopsin) of the cones (but see p. 108).

The inner portion of the cone is bulged, and unlike the rod is directly continuous with its nucleus, the cone granule staining differently from the rod granule, and situated just on the inner side of the external limiting membrane (Figs. 95, 101, 120). Striation, etc., is like that of the rods. The shape of the cones varies greatly, depending on which part of the retina they come from (see Macular Cones).

The stout cone fibre runs from the nucleus to end in a *pedicle* provided with lateral processes which arborise with the dendrites of the bipolar cells in the outer molecular layer.

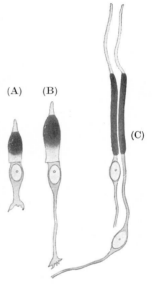

The visual cells with their nuclei and processes are not vascularised but get their nourishment from the choriocapillaris.

According to Østerberg there are 147,300 cones per mm² at the foveola. At the point where the rods commence, that is at 130 μm from the centre of the fovea, there are 74,800 cones per mm²; 3 mm farther 6,000 cones per mm², and 10 mm from the fovea about 4,000. There is a ring-shaped zone 5–6 mm from the fovea where the rods are most numerous (160,000 per mm²). Actually they are densest directly below the disc, i.e. 170,000 per mm². From here to the periphery the rods become less dense, but are more plentiful in the upper nasal portion of the retina than in the lower temporal (23,000 to 50,000 per mm²). The total number of cones is about 6·3–6·8 millions while the rods number 110 to 125 millions in the human retina. For the most recent surveys on photoreceptor distribution see Østerberg (1935), Hogan (1971) and Rodieck (1973).

FIG. 113.—HUMAN CONES FROM DIFFERENT AREAS OF THE RETINA.

A = from near the ora serrata. B = from midway between ora and disc. C = from the fovea centralis.

(After Greeff.)

Note.—The outer member in A and B ought to be longer.

Differential Staining of the Rods and Cones.—Kolmer (1936), an eminent early exponent of differential staining of the neuro-epithelium, after stating that he did not believe that there are transition forms between rods and cones, wrote:

"By means of certain stains, for instance Unna's Orcein-polychrome methylene blue-tannin stain, I succeeded in the human and many animals in colouring the outer limbs of the cones deep blue, while the rods were entirely uncoloured—which indicates a physico-chemical difference between the two.

"With Mallory's stain and often with Heidenhain's azan a distinct difference is seen in the cone and rod nuclei, for the former stain red with fuchsin while the latter stain orange.

"The above differences can already be made out in cyclostomes, for instance in *Petromyzon*, as distinctly as in the human.

"That the cones are made of different material from the rods I was also able to demonstrate in man and the primates in the following way. After fixation in chrome-containing fluids and treatment with nascent chlorine, Unna's epithelial stain coloured the inner and outer portions of cones a deep blue (with Wasserblau), while the inner and outer portions of the rods were coloured red (with safranin).

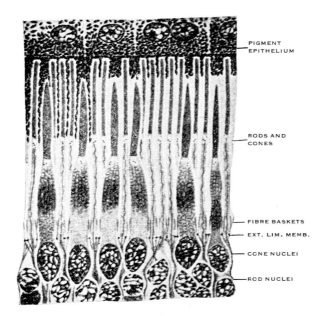

PIGMENT
EPITHELIUM

RODS AND
CONES

FIBRE BASKETS

EXT. LIM. MEMB.

CONE NUCLEI

ROD NUCLEI

Fig. 114.—Vertical Section of Retina, stained Molybdic Acid Hæmatoxylin.

(*From the Kurzes Handbuch.*)

"Shaffer, indeed, showed as early as 1890 that after fixation by Kulschitsky's fluid and staining in a similar way to Weigert's method for medullated nerve fibres (see Fig. 108), he coloured the cones and cone fibres electively in the human retina.

"Also in many fishes the chemical differences between the rods and cones are striking. Thus in *Brosmius*—a shellfish-like fish—the rods cut easily while the larger cones, due to their extremely large albumen content, become so hard with similar fixation that they, like the lens nucleus, jump out of the section during cutting.

"It seems to me that the above criteria, demonstrated in an extensive range of vertebrates, are quite sufficient to distinguish (with but few exceptions) between rods and cones."

The author (Eugene Wolff) succeeded, in the human, in colouring the inner portions of the cones red with Mallory's triple stain after Zenker fixation, while the corresponding portion of the rod stained blue. This was done both in vertical and in flat sections. This method of staining proved especially interesting in the macular region, where the inner limbs of the rod-like cones stained red (Figs. 106, 107, 109, 110).

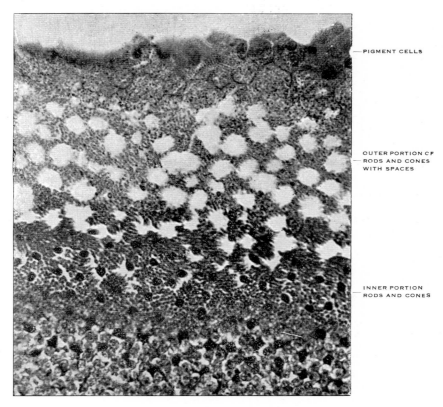

FIG. 115.—FLAT (ALMOST TANGENTIAL) SECTION OF THE OUTER PORTION OF THE RETINA TO SHOW THE SPACES BETWEEN THE OUTER PORTIONS OF THE RODS AND CONES.
(*From the Proc. Roy. Soc. Med.*, 1938, **31**, 1101.)

In another eye where the sections stained with Mallory's triple stain were inadvertently left washing for a long time, the outer elements of the cones stained reddish brown while the corresponding part of the rod stained blue. Perhaps more interesting from a historical point of view, are the old observations by Schultze (1873) of a discoid serial pattern in the outer segments of photoreceptors, thus foreshadowing the classical electron microscopy of Sjöstrand (1948, etc.). Moody (1964) has reviewed the history of these developments.

The Ultrastructure of Photoreceptors.—Electron microscopic observations of the rod and cone processes have now accumulated for almost two decades. While the amount of detailed description now available (see Rodieck, 1973) is great, it must be said that the functional significance of these details is still largely obscure. The basic structure of both rod and cone *outer segments* (Figs. 117, 118) is a highly regular series of lamellæ, 600–1200 in number, packed in a columnar manner at a spacing of 24 to 30 per μm. These discoid structures are about 5·5 to 6·5 nm thick centrally, and rather more at their peripheries (7–8 nm). The space between discs

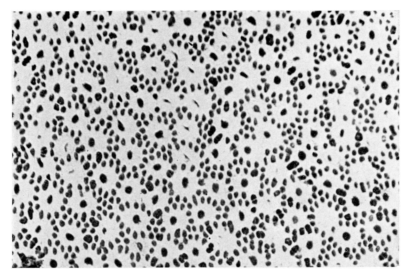

Fig. 116.—Transverse Section across Rod and Cone Processes in Human Retina ($\times$ 3,150). The larger cone processes are within rings of rod processes.

(*By courtesy of Dr. John Marshall and Mr. P. L. Ansell, Institute of Ophthalmology, London.*)

is about 20 nm. The main difference in cone processes is that the discs have a greater diameter in the basal region of the "cone". Each disc is a flattened membranous bag, the thin intradisc space being less electron dense. The membrane is of "unit" construction; a small amount of the cytoplasm of the inner segment of the photoreceptor encloses the discs, and in this microtubules are often visible. The *inner segment* is connected to the outer by a short region of relatively featureless cytoplasm, but this is crossed by a connecting *cilium* extending from the region of the proximal discs (Fig. 118) to the "ellipsoid" of the inner segment. The latter is divided into the *ellipsoid* and a basal part, the *myoid* (Fig. 105). The cilium displays the usual features—a basal body (Fig. 117) and an annulus of nine doublets. The inner segment contains many mitochondria, Golgi apparatus, and a granular endoplastic reticulum. Free ribosomes and neurotubules also exist. The inner segments are related to the external limiting lamina, which separates them. The

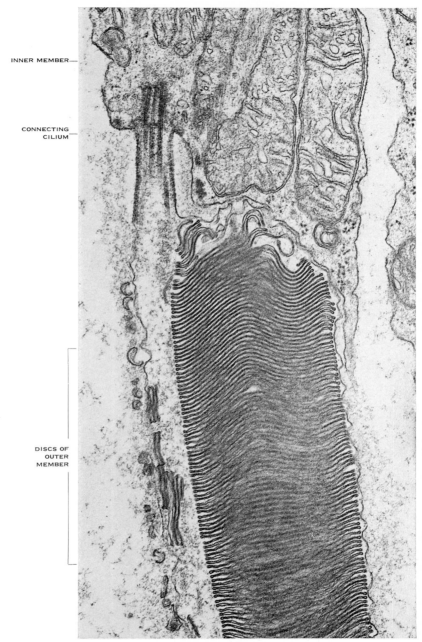

INNER MEMBER —

CONNECTING CILIUM —

DISCS OF OUTER MEMBER

Fig. 117.—Electron Micrograph of Junction between Outer and Inner Members of a Human Rod Process (× 59,200).
See text for details.

(*By courtesy of Dr. John Marshall and Mr. P. L. Ansell, Institute of Ophthalmology, London.*)

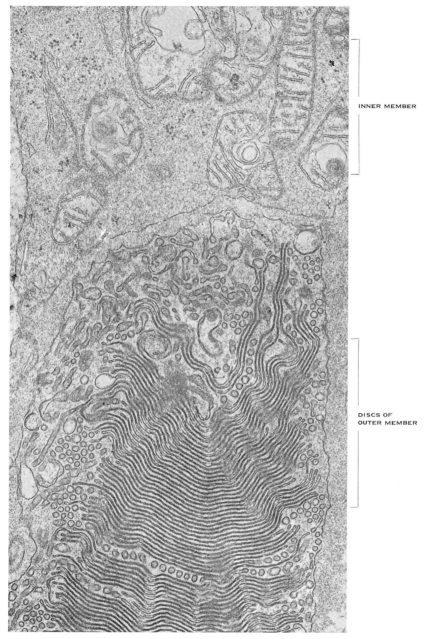

INNER MEMBER

DISCS OF
OUTER MEMBER

FIG. 118.—ELECTRON MICROGRAPH OF JUNCTION BETWEEN OUTER AND INNER MEMBERS
OF A HUMAN CONE PROCESS (×54,400).
See text for details.

(By courtesy of Dr. John Marshall and Mr. P. L. Ansell, Institute of Ophthalmology, London.)

spaces between the ellipsoids of the inner segments are filled with a mucopoly-saccharide.

The mode of action of the rod and cone processes is not yet clear, but the repetitive piles of discoid membranes have suggested to some the role of a photo-multiplier. The myoids contain refractile droplets of a coloured lipid which may act as light filters.

An *outer fibre*, thicker in cone photoreceptors, connects the whole process to its soma or cell body, which contains the nucleus of the cell. The *inner fibre* (*vide*

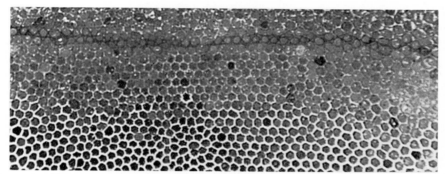

FIG. 119.—SECTION THROUGH EXTERNAL LIMITING MEMBRANE OF HUMAN RETINA (× 3,750).

(By courtesy of Dr. John Marshall and Mr. P. L. Ansell, Institute of Ophthalmology, London.)

infra) connects the soma, through a complex synaptic arrangement with bipolar nerve cells and other elements of the inner nuclear layer. The somata of the cones are closer to the external limiting membrane and tend to form a single tier, those of the rod receptors being in general more numerous and arranged in several tightly packed rows. At the macula and fovea these arrangements are modified (p. 38).

It has been suggested that the lamellar discs in photoreceptor outer segments may not be entirely independent of each other or the cell membrane. A recent study combining freeze-fracture technique and electron microscopy negates such suggestions (Leeson, 1970).

For further remarks upon the "space" between rod and cone outer segments and the pigment epithelium, see pp 104, 426.

3. **The External Limiting Membrane.**—The external limiting membrane of the retina has the form of a widely fenestrated membrane, extending from the ora serrata to the edge of the optic disc.

Through the holes in the net pass the processes of the rods and cones. In a section at right angles the membrane appears as a series of dots (Fig. 120); if the section is slightly oblique, it may appear as a line. Its true form can only be appreciated in a flat section parallel to the surface. Such a section shows clearly that the diameter of each aperture in the net depends on the structure which

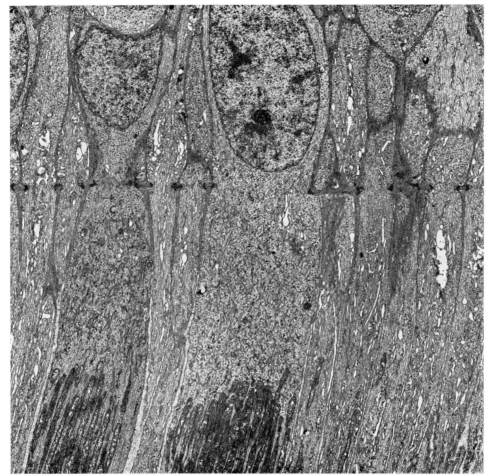

FIG. 120.—RETINAL SECTION (RHESUS MACAQUE) TO SHOW EXTERNAL LIMITING MEMBRANE
(× 7,500).
Nuclei of photoreceptors above. The "membrane" is seen to be a series of tight junctions between
photoreceptor processes.

(*By courtesy of Dr. John Marshall and Mr. P. L. Ansell, Institute of Ophthalmology, London.*)

passes through it. Thus a rod has a small aperture, while a cone (Fig. 119) has a
much larger one.

In the macular region the holes are all more or less of the same size except at
the fovea, where the cones are exceptionally fine and the holes correspondingly
small. At the fovea, also, the greater length of the cones pushes the external
limiting membrane inwards and causes a posterior concavity which is called the
fovea externa.

Light microscopy suggested that the external limiting membrane was formed by the apposition of terminal expansions of the fibres of Müller's cells (p. 124). Arey (1932) suggested, however, that it consists of junctions known as "terminal bars" between the cell membranes of the rod and cone processes and Müller's cells. Electron microscopy has largely confirmed and amplified this view (Sjöstrand, 1958, Spitznas, 1970), various forms of tight junction, desmosomes and maculæ adherentes, being described between the inner segments of rod and cone cells and the processes of Müller's cells.

Anteriorly at the ora serrata the external limiting membrane ends at the same level as the pigment epithelium by becoming continuous with the cement substance between the pigmented and nonpigmented portions of the ciliary epithelium (Wolfrum).

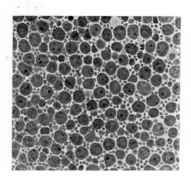

Fig. 121.—Tangential Section of external Nuclear Layer of Human Retina (× 2,775).
(By courtesy of Dr. John Marshall and Mr. P. L. Ansell, Institute of Ophthalmology, London.)

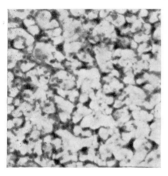

Fig. 122.—Flat Section of the Outer Plexiform Layer × 1,000. (Phosphotung. Hæm.)
Avascular and much looser in texture than the inner nuclear layer (compare Fig. 129).
(Wolff's preparation.)

4. **The Outer Nuclear Layer.**—This consists essentially of the nuclei of the rod and cone cells. The rod granule is round, and consists of practically nothing but nucleus with very little protoplasm around it. The cone granule is larger, oval, and stains differently. As the cone fibres are very short, the granules lie as a single layer situated close to the external limiting membrane (Figs. 95, 105).

Occasionally, most commonly in the macular region, cone nuclei may be found on the outer side of the external limiting membrane (Extruded Nuclei).

The rod and cone inner fibres continue into the outer plexiform layer to end among dendrites of the bipolar cells. The rod fibre ends in a small knob, while the cone fibre terminates in a conical swelling with lateral processes. These are known as rod spherules and cone pedicles (Fig. 128). They are the expanded terminations of the rod and cone inner fibres, which form complex synapses with the dendrites of bipolar neurons and the processes of horizontal cells, whose somata are in the inner nuclear layer. These highly complex neurono-photoreceptor connections form a dense neuropil usually known as the external plexiform (molecular) lamina.

5. **The External Plexiform Lamina.**—The connections in this lamina between rod spherules and cone pedicles with the dendrites of bipolar and horizontal cells have long been known through the classical studies of Cajal (1896), Polyak (1941)

and others. The facts that large numbers of photoreceptors except cones at the fovea (p. 138) converge upon single bipolar cells, and that horizontal neurons link together groups of photoreceptors over considerable areas of the retina, are both well-established. With the advent of electron microscope technique finer

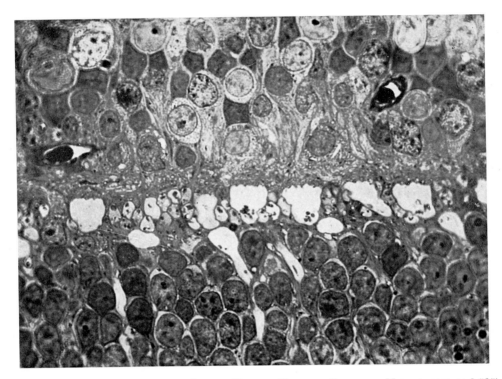

FIG. 123.—THE OUTER PLEXIFORM LAYER (RHESUS MONKEY, ELECTRON MICROGRAPH, × 3,525).

Between the photoreceptor nuclei below and those of the outer nuclear lamina above, i.e. in the external plexiform layer, are cone pedicles (pale profiles).

(By courtesy of Dr. John Marshall and Mr. P. L. Ansell, Institute of Ophthalmology, London.)

details have merely furthered these studies (see Missotten, 1965, Boycott and Dowling, 1969, Hogan *et al.*, 1971 and Rodieck, 1973, for excellent resumés of such work.) The spherule and pedicle (Fig. 128) are in their structure complex synaptic invaginations, and in both cases dendrites of bipolar and horizontal neurons are involved. The invaginated photoreceptor termination shows in both forms organelles of synaptic significance, including synaptic vesicles, ribbons, microtubules and mitochondria. Rod spherules make contacts with two to seven dendrites (on average four), whereas cone pedicles display about 25 invaginations containing "triads" of horizontal and bipolar dendrites. In addition simpler contacts are made by bipolar dendrites upon the cell membrane of the pedicles—up to 500 in each. The pedicles also display lateral "interreceptor" contacts with adjacent cone and rod receptors (Fig. 128). Reconstructions from serial sections of these complex synaptic arrays have been made by Missotten (1965, 1966) and by Dowling and Boycott (1966).

The functional significances of this elaborate network of cross-connections are still largely subjects of speculation. As we shall see below similar cross-connections are established in the internal plexiform lamina. Whatever else, it is abundantly apparent that simple "through" pathways, from the photoreceptors to the ganglion cells and their optic nerve fibres certainly cannot exist for the majority of the retina; but then, the light microscopic observation—that rods and cones greatly outnumber bipolar cells and they in their turn the ganglion cells—has long since pointed in the same direction. It is now even more evident that there

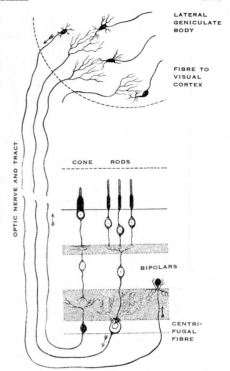

FIG. 124.—SCHEME TO SHOW THE COURSE OF THE VISUAL FIBRES FROM THE RODS AND CONES TO THE LATERAL GENICULATE BODY.

(*Greeff and Cajal modified.*)

Note that in this light microscopic study cones and bipolars are shown with a 1:1 ratio. Contrast with Figs. 123, 128.

exists in the retina a most intricate arrangement of cross-connections making possible extensive interactions between the pathways excited by the photoreceptors. How far the horizontal neurons in fact function in this manner is still uncertain. It is interesting to note that electrophysiological data suggest that the horizontal and bipolar cells display graded activity.

6. **The Inner Nuclear Layer.**—This consists of the following elements, principally cell somata:

(*a*) The bipolar neurons.

(*b*) The horizontal neurons.

(*c*) The amacrine neurons.

(*d*) The somata of the cells of Müller.

(*e*) Capillaries of the central retinal vessels.

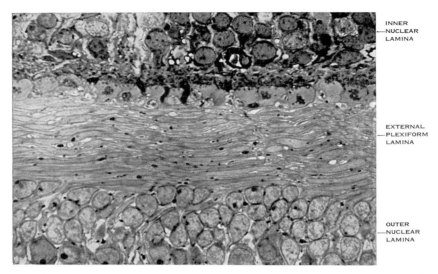

FIG. 125.—SECTION OF OUTER (BELOW) AND INNER NUCLEAR LAYERS AND INTERVENING EXTERNAL PLEXIFORM LAMINA OF HUMAN RETINA NEAR THE MACULA (× 3,225).

(*By courtesy of Dr. John Marshall and Mr. P. L. Ansell, Institute of Ophthalmology, London.*)

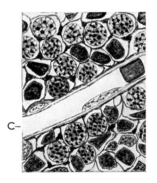

FIG. 126.—FLAT SECTION OF THE INNER NUCLEAR LAYER (× 1,000).

The nuclei of the fibres of Müller stain darker and are more angular than the bipolar nuclei. Note the capillary (C) with a deformed blood corpuscle; and the neuroglial surround to the cells.

(*Wolff's preparation.*)

The bipolar cells are neurons of the first order. They have their nuclei in the inner nuclear layer and their dendrites arborize in the outer molecular layer with the rod and cone fibres, as we have seen.

The bodies of the bipolar cells resemble the granules of the outer nuclear layer, and consist almost entirely of nucleus with very little surrounding protoplasm. The whole layer, therefore, on ordinary microscopic section resembles the outer nuclear layer but is generally much thinner. As we approach the macula this layer gradually becomes thicker and then thins again towards the fovea, where it practically disappears.

Although it is difficult to distinguish different forms of bipolar neuron with electron microscopy, with the light microscope at least three varieties have been identified: *rod bipolars*, which have comparatively large somata and a wide, profuse arborization of dendrites, connecting only with rod spherules; *midget bipolars*, which are relatively small and make contacts only in the triads of cone pedicles; and *flat bipolars*, whose dendrites form light contacts with cone pedicles only,

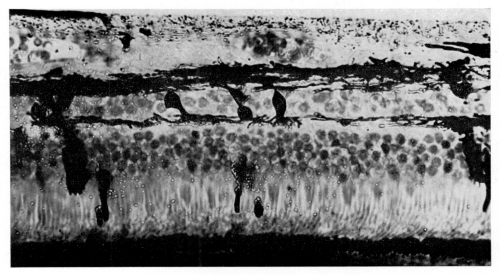

FIG. 127.—HORIZONTAL CELLS OF PRIMATE RETINA.
(*Photomicrograph provided by Dr. John Marshall.*)

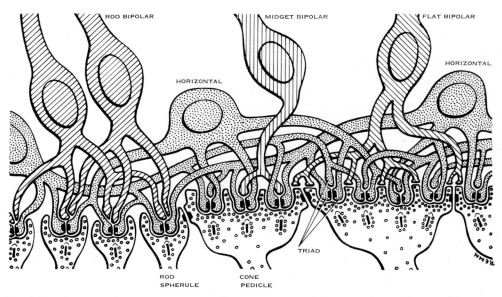

FIG. 128.—SYNAPTIC JUNCTIONS BETWEEN PHOTORECEPTORS, HORIZONTAL AND BIPOLAR NEURONS.
(*Modified after Dowling and Boycott, 1966.*)

In the diagram note the triads—synaptic complexes between all three of these retinal elements.

but not with their triads (Fig. 128). The axons of all three types of bipolar extend into the internal plexiform layer and into the ganglion cell lamina to make synaptic contacts with the dendrites and somata of the ganglion cells. The rod bipolar axons branch little and form synapses chiefly with the somata of up to four ganglion cells. The axons of midget bipolar neurons synapse with a single midget ganglion cell (*vide infra*). The flat bipolar cell axons make synaptic contacts with a number of ganglion cells of all types. Thus, only the midget bipolar neurons provide unitary pathways from one cone photoreceptor to one ganglion cell. (For ultrastructural details of bipolar neurons see Missotten, 1965. For further details of the synapses of bipolar neurons see Dowling and Boycott, 1966.)

The Horizontal Neurons are flat cells whose processes spread horizontally—that is, parallel to the surface of the retina. They are placed next the outer plexiform layer (Figs. 95, 96, 127). They have one long process, or axon, often as long as 1 mm, and a considerable number of short dendrites with branching terminals. The distribution of these processes in the external plexiform layer has already been partly described. Their long processes display no organised orientation in the retina. Two types, A and B, have been demonstrated in light microscopic studies (Boycott and Dowling, 1969). Type A horizontal cells have seven groups of dendrites which synapse in the triads of seven cone pedicles. Type B horizontal cell dendrites are confined to rod receptors. The long processes of these cells may form contacts with distant groups of rods. It is doubtful whether one should refer to the processes or neurites of horizontal cells as axons or dendrites; their electrotonic characteristics are graded and conduction may be bidirectional.

The Amacrine Neurons have a piriform body and a single process which passes inwards and ends in the inner plexiform layer. (Some may make connection with the centrifugal fibres of the optic nerve.) They are placed next the inner plexiform layer (Figs. 95, 98). A considerable variety of types have been identified in light microscope preparations (Boycott and Dowling, 1969). These have been named *stratified* (unistratified and bistratified) and *diffuse* (narrow field diffuse, wide field diffuse, and stratified diffuse), the chief criterion of differentiation being in the mode of arborization of their single process. These types have as yet not been characterised by any ultrastructural details. Their processes form complex connections with the axons of bipolar neurons and the dendrites and somata of ganglion cells, as will be described with the ganglion cells.

Since their cell bodies are in the internal nuclear layer the complex gliaform elements known as the *"fibres"* or *cells* of *Müller* will be described in their entirety here. Whatever other junctions they may perform these cells appear structurally to be well adapted to a supportive role—in the physical sense. Their processes extend from the cell somata through all retinal laminæ except the pigmented epithelium and the zone containing the outer segments of the photoreceptors, which project through the so-called external limiting membrane (Fig. 82, p. 133), itself formed from the junctions between the rod and cone processes with the expanded terminations at the peripheral ends of the Müller cells. Centrally, towards the vitreous, the "fibres" of these cells contribute similarly to the internal limiting lamina (p. 133). In the plexiform layers the major processes produce side branches forming a profuse, horizontally extended reticulum, while in the nuclear layers and amongst the ganglion cells secondary branches form a reticulum around the cell somata. In the vascularized layers of the retina the processes form wide areas of contact with capillaries, a basement membrane intervening. In total the cells of Müller occupy almost all the space between the other elements in the retina. Electron microscopy demonstrates fine fibrils in their cytoplasmic processes and microvilli at their vitreal extremities. (For further details see Pedler, 1963, Hogan and Feeney, 1963, Dowling and Boycott, 1966.)

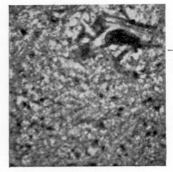

CAPILLARY WITH —ENDOTHELIAL NUCLEUS

FIG. 129.—FLAT (HORIZONTAL) SECTION OF THE INNER PLEXIFORM LAYER (× 1,000).

Vascularised and much denser in structure than the outer plexiform layer (compare Fig. 122).

(*Wolff's preparation.*)

Other forms of glial cells also occur in the retina (Fig. 131). These have been classified as (*a*) retinal astrocytes, which, as in the brain, make contacts with capillaries, as do (*b*) the perivascular glial cells, but not (*c*) the microglial cells, which are phagocytes (consult the papers of Walter, 1959, 1961). In general these accessory glial cells are confined to the more internal retinal layers, some astrocytes reaching as far as the outer plexiform lamina.

7. **The Inner Plexiform (Molecular) Layer.**—This consists essentially of the arborization of the axons of the bipolar cells with the dendrites of the ganglion cells. Comprising it also are:

(*a*) Processes of the amacrine cells.
(*b*) Fibres of Müller cells.
(*c*) Branches of the retinal vessels.
(*d*) A few scattered nuclei.

The inner molecular zone forms a reticulum which is divided into several substrata by the horizontally coursing processes of the amacrine cells and the dendrites of the stratified ganglion cells. (This subdivision into layers is better seen in some animals, especially birds, than in man.)

It has practically the same thickness everywhere in the retina, except at the fovea centralis, where it is absent.

The nuclei present in this layer are those of the endothelium of the vessels (Fig. 129) or possibly those of displaced ganglion (Fig. 95) or amacrine cells.

This layer consists of the junctions between the first and second order sensory neurons of the visual pathway, and contains complex synapses between bipolar,

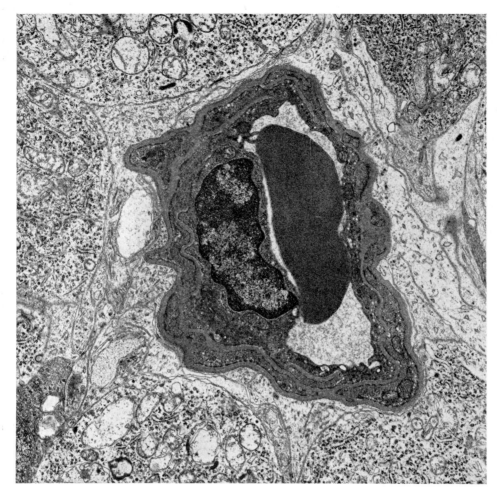

FIG. 130.—ELECTRON MICROGRAPH OF A CAPILLARY AND SURROUNDING NEURONAL AND NEUROGLIAL ELEMENTS IN THE INTERNAL PLEXIFORM LAMINA OF HUMAN RETINA (× 15,700).
A fibre of Müller approaches the capillary from the right.

(*By courtesy of Dr. John Marshall and Mr. P. L. Ansell, Institute of Ophthalmology, London.*)

ganglion and amacrine cells. The details of these can be better described when the ganglion cells have been considered (see p. 128).

8. **The Ganglion Cell Layer.**—This consists essentially of the ganglion cells of the retina. In it are also found:

       (*a*) Fibres of Müller cells.

       (*b*) Neuroglial cells.

       (*c*) Branches of the retinal vessels.

The ganglion cells of the retina are multipolar nerve cells, but some are in fact bipolar, with a single dendrite. They have a clear, round, or slightly oval nucleus with a well-marked nucleolus. Nissl granules are well developed (Fig. 132). The cells vary greatly in size and shape. Generally large, they may reach up to 30 μm in diameter, but may be much smaller, especially in the macular region. They may be round, piriform, or oval.

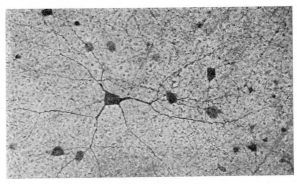

FIG. 131.—PHOTOMICROGRAPH OF A GANGLION CELL.

(Courtesy of Dr. John Marshall, Institute of Ophthalmology, London.)

From the rounded internal pole of the cell the axon emerges and turns horizontally into the nerve fibre layer. From the opposite extremity, which adjoins and projects into the inner plexiform layer, one or more dendrites, which are thicker than the axon, emerge and branch widely in this layer. The processes of the ganglion

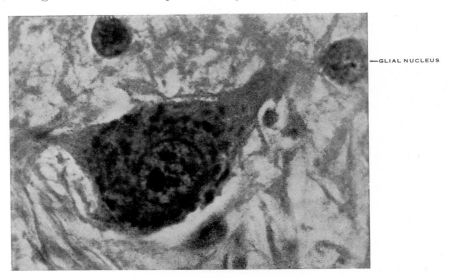

—GLIAL NUCLEUS

FIG. 132.—GANGLION CELL OF RETINA (ZENKER. BORELL'S METH. BLUE. × 2,000).
To show Nissl's granules. Also note nucleus and nucleolus.
(Wolff's preparation.)

cells may be *stratified* when they run horizontally in one to three layers, or *diffuse* when they branch like a tree and end anywhere in the inner plexiform layer (Fig. 128).

The ganglion cells are neurons of the *second order* and correspond to cells in the *nucleus gracilis* and *cuneatus*. Their axons synapse with cells in the lateral geniculate body (Fig. 124), superior colliculus, etc. (p. 358). In the retina generally the ganglion cells form a single row, but on the temporal side of the disc we find two layers. As we approach the macula they increase in depth, so that up to eight layers may be formed at its margin. They decrease again towards the fovea, where they disappear entirely (Figs. 147–149).

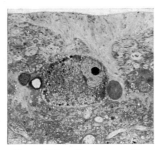

FIG. 133.—GANGLION CELL OF HUMAN RETINA (× 1,000).

(Preparation by Dr. John Marshall, Institute of Opthalmology, London.)

Towards the ora serrata the ganglion cells are sparser and gradually make their way into the nerve fibre layer.

The classical observations of Cajal (1911) and Polyak (1941) on ganglion neurons and other retinal elements has been carried much further by Boycott and Dowling (1969), who have recognised two main types, (*a*) *Monosynaptic*, or *midget* ganglion cells, and (*b*) *Polysynaptic* ganglion cells, the latter subdivided into *unistratified, diffuse, large diffuse,* and *stratified diffuse.* This classification obviously depends primarily upon the arrangements of dendrites and their synapses.

Midget ganglion neurons predominate in the central retina and are linked to cone receptors by a single midget bipolar neuron; their dendrites spread little. This does not imply, however, that a single cone cell discharges *only* to a single train of midget bipolar and ganglion cells, because some of the cones are also connected to flat bipolar cells.

Polysynaptic ganglion neurons are less numerous centrally and become more and more predominant towards the peripheral retina. All have much wider dendritic fields than the midget cells, some (as their names indicate) forming one or more widespread "strata" of dendrites, the most widely extended being the unistratified cells, which may synapse with hundreds of bipolar cells. The large diffuse type is characteristic of the central retina.

The connections between the bipolar axons, the neurites of amacrine neurons, and the dendrites and somata of the ganglion cells are complex. (For further details see Dowling and Boycott, 1966.) They will be discussed further in the section on the visual pathway (p. 374).

The ultrastructural appearances of ganglion cells conform with those of similar cells elsewhere in the central nervous system. (Fine, 1963.)

9. **The Stratum Opticum or the Nerve Fibre Layer.**—This consists essentially of the axons of the ganglion cells which pass through the lamina cribrosa to form the optic nerve.

(It must always be remembered that these are the axons of *secondary* sensory neurons, corresponding to neurons entirely within the brain or spinal cord in other sensory pathways.)

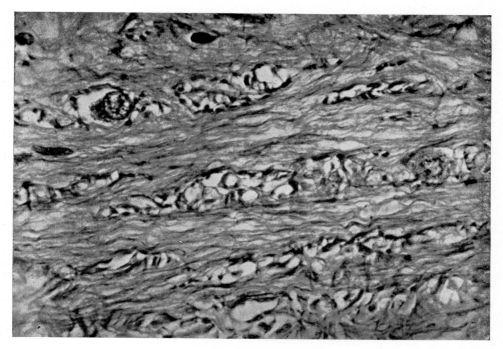

FIG. 134.—FLAT SECTION OF NERVE FIBRE LAYER OF RETINA.

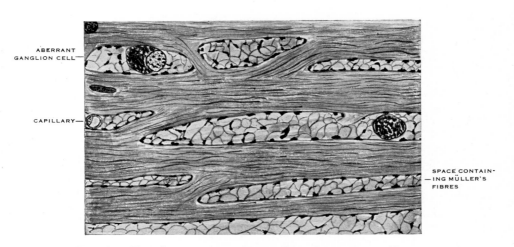

FIG. 135.—FLAT SECTION OF THE NERVE FIBRE LAYER OF THE RETINA.

(*Wolff's preparation.*)

But there are also:

     (*a*) Centrifugal fibres.

     (*b*) Fibres of Müller cells.

     (*c*) Neuroglial cells.

     (*d*) Retinal vessels.

The nerve fibres are arranged in bundles which run parallel to the surface of the retina. This structure can be made out with ordinary stains, and makes it obviously different from that of the plexiform layers. The bundles interweave with each other, forming a network in whose meshes are the processes of Müller

PAPILLA PAPILLO-MACULAR BUNDLE FOVEA

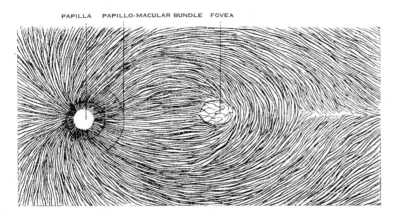

FIG. 136. — THE NERVE FIBRE LAYER OF THE RETINA (SURFACE VIEW OF THE PAPILLO - MACULAR REGION).

(*From Poirier, after Dogiel and Greeff.*)

and other glial cells. The fibres all converge towards the optic disc. Those from the nasal side reach it without interruption; those from the temporal side do not pass through the macula, but have to go round it. The fibres above the horizontal meridian pass above the macula and those below under it.

Thus we find to the lateral side of the macula a sort of raphé from which the nerve fibres arise in a pennate manner (Greeff, 1900) (Fig. 136). Those just to the lateral side of the macula encircle this structure closely, while the more lateral ones pass above and below in ever-increasing arcs.

The fibres from the macula itself pass straight in towards the temporal side of the disc and constitute the important *papillo-macular bundle*.

The nerve fibre layer is thickest around the margins of the optic disc, 20–30 μm, and here differs in the different quadrants. Thus it is thinnest directly lateral, i.e. in the region of the papillo-macular bundle. Next in thickness are the upper and lateral quadrant and the lower and lateral quadrant, then the most medial part of the edge of the disc, and finally the thickest parts are the upper and medial quadrant and the lower and medial quadrant. *The relative thickness most probably determines at which part of the disc papillœdema commences. The swelling is first visible in the thicker parts, that is, at the upper and medial lower and medial quad-*

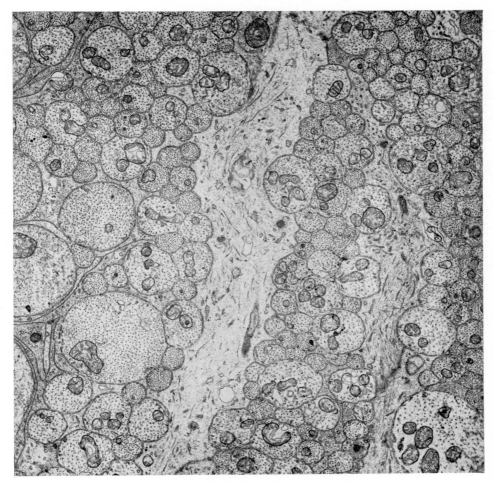

FIG. 137.—ELECTRON MICROGRAPH SHOWING AMYELINATE NERVE FIBRES IN THE NEUROFIBROUS
STRATUM OF HUMAN RETINA (× 19,500).
A fibre of Müller extends almost vertically through the field.
(*By courtesy of Dr. John Marshall and Mr. P. L. Ansell, Institute of Ophthalmology, London.*)

*rants; next comes the medial edge, then the upper and lower lateral quadrants, while
the last part of the disc to show visible swelling will be directly lateral.*

From the disc the nerve fibre layer becomes thinner as we pass towards the
periphery, and near the ora serrata is invaded by the sparse ganglion cells—the
two layers becoming one. As has been said, it is thinner on the lateral side of the
disc than in the other quadrants, and as we pass towards the macula it becomes
thinner still. At the bottom of the fovea it seems to disappear entirely, although
Dogiel, using methylene blue, showed that even here a fine network of fibres exists.

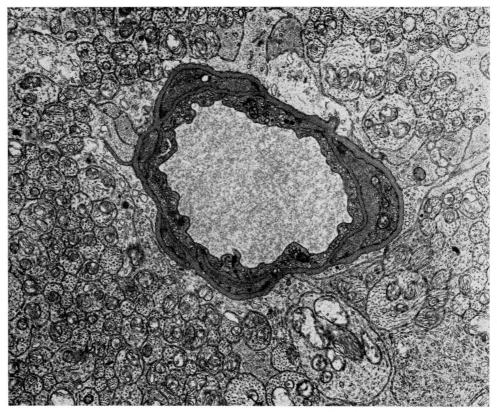

FIG. 138.—ELECTRON MICROGRAPH OF A CAPILLARY IN THE NERVE FIBRE LAYER OF HUMAN RETINA
($\times 30,000$).

The capillary endothelium is thin, and pericytes lie outside this.

(By courtesy of Dr. John Marshall and Mr. P. L. Ansell, Institute of Ophthalmology, London.)

The nerve fibres are non-medullated (except when the so-called congenital opaque fibres are present) (Fig. 137). They vary from 0·5 to 2 μm in diameter but larger fibres occur. The cytoplasm of the axons contains microtubules, fine fibrils, mitochondria, and occasional vesicles. Individual fibres are separated by neuroglial processes, but many fibres directly adjoin each other and may show actual contact junctions.

The Centrifugal Fibres are thicker than the centripetal (Ramon y Cajal, 1893). They pass through the ganglion cell layer and inner plexiform layer, and end by ramifying in the inner plexiform layer around an amacrine cell or among the elements of the inner nuclear layer (Fig. 124). Cajal made these observations in the

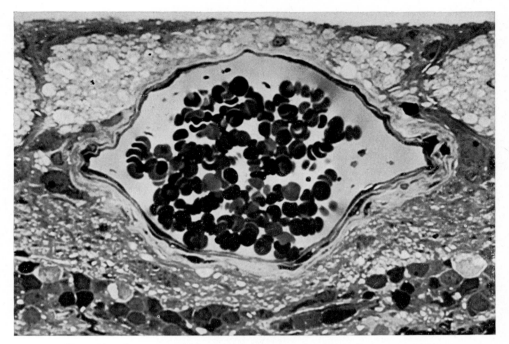

FIG. 139.—SECTION OF HUMAN RETINA SHOWING A SMALL VESSEL (× 1,320).

Note the thinning of the internal limiting membrane (above) where the vessel lies close to it. The vessel extends across the nerve fibre, ganglion cell, and internal plexiform strata, seen in this order from above downwards.

(*By courtesy of Dr. John Marshall and Mr. P. L. Ansell, Institute of Ophthalmology, London.*)

avian retina. The occurrence of centrifugal axons, derived from neurons elsewhere in the central nervous system, has been confirmed in flat preparations of the human and simian retinæ (Honrubia and Elliot, 1970). Such axons may reach the external plexiform layer; it is uncertain whether they terminate on vessels or neurons.

In the stratum opticum the glial fibres form a kind of membrane (limitans perivascularis of Krückmann) around the vessels (see p. 184 and Figs. 146, 167).

The retinal vessels are found mainly in the nerve fibre layer, but may also lie in part in the ganglion cell layer (Fig. 169). They do not as a rule project on the inner surface of the retina, but rarely may do so very slightly.

10. **The Internal Limiting Membrane.**—At the junction of retina and vitreous is a membrane which forms both the inner limit of the retina and the outer boundary of the vitreous (Figs. 95, 96, 141, 145). It has, therefore, been called with equal justification the internal limiting membrane of the retina and the hyaloid membrane of the vitreous. Here the former term will be used. According to

Redslob (1939), the outer limiting membrane has a double contour. The outer, he holds, is formed by the feet of the fibres of Müller, and is thus the true internal limiting membrane, while the inner is the hyaloid membrane. It is quite true that with the denser stains a double contour can often be made out as seen in Fig. 145.

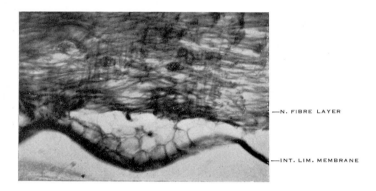

—N. FIBRE LAYER

—INT. LIM. MEMBRANE

FIG. 140. — VERTICAL SECTION OF INNER PART OF RETINA.

The internal limiting membrane has become detached as an artefact and so the normal reticulum formed by the foot-pieces of the fibres of Müller on its outer surface has become visible (see Fig. 144).

The inner portion may even separate from the outer and cells may be seen between the two. But if we follow this method of description we must always in illustrations label the membrane with both names (which is complicated) and call the membrane, which separates the *outer* part of the disc from the vitreous, the hyaloid,

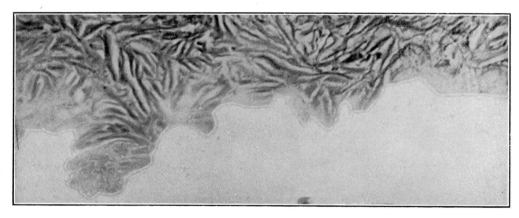

FIG. 141.—FLAT SECTION OF THE INTERNAL LIMITING MEMBRANE.

The inner portion is homogeneous (glass-like); the outer shows the characteristic mosaic.

(*Trans. O.S.U.K.*, 1937.)

since there are no fibres of Müller here. Also the internal limiting membrane will be absent where a large vessel comes close to the hyaloid (as in Fig. 139).

At the outset it must be emphasised that the membrane stains like collagenous tissue. Thus with Mallory's triple stain it is coloured blue (Fig. 142).

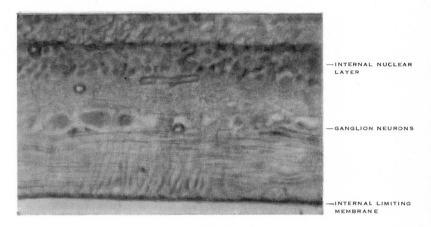

—INTERNAL NUCLEAR
LAYER

—GANGLION NEURONS

—INTERNAL LIMITING
MEMBRANE

Fig. 142.—Vertical Section of Retina. (Zenker. Mallory.)
The internal limiting membrane stains blue; fibres of Müller stain reddish.

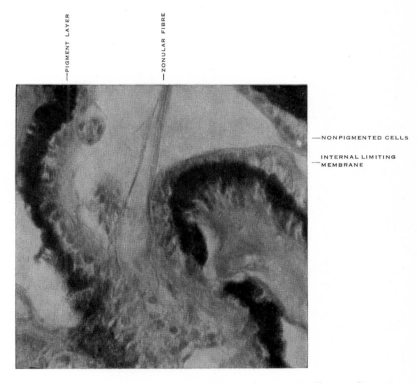

PIGMENT LAYER

ZONULAR FIBRE

—NONPIGMENTED CELLS

INTERNAL LIMITING
—MEMBRANE

Fig. 143.—Coronal Section of Ciliary Valley. (Zenker. Mallory's Triple Stain.)
To show the attachment of a zonular fibre to the limiting membrane, both of which stain blue.

In an ordinary section of the retina this membrane appears as a thin line some 1–2 μm thick, perfectly smooth towards the vitreous but having marked irregularities towards the retina. Electron microscopy (Pedler, 1961, Hogan, 1963) shows that this sinuous contour is due to the adaptation of a basement membrane to the microvilli of the processes of Müller cells (p. 125) and to other glial elements.

In a flat section of the retina the membrane appears in two parts: (a) a homogeneous portion, and (b) a curious and rather characteristic mosaic which seems to be due to the irregularities on the retinal aspect. Sometimes on the surface of this mosaic (or lying loose where the membrane has become detached as an artefact, which happens quite frequently, especially in paraffin sections) (Figs. 140, 144, 167), one sees a honeycomb of fibres, forming, no doubt, the material which binds the foot-pieces of the fibres of Müller together (Van der Stricht, 1922).

A very interesting and instructive picture is often seen if one examines a section of the retina where a large vessel comes close to the membrane. Here, opposite the vessel, the membrane is very thin. *It is smooth both on its retinal and vitreous aspects and no fibres of Müller go to it* (Fig. 139).

Further, when it is remembered that the fibres of Müller stain red with Mallory's triple stain, as does neuroglia, it becomes clear that the membrane, which is labelled the internal limiting membrane in all or nearly all modern textbooks of anatomy, cannot be formed by the apposition of the bases of the fibres of Müller as is usually and classically described (see also Salzmann, 1912; Kolmer, 1936). The feet of the fibres of Müller are in fact only attached to this membrane.

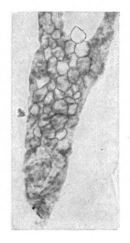

FIG. 144.—To show the Network (dark staining) of Fibres lying on a detached (light staining) Internal Limiting Membrane. (Flat Section. Zenker. Mallory's Triple Stain.)

(Trans. O.S.U.K., 1937.)

The internal limiting membrane is a typical glass-like (hyaloid) membrane. It is present at the fovea but is gradually lost at the nerve head where it is continuous with the neuroglia forming the central connective tissue meniscus of Kuhnt (Fig. 30).

On the basis of the electron microscopic studies cited above the internal limiting membrane is now considered to be an amalgam. The "membrane" proper is a PAS-positive layer, about 1–2 μm thick, which is regarded as the basement membrane of the vitreous aspect of the retina. To this are attached, externally and internally, the cells of Müller and the collagen fibrils of the vitreous. It is usually absent where capillaries of the retina adjoin the vitreous.

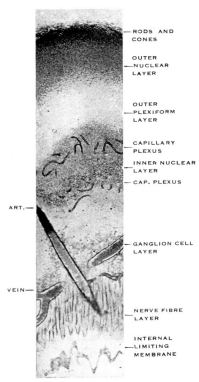

RODS AND CONES

OUTER NUCLEAR LAYER

OUTER PLEXIFORM LAYER

CAPILLARY PLEXUS

INNER NUCLEAR LAYER

CAP. PLEXUS

ART.—

GANGLION CELL LAYER

VEIN—

NERVE FIBRE LAYER

INTERNAL LIMITING MEMBRANE

FIG. 168.—FLAT (ALMOST TANGENTIAL) SECTION OF THE RETINA TO SHOW ITS VASCULARIZATION. (ZENKER. MALLORY'S TRIPLE STAIN.)

Note.—The main vessels lie in the nerve fibre and ganglion cell layers. The capillary plexus in the ganglion cell layer is not visible here, but the plexuses at the inner and outer parts of the inner nuclear layer are well shown.

epithelium varies in thickness and thus is not equally dark all over. A finer mottling is also often seen since the pigment tends to collect at the periphery of each pigment epithelial cell (Figs. 99, 100). The pigment of the retinal pigment epithelium (when viewed on the flat) tends to collect towards the periphery of the cell, leaving the central nuclear portion relatively free of pigment. It is probable that the darker the fundus the more the central portion is invaded. In not too highly pigmented fundi, therefore, the pigment forms a network, the individual holes of which are constituted by a single living epithelial cell. Now the diameter of a hexagonal cell is about 16 μm; this multiplied by 15, which is the magnification given by the direct method of ophthalmoscopy, makes 240 μm, i.e. about 0·25 mm. This is within visual limits (Wolff, 1938).

If the pigment in the pigment epithelium is less marked, and that of the choroid profuse, a tessellated fundus is produced. This consists of dark areas surrounded by red, apparently anastomosing (see p. 93) bands, produced by the choroidal vessels, for the most part the veins. These bands are not sharply defined as they are to a certain extent obscured by the pigment.

The less pigment there is in the pigment epithelium and the choroid the more the sclera shows through and the fairer will be the fundus.

In very fair people, and more so in albinos, in whom there is little or no pigment, the choroidal vessels can be seen distinctly. The vessels are broader and less sharply defined than the retinal vessels which run superficial to them. Moreover, they appear flat and ribbon-like, and show no light reflex. Also, unlike the retinal vessels, which branch dendritically and do not anastomose, the choroidal vessels *appear* to form a dense network (see p. 94), except anteriorly, where the *straight* vessels pass towards the ora serrata.

The Optic Disc is pink, owing to the numerous capillaries which it contains (Fig. 300). It must be emphasised, as it is curiously often forgotten, that the white element in its colour is due to the *lamina cribrosa*, and not to the nerve fibres of the "papilla", which are of course nonmedullated.

The optic disc under normal conditions lies in the same plane as the retina, and does not therefore form a projection as the name "papilla" would lead one to suppose.

The optic disc is excavated by a funnel-shaped depression, called the physiological cup, which varies much in form and size. It is most often not in the centre of the disc but displaced slightly to the temporal side. It tends to be absent in high hypermetropia. Its colour is whiter than the rest of the disc, because there are fewer vessels and nerve fibres obscuring the lamina cribrosa. Very often the holes in this membrane for the passage of the nerve fibres can be seen as grey dots. *They become more evident in glaucoma and atrophy of the disc.*

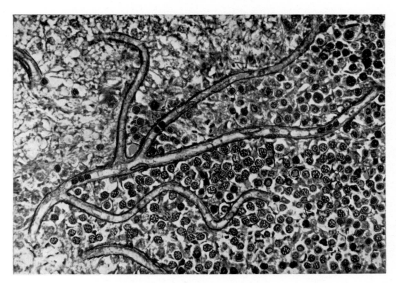

FIG. 169.—FLAT SECTION OF THE CAPILLARY PLEXUS IN THE INNER NUCLEAR LAYER.
(*Wolff's preparation.*)

The optic disc is pinker in colour to the medial side of the physiological cup than to the lateral. This is due to the greater thickness of nerve fibres and more capillary vessels. For the same reason the medial edge of the disc tends to be less well-defined than the lateral.

The Retinal Vessels climb up the medial side of the physiological cup. The arteries are easily distinguishable from the veins. The arteries are narrower, of a brighter red colour, and have a well-marked light streak or reflex along their axes. The light streak along the veins is much less marked. It is the image of the source of light used in the ophthalmoscopic examination.

When the scleral canal is straight, the end of the arteria centralis is seen in optical section, and the branches appear to come off at 180°.

If the intra-mural portion of the optic nerve is directed laterally as well as forwards (temporally oblique scleral canal) the nasal border of the physiological cup is steep or overhanging. The arteria centralis is usually invisible, and its first divisions make an angle which is open towards the temporal side.

If the scleral canal runs forwards and medially (nasally oblique canal) the artery can be seen for some distance and the central vessels appear displaced towards the temporal side.

It should be noted carefully that as the disc is on the same plane as the retina, the light streak is not normally lost as the vessels pass over the edge of the disc. With the slightest amount of swelling of the disc (as in papilloedema) the vessels bend over its edge, and the image of the source of light is thrown beyond the pupil. It thus does not reach the examining eye, and the bent portion of the vessel appears dark. In this way we get the loss of light reflex so important in the diagnosis of papilloedema.

As the vessels pass out into the retina the nasal vessels run a more or less direct though sinuous course, while the temporal ones are arcuate.

It will be noted that although an artery is accompanied by the corresponding vein, they never or almost never run next to each other for this would cast too much of a shadow on the rods and cones.

Arterial pulsation cannot be observed with an ordinary monocular ophthalmoscope, but is visible with binocular instruments of higher magnification. When seen ordinarily it has a pathological significance. Venous pulsation is normally visible.

The *connective tissue* or *scleral ring* is the white ring or part of a ring often seen next to the disc. This may be due to the border tissue not covered by the epithelium or to the side wall of an oblique scleral canal.

The Choroidal Ring is a dark ring (or portion of a ring) outside the scleral ring. It is produced by a heaping up of the retinal pigment epithelium; hence "choroidal" is a misnomer (Elschnig).

The Macula appears as a small oval area devoid of vessels, of a deeper red than the rest of the fundus, and often slightly stippled with pigment.

The retinal reflexes, which usually change their position with the slightest movement of the eye or ophthalmoscope, are fixed in the macular region.

The oval macular reflex comes from the wall which surrounds the macula. The fovea forms a small concave mirror, and so produces the bright foveal reflex (which at times may be so bright as to deserve the name of bull's-eye lantern reflex).

The region of the clivus is, however, darker than the surrounding retina, because light falling on it from the ophthalmoscope is not reflected back through the pupil; also the retina here is very thin and the pigment epithelium much denser.

For further details of fundal appearances appropriate monographs should be consulted (e.g. Ballantyne and Michaelson, 1962). Apart from direct ophthalmoscopy a number of other techniques for examining the fundus, and especially its vessels, have been elaborated. Consult Wise, Dollery and Henkind (1973) and

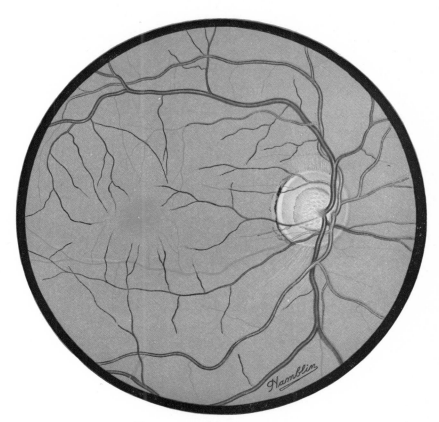

FIG. 170.—THE NORMAL FUNDUS.

(Direct image of the right eye.)

The central vessels climb up the nasal side of the physiological cup. The central artery appears as a single stem which is just visible here and then divides into two branches which appear to separate at an angle of 180°. (Often the stem is invisible where the scleral canal is quite straightforward, or it may be seen for some distance in a very oblique canal; more rarely it appears as two or more trunks.)

The central vein, on the other hand, appears as two trunks, since its formation (seen hazily) is in the lamina cribrosa. It is lateral to the artery.

As the vessels pass over the edge of the disc they do not lose their light streak.

The macula is seen as an area darker red than the rest of the fundus. Its centre (the fovea), seen as a whitish reflex, lies below the centre of the disc.

At the edge of the disc are a pigmented "choroidal" crescent and a scleral ring.

The normal striation which is often seen above and below the disc and due to the *non-medullated* nerve fibres has come out much too prominently in the figure.

classical texts such as Duke-Elder (1932), Duke-Elder and Wybar (1961) for details. Fluorescence fundus photography (Rosen, 1969), is of particular interest, providing dynamic sequential studies of the retinal circulation.

THE ANTERIOR AND POSTERIOR CHAMBERS

The space in front of the lens and suspensory ligament is divided into two by the iris (Fig. 21) but both parts of the cavity are freely continuous through the pupil.

In front of the iris is the anterior chamber, behind it the posterior chamber.

The Anterior Chamber is bounded in front by the cornea and a small portion of the sclera.

The amount of sclera entering into the formation of the anterior chamber is about 2 mm above, 1·5 mm below and 1 mm at the sides. Rochon Duvigneaud, measuring from the limbus to the angle, finds 2·25 mm, 2 mm and 1·25 mm; while Lagrange finds (from limbus to a point opposite the attachment of the iris) 1·75 mm, 1·45 mm and 1 mm as the corresponding figures.

Behind is the iris, a part of the ciliary body, and a variable area of the anterior surface of the lens exposed by the pupil.

At the periphery of the anterior chamber is its so-called *angle*, and here is the trabecular tissue usually known as ligamentum pectinatum iridis, with the spaces of Fontana and the adjacent sinus venosus scleræ (canal of Schlemm). The anterior chamber is about 3·5 mm deep centrally and is narrowest not at the angle but slightly central to this (Fig. 47).

(For recent estimates of anterior chamber dimensions see Aizawa, 1958 and Weekers *et al.*, 1961, 1963.)

The Posterior Chamber is somewhat triangular on section, the apex of the triangle being where the edge of the iris rests on the lens. The base is formed by the ciliary processes and the valleys between them, in which are the recesses of Kuhnt. The posterior wall is formed by the lens and its zonules (suspensory ligament) and the anterior by pigment epithelium of the iris. Sometimes the lenticular zonules are regarded as part of the posterior chamber, whose posterior limit is then at the vitreous humour.

The posterior chamber is frequently divided, somewhat arbitrarily, into three zones or regions:

(*a*) The posterior chamber proper, between the iris and the zonules of the lens. This contains aqueous humour derived from the ciliary processes at the front of the ciliary body.

(*b*) The zonular region, consisting of the aggregations of collagenous fibrils which form the zonules (p. 168).

(*c*) The retrozonular space, the so-called canal of Petit (p. 169), between the posterior aspect of the zonular fibres and the anterior aspect of the vitreous humour.

The aqueous humour is produced by the ciliary processes, secreted into the posterior chamber, circulates through the pupil, and is removed through the trabecular tissue of the iridocorneal angle, returning to the venous system via the scleral venous sinus.

For its detailed composition and the factors governing its formation and absorption suitable physiological texts should be consulted (e.g. Davson, 1969). Being the intermediary pathway between the blood and the avascular tissues of the eyeball (lens and cornea), it contains many substances in solution. It is, however, very dilute, containing less than a tenth of the solutes of blood, the chief difference being in a much lower protein content, particularly gamma globulin. It has a higher ascorbic acid content than blood plasma. It is a factor in the maintenance of intraocular pressure and hence of the optical shape of the eyeball.

The Lens

The lens of the eye is a transparent bi-convex body of crystalline appearance placed between the iris and the vitreous.

The diameter of the lens is 9–10 mm. Its axial diameter varies markedly with accommodation. By direct measurement it is about 3·5 to 4·0 mm at birth, about 4 mm at 50 years, increasing slowly to 4·75 to 5·0 mm in extreme old age. In contrast its equatorial diameter, 6·5 mm at birth, is 9–10 mm in the second decade and changes little thereafter.

Like all lenses, that of the eye presents for examination two surfaces, anterior and posterior, and a border where these surfaces meet, known as the equator (equator lentis).

The anterior surface, less convex than the posterior, is the segment of a sphere whose radius averages 10 mm (8·0 to 14·0 mm).

It is in relation in front, through the pupil, with the anterior chamber of the eye, with the posterior surface of the iris, the pupillary margin of which rests on the anterior surface, with the posterior chamber of the eye, and with the ciliary processes.

The centre of the anterior surface is known as the anterior *pole*, and is about 3 mm from the back of the cornea.

The posterior surface, more curved than the anterior, presents a radius of about 6 mm (4·5 to 7·5 mm). It is usually described as lying in a fossa lined by the hyaloid membrane on the front of the vitreous, but it is separated from the vitreous by a slight space filled with primary vitreous (p. 177). This retrolenticular space was described by Berger (1882), and is confirmed by the slit-lamp (see p. 247).

The Equator of the lens forms a circle lying 0·5 mm within the ciliary processes. The equator is not smooth, but shows a number of dentations corresponding to the zonular fibres (Fig. 171). These tend to disappear during accommodation when the zonular fibres are loose.

The refractive index of the lens (1·39) is only slightly more than that of the

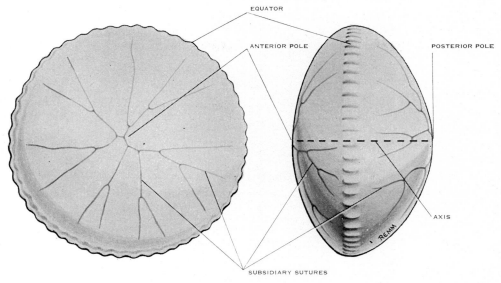

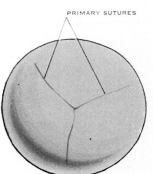

FIG. 171.—THE LENS.
Adult lens above, fetal lens below.

aqueous and vitreous humours (1·33), and hence, despite its smaller radii of curvature, it exerts much less dioptric effect than the cornea. The dioptric contribution of the lens is about 15 out of a total of about 40 dioptres for the normal eye. At the time of birth the accommodative power is 15 to 16 dioptres, diminishing to half of this at about 25 years and to 1 to 2 dioptres at 50.

Structure of the Lens

The lens consists of:

1. The lenticular capsule.
2. The lenticular epithelium.
3. The lens cells or fibres.

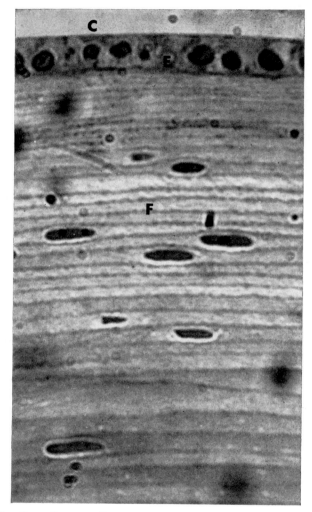

FIG. 172.—THE LENS CAPSULE, EPITHELIUM AND FIBRES (PHOTOMICROGRAPH, × 500).
(By courtesy of Dr. C. Pedler, Institute of Ophthalmology, London. Preparation by Mrs. R. Tilly.)

The Capsule of the lens forms a transparent, homogeneous, highly elastic envelope, which is really a particularly thick basement membrane. It is PAS-positive. It contains no true elastic tissue, and its elasticity must reside in the disposition of the fine fibrils which can be seen in places to form it. These fibrils, probably composed of a form of collagen, have a striation period of about 60 nm, which is different from that of the fibrils of the zonules, though these fuse with it at their attachments. Ultrastructurally the capsule has a lamellated appearance.

Much of the capsule, however, has an almost homogeneous structure. (See Cohen, 1965.)

When cut or ruptured its edges roll out and then curl up, so that the outer surface is innermost. It is much thicker in front than behind, and the anterior and posterior portions are thicker towards the periphery (equator), just within the

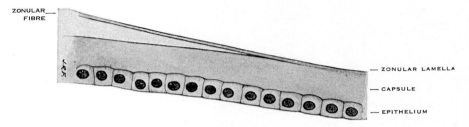

ZONULAR FIBRE

ZONULAR LAMELLA

CAPSULE

EPITHELIUM

FIG. 173.—LENS CAPSULE AND ZONULAR LAMELLA.

attachment of the suspensory ligament, than at the poles. It is this difference in the thickness of the central and peripheral parts of the anterior capsule which Fincham believes is responsible for the hyperbolic form of the anterior surface of the lens during accommodation.

Salzmann (1912) gave the following data for capsule thickness at different ages

Age	Anterior pole	Equator	Posterior pole
2·5 years	8 μm	7 μm	2 μm
35 years	14 μm	1·7 μm	4 μm
71 years	14 μm	9 μm	2·3 μm

Fincham (1925, 1937) recorded figures of 2·8 μm at the posterior pole and 15·5 μm at the anterior (Fig. 174). The maximum anterior and posterior capsular thicknesses were recorded as 14·8 μm and 22·5 μm (Salzmann—23 μm and 21 μm). Fincham's views on the effect of these variations on the moulding of the lens in accommodation have not been superseded.

The Lenticular Epithelium (Figs. 172, 173, 175).

This consists of a single layer of cubical cells spread over the front of the lens deep to the capsule. There is no corresponding posterior epithelium, since the posterior cells were used up in filling the central cavity of the lens vesicle.

If we trace the cells of the anterior epithelium towards the equator we find that they gradually become columnar and, elongating, are eventually

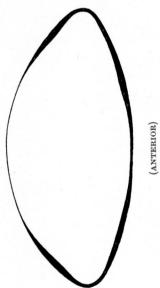

(ANTERIOR)

FIG. 174.—VERY SCHEMATIC ANTERO POSTERIOR SECTION OF THE LENS CAPSULE TO SHOW RELATIVE THICKNESS OF VARIOUS PORTIONS (FINCHAM).

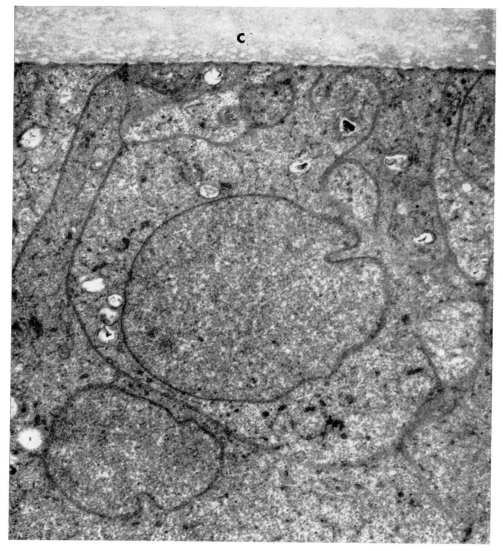

FIG. 175.—THE LENS CAPSULE (C) AND EPITHELIUM (RHESUS MONKEY, ELECTRON MICROGRAPH, ×20,000).

(By courtesy of Dr. C. Pedler, Institute of Ophthalmology, London. Preparation by Mrs. R. Tilly.)

converted into lens fibres. In Fig. 177 all the stages of development of the lens fibres can be seen.

It will be noted that the base of the cell, i.e. the part in contact with the capsule, becomes the posterior part of the lens fibre, while the opposite end grows into the anterior portion of the lens fibre. The nuclei form a somewhat S-shaped nuclear zone at the equator (see also p. 439).

In the central area of the lens the epithelial cells are polygonal in tangential section, with a width of about 15 μm and a depth of only 6 μm. Although they are slowly multiplying, mitoses are rarely visible. They are smooth on both aspects, basally where they adjoin the capsule, their basement membrane, and also over their apices, which are con-tiguous with the most anterior lens fibres. Peri-pheral to this the cells become narrower but more elongated, and their basal and adjacent aspects are reciprocally folded. Mitoses are more fre-quently observed in this zone. At the equator division is most active and the elongation accentu-ated, forming new lens fibres, or cells as they should be called, because they are nucleated.

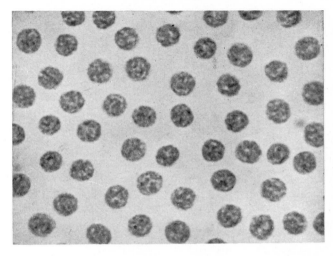

Fig. 176.—Portion of Anterior Capsule of Lens viewed on the flat to show the Nuclei of the Epithelium.

Electron microscopy reveals no unusual features in these cells. Various forms of junctional complex, particularly occluding zonules and adherent maculæ, occur between them and adjacent lens fibres (Fig. 175). It is appropriate to add here that the amorphous "cement substance" described by light microscopists as existing between adjoining lenticular cells and fibres is not confirmed by the findings of electron microscopy. (See Cohen, 1965.) (Fig. 182).

The Lens Cells or Fibres.—All but the oldest lens "fibres" are in reality elon-gated, nucleated *cells*. Each element is a very long hexagonal prism, flattened in such a way that two of its sides are much wider than the rest (Fig. 178). These two sides remain parallel through much of the length of the cell but converge at its extremities (i.e. near the sutures—*vide infra*). The earlier formed fibres are naturally those in the central core or nucleus of the lens, and these gradually lose their nuclei and become true *fibres*.

The first lens fibres were formed from the posterior epithelium and ran from the back to the front of the vesicle. But the later ones are derived from the equatorial portion of the anterior epithelium.

Here, as we have seen, we find all stages in the formation of a lens fibre from its cell (Fig. 177).

The newest lens fibres are laid on externally to the older deeper ones, and so the lens acquires a laminated structure. On equatorial section the laminæ are cut transversely, forming the radial lamellæ of Rabl (Fig. 178), while anteroposterior section shows them as long fibres placed one on the other in concentric layers. The fibres belonging to each lamina are of the same length.

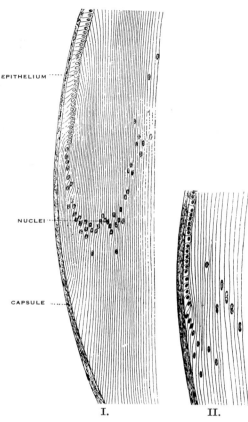

FIG. 177.—MERIDIONAL SECTION OF THE EQUATORIAL REGION OF THE LENS.
I. New-born.   II. Old man.

(*From Poirier, after Otto Becker.*)

The superficial (youngest) fibres, too, are nucleated, their nuclei lying near the equator, and arranged so as to form a letter S in meridional section. Moreover, their sides are quite smooth. The nuclei are at first rounded or slightly oval. As the fibre ages the nucleus becomes longer, often narrower at its middle, and then breaks down into granules.

The deeper, older fibres lose their nuclei, become less succulent as it were, and their edges become serrated, the serrations of one fitting into those of its neighbour. Thus the oldest fibres are irregular in thickness and their contours serrated due to shrinkage. Outside these fibres we see cross-sections of fibres having four, five, or six sides. They are of irregular thickness, but get thinner towards the periphery. Finally, at the periphery itself is a concentrically striped layer. This appearance must not lead one to think that the whole lens has a concentrically layered structure; for if so this appearance ought to be found in equatorial as well as meridional sections.

Although the first-formed lens fibres go from pole to pole, of the later ones none do.

In the infantile lens, each starts and finishes on the anterior and posterior Ys respectively in such a way that the nearer the axis of the lens it commences the farther away it ends (Fig. 395).

The fibres formed later, for instance the superficial ones of the adult lens, start and finish on the more complicated stellate figures, conforming, however, to the above rule (pp. 167, 168).

Two of the sides of the hexagonal lens fibres are longer than the remainder, and adhere much less firmly to the neighbouring fibres than do the short sides. It follows that if we treat the infantile lens with alcohol, which dissolves the cement substance, it will first of all divide into three sectors, and then each of these will separate into laminæ like the layers of an onion.

It is possible only to give average dimensions for the lens cells, especially in regard to their length. In the cortical zone they are about 7 μm wide and about 5 μm in the nuclear region, thinning out to 2 μm near the sutures. Their length is 8 to 12 mm. The total number of cells and fibres is over 2000 in the adult lens.

By electron microscopy the most superficial cells are seen to contain the usual organelles of epithelial cells; the cytoplasm is fibrillar. As the cells "age" the cytoplasm becomes progressively more homogeneous. The outlines of the cells also show ageing changes. In their early stages the fibres show reciprocal interlocking indentations only on their shorter sides or edges. Later, these sides become smoother, and indentations appear on the long flat aspects of the tape-like fibres (Figs. 181, 182). These indentations are presumably an adhesional mechanism between cells; no clear evidence of junctional complexes has been adduced. The interdigitations may permit a small degree of movement between the lens fibres in accommodational changes of shape.

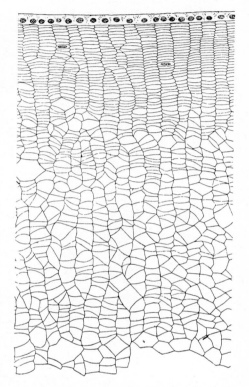

FIG. 178.—PERIPHERAL PORTION OF AN EQUATORIAL SECTION OF THE HUMAN LENS TO SHOW THE RADIAL LAMELLÆ.

(*From Rabl.*)

New lens fibres are laid on throughout life, and as the central portion which corresponds to the keratin layer of the skin cannot be shed, the lens keeps on growing. This, however, is not proportional to the number of fibres, for the older ones, as we have seen, shrink. At the 65th year the lens is said to be one-third larger than at 25.

The consistency of the lens varies, the more superficial portion or *cortex* being softer than the central part or *nucleus*. The nucleus increases with age. The lens becomes flatter with age, but its refractive power is retained by an increase in the refractive index of the nucleus. (Consult Norman *et al.*, 1974.)

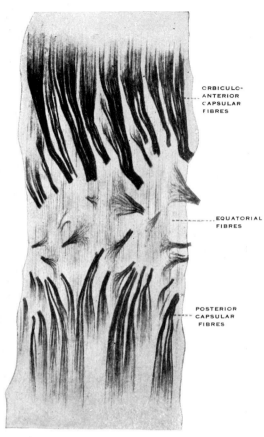

ORBICULO-
ANTERIOR
CAPSULAR
FIBRES

EQUATORIAL
FIBRES

POSTERIOR
CAPSULAR
FIBRES

Fig. 179.—Equatorial Zone of the Lens Capsule
with the insertion of the Zonular Fibres.

(*From Salzmann.*)

The sclerosing of the nuclear portion, which starts in earliest youth, continues with increasing speed with age, while new nucleated fibres are laid on around. These in turn lose their nuclei, to be surrounded again by younger nucleated fibres.

As stated before, some new fibres are laid on throughout life, but more slowly with advancing age; hence there are more nucleated fibres in the young than in the old.

Hence also, the nuclear bow which in young embryos extended right across the lens shows a greater and greater gap with advancing age (Figs. 25, 382).

In a well-stained meridional section through the normal adult lens we see at its centre a relatively narrow area of axially directed fibres which become more and more convex outwards as we pass laterally.

The colour of the lens, too, changes with age. In the infant and young adult it is usually stated to be quite colourless but, according to Hess, a *very faint* yellow tinge can be made out even here. After about thirty-five years the central portion gets a definite yellow tinge, which becomes darker and more extensive as time goes on. In the old man the lens often has an amber colour.

One other point of practical importance must be mentioned. In old people the lens often appears grey when viewed by indirect illumination. *This appearance may easily be mistaken for a cataract by the uninitiated.*

The Ciliary Zonule
(Zonule of Zinn, Suspensory Ligament of the Lens)

The Ciliary Zonule consists essentially of a series of fibres passing from the ciliary body to the lens. It holds the lens in position and enables the ciliary muscle to act on it. The lens and zonule form a diaphragm which divides the eye into a smaller anterior portion which contains aqueous and a larger posterior portion filled with vitreous. As a whole the zonule forms a ring which is roughly triangular on meridional section. The base of the triangle is concave, and occupies the equator and portions of the anterior and posterior surfaces of the lens. The apex is elongated, curved, and follows the posterior border of the ciliary processes and then the orbiculus ciliaris to the ora serrata.

The anteroexternal side forms part of the posterior boundary of the posterior chamber and then follows the whole of the inner surface of the corona ciliaris. The posterointernal border is in close contact with the anterior limiting layer of the vitreous. The zonular fibres do not fill this triangle uniformly. They are collected mainly into anterior and posterior layers lying along the anterolateral and posteromedial sides of the triangle. The space between these layers is known as the canal of Petit, but actually it is subdivided into larger and smaller spaces by the crossings of the zonular fibres.

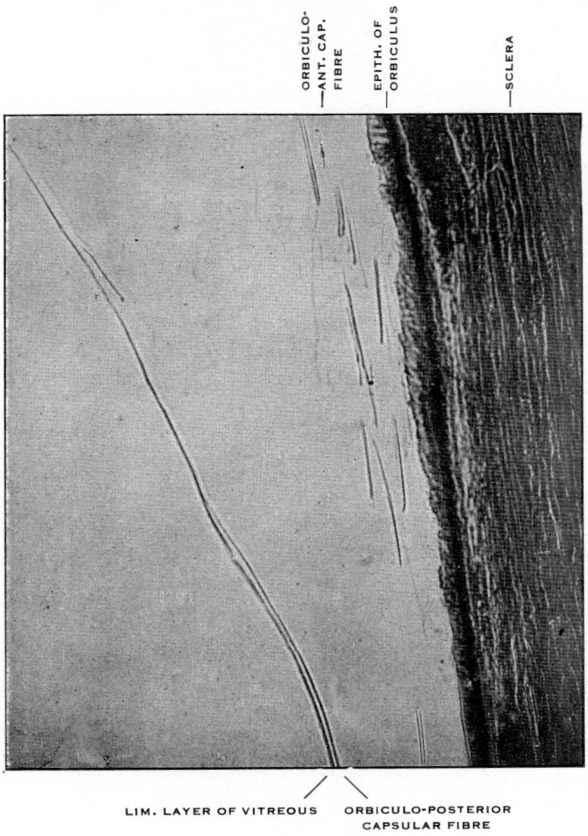

Although the above is now the usual description, Petit himself thought that the hyaloid membrane split at the ciliary body, the anterior portion forming the suspensory ligament, the posterior continuing over the front of the vitreous, and that he had injected the space between the two. It was Hannover who actually showed that one could inject the space between the anterior and posterior portions of the suspensory ligament.

FIG. 180.—ANTEROPOSTERIOR SECTION TO SHOW SOME FIBRES OF THE ZONULE AND THE LIMITING LAYER OF VITREOUS.

The zonule consists of fibres which are transparent, straight for the most part, stiff in appearance and inextensible. Viewed along their length they appear roughly rounded or flattened and faintly grooved. The cross-section has an

A.E.—12

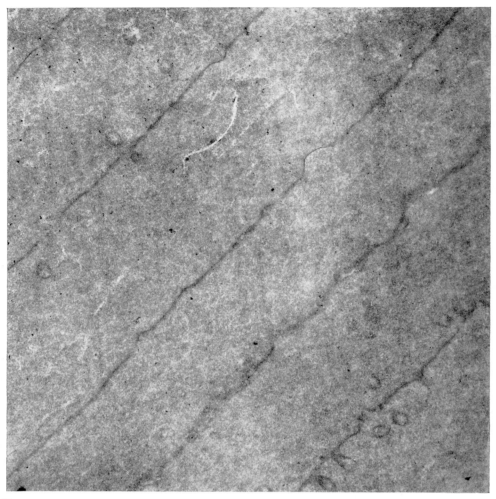

Fig. 181.—Lens Fibres in Longitudinal Section (Rhesus Monkey, Electron Micrograph, × 13,500).

(By courtesy of Dr. C. Pedler, Institute of Ophthalmology, London. Preparation by Mrs. R. Tilly.)

irregular outline corresponding to the grooves and indicating the composite nature of each fibre. Although individual zonular fibres are of very even calibre, electron microscopy and phase-contrast microscopy (Pappas and Smelser, 1958, Garzino, 1953) demonstrate considerable variations between fibres in the same and different species. By phase-contrast three types of fibre were identified, one about 1 μm in diameter, sinuous and usually near the vitreous, a second type which was thin and flat, and a third one even thinner and pursuing a circular course. The fibres are composed of microfibrils with a diameter ranging from 8 to 40 nm (Hogan,

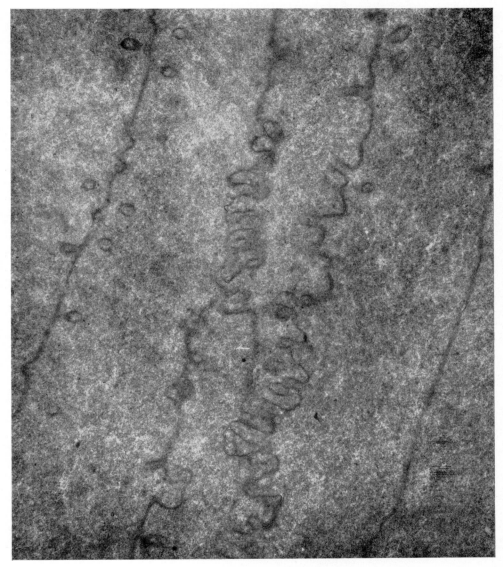

Fig. 182.—Lens Fibres Cut in Longitudinal Section. (Rhesus Monkey, same as Fig. 181, Electron Micrograph, ×11,000).

These older fibres show the highly tortuous interdigitations between adjacent surfaces. There is no "amorphous substance" to be seen between the fibres.

(By courtesy of Dr. C. Pedler, Institute of Ophthalmology, London. Preparation by Mrs. R. Tilly.)

Alvarado and Weddell, 1971). Microfibrillary periodicity is 11 to 18 nm, as in the vitreous.

On ordinary histological examination the fibres appear homogeneous, but actually each consists of extremely fine fibrils so closely united that it requires maceration in alcohol, permanganate of potash, etc., to demonstrate this. Only at times can a faint longitudinal striation be made out in the stained section.

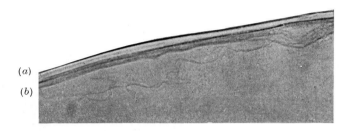

(a)

(b)

Fig. 183.—To show the relation of an Orbiculo-posterior Capsular Fibre (a) and the Anterior Limiting Layer of Vitreous (b); (Ant.-post. Section).

Note fibrillar appearance of latter.

The composite nature of each fibre is again seen at its attachments. To the side of the lens it breaks up in a fan-shaped manner into a series of extremely fine fibrils (Fig. 179), which become continuous with the zonular lamella; to the side of the ciliary body it may do this too or give off its fibrils like the barbs of a feather but on one side of the fibre only (Fig. 184).

Among the fibres, or attached to them, one may find white cells which are probably endothelial cells or wandering leucocytes.

In the zonule, Main and Auxiliary Fibres may be distinguished.

The Main Fibres may be classified as follows:

1. *The orbiculoposterior capsular fibres* are the most posterior and also the innermost fibres of the zonule. They take origin from the ora serrata. As regards their thickness they are of the second order. They lie throughout their extent in close contact with the anterior limiting layer of the vitreous, which, exercising a pressure on them, causes their forward convexity. They are inserted together with the vitreous (ligamentum hyaloideocapsulare of Wieger) to the posterior lens capsule. In meridional sections they may easily be taken for a hyaloid membrane (Figs. 180, 183), but they are hyaline in nature and discontinuous in a section, whereas the limiting layer of the vitreous is fibrillar and continuous. Also, if one looks at oblique meridional (tangential) sections in which the posterior attachments of these fibres are cut it may appear as if they have their origin in the vitreous, which is not the case.

2. *The Orbiculoanterior capsular fibres* are the thickest and strongest of the zonular fibres; they arise from the orbiculus ciliaris, a great number from a slight ridge known as the posterior zonular border which lies 1·5 mm in front, and imitates the indentations, of the ora serrata. They are inserted into the anterior capsule of the lens. They receive supporting (auxiliary) fibres along their whole

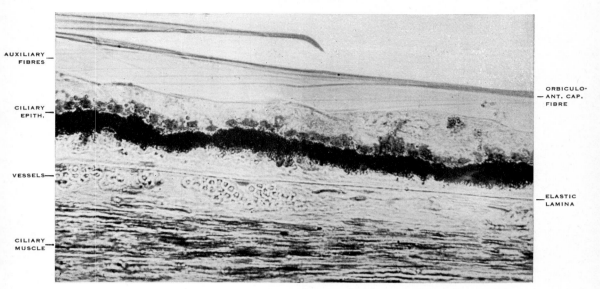

AUXILIARY FIBRES

CILIARY EPITH.

VESSELS

CILIARY MUSCLE

ORBICULO-ANT. CAP. FIBRE

ELASTIC LAMINA

Fig. 184.—Meridional Section of Orbiculus Ciliaris with Orbiculoanterior Capsular and Auxiliary Fibres.

course. They lie in the valleys between the taller ciliary processes at whose sides they form well-marked bundles (Figs. 62, 185). They are attached to the valleys and the sides of the processes by their supporting fibrils. Some cross the heads of the ciliary processes, which they depress like a finger on the string of a harp (Rochon-Duvigneaud).

3. *The Cilioposterior capsular fibres* are the most numerous zonular fibres. As regards their thickness they are of the third order. They arise from the valleys and less from the sides of the ciliary processes, pass posteriorly, cross the anteriorly directed fibres, and are inserted into the posterior capsule, anterior to the insertion of the orbiculoposterior capsular fibres. In posterior dislocation of the lens these fibres pull on the ciliary processes.

4. *The Cilioequatorial fibres* are really only present in youthful eyes. They arise from the ciliary valleys, a few from the orbiculus, and run to the equator of the lens. Sometimes they occupy the whole interval between the anterior and posterior groups of fibres. With age these fibres largely disappear and only a few sparse bundles eventually remain. Their thickness is much that of the previous group.

The Auxiliary Fibres.—Some of these strengthen the *main* fibres and help to anchor the individual portions of the zonule; others hold the various portions of the ciliary body together. The auxiliary fibres are for the most part very fine. They run as a rule from without inwards and forwards. But from the posterior part of the corona ciliaris fibres run from without backwards and inwards to the orbiculoanterior capsular fibres, crossing the auxiliary fibres that run anteriorly.

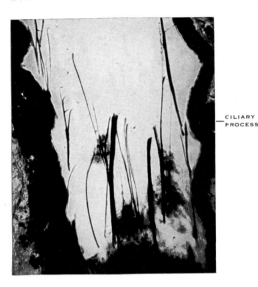

CILIARY
PROCESS

FIG. 185.—CORONAL SECTION OF A CILIARY VALLEY TO SHOW ORBICULOANTERIOR CAPSULAR FIBRES.

The zonular fibres here, therefore, have a double attachment which makes for strength; and so always or nearly always the zonular fibres break just beyond this area.

Over the orbiculus ciliaris the auxiliary fibres run almost parallel with the inner surface of the ciliary body, but more anteriorly they become more and more vertical while the most anterior ones are almost perpendicular to the surface.

The Orbiculociliary fibres run from the orbiculus to the posterior ciliary processes, whose forward movement they tend to prevent.

The Interciliary fibres tend to prevent the separation of two neighbouring processes (Fig. 186).

The great majority of zonular fibres have a meridional or radial direction. Salzmann describes some *circular zonular fibres* which, lying on the anterior limiting membrane of the vitreous, are often hidden in the folds of this layer.

The zonular fibres are firmly attached to the ciliary epithelium and if they are torn away some of the epithelium comes away with them. The exact method of insertion is still much disputed. They appear, however, to run into the internal limiting membrane of the ciliary body (*q.v.*) (Fig. 143). This interpretation is confirmed by electron microscopy.

Also Garnier demonstrated that in the new-born child the number of zonular fibres is much larger than in the adult; that fibres pass to the anterior capsule from the most anterior ciliary process and even from the angle of the posterior chamber. In childhood these last disappear, so that in the adult the anterior ciliary process lies free and sends no fibres to the anterior capsule.

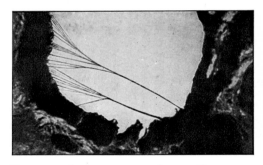

FIG. 186.—CROSS-SECTION OF CILIARY VALLEY TO SHOW INTERCILIARY FIBRES.

In old age a large number of zonular fibres disappear, but in the process some fibres are much thickened.

Macroscopic Appearances.—The zonular fibres can be seen with the naked eye and better with a magnifying loupe. To do this, divide the eye equatorially, remove the vitreous, place the anterior part on a slide, remove the cornea as peripherally as possible, pull out the iris and illuminate the perilental space from below.

Looked at in this way each ciliary process is seen to be flanked on each side by a bundle of zonular fibres. As there are seventy processes, there are one hundred and forty bundles.

These bundles (consisting of orbiculoanterior capsular fibres) are seen to run to the anterior capsule; they appear, however, to arise from the valleys between the processes. But, as we have seen, they come from farther back; in fact, from the orbiculus ciliaris.

If the preparation be now reversed the zonule can be seen from behind. In the anterior part of the orbiculus the (orbiculoanterior capsular) fibres give rise to a fine silky meridional striation (better seen in the hardened than in the fresh specimen) which extends into the ciliary valleys leaving the processes free (Salzmann). From the ciliary processes again fibres are seen to run to the posterior capsule. These are the cilioposterior capsular fibres; for the orbiculoposterior capsular fibres have been removed with the vitreous. (If the vitreous had not been removed in the preparation the spaces between the zonular fibres would be filled in and therefore they would not be so clearly visible.)

The zonular fibres can also be seen in the living (especially with the help of a slit-lamp) in cases of coloboma of the iris and dislocation of the lens.

THE VITREOUS

The vitreous humour is a perfectly transparent, colourless, gelatinous mass of a consistency somewhat firmer than egg-white, which fills the posterior four-fifths of the globe. Its shape is that of the cavity in which it lies, that is, of the space behind the diaphragm formed by the lens and ciliary zonule. Thus it has the form of a sphere flattened frontally and indented anteriorly by a saucer-shaped depression known as the patellar fossa which lodges the lens. At the sides it supports the ciliary body (covered by the zonule) and the retina. Through its central region runs the hyaloid canal, which in the fetus lodges the hyaloid artery; it is a vestige, therefore of embryonic development (p. 451).

The vitreous lies in contact with, but only slightly adherent to, the retina. It is, however, attached to the edge of the optic disc, and to the ciliary epithelium in a zone 2 mm broad immediately anterior to the ora serrata. This area is known as the *base* (Salzmann) or origin (Wolfrum) of the vitreous, for it is here that, as the result of fixation of hardening fluids, or under pathological conditions, the vitreous remains adherent. Even severe injuries do not tear the living vitreous from this situation, and when it does give way it takes part of the ciliary epithelium with it (Salzmann). Also, as will be seen later, all vitreous fibrils can be traced back to this region. The vitreous attachment, at its base, extends posteriorly for about 4 mm on to the retina.

From the ora to the lens the vitreous is convex forwards. This portion is in contact all the way with the posterointernal fibres of the zonule. It is held away from the orbiculus ciliaris by the zonular fibres. More anteriorly the ciliary processes although separated by zonular fibres press on and form radial grooves in this portion of the vitreous (Fig. 24).

The vitreous is adherent to the lens in a circle some 9 mm in diameter, while posteriorly within the circle of adhesion the capillary space of Berger (see p. 247) appears to separate the lens from the vitreous. This adhesion is firm only in youth and weakens in later decades, so that separation of the lens from the vitreous in intracapsular cataract operations is usually easy. There is also usually an attachment, 3 to 4 mm in diameter, over the macula, but this also is firmer in fetal, postnatal and adolescent individuals.

The hyaloid canal (canal of Cloquet or Stilling) starts in front of the disc as a funnel-shaped area (area of Martegiani), passes through the vitreous as a narrow canal 1–2 mm wide, and expands again anteriorly in the patellar fossa of the vitreous. It is probable that in the adult the canal does not run a direct sagittal course as is usually depicted. It probably sinks with gravity and moves about with movements of the eye and head. Its walls are formed of a condensation of the vitreous and not by an actual membrane (Ida C. Mann, 1927, Busacca *et al.* 1957, and Goldmann, 1954).

MICROSCOPIC STRUCTURE OF THE VITREOUS

It is extremely difficult to get a satisfactory microscopic preparation of the vitreous. This is due to the following facts: it contains a higher percentage of water than any other tissue in the body; it is very liable to artefacts, and it stains badly with ordinary dyes.

They eye must be fixed as a whole without opening. One of the best earlier fixatives was the acetone fluid of Szent-Györgi (1914). The eye should be embedded in celloidin and stained preferably with Held's phospho-molybdic acid hæmatoxylin. Malloy's triple stain folling fixation with Zenker's fluid also gives good results. Dissecting microscopy, darkfield illumination, phase-contrast and electron microscopy have all added further information.

The limiting layer is simply a condensation of the vitreous and not a hyaloid membrane, but it does act as a fragile envelope. It is present everywhere, except just in front of the origin of the vitreous (zonular cleft of Salzmann) and at the area of Martegiani. It is divided by Salzmann into anterior and posterior limiting layers.

The Posterior limiting layer or hyaloid extends posteriorly from the base of the vitreous, in contact with the retina, to the optic disc, where it is firmly attached to the internal limiting membrane of the retina. It is itself not a true membrane, being rather a condensation of collagen fibres attached at places to the basement membrane of the cells of Müller (see p. 124).

The Anterior limiting layer or hyaloid starts about 1·5 mm from the ora, just anterior to the mass of fibrils passing into the vitreous from its origin or base but continuous with the most anterior of these.

It passes inwards to the posterior aspect of the lens, to which it is attached in the form of a ring some 9 mm in diameter. This attachment is known as the ligamentum hyaloideo-capsulare of Wieger.

Up to this point the anterior limiting layer is narrow, well defined, and has a constant thickness. Traced inwards from here it becomes thinner through its fibrils peeling off into the vitreous, and almost (but not quite) disappears at the middle of the patellar fossa.

From its start to its attachment to the lens the anterior limiting layer is in contact with and, in fact, adherent to, the most posterior (the orbiculoposterior capsular) fibres of the zonule. It thus comes about that if the vitreous is removed with forceps the posterior zonular fibres are usually removed with it; on the other hand, if the vitreous is merely allowed to flow away some vitreous remains attached to the zonular fibres (Garnier).

Busacca *et al.* (1957) maintain emphatically that the so-called "hyaloid" membrane exists only anteriorly; from its attachment at the ora serrata it clothes the back of the zonule and of the lens, being adherent to both. They base their views on histological as well as biomicroscopical appearances. Behind this anterior "hyaloid" membrane, and over the posterior convexity of the vitreous, as well as along the hyaloid canal, there is a condensation of vitreous that, while perhaps acting physiologically as a membrane, has no *anatomical* structure, and differs absolutely from the "anterior hyaloid". This surface condensation encloses the definitive vitreous. *Behind* their "hyaloid" membrane the retrolental space consists of the anterior end of the hyaloid canal, expanded into a funnel, containing what they call "hyaloid" vitreous. This is the "primitive" vitreous discussed on p. 452.

The anterior limiting layer is not a hyaloid membrane, for a hyaloid membrane must be transparent, homogeneous, with sharp contours.

But the anterior limiting layer has more the structure of connective tissue and shows a striation due to its constituent fibrillæ parallel with the surface. It is the close relation of the hyaline zonular fibres which is at any rate partly responsible for the error of calling the anterior limiting layer a hyaloid membrane (Figs. 180, 183). But the zonular fibres are not continuous in a section, whereas the anterior limiting layer is.

The anterior and posterior hyaloid "membranes" constitute the *cortex* of the vitreous, formed of a condensation of collagen fibrils, cells, proteins and a mucopolysaccharide interfibrillar substance (Balazs, 1961). They are interrupted by the vitreous *base*, where the fibrils of collagen are attached to the ciliary epithelium.

The main mass of the vitreous appears under the microscope as a reticulum of extremely fine fibrils, in the meshes of which presumably a fluid is present during life. It would seem that in the adult human eye these fibrils, probably for the most part at any rate, only cross each other without forming any actual connections. The fibrillary structure is the same as in the cortex, but the arrangement is less dense.

At more or less regular intervals there occur on the fibrils somewhat spherical thickenings, which stain better than the fibrils themselves.

The swellings have been regarded as granular deposits (artefacts) from the fixative or stain, as optical cross-sections of the fibrils, or as junctional points between the fibrils. As stated above, they are probably actual thickenings of the fibrils.

The Zonular Cleft lies between the origin or base of the vitreous and the commencement of the anterior limiting layer. It is circular in form in close relation to some of the zonular fibres and marks a place where the vitreous nucleus comes to the surface, i.e. is not covered by a limiting layer.

The Vitreous as seen with the Ultra-microscope.—While the above description is what one finds by ordinary histological methods, the ultraviolet microscope studies of Baurmann (1923–26), Comberg (1924), Heesh (1926), Redslob (1927–32), and Duke-Elder (1927), have led them to the following conclusions. Macroscopically the vitreous has the appearance of a colourless transparent jelly. Microscopically absolutely fresh vitreous has no structure at all. With the ultra-microscope perfectly fresh vitreous is optically empty. Soon, however, fibrillæ of colloidal dimensions, such as are seen in soap gels, appear. When the vitreous has been standing for some time the fibrillæ break up into separate particles.

Thus the appearances seen with various fixatives they suggest are artefacts: the vitreous has no structure in the ordinary sense of the word. The appearance seen with the slit-lamp is due to the fact that the fibrillæ become evident when large numbers of them are arranged in a direction perpendicular to the incident light as obtains near the surface of the vitreous. The optical effect of this arrangement is that of a waved or moiré appearance, suggestive of marcelled hair or watered silk. Where the arrangement of the fibrillæ is haphazard the vitreous appears optically empty. A similar appearance is seen when any gel of like constitution is examined by the slit-lamp in a glass vessel which is gently shaken. This appearance, it must be remembered, is an optical illusion, for the fibrillæ are far too small, being somewhat of the size of molecules, to be seen with the slit-lamp.

The vitreous humour consists of 98·5 per cent of water, with traces of albumen, NaCl, etc. It has in fact practically the same composition as the aqueous, except that it contains in addition a small amount of residual protein of the collagen-gelatin type (called vitrein by Friedenwald) and hyaluronic acid which is a viscous polysaccharide (Pirie, 1949).

But while many of the properties of the vitreous are those of a gel, there are a number of facts which suggest that this cannot be the whole explanation of its structure. There is the constancy of the microscopic appearances which is against their being artefacts; there is the firm attachment at the origin or base; then there is the difference between the central and peripheral portions and the changes with age. Also there are certain pathological considerations which speak for a definite structure of the vitreous; important among these is the definite arrangement in rows of the blood corpuscles which distinguishes an intra-vitreous from an extra-vitreous hæmorrhage in the region of the ora serrata.

The vitreous cells or hyalocytes occur in the vitreous cortex, more abundantly in late embryonic and fetal life. By light microscopy they are fusiform or stellate, with dark-staining nuclei. By phase-contrast the living cells have been seen to contain slow-moving granules near their nuclei (Hamburg, 1959). They are PAS-positive, but contain no hyaluronidase. Hyaluronic acid is, however, concentrated in the cortex of the vitreous, and perhaps the cells are involved in mucopolysaccharide production. They differ from histiocytes and glial cells in their staining features. Electron microscopy has added little to our knowledge of these cells. Macrophages have also been described in the vitreous.

THE "LYMPHATIC" DRAINAGE OF THE EYE

There is no clear evidence for the occurrence of recognisable lymph channels or nodes in orbital tissues, including the eyeball. Only in the eyelids are true lymphatics observed (p. 198).

The aqueous humour may be regarded as the lymph of the eye, although its composition is not that of lymph in the body generally: it contains less albumen, and does not clot unless pathologically altered.

There are three main theories with regard to the formation of the aqueous:
    (*a*) That it is a *filtrate* from the ciliary vessels.
    (*b*) That it is *secreted* by the ciliary epithelium (see p. 77).
    (*c*) That it is a dialysate through the endothelium of the capillaries of the ciliary body (Duke-Elder).

These theories do not, in fact, conflict and all these mechanisms appear to be involved (see Davson, 1963).

However formed, the aqueous passes from the ciliary body into the recesses of the posterior chamber and thence anteriorly or posteriorly. Current views are that about 50 microlitres per minute of aqueous are produced. Of this, less than 3 microlitres enter and leave the anterior chamber by flow; the remaining 47 escape by diffusion and filtration (Adler, 1959, quoting Kinsey and others).

Anterior Drainage.—From the recesses the aqueous flows into the posterior chamber, then through the pupil into the anterior chamber. From here it may pass at the angle through the spaces of Fontana into the sinus venosus scleræ, and thence to the aqueous veins and anterior ciliary veins. Another way open to it is via the crypts of Fuchs, where we remember the anterior epithelium and anterior border layer are wanting, directly into the iris. From here the flow is partly into the ciliary veins, partly into the suprachoroidal lymphatic space. From the latter the drainage is via the perivascular lymphatics around the venæ vorticosæ through the sclera to Tenon's space.

Posterior Drainage.—From the posterior chamber again the lymph passes backwards through the slit-like spaces of the suspensory ligament into the canal of Petit, around the equator of the lens. From here it might pass into the post-lental space of Berger, and then down the hyaloid canal to the optic disc, but no lymphatic channels have been substantiated here.

CHAPTER III

THE OCULAR APPENDAGES

THESE comprise the eyelids (palpebræ), the eyebrows (supercilia), the conjunctiva, and the lacrimal apparatus.

THE EYELIDS OR PALPEBRÆ

The eyelids are movable folds which act as shutters protecting the eye from injury or excessive light. They thus aid the pupil in regulating the amount of light which reaches the retina. Only when they are shut can the visual cortex really be at rest.

But essentially the lids perform a dual function concerning tears: (1) by blinking, the upper lid acts like a swab to spread a film of tears over the cornea, and this "blinking reflex" is fired off rhythmically by evaporation and by certain other factors; (2) where excessive tears are present, blinking empties the conjunctival sac by its pumping effect on the lacrimal sac (p. 240).

The upper eyelid extends above to the eyebrow, which separates it from the forehead—the lower passes usually without line of demarcation into the skin of the cheek. Often, however, especially in the old, two sulci, the naso-jugal and malar folds, occur just beyond the orbital margin, and limit it below.

At the sulci the skin is tied to the periosteum (on the medial side, at the naso-jugal fold, the band of fascia passes to the interval between the orbicularis oculi and

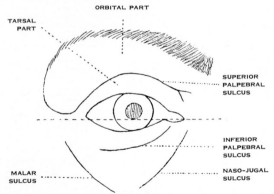

FIG. 187.—THE SURFACE ANATOMY OF THE EYELIDS. (L. W.)

the levator labii superioris). The furrows mark the line of junction between the loose tissues of the lid and the denser tissues of the cheek; and because the skin is tied down tend to limit effusions, and, especially in the old, fat which has escaped from the orbit.

The upper eyelid is much the more mobile of the two, being served by a special elevator muscle (levator palpebræ superioris). When the eyes are open and looking straight ahead, it just covers the upper part of the cornea; when they

181

are closed it covers the whole. The lower lid, on the other hand, is just below the cornea when the eye is open and rises only slightly when it shuts (see also table on p. 183).

When the eye is open an elliptical space, the palpebral fissure, remains between the lid margins, which meet in the medial and lateral "angles" or canthi of the eye.

The lateral canthus is acute. It measures about 60° when the eye is widely open, and about 30–40° normally. The lateral angle is often continuous with a groove which passes laterally and downwards from it, that is a continuation of the line of the margin of the upper eyelid. It is around this groove that the furrows of the "crow's foot" are placed. The lateral canthus is some 5–7 mm from the orbital margin and about 1 cm from the frontozygomatic suture (Fig. 18).

The medial canthus.—The lower boundary is horizontal, while the upper passes downwards and medially—as do, therefore, the corresponding canaliculi. The medial angle is continued medially by the *ridge* produced by the medial palpebral ligament (Fig. 18).

The lateral angle is placed directly against the globe. The medial, more rounded, is separated from it by a little bay—the tear-lake (lacus lacrimalis). In this is a yellowish elevation, the *lacrimal caruncle*, lateral to which is a reddish semilunar fold, the *plica semilunaris*.

The Lacrimal Caruncle is a small area of skin containing large modified sweat glands, and sebaceous glands that open into the follicles of fine hairs (see also p. 219).

The Plica semilunaris represents the third eyelid, membrana nictitans, of the lower animals. It often contains plain muscle tissue supplied by the sympathetic (see also p. 220).

At a point in the lids corresponding to the plica semilunaris is a small elevation known as the *lacrimal papilla*, the centre of which is pierced by a hole, the *punctum lacrimale*, which, as we shall see, serves to carry the tears into the lacrimal channels.

The puncta divide the lid margins into *ciliary* and *lacrimal portions*.

Most normal eyes are practically the same size. When we speak therefore of eyes appearing small or large, we usually refer, not to their actual size, but to the amount visible, which depends on the size of the palpebral fissure.

With the eyes open the lateral angle is about 2 mm above the medial, and thus the axis of the fissure is not horizontal, but slopes from medially upwards and laterally.

An increase in this obliquity is characteristic of the Mongolian races. Moreover, these races have a fold passing from the medial end of the upper lid to the lower, hiding the caruncle—a condition known as *epicanthus*.

Epicanthus occurs normally in the human fetus, but usually disappears with the development of the bridge of the nose. It is also seen in congenital ptosis

(Pockley, 1919). Indeed, it has been regarded as dependent upon the flatness of the nasal bones; but Duckworth (1904) points out that in the Negroid races, whose nasal bones are even flatter than those of the Mongols, it is usually absent.

When the eyes are open, too, the palpebral fissure, which measures about 30 mm by 15 mm (see table below), is seen to be asymmetrical. Its greatest width above the line joining the two angles is on the medial side, while below it is on the lateral side.

When the eyes are shut the lateral angle drops till it lies lower than the medial and the fissure becomes sinuous, concave upwards in its central portion. The roots of the lashes give the shape of the fissure except in the lacrimal portion where it is horizontal. In its lateral part the fissure slopes downwards.

The portions of the eye that are normally visible in the palpebral opening are the cornea, the iris and pupil, a triangle of sclera to the lateral side and a crescent of it to the medial, the caruncle and the plica.

The most exposed portion of the globe is a zone just below the centre of the cornea; for this remains relatively uncovered even when the lids are almost shut. *Hence it is the common site of those congestive or degenerative changes which result from exposure.* At the approach of danger the eyes tend to turn up. Here the exposed portion will be below, and it is thus this region which will be most *affected by injuries due to burns and caustics, and is also the site of ulceration seen sometimes in the coma vigil of typhoid and other severe illnesses.*

The following table shows some of the characteristics of the palpebral opening and its relation with certain parts of the globe.

	Length	*Height*	*Pupil*	*Cornea*	*Lacus and Plica lacrimales*	*Position of Transverse Axis*
Newborn	18·5– 19 mm	10 mm	Touches free border of lower eyelid	Upper border at level of free margin of upper eyelid	Not visible	Middle of pupil
Infant	24– 25 mm	13 mm	Equidistant from free borders of eyelids	Upper and lower borders covered to same extent	Slightly visible	Below middle of pupil
Adult	28– 30 mm	14– 15 mm	Near free border of upper eyelid	Lower border at level of free margin of lower eyelid	Visible	Lower border of pupil
Old age	28 mm	11– 12 mm	Touches free margin of upper eyelid	Lower border a little distance from free margin of lower eyelid	Very visible	Near lower border of cornea

Here we see that the portion of the globe visible between the eyelids is lower as age increases.

The palpebral margin of the lid is about 2 mm broad, with anterior and posterior borders.

From the anterior rounded border project the eyelashes (cilia), stiff hairs arranged in two or three rows. The upper lashes are longer and more numerous and curl upwards, while the lower ones turn downwards, so that they do not interlace when the eyes are shut. The lashes are as a rule darker than the hair, and

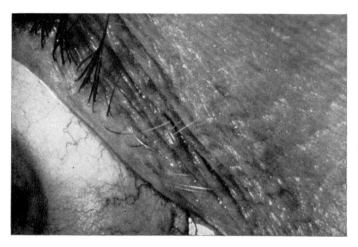

FIG. 188.—SKIN OF NASAL PORTION OF THE RIGHT UPPER EYELID.
Note almost devoid of hairs (apart from lashes).

do not become grey with age, although they may do so after some diseases (e.g. alopecia areata). It takes about ten weeks for the replacement of a lash to grow to its full size. The lashes are longest and most curled in childhood.

The Follicles of the Lashes.—Although generally like those of hairs elsewhere, the lashes have no arrector muscles. They pass into the lid obliquely in front of the palpebral muscle (of Riolan) to reach the tarsus. The lashes are very sensitive, being richly supplied with nerves. Young lashes are knob-shaped, and a persistence of this condition is seen in many chronic inflammatory conditions. Each lash remains about five months.

The Posterior Border of the lid margin is sharp and placed against the globe. Just in front of it can be seen the small orifices of the tarsal glands. Between these and the eyelashes is a thin grey line, where the lid can be quite easily split into an anterior and a posterior portion.

The free margins of the lids have the above characteristics in the *ciliary* portion, i.e. up to the puncta. To the medial side of these, i.e. in *the lacrimal portion,* there are as a rule no cilia or tarsal glands. Rarely after the age of ten years lashes are found on the lacrimal portion of the lid margins. This portion is rounded, hence has no borders. In its thickness is the lacrimal canaliculus.

The Structure of the Lids.—The tissues of the palpebræ are, from anterior (cutaneous) to posterior (conjunctival) aspects as follows:

1. The skin.
2. A layer of subcutaneous areolar tissue.
3. A layer of striated muscle (orbicularis oculi).
4. The submuscular areolar tissue.
5. The fibrous layer—including the tarsal plates.
6. A layer of nonstriated muscle.
7. The mucous membrane or conjunctiva.

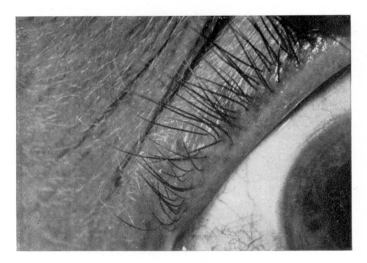

FIG. 189.—SKIN OF LATERAL PORTION OF UPPER EYELID.
Note numerous hairs (in addition to lashes).

1. *The Skin* of the eyelids is about the thinnest in the body. It is less than 1 mm in thickness and almost transparent. Hence it forms folds, and is easily wrinkled. A well-marked fold is often seen on the lateral side of the upper lid in old people. It may overhang the lid margin. The skin also is very elastic so that it recovers rapidly after being distended by fluids, etc. When the eye is open the upper lid is marked at the upper border of the tarsal plate by a sulcus, the mouth of which gets nearer the lid margin the wider the eye is opened. This furrow is produced by the pull of the tendon of levator palpebræ superioris (p. 260). The skin of the upper lid is thus furrowed when the eye is open—the skin of the upper lid is wholly in view only when the eye is closed. The corresponding furrow in the lower lid is ill-marked and often broken up.

A.E.—13

Also, as has been mentioned before, furrows exist at times—especially in the old—just beyond the lower orbital margin; these are emphasised when the lower lids are puffed out with fat escaped from the orbit (see also p. 271). They are due to attachment of the skin to the orbital margin. It is also attached at the medial and lateral canthi to the medial and lateral palpebral ligaments, especially the former.

It should be carefully noted that the nasal portion of the eyelid (Fig. 188) differs quite markedly from that of the temporal side (Fig. 189). It is smoother, shinier, and greasier. Also it has practically no hairs and those that are present are very feeble and have only rudimentary sebaceous glands attached to them. On the other hand, the skin here is well provided with those unicellular sebaceous glands which occur normally in the basal layer of the human epidermis (Wolff, 1951) (Fig. 190).

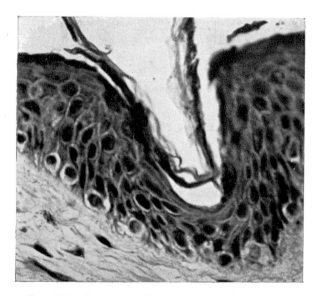

FIG. 190.—SECTION OF SKIN FROM THE NASAL SIDE OF THE EYELID TO SHOW NUMEROUS UNICELLULAR SEBACEOUS GLANDS IN THE BASAL LAYER OF THE EPIDERMIS.

Structure. — The epithelium forms a relatively thin layer. The stratum corneum is well developed. The stratum granulosum is present; the stratum mucosum consists of three or four layers of cells. Then comes the stratum germinativum resting on a basement membrane.

At the lid margin the epithelium becomes modified as we trace it from the anterior to the posterior border. It thickens and contains some 7–10 layers of cells. The dermis is denser and richer in elastic fibres; it becomes folded to form papillæ which become higher and narrower, and the basement membrane is correspondingly wavy.

The mucocutaneous junction lies at the level of the posterior margin of the openings of the tarsal glands, i.e. at the junction of "dry" and "moist" portions where the marginal strips of tear fluid end in a sharp line (see p. 233).

The hairs on the lids, although comparatively large in the fetus, are more like down in the adult, and have small sebaceous glands connected with them.

The sweat glands, although numerous, are of small size.

There are always, in the skin of the eyelids, in the connective tissue tracts

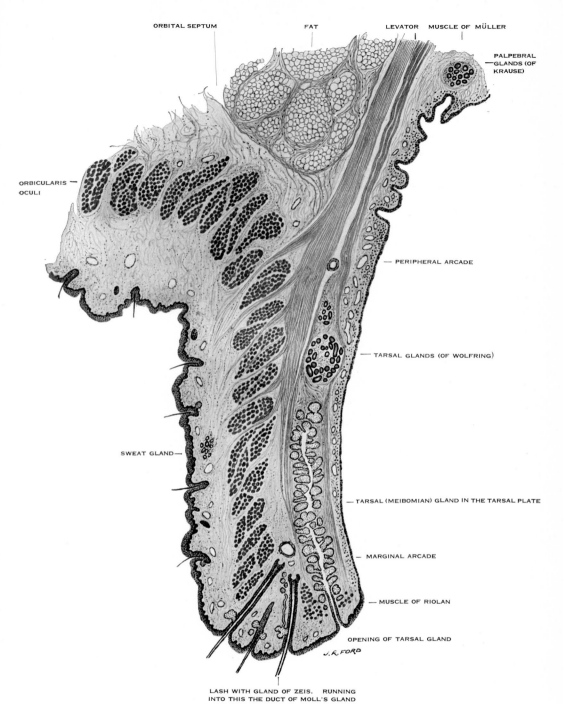

ORBITAL SEPTUM   FAT   LEVATOR   MUSCLE OF MÜLLER

PALPEBRAL GLANDS (OF KRAUSE)

ORBICULARIS OCULI

PERIPHERAL ARCADE

TARSAL GLANDS (OF WOLFRING)

SWEAT GLAND

TARSAL (MEIBOMIAN) GLAND IN THE TARSAL PLATE

MARGINAL ARCADE

MUSCLE OF RIOLAN

OPENING OF TARSAL GLAND

J. R. FORD

LASH WITH GLAND OF ZEIS. RUNNING INTO THIS THE DUCT OF MOLL'S GLAND

FIG. 191.—VERTICAL SECTION THROUGH THE UPPER LID.

(*Wolff's preparations.*)

187

which accompany the vessels, and in the hair follicles, large pigment cells with processes. These cells are found in the skin in most of the body in variable numbers, while here they are more abundant. They are more numerous in brunettes than blondes. The pigment is golden yellow or brown. These melanocytes may wander and so determine the changes more or less marked in the coloration of the eyelids seen in the same individual in different states of health.

2. *The Subcutaneous Areolar Layer* consists of loose connective tissue containing no fat; so the skin can easily be lifted off the underlying muscle and also be distended with œdema or blood. It is absent near the ciliary margin, at the palpebral furrows, and at the medial and lateral angles where the skin is adherent to the palpebral ligaments.

3. *The Layer of Striated Muscle.*—This is the *palpebral part* of the orbicularis palpebrarum, supplied by the facial nerve. The muscle fibres are arranged concentrically around the palpebral opening. The fibres are placed obliquely in relation to each other and overlap as do tiles on a roof. The part of this muscle which lies next and occupies nearly the whole thickness of the lid margin is called the *ciliary part* (muscle of Riolan) (Fig. 191). It is traversed successively by the follicles of the lashes, the glands of Moll, and the excretory ducts of the tarsal glands (Fig. 194) (see also p. 202).

4. *The Submuscular Areolar Tissue* resembles the subcutaneous layer. It lies between the orbicularis and the tarsal plate, and communicates above with the sub-aponeurotic stratum of the scalp, the so-called "dangerous area" of the surgeons. Hence pus or blood can make its way into the upper lid from the dangerous area (see also p. 206). It is through this plane, which is reached by entering the knife at the grey line, that the lid may, with the greatest ease, be split into anterior and posterior portions. This space is traversed by the fibres of the levator, some of which pass on to the skin through the orbicularis, while others gain attachment to the lower third of the tarsus. The main nerves to the eyelids also lie in this areolar tissue; *hence, when injecting a local anæsthetic to anæsthetize the lids, it is necessary to inject deep to the orbicularis.*

In the lower lid this tissue lies in a single small space (the preseptal space) in front of the septum orbitale. In the upper lid the space in which the tissue lies is divided by the levator into the pretarsal and preseptal spaces.

The pretarsal space is small. It contains the peripheral arterial arcade (Figs. 191, 253). It is bounded anteriorly by the levator tendon and the orbicularis; posteriorly by the tarsal plate and the muscle of Müller. Its upper end corresponds to the place where the muscle of Müller arises from the levator. Its lower limit is formed by the attachment of the fibres of the levator to the front of the tarsal plate. On vertical section the space is fusiform.

The preseptal space is triangular on vertical section. It is bounded in front by the orbicularis, behind by the septum and those tendinous fibres of the levator which pierce the orbicularis. Above is the preseptal cushion of fat.

The preseptal cushion of fat is a well-defined agglomeration of fat different from the subcutaneous fat. It is for the most part in front of the septum and behind the orbicularis. Crescent-shaped, it lies along the orbital margin which it may overlap at times. Its lower, thicker border is parallel to the upper palpebral furrow. The fat is adherent to the orbicularis and the epicranial aponeurosis and this, according to Charpy, separates the preseptal space from the dangerous area of the scalp.

The pre-muscular and retro-muscular spaces communicate between the fibres of the orbicularis, but are separated by the septum and tarsal plates from the orbit. Also infiltrations of the eyelids do not extend on to the cheek and forehead.

5. *The Fibrous Layer*. The fibrous layer may be regarded as the framework of the lids. It consists of a thickened central portion, the tarsal plates, and a thinner peripheral part known as the palpebral fascia or septum orbitale. Although the term septum orbitale is usually applied to the palpebral fascia only, it is the whole fibrous layer which, when the eyes are shut, forms a septum to the orbital opening, incomplete only at the palpebral fissure.

The Tarsal Plates—one for each of the lids—form the skeleton of the lids, giving them their shape and firmness. They are often called the tarsal cartilages, but consist of dense fibrous and some elastic tissue, found mainly around the acini, in which are embedded the tarsal glands. They contain no cartilage. The lateral ends are 7 mm from Whitnall's tubercle. The medial ends terminate at the lacrimal puncta, some 9 mm from the anterior lacrimal crest.

The tarsus is well delimited from the surrounding tissues, but laterally at the palpebral margin its connective tissue is closely united with that of the follicles of the lashes to form a characteristic thickening at the margin of the lid (ciliary mass of Whitnall).

The superior tarsus, which is shaped like a transverse crescent, is much larger than the lower, being 11 mm in height at its middle. The corresponding measurement in the lower tarsus, which is somewhat oblong in form, is 5 mm.

Each tarsus, some 29 mm long and 1 mm thick, may be described as having an anterior and posterior surface, a free and attached border, and a medial and lateral extremity.

The anterior surface of the tarsus is convex, and is separated from the orbicularis by loose areolar tissue, so that the muscle moves freely on the tarsus.

The posterior surface, which is concave, clothed by and adherent to the conjunctiva, moulds itself on the globe of the eye.

The free border, forming the margin of the lid, is thick, almost horizontal, and co-extensive with the ciliary portion of the lid margin; *the attached border* is thin, and gradually runs into the septum orbitale, with which it is held by some to be continuous, except where it is pierced by the levator in the upper lid and the prolongation of the inferior rectus in the lower (see below). The superior border of the upper tarsus gives attachment to the nonstriated superior palpebral muscle (Figs. 191, 192, 253), while similarly to the inferior border of the lower tarsus the inferior palpebral muscle is attached.

The extremities of the tarsal plates are attached to the orbital margin by strong fibrous structures known as the medial and lateral palpebral ligaments.

The Medial Palpebral Ligament is a somewhat triangular band which is attached to the frontal process of the maxilla from the anterior lacrimal crest to near its suture with the nasal bone (Figs. 18, 224, 275, 276).

The ligament has a lower free border (under which some of the fibres of the orbicularis insinuate themselves), while above it is adherent to and continuous with the periosteum.

At the base of the triangle, that is, at the anterior lacrimal crest, the ligament divides into anterior and posterior portions. The posterior portion is continuous with the lacrimal fascia, and thus helps to roof over the upper part of the lacrimal sac.

The anterior portion is continued at the medial canthus into two bands, which pass across the lacrimal fossa (but not in contact with the sac), to attach it to the medial extremities of the tarsal plates. These bands make an angle open laterally with the lacrimal fascia. They form with the main ligament a letter Y placed on its side. The two branches, which correspond to the lacrimal portions of the lid margins, and in fact are tubular, contain the lacrimal canaliculi, enclose the caruncle, and delimit the medial canthus.

The anterior surface of the ligament is free and adherent to the skin. It looks forwards and laterally; the two branches look forwards and medially and thus make with it an obtuse angle open forwards.

A deep or reflected portion of the medial palpebral ligament is usually described. This is said to arise from the main ligament as it crosses the sac and is attached behind the sac. Some authorities, however, have regarded this reflected part of the ligament as merely a thin fascial expansion. (Whitnall, 1932.)

When the lateral canthus is pulled laterally and upwards the medial palpebral ligament forms a well-marked prominence. It should be carefully noted that this prominence lies almost entirely on the frontal process of the maxilla.

A finger placed in the lacrimal fossa lies under the medial angle of the eye.

According to some the medial canthus corresponds more or less to the anterior lacrimal crest. Also, if a vertical incision is made 2 mm medial to the medial canthus, *the whole of the dissection to expose the sac is made under the lateral lip of the wound.*

It follows from this, and from what has been said above, that the lower prominent portion of the medial palpebral ligament does not lie in front of the lacrimal sac, at any rate not for more than a millimetre or two, and a probe pressed backwards below its prominence hits the bone and not the sac.

The Lateral Palpebral Ligament is attached to the orbital tubercle on the zygomatic bone 11 mm below the frontozygomatic suture. It is some 7 mm long and 2·5 mm broad. It consists of fibrous tissue which is not very dense. Indeed, it is rather a descriptive verbiage than an anatomical reality; it does not exist in the sense of the strong and well-developed medial palpebral ligament. It is no more than the areolar tissue of the septum orbitale behind the lateral palpebral raphé.

It lies deeper, and does not form a prominence as does the medial palpebral ligament. Its anterior surface is fused with the preciliary fibres of the orbicularis. Superficial also to this ligament are a few lobules of the lacrimal gland and the lateral palpebral raphé formed by the orbicularis and strengthened by the septum orbitale.

The posterior surface is in front of the lateral check ligament, separated from it, however, by a lobule of the lacrimal gland (Fig. 254). Its upper border is united with the expansion of the levator (Fig. 277); its lower border with an expansion from the inferior oblique and the inferior rectus.

THE PALPEBRAL FASCIA OR SEPTUM ORBITALE (Figs. 192, 193, 275)

The palpebral fascia or septum orbitale is attached to the orbital margin at a thickening called the arcus marginale, which is formed where the periorbita is continuous with the periosteum; centrally it is generally held to be continuous with the tarsal plates, except where it is pierced by the fibres of the levator in the upper lid and the expansion from the inferior rectus in the lower. But the continuity of the septum, with the tarsus between the fibres of the levator, can only be made out with difficulty by dissection under water and is denied by many observers.

A portion of the septum is also carried forwards with the fibres of the levator, and a portion reflected back along its upper surface. (Fig. 191).

The palpebral fascia must not be regarded as a fixed and rigid structure. It is a floating membrane, which takes part in all the movements of the lids, and has been regarded (though this is doubtful) as the deep fascia of the palpebral portion of the orbicularis. It consists of two layers, the fibres of which, running in arcades, cross each other more or less at right angles.

The septum is thicker and stronger on the lateral side than on the medial and in the upper lid than in the lower. In the upper lid, in fact, two tendon-like thickenings can be seen starting from the lateral side and gradually becoming lost as we trace them medially.

It is the weak portions of the septum orbitale which determine the site of herniæ of the orbital fat which lies just deep to it. These herniæ are seen frequently, especially in old people.

The attachment of the septum while more or less following the orbital margin does not do so exactly. It does, however, mark the junction of periorbita and periosteum (Fig. 193).

Starting on the lateral side we find the septum attached to the orbital margin in front of the lateral palpebral ligament which goes to Whitnall's tubercle, being separated from it by loose connective tissue containing a lobule of fat. From here the line of attachment runs upwards, crosses the frontozygomatic suture, and then follows the posterior lip of the upper orbital margin to the supraorbital notch

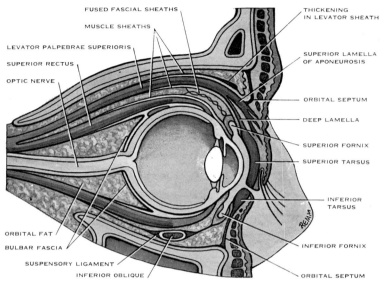

FIG. 192.—VERTICAL ANTEROPOSTERIOR SECTION OF THE ORBIT.

which it bridges over, converting it into a foramen. Again following the supraorbital margin, the attachment of the septum passes in front of the pulley of the superior oblique and then, leaving the bone, bridges over the upper and medial angle of the orbital opening with its vessels and nerves, to become again attached to the bone behind the upper part of the posterior lacrimal crest. It now runs down on the lacrimal bone behind Horner's muscle and thus behind the lacrimal sac and the medial palpebral ligament and in front of the medial check ligament (Fig. 224). The line of attachment crosses the lacrimal sac (or rather the fascia covering it) about its middle, to reach the anterior lacrimal crest at about the level of the lacrimal tubercle. From here it follows the lower orbital margin to the point where the zygomatic portion starts ascending. Here the attachment leaves the margin and lies actually a few millimetres from it on the facial aspect of the zygomatic bone; so that here the septum forms an osteofibrous pocket, the premarginal recess of Eisler, which contains fat. The line of attachment again reaches the lateral orbital margin just below the level of Whitnall's tubercle.

It will be noted that on the lateral side the septum is superficial, lying anterior to the lateral palpebral ligament, while on the medial side it is deep, lying behind the lacrimal part of the orbicularis oculi (Horner's muscle).

Where the lacrimal muscle of Horner diverges to reach the upper and lower eyelids the portions of the septum belonging to the upper and lower eyelids meet behind the caruncle and plica. The inferior medial palpebral artery runs here in a plane between the caruncle and the muscle.

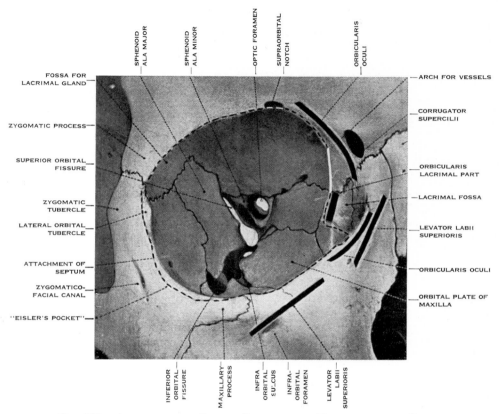

FIG. 193.—ATTACHMENT OF SEPTUM ORBITALE AND MUSCLES AROUND ORBIT.

Relations.—In the upper eyelid the septum is mainly in contact with orbital fat (continuous with the upper and lateral mass of perimuscular fat). This separates the septum from the lacrimal gland, the levator and the tendon of the superior oblique. On the medial side the septum is in contact with that portion of the orbital fat which tends to pass out of the orbit between the pulley of the superior oblique and the medial palpebral ligament, pushing the palpebral fascia in front of it (Fig. 257).

In the lower eyelid the septum lies in contact with those portions of the orbital fat which tend to escape through three orifices and also with the expansion of the inferior rectus and inferior oblique (Figs. 192, 253).

In the lower lid there is only one space, bounded behind by the septum orbitale and the tarsal plate, and in front by the orbicularis.

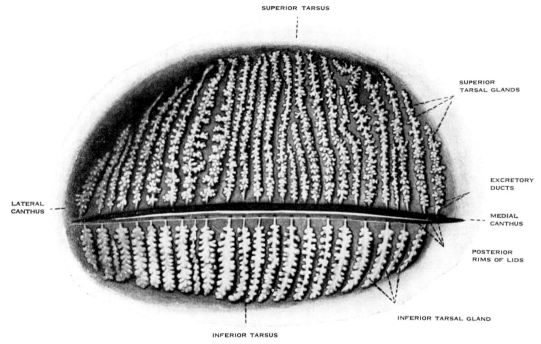

FIG. 194.—THE POSTERIOR SURFACE OF THE TWO EYELIDS WHICH HAVE BEEN MADE TRANSPARENT BY SODA-GLYCERINE TO SHOW THE TARSAL GLANDS (OF MEIBOMIUS).
(*From Sobotta.*)

The Septum Orbitale is pierced by the following structures:

(*a*) The lacrimal vessels and nerves.

(*b*) The supraorbital vessels and nerves.

(*c*) The supratrochlear nerve and artery.

(*d*) The infratrochlear nerve.

(*e*) The anastomosis between the angular and ophthalmic veins.

(*f*) The superior and inferior palpebral arteries above and below the medial palpebral ligament.

(*g*) The levator palpebræ superioris in the upper lid and in the lower by a prolongation of the inferior rectus. It must be pointed out that many hold that the lower border of the septum and the upper border of the tarsus are not continuous between the fibres of the levator. The muscle would then pass between these two structures.

6. *The Layer of Nonstriated Muscle Fibres*, the palpebral muscle (of Müller), lies just deep to the septum orbitale in both upper and lower lids, and, running for

the most part vertically, takes origin among the fibres of the levator in the upper lid and the prolongation of the inferior rectus in the lower. It is attached to the orbital margins of the tarsal plates (Figs. 191, 192, 253).

The inferior palpebral muscle is sometimes visible through the conjunctiva. The muscle is supplied by sympathetic nerve fibres, and when in action widens the palpebral fissure. Fibres of nonstriated muscle are also found across the inferior orbital fissure and usually in the capsule of Tenon. The whole system represents the retractor bulbi of some mammalia (see pp. 22, 270).

7. *The Conjunctiva* which lines the lids is called the palpebral conjunctiva. It is firmly adherent to the tarsus (see also p. 206).

THE GLANDS OF THE LIDS

Apart from the glands of the skin, which have already been considered, and those of the conjunctiva, there are a variety of tarsal glands, commonly named eponymously after Meibomius, Moll, and Zeis.

TARSAL PLATE

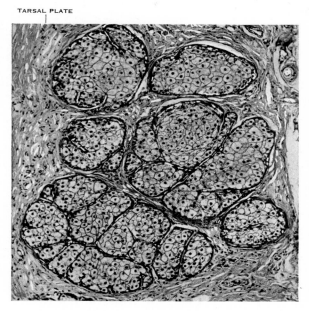

FIG. 195.—LOBULES OF A TARSAL (MEIBOMIAN) GLAND.

(Wolff's preparation.)

1. **The Tarsal Glands** (Meibomian Glands) are long sebaceous glands which are unusual in not being connected with hairs; this, however, is due to the fact that they take the place of a row of lashes (see p. 494). They are situated actually *in* the tarsal plates and run from their attached to their free margins (Fig. 191). The upper ones are therefore the longer. They are arranged vertically parallel with each other, about twenty-five in the upper lid and twenty in the lower. Each consists of a central canal, into the sides of which open numerous rounded appendages which secrete sebum. The small orifices of the canals, whose number corresponds to that of the glands, can be seen on the margin of the lid just in front of its posterior border (Figs. 191 and 194).

It is here that the sebaceous material is poured *to prevent the overflow of tears, to ensure an airtight closure of the lids, to prevent the tears from macerating the skin and after blinking to leave an oily film* (p. 242) *over the moistened cornea to retard evaporation of the underlying tears.* Each duct is lined by four layers of cells situated on a basement membrane. The mouth of the duct is lined by six layers of cells, of which the deepest are cylindrical. Keratinisation increases towards the lid margin. The acini are usually globular, 10–15 in number and placed irregularly round the central canal till near its orifice and so resemble a chain of onions. The

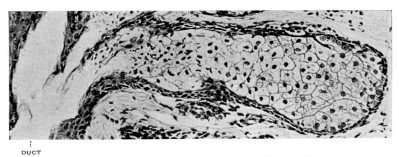

DUCT

FIG. 196.—SECTION OF A SACCULE OF A TARSAL GLAND.

Note that nuclei in gland become darker and then break up towards the duct.

Meibomian glands can be seen easily, showing through the conjunctiva as yellow streaks.

2. **The Tarsal or Ciliary Glands (of Moll)** consist of unbranched spiral or sinuous tubules which begin in a simple spiral and not in a glomerulus as do ordinary sweat glands. They may be considered as sweat glands which have become arrested in their development. They are some 1·5 to 2 mm long and placed obliquely in contact with and parallel to the bulbs of the cilia. They are more numerous in the lower lid, but even here there is not one to every lash.

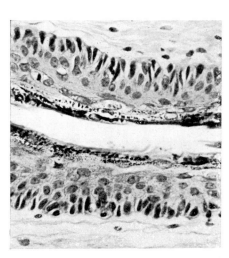

FIG. 197.—LONGITUDINAL SECTION OF A TARSAL DUCT.

Each has a fundus, a body, an ampullary portion and a neck. The cavity is singularly large (Figs. 198, 199, 222) but gets narrower at the neck. The duct passes through the dermis and epidermis and may terminate separately between two lashes or between the lash and its epithelial covering or into the duct of a sebaceous gland of Zeis (Fig. 191).

Structure.—The structure of a ciliary gland of Moll is like that of an ordinary sweat gland. The secretory portion is lined by a layer of cylindrical cells which contain secretory granules and fatty granulations; and between these cells and the basement membrane is placed an ill-defined layer of longitudinal or obliquely placed cells and fibres which are muscular (myo-epithelial) in character.

The duct is lined by one or two layers of cells, the most superficial of which are cylindrical. There are no muscle fibres.

3. **The Sebaceous Glands of Zeis** are modified sebaceous glands which are attached directly to the follicles of the eyelashes (Figs. 191, 198, 201). Each is reduced to a simple cul-de-sac or to two or three lobules only (in general there are

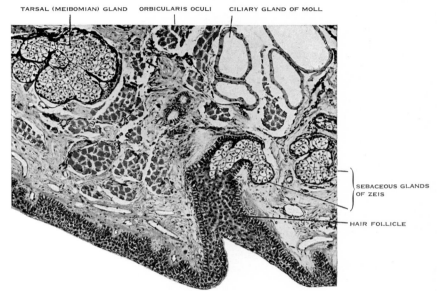

FIG. 198.—SECTION OF THE LID MARGIN TO SHOW THE THREE TYPES OF GLANDS.
(*Wolff's preparation.*)

10 to 20 or more). Usually there are two to each cilium. Each gland consists of epithelium placed on a basement membrane. Next to this membrane is a layer of small cubical cells which are actively dividing. The cells resulting from this division enlarge, become polygonal and filled with sebaceous granules. The nuclei, which at first enlarge, become rounded, paler, and usually contain one well marked nucleolus, diminish in size, stain more densely, become star-shaped, and disappear. The degenerative cells lose their cell walls and are pushed towards the centre of the gland and then towards the secretory duct. The sebum passes out between the lash and its epithelial covering. The purpose of this oily secretion, as elsewhere in the body, is to prevent the hair (eyelash in this case) from becoming dry and brittle.

THE BLOOD-VESSELS OF THE LIDS

Arteries.—The blood supply to the lids is derived mainly from the *ophthalmic* and *lacrimal* arteries by their *medial* and *lateral palpebral* branches.

The medial palpebral arteries—superior for the upper lid, inferior for the lower—pierce the septum orbitale above and below the medial palpebral ligament (Fig. 213).

Each anastomoses with the corresponding lateral palpebral artery from the lacrimal to form the *tarsal arches*, whose plane in the lids is in the submuscular areolar tissue (i.e. between the orbicularis and the tarsal plate), close to the lid margin (Figs. 191 and 214).

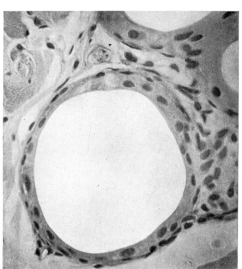

FIG. 199.—SECTION OF CILIARY GLAND (OF MOLL).

The Tarsal Arches (*Arcades*) receive anastomosing twigs from the superficial temporal, transverse facial, and infraorbital arteries.

In the upper lid a *second arterial arch* is formed from the superior branch of the medial palpebral. It is called the arcus tarseus superior and is situated in front of the upper margin of the tarsal plate (Figs. 191 and 214).

From the arches, branches pass forward to supply the orbicularis and skin, backward to the conjunctiva and tarsal glands.

The Veins of the lids are larger and more numerous than the arteries. They are arranged in pretarsal and post-tarsal sets, and form a dense plexus (which can be seen in the living) in the region of the upper and lower fornices of the conjunctiva.

Some of them empty into the veins of the forehead and temple, others pass through the orbicularis to reach radicles of the ophthalmic vein.

Lymphatics.—Like the veins, the lymphatics are arranged in *pre- and post-tarsal plexuses*, connected, however, by cross-channels. According to Fuchs the former have many valves, the latter none.

The *post-tarsal* drain the conjunctiva and tarsal glands; the *pretarsal* the skin and skin structures.

Both groups drain as follows: those for the lateral side run into the preauricular and parotid nodes; those from the medial side into the submandibular lymph glands.

Nerves.—*Motor.*—The orbicularis is supplied by the facial, the levator by the upper division of the oculomotor, and nonstriated muscle by sympathetic nerves.

Sensory.—The upper lid is supplied mainly by the supraorbital. On the medial side the supra- and infratrochlear, and on the lateral side the lacrimal branches

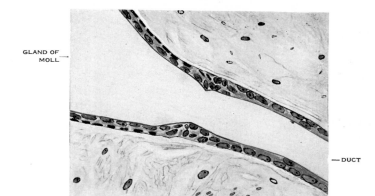

FIG. 200. — JUNCTION OF CILIARY GLAND (OF MOLL) AND DUCT.

Note funnel-shaped termination of gland.

—DUCT

of the ophthalmic division of the trigeminal assist. The lower lid has its supply from the infraorbital, with minimal overlap near the angles by lacrimal and infratrochlear nerves.

The plane of the main branches of the nerves is between the orbicularis and the tarsal plate. From here branches pass forwards to the skin, backwards to the conjunctiva and tarsal glands.

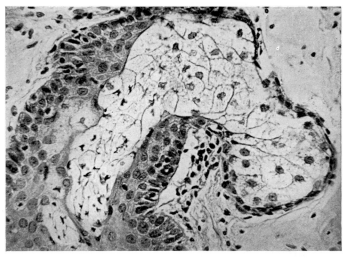

FIG. 201. — SECTION OF CILIARY GLAND (OF ZEIS).

Note how nuclei in gland become dark and then break up as we trace them to hair follicle.

HAIR FOLLICLE

THE PALPEBRAL AND NEIGHBOURING MUSCLES

The Orbicularis Oculi is the sphincter of the eyelids. It forms an elliptical sheet, which surrounds the palpebral fissure, covers the lids, and spreads out for some distance on to the forehead, temple, and cheek.

It consists of two main parts:

(a) Palpebral.
(b) Orbital.

The Palpebral Portion is the central part of the muscle. It is confined to the lids, consists of pale muscle fibres, and may itself be divided into pretarsal and preseptal strata. The junction of the two, the thinnest portion of the muscle, lies at the upper- and lower-lid furrows.

It diverges from the medial palpebral ligament and the neighbouring bone, and passes across the lids in a series of half ellipses, which meet outside the lateral canthus in the lateral palpebral raphé. This consists of inter-digitating muscle fibres strengthened by the septum orbitale (Whitnall).

The Orbital Portion has a curved origin from the medial side of the orbit: from the medial region of the upper orbital margin medial to the supraorbital notch; from the maxillary process of the frontal bone; from the frontal process of the maxilla; from the medial palpebral ligament, and from the lower orbital margin medial to the infraorbital foramen. The origin is by muscular or short tendinous fibres, and is not continuous. From this origin the peripheral fibres sweep across the orbital margin in a series of concentric loops, while the more central ones form nearly complete rings.

Relations.—*The Palpebral Portion* of the orbicularis has a layer of areolar tissue containing *no fat* both in front and behind. The anterior, subcutaneous layer, separates it from the skin. The posterior, submuscular areolar layer, which separates it from the tarsal plates and palpebral fascia, contains the main vessels and nerves of the lids and fibres of the levator. This portion of the muscle is only adherent to the dermis at the medial and lateral canthi.

The fibres of the levator pass through the palpebral portion to reach the skin (Fig. 191).

The Orbital Portion spreads upwards on to the forehead, where it takes part in the formation of the eyebrow and covers the corrugator supercilii laterally on to the temple, where it covers the anterior part of the temporal fascia, and downwards on to the cheek, where it lies on the zygomatic bone and the origin of the elevator muscles of the upper lip and ala of the nose.

Anteriorly it is separated from the skin, *not* by areolar tissue, but by a layer of *fat*, to which it is adherent, and so acts on the skin, which actually receives only the following fibres, mostly from the periphery of the muscle:

(a) *The Musculus Superciliaris* (Merkel), a depress of the medial end of the eyebrow (Arlt), comprises some of the upper medial peripheral fibres which pass to the skin of the medial portion of the eyebrow.

(b) *The Musculus Malaris* (Henle) consists of some of the medial and lateral lower peripheral fibres which are attached to the skin of the cheek. Also Merkel has described some fibres which are attached to the skin round the medial canthus, which produce a series of fine lines on the medial part of the lids, especially in those who have small eyes and are subject to frequent blinking (Poirier).

A third part of the orbicularis oculi is usually described as a recognisable entity. It is the **pars lacrimalis**, also variously called the *tensor tarsi* or Horner's muscle. (Early descriptions were recorded by Duverney, 1749, and Gerlach, 1880.)

It consists of a thin layer of fibres which arises behind the lacrimal sac from the upper part of the posterior lacrimal crest (Figs. 223, 224), and from the lacrimal fascia. The muscle passes laterally and forwards, and divides into two

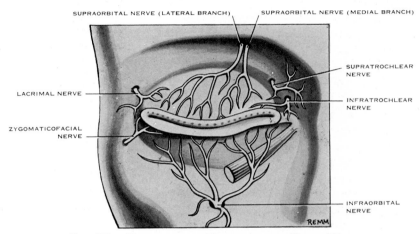

FIG. 202.—NERVES OF THE EYELIDS OF THE RIGHT EYE.

slips, which surround the canaliculi and become continuous with the pretarsal fibres and the ciliary part (of Riolan) of the orbicularis oculi in both lids.

The *pars ciliaris* (muscle of Riolan) of the orbicularis consists of very fine striated muscle fibres which lie in the dense tissue of the lids near their margin. The ciliary glands (of Moll) separate them from the palpebral portion of the orbicularis (Fig. 191).

A part of the muscle lies superficial to the tarsal (Meibomian) glands and a part (the subtarsal portion) deep to them (Figs. 191, 207).

Medially the pars ciliaris is continuous with the pars lacrimalis (Fig. 223).

Actions.—The orbicularis is the sphincter muscle of the eyelids. Its two parts have each a dilator muscle in opposition.

The Palpebral Part is used in closing the eye without effort. Usually it is an involuntary movement, as in blinking, which goes on continuously almost without our being aware of it. People also blink their eyes when they want to see more clearly, often when they are thinking rapidly, to get, as it were, a sharper mental picture of the situation. The eyes are closed reflexly when there is any danger to them, and curiously enough on hearing a loud noise.

A.E.—14

The Orbital Part is used to close the eyes tightly. When this region of the muscle is in action the skin of the forehead, temple and cheek is drawn towards the medial side of the orbit, the eyelids being firmly closed. Radiating furrows are formed, especially on the lateral side and below the eye. In the young they are only seen when the muscle is acting; later they become permanent, and have received the name of "crow's feet". The muscle comes into play in sudden, short-lived conditions, bringing an increased supply of blood to the head and eye, and giving rise to a strong expiratory effort. Thus it is seen in action in crying children, in coughing, in blowing the nose, sneezing, and *excessive* laughing. Charles Bell thought that the eye was shut tightly to lessen the vascular dilatation which accompanies these efforts, and thus act as a protective bandage. *This action of the orbicularis can be greatly curtailed by drawing the lateral canthus laterally or dividing it.*

One part of the orbicularis may be paralysed without the other. The orbicularis also holds the lower lid in contact with the globe, since in paralysis of the muscle it falls away and epiphora results.

The normal, rhythmical, blinking reflex (palpebral portion of orbicularis) is fired off by dryness of the cornea, and the lids, especially the upper, spread a film of tears over the surface to moisten it. Blinking, moreover, has a further use —to pump away excessive tears (see p. 237). Contraction of the orbital portion of orbicularis depresses the eyebrow—a common defence, this, against excessive light from above. The relaxed palpebral portion meanwhile allows the lids to remain open. Only when both parts contract together are the eyelids "screwed up".

The two parts of the muscle exercise different effects on the *volume of the conjunctival sac*. The palpebral part, in closing the lids gently, does not diminish the volume of the sac, so that "an eye brimful of tears" is pumped empty by blinking, and no tears spill. "Screwing up the eye" by the orbital fibres compresses the conjunctival sac, and causes an eye brimful of tears to spill down over the cheek. The full contraction of the orbital portion, pressing the thickened lids tight against the globe and orbital outlet, is more strongly protective against external violence than is mere blinking.

The palpebral portion, which closes the lids gently into marginal apposition, is opposed by levator palpebræ superioris. The orbital portion is opposed by frontalis (occipitofrontalis).

Nerve-supply.—The orbicularis is supplied by the *facial nerve*. The upper part of the muscle is supplied by the temporal and upper zygomatic branches of the facial, the lower by the lower zygomatic branches. These branches enter the muscle from the lateral side and on its deep surface.

The former cross the zygoma, as several branches, 2 cm behind the frontal, run a little above the lateral canthus, and then parallel with the supraorbital margin (see Fig. 291).

The lower zygomatic branch (or branches) reaches the lower part of the muscle by crossing the cheek. As these nerves actually penetrate into the muscle they divide into many branches (Fig. 275).

The Corrugator supercilii (Fig. 198) is a small, darkly coloured muscle situated at the medial side of the eyebrow under cover of the frontalis and orbicularis. *Arising* from the medial end of the superciliary ridge, it passes upwards and laterally, and then through the overlying muscles (Fig. 275), to be *inserted* into the skin of the eyebrow about its middle. It is responsible for the gaping of a vertical wound of the eyebrow.

Action.—The corrugators pull the eyebrows towards the root of the nose, making a projecting roof over the medial angle of the eye and producing characteristic vertical furrows in the middle of the lower part of the forehead and a dimple at its point of insertion.

The muscle is used primarily to protect the eye from the glare of the sun by forming a projecting shelf above it. It is well developed in those farm children who go about in the open without hats. These acquire permanent vertical furrows between the eyebrows quite early in life. In relation to facial expression it is *par excellence* the muscle of "*trouble*". It is used to express opposition to anything uncomfortable, and is seen in action in the crying child, in sorrow and pain, in frowning, and in retrospect on difficulty.

Nerve-supply.—The facial nerve, superior zygomatic branch.

The Occipitofrontalis consists of the two occipital and two frontal muscles, united together by the large, thin, epicranial aponeurosis, which extends over much of the cranium.

Each *occipital muscle*, small and of a quadrilateral form, arises from the lateral two-thirds of the highest nuchal line of the occipital bone and its extension on to the mastoid process, immediately superior to the attachment of sternocleidomastoid. The muscle's fibres pass thence into the epicranial aponeurosis.

The frontalis, also somewhat quadrilateral in shape, *arises* by a convex upper border from the epicranial aponeurosis midway between the coronal suture and the orbital margin. It is *inserted* into the skin of the eyebrows, mingling with the fibres of the orbicularis and the corrugator. Above, there is a distinct triangular interval between the two frontal muscles. Below, the medial fibres are joined and intermingle with the procerus, but it must be remembered that the latter muscle is running upwards, and is the antagonist of this medial part of frontalis.

Action.—The frontalis raises the eyebrows and draws the scalp forwards, throwing the forehead into a number of transverse wrinkles. These furrows are convex upwards on either side, joined by a piece in the centre, usually convex downwards. The lines are often absent in the triangular interval between the two muscles above. The occipitalis draws the scalp back. By the alternate contraction of the two muscles the scalp may be drawn forwards and backwards, but this can scarcely be regarded as its common use.

Occipitofrontalis is thus the opponent of the orbicular portion of orbicularis oculi; it is especially used in gazing upwards, to *elevate the eyebrows* above the line of vision. Note that levator palpebræ superioris is the true elevator of the upper *lid*, and so opposes the palpebral portion of the orbicularis.

More light thus reaches the eye, and more therefore is reflected from it, making it brighter and animating the gaze. The frontalis is brought into action when vision is rendered difficult, either by the distance of the object or the absence of sufficient light.

From the point of view of facial expression, the frontalis, as Duchenne has so well described it, is the muscle of "attention". It is used in expressing surprise, admiration, fear and horror, in all of which the element of "attention" is present. If the eyebrows are raised, the lids being half-closed, the appearance of forced attention results.

Nerve-supply.—Facial nerve, posterior auricular and temporal branches.

Musculus Procerus.—The two muscles so named, close together on each side of the midline, occupy the bridge of the nose and the interval between the lower fibres of the two frontales. The muscles are attached inferiorly to the nasal bones near the lateral nasal cartilages (and to the adjacent cartilage) and pass upwards to blend with the dermis of the forehead at and above the bridge of the nose (Fig. 275).

They pull the skin of this region downwards, producing transverse furrows in the lower part of the forehead and root of the nose. It is for this reason that the somewhat sinuous wrinkles of the forehead are convex upwards on each side, due to the frontales, and tend to be convex downwards in the middle.

The procerus is closely associated with the corrugator supercilii. It increases the prominence of the eyebrows as a protection when the eyes are exposed to bright light. From the point of view of facial expression Duchenne calls it the muscle of "aggression" or "menace". Associated with other muscles it expresses painful and similar emotions.

Nerve-supply.—Facial nerve, superior buccal branch.

The frontalis, orbicularis oculi, corrugator supercilii, and procerus have been called by Howe (1907) the *accessory muscles of accommodation*, since they appear to contract when vision is carried out under difficulties. It is possible that the attachment of the frontalis to the occipitalis may explain certain cases of occipital headache due to eye-strain (see also p. 317).

THE EYEBROWS

Each eyebrow is a transverse elevation studded with hairs, and situated at the junction of the forehead and upper lid. In structure it resembles the hairy scalp. It consists of skin, subcutaneous connective tissue, a muscular stratum, sub-muscular areolar tissue, and pericranium. The latter is adherent to the more or less prominent part of the frontal bone to which the region owes its shape. The influence of the size of the frontal sinuses in this is obvious (p. 26).

1. **The Skin** is thick, very mobile, and richly supplied with sebaceous glands. Like that of the scalp, it is closely adherent to the superficial fascia.

The hairs of the eyebrow are hard but silky. Taken as a whole eyebrows are comma-shaped. The *head* of the comma, the hairs composing which run upwards, is placed typically *under* the medial end of the orbital margin. The *body* of the comma lies along the orbital margin, and the hairs composing it run horizontally outwards. The *tail* of the comma usually lies somewhat above the lateral orbital margin, whose prominence can be made out *below* it. Many variations exist. The higher the eyebrow the more curved does it become, the lower its position the more horizontal. Many muscles of facial expression are attached to the mobile skin of the eyebrows, so that they may be raised, lowered or drawn towards the midline.

Usually the space between the eyebrows is smooth and hairless—hence the term *glabella*. Frequently the eyebrows are continuous across the midline.

2. **The Subcutaneous Tissue**, like that of the scalp, contains little fat and much fibrous tissue. It is strongly connected to the dermis on the one hand, and to the underlying muscles on the other. Thus, in movements of the eyebrow, the skin, subcutaneous and muscle layers move on the submuscular areolar layer.

3. **The Layer of Muscles.**—This is constituted by the vertical fibres of the frontalis, the arched horizontal fibres of the orbicularis, and the oblique darker coloured corrugator supercilii.

4. **The Submuscular Areolar Layer.**—This is a continuation of the "dangerous" area of the scalp, and since the frontalis is *not* attached to the orbital margin, it is further continued into the upper lid in the plane between the septum orbitale and the orbicularis.

But a deep part of the epicranial aponeurosis may be attached to the orbital margin, cutting off the dangerous area from the lids.

The *arterial supply* of the superciliary region is from the supraorbital and superficial temporal arteries (*q.v.*), the *venous drainage* to the same veins and also the angular vein (p. 414).

The lymphatic capillaries converge towards the submandibular and parotid nodes.

THE CONJUNCTIVA

The conjunctiva is a thin, translucent mucous membrane which derives its name from the fact that it joins the eyeball to the lids.

It lines the posterior surface of the lids, and is then reflected forwards on to the globe of the eye. Its epithelium becomes continuous anteriorly with the epithelium of the cornea.

It thus forms a complex space, the conjunctival sac, which is open in front at the palpebral fissure, and only closed when the eyes are shut.

Although all parts of the conjunctiva are continuous with each other, it is divided for purposes of description into three regions; palpebral conjunctiva (lining the eyelids), bulbar conjunctiva (attached to the eyeball), and the conjunctival fornix, where the palpebral and bulbar regions are continuous.

1. **The Palpebral Conjunctiva** of the lids may itself be subdivided into *marginal*, *tarsal* and *orbital* zones.

The conjunctiva of the margin of the lid is actually a transition zone between skin and conjunctiva proper (see p. 208). The structure of the marginal zone is continued on to the back of the lid for about 2 mm (Parsons) to a shallow groove known as the subtarsal fold, at which the perforating vessels pass through the tarsus to reach the conjunctiva.

The puncta open on to the marginal portion of the conjunctiva, and through them the conjunctival sac becomes directly continuous with the inferior meatus of the nose via the lacrimal passages.

Thus disease from the conjunctival sac may spread to the nose and vice versa.

The tarsal conjunctiva is thin, transparent, adherent and very vascular.

The vascularity gives the region its reddish or pinkish colour, and accounts for the fact that it is examined in cases of suspected anæmia.

As the conjunctiva is transparent, the tarsal glands can be seen through it as yellowish streaks.

The tarsal conjunctiva is intimately adherent to the superior tarsus; in fact, it is almost impossible to separate the two by dissection; for this reason too it is impossible to cover up gaps in the tarsal conjunctiva, as one can with the bulbar portion, simply by dissecting up neighbouring flaps and drawing them over the bare area. Unlike the upper tarsal conjunctiva, which is closely adherent to the tarsus in almost its whole extent, the lower is only so adherent for half the width of the tarsus.

The Orbital Zone of the conjunctiva of the upper lid lies between the upper border of the tarsal plate and the fornix. It lies loosely over the underlying nonstriated muscle of Müller (Fig. 191). Its surface is thrown into horizontal folds. They are folds of movement, and are deepest when the eyes are open and almost disappear when the eyes are shut. The folds appear after birth.

If the area just above the superior tarsal plate be examined with a loupe it will be found marked by a series of shallow grooves, which divide it up into a mosaic of low elevations (Stieda's plateaux and grooves). These elevations are not true papillæ, although they may become so in inflammation. This area may encroach on the conjunctiva tarsi, but never beyond the middle of the tarsus.

2. **The Conjunctival Fornix** is a continuous circular cul-de-sac, which is broken only (on the medial side) by the caruncle and the plica semilunaris.

It is divided for purposes of description into superior, inferior, lateral and medial regions.

The Superior Fornix reaches to the level of the orbital margin some 8–10 mm from the limbus.

The Inferior Fornix extends to within a few millimetres of the inferior orbital margin, 8 mm from the limbus.

The Lateral Fornix is placed at a depth of 5 mm from the surface, i.e. 14 mm from the limbus, and extends to just behind the equator of the globe.

The Medial Fornix is the shallowest, and is merely represented by the medial ends of the superior and inferior recesses.

The fornix conjunctivæ is in contact with and adherent to loose fibrous tissue, which is derived from the fascial expansions of the sheaths of the levator and recti muscles, and which is easily distensible.

In it are the conjunctival glands of Krause and nonstriated muscle of Müller. By means of this fibrous tissue the levator and recti can act on the fornix, deepening it when they contract.

Centrally, the fibrous tissue becomes continuous with the tarsus.

In the intertendinous interval, that is, in the diagonal regions of the fornix, the conjunctiva is in contact with the orbital fat, and it is in this region that infiltrations and hæmorrhage, such as arise in fracture of the base of the skull, reach the conjunctiva and may extend to the cornea.

The fornix is well supplied with vessels, and a rich venous network can be especially well seen in the inferior fornix, where also the whitish aponeurotic expansion from the inferior rectus and inferior oblique may be visible through the conjunctiva.

A knife passed through the upper fornix will enter the fibrous tissue between the levator and superior rectus, while through the inferior fornix the knife will hit the interval between the inferior palpebral muscle and the inferior rectus, and if pushed on the aponeurotic expansion from the inferior rectus and inferior oblique (Figs. 192 and 253).

3. **The Bulbar Conjunctiva** is thin, and so translucent that the sclera appears white as seen through it—hence the expression "the white of the eye".

It lies loosely on the underlying tissues, so that it can easily be moved apart from them. This movement takes place slightly with all movements of the eye; it is made evident in the living by pressure on the conjunctiva through the lower lid, and the operator knows how easy it is to pick up a fold of bulbar conjunctiva with forceps.

The bulbar conjunctiva is at first in contact with the tendons of the recti muscles covered by the fascia bulbi (Tenon's capsule).

Thus, in exposing these tendons, for instance in tenotomy, we must divide the conjunctiva, then the bulbar fascia before they are reached.

In front of the insertion of the recti tendons the bulbar conjunctiva lies on the anterior part of the bulbar fascia. Up to a point about 3 mm from the cornea the conjunctiva is separated from the bulbar fascia by loose areolar tissue, in which we find the subconjunctival vessels, and between it and the sclera is the loose epi-scleral tissue in the anterior portion of Tenon's space. In this *episcleral* space are the anterior ciliary arteries, forming the pericorneal plexus, and the tendons of the recti.

At about 3 mm from the cornea, the conjunctiva, fascia bulbi, and sclera become much more closely united. For this reason, although it is more difficult

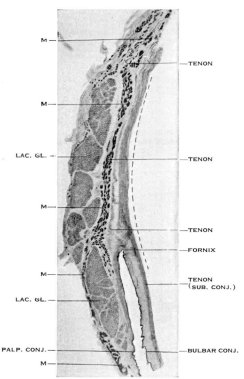

to raise a fold of conjunctiva close to the cornea, a much firmer hold can be obtained here with forceps than else-where.

At the point of union the conjunctiva is sometimes raised by a slight ridge, which becomes very apparent in in-flammatory conditions. This portion of the conjunctiva is known as the *limbal conjunctiva*. At the limbus in the angle between the epithelium and the sclera, the dermis of the conjunctiva, fascia bulbi, and the episclera are fused into a dense tissue.

The Structure of the Conjunctiva varies fundamentally in its different regions. On this depends the limitation of certain pathological processes to definite areas (Parsons).

Only in the new-born is the conjunc-tiva really normal, for owing to its exposed condition slight pathological changes are apt to take place from the earliest age.

Fig. 203.—Meridional Section Upwards and Outwards through the Soft Parts surround-ing the Eye.

M = unstriped muscles.
(*From Hesser.*)

The conjunctiva, like all other mucous membranes, consists of two layers—the epithelium and the sub-mucosal lamina propria.

The Epithelium.—The greater por-tion of the free margin of the lid is covered by keratinised stratified epithelium.

The mucocutaneous junction (Figs. 207, 208, 209) lies at the level of the pos-terior margin of the openings of the tarsal glands, i.e. at the junction of "dry" and "moist" portions where the marginal strips of tear fluid end in a sharp line. Here the eleidin and keratin layers of the skin end quite sharply, giving place to about five layers of non-keratinised squamous epithelium, the most superficial cells of which still retain their nuclei. The deeper portion of the epithelium does not alter at all at the mucocutaneous junction. It retains the same papillary structure.

At this point, then, the mucous membrane is much like that of the mouth, i.e. the deepest layer consists of high cylindrical cells as in the epidermis; this is followed by several layers of polyhedral cells, while the most superficial cells are flattened but still retain their nuclei. As we travel backwards (Fig. 207) the number of layers of squamous cells is gradually reduced and replaced by columnar and cubical ones. The total number of layers is also reduced, but the deepest layer remains cylindrical. Also in this region goblet cells, which, however, never reach the muco-cutaneous junction, begin to appear and are particularly numerous just beyond the subtarsal fold.

The epithelium of the tarsal conjunctiva of *the upper eyelid* consists, as classically described, of two layers. The deeper layer is composed of *cubical* cells whose oval nuclei lie with their axes parallel to the surface. The superficial layer consists of tall *cylindrical* cells, whose oval nuclei lie near the base of the cells and have their long axis at right angles to the surface.

As the fornix is approached, there is a tendency for a third layer of polyhedral cells to be inserted between the other two. So that at the fornix, although generally the structure is like that of the palpebral conjunctiva, we often find three layers instead of two.

The epithelium of the tarsal conjunctiva of *the lower eyelid* differs from the upper in having three or four layers of cells over nearly the whole of its extent; a two-layered arrangement as in the upper is only rarely present; sometimes five layers may be found. When four layers are present the basal cells are cubical as in all the tarsal conjunctiva (save the juxtamarginal zone), the next layer is polygonal, superficial to this are elongated wedge-shaped cells, their narrow ends jutting between the cells of the most superficial layer which are cone-shaped.

From the fornix to the limbus the epithelium becomes less and less glandular with a disappearance of the goblet cells, and more like that of the epidermis, but it never becomes keratinised.

More and more polyhedral layers are added between the superficial and deep cells. The superficial cells become flatter, while the deep cells grow taller. At the limbus the epithelium is definitely stratified with the formation of papillæ, which give the deep aspect of the epithelium a characteristic wavy outline (Fig. 28). Here the deepest or basal cells form a single layer of small cylindrical or cubical cells, with a large, darkly staining nucleus and little protoplasm. It is this fact that produces the *dark line* or seam seen under the low power of the microscope, and characteristic of the limbal conjunctiva (Figs. 25, 28). Moreover, the basal cells often contain pigment granules. There are several layers of polygonal cells, and superficially one or two layers of flattened cells with oval nuclei parallel to the surface. The polygonal cells differ from those of the cornea in having no prickles between them.

Goblet Cells occur in all regions of the conjunctiva, including the plica semilunaris (Fig. 217). They are large, oval, or round cells which look like fat-cells. The nucleus is flattened, and is near the base of the cell (Fig. 204).

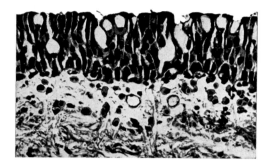

FIG. 204.—SECTION OF THE PALPEBRAL (ORBITAL) CONJUNCTIVA TO SHOW GOBLET CELLS.

They are said to be formed from the deepest layer of the conjunctiva, i.e. from the cylindrical cells, and then to pass towards the surface, tending, however, to remain attached to the basement membrane by a pointed process.

At first rounded, they grow larger and more oval as they approach the surface,

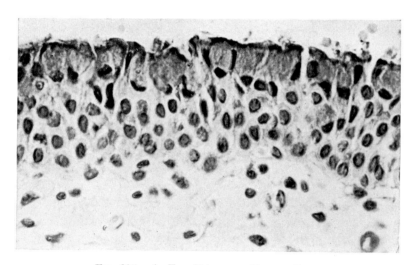

FIG. 205.—AS FIG. 204 UNDER HIGHER POWER.

where they resemble the goblet cells of the large intestine, but differ from these in being destroyed once they have discharged their contents.

The superficial goblet cells, too, have a stoma, through which the content of the cell, mainly mucin, is discharged. The goblet cells are true, unicellular mucous glands, moistening and protecting the conjunctiva and cornea, so that even extir-

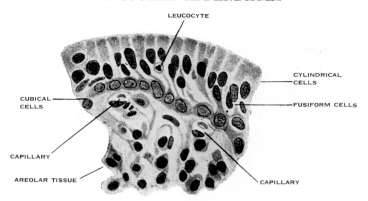

Fig. 206.—Epithelium of Conjunctiva of Upper Eyelid at upper end of Tarsus (Virchow).

pation of the lacrimal gland becomes innocuous, whilst on the other hand xerosis of the conjunctiva, involving their destruction, leads to desiccation, in spite of a copious flows of tears.

Although goblet cells occur normally in the conjunctiva they are greatly increased in inflammatory conditions.

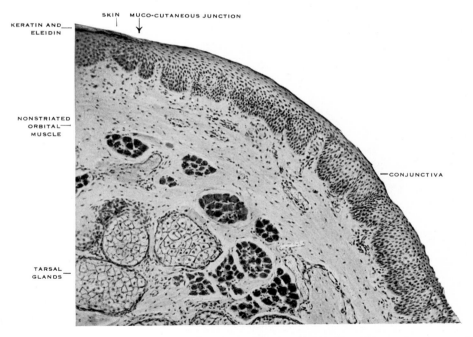

Fig. 207.—Vertical Section of Posterior Edge of Lower Lid Margin (low power).

Note how the layers of squamous cells diminish in number when traced to the right.

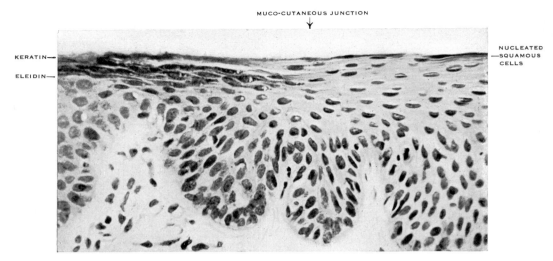

FIG. 208.—VERTICAL SECTION OF THE MUCO-CUTANEOUS JUNCTION OF THE LOWER EYELID.

Note sudden termination of keratin and eleidin layers at arrow. To the right are nucleated squamous cells.

Kessing (1966) from studies of the whole conjunctiva has mapped out the density of goblet cells. He finds them to be most dense nasally, least dense in the upper temporal fornix, and absent from the bulbar conjunctiva to the nasal and temporal sides of the limbus.

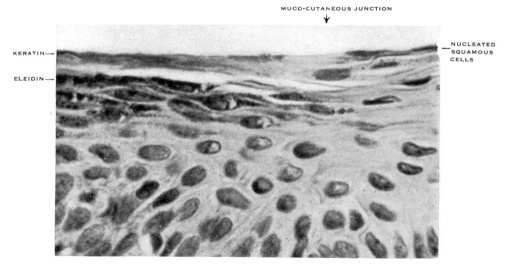

FIG. 209.—AS FIG. 208, BUT ACTUAL JUNCTION UNDER HIGHER POWER (OIL IMMERSION).

Melanocytes are present in the conjunctiva of the coloured races. In the white races the cells are present but not usually pigmented. The melanin can, however, always be brought out by the Dopa reaction or silver stains (Fig. 212).

These cells are found at the limbus, at the fornix, in the plica and caruncle, and at the site of perforation of the anterior ciliary vessels. (Montagna, 1967.)

THE CONJUNCTIVAL GLANDS

Associated with the conjunctiva are a number of small glands differentiated both histologically and topographically into differing types. These are known collectively as the conjunctival glands and distinguished only by eponymous names for the present.

The glands of Krause are accessory lacrimal glands having the same structure as the main gland. They are placed deeply in the subconjunctival connective tissue (mainly) of the upper fornix between the tarsus and the inferior lacrimal gland, of which they are offshoots. There are some 42 in the upper and 6 to 8 in the lower fornix (Krause, 1867). They are thus largely on the lateral side. Their ducts unite into a rather long duct or sinus which opens into the fornix. Similar glands are found in the caruncle.

The Glands of Wolfring or Ciaccio are also accessory lacrimal glands, but larger than the glands of Krause. There are 2 to 5 in the upper lid situated actually in the upper border of the tarsus about its middle between the extremities of the tarsal glands or just above the tarsus. There

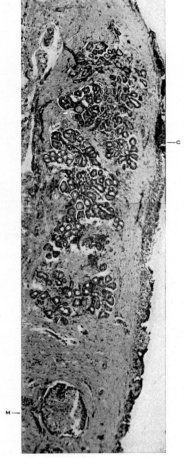

FIG. 210.—GLAND OF WOLFRING OR CIACCIO SITUATED IN UPPER PART OF TARSAL PLATE.

C = conjunctiva.
M = acinus of tarsal gland.

are two glands in the inferior edge of the lower tarsus. The excretory duct is large and short and lined by a basal layer of cubical cells and a superficial layer of cylindrical cells like the conjunctiva on which it opens.

Henle's "Glands" occur in the palpebral conjunctiva between the tarsal plates and the fornices. They are probably not true glands, but folds of mucous membrane cut transversely. They resemble Lieberkühn's crypts in the large intestine, and are lined by epithelium, which is like that of the surrounding conjunctiva.

The Glands of Manz are saccular or utricular glands found at the limbus in the

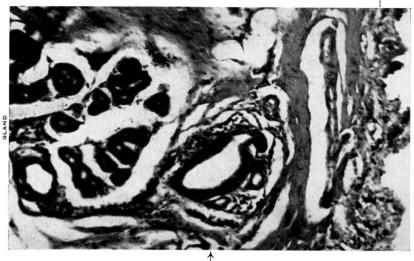

FIG. 211.—GLAND OF CIACCIO OR WOLFRING AND ITS DUCT (ARROW).

pig, calf and ox. They have also been described in the human but this is not generally accepted.

The Conjunctival Submucosa has a superficial lymphoid layer and a deeper
fibrous layer. Both end at the limbus; neither layer passes over the cornea. The
lymphoid layer is not present at birth, but is formed first in the region of the
fornix at 3 to 4 months. It is the formation of this lymphoid layer, together with a general increase in the surface area of the conjunctiva, that produces the folds in the upper part of the palpebral conjunctiva at the fifth month.

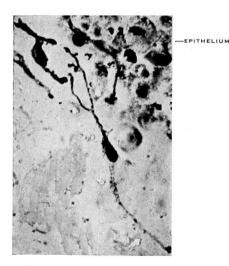

FIG. 212.—FLAT SECTION AT LIMBUS TO SHOW SUBCONJUNCTIVAL MELANOCYTES (STAINED BIELCHOWSKY).

The Lymphoid Layer is thin, but most developed in the fornix, being here 50–70 μm in thickness (Villard). It consists of a fine connective tissue reticulum, in the meshes of which the lymphocytes lie. This layer ceases at the subtarsal fold, so that the lymphocytes which are normally present under the conjunctiva in large numbers are not found in the marginal conjunctiva (Fig. 191).

Although nodules of lymphocytes are found in the human conjunctiva, especially towards the angles, they usually diminish at the periphery, and do not form true follicles such as are found especially in the lower fornix of the dog, cat, rabbit, etc. Pathological development of these nodules leads to the formation of undulations on the surface—pseudopapillæ (Parsons).

The Fibrous Layer is generally thicker than the lymphoid, but is almost non-existent over the tarsus, with which it is continuous. In it are found the vessels and nerves to the conjunctiva, the nonstriated palpebral muscle, and Krause's glands.

Conjunctival Papillæ.—True papillæ are found only at the limbus (Fig. 28) and at the lid margins.

Those near the limbus are finger-like extrusions of submucosal tissue, the interspaces of which are filled with epithelium, whilst the surface of the epithelium remains flat.

Arteries.—The arterial supply of the conjunctiva comes from three sources.

        1. The peripheral arterial arcades.
        2. The marginal arterial arcades.
        3. The anterior ciliary arteries.

Of these, so far at any rate as the upper lid is concerned, the peripheral arcade supplies by far the greatest area, i.e. almost the whole of the tarsal conjunctiva, the fornix, and the bulbar conjunctiva up to 4 mm from the cornea.

The Peripheral Arcade in the upper lid is situated at the upper border of the tarsus, between the two portions of the levator (Figs. 191, 192, 214). It gives off the peripheral perforating branches, which pass above the tarsal plate and pierce the palpebral muscle to reach the conjunctiva, under which it sends branches upwards and downwards.

The descending branches supply nearly the whole of the tarsal conjunctiva. They run perpendicularly to the lid margin, and anastomose with the much shorter branches of the marginal artery which have pierced the tarsus at the subtarsal fold.

The ascending branches pass upwards to the fornix, then bending round this, descend under the bulbar conjunctiva as the posterior conjunctival arteries (Fig. 214). They pass towards the cornea, at 4 mm from which they anastomose with the anterior conjunctival arteries, branches of the anterior ciliaries. The posterior conjunctival vessels are mobile, moving with the bulbar conjunctiva.

The peripheral arcade of the lower lid is, when present, placed in front of the inferior palpebral muscle of Müller and then generally behaves as does that of the upper lid. But it is inconstant and may come from other arteries beside the lacrimal, for instance, the transverse facial or superficial temporal.

It is often absent, in which case the conjunctiva of the lower lid, the lower fornix, and inferior portion of the bulbar conjunctiva get their blood-supply from the marginal arcade or from the muscular arteries to the inferior rectus.

The Marginal Arcade sends its perforating branches through the tarsus to reach the deep surface of the conjunctiva at the subtarsal fold. These branches divide into *marginal* and *tarsal* twigs.

The marginal arterioles run perpendicularly to the lid margin, forming a very vascular zone; the tarsal arterioles run perpendicularly to meet the corresponding branches from the peripheral arcade.

The tarsal conjunctiva is well supplied with blood, hence its red colour. The colour diminishes as we pass towards the fornix and the bulbar conjunctiva is colourless except when its vessels are dilated.

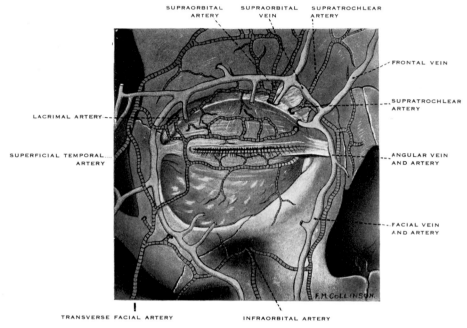

FIG. 213.—THE BLOOD-SUPPLY OF THE EYELIDS.

The Anterior Ciliary Arteries come from the muscular arteries to the recti (Figs. 86, 214, 215). Each muscular artery gives off two anterior ciliaries, except that to the lateral rectus, which supplies only one.

The anterior ciliary arteries pass forwards on a deeper plane than the posterior conjunctival. They are, however, visible, but appear darker than the superficial vessels. Some 4 mm from the cornea-scleral junction they bend towards the interior of the eye and pierce the sclera to join the circulus iridis major, which they help to form (Fig. 86). The hole in the sclera is often marked by pigment.

At the bend the anterior ciliaries give off the *anterior conjunctival arteries*, which pass forwards at a deeper level than the posterior conjunctival vessels (Fig. 214). They do not move with the conjunctiva. They pass forwards and, anastomosing with each other, form a series of arcades parallel to the corneal margin which more anteriorly gives place to the pericorneal plexus, while posteriorly they send twigs which anastomose with the posterior conjunctival arteries.

The pericorneal plexus is arranged in two layers: a superficial *conjunctival* and a deep *episcleral* (Figs. 25, 28).

The superficial portion is injected in superficial affections of the cornea, while the deeper portion is hyperæmic in diseases of the iris, ciliary body, or deep portion of the cornea.

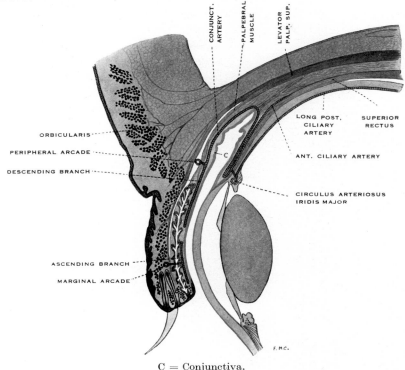

C = Conjunctiva.

FIG. 214.—SECTION OF THE UPPER LID AND ANTERIOR PORTION OF THE EYE TO SHOW THE BLOOD-SUPPLY TO THE CONJUNCTIVA.

It is the dilatation of the deeper vessels which gives rise to the characteristic rose-pink band of "ciliary injection". It will be noted that the redness disappears on pressure, but the vessels do not move with the conjunctiva.

In conjunctivitis the bulbar conjunctiva becomes brick-red, due to hyperæmia of the close network of small superficial vessels which, derived from the posterior conjunctival, are normally almost invisible. The redness increases towards the fornices and diminishes towards the cornea; it does not fade on pressure. The vessels move with the conjunctiva.

All the above facts are explained by the anatomical arrangements of the vessels. Thus we see that although joined by anastomoses the area supplied by the palpebral arcades on the one hand and that which gets its blood-supply from the

A.E.—15

anterior ciliaries on the other hand are more or less sharply differentiated, and in affections of the conjunctiva the vessels of the former area are injected, the redness increasing towards the fornix, while in deep inflammation, that is, of the iris and ciliary body, the network of vessels around the cornea coming from the anterior ciliaries forms a characteristic rose-pink band.

In interstitial keratitis the new vessels that invade the substantia propria of the cornea come from the anterior ciliaries as these are passing through the sclera to reach the iris and ciliary body. They are thus, since the sclera is opaque, only visible up to the limbus.

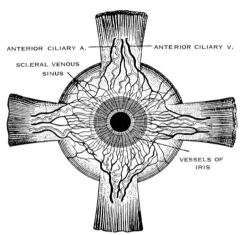

ANTERIOR CILIARY A. — ——— ANTERIOR CILIARY V.

SCLERAL VENOUS SINUS

VESSELS OF IRIS

FIG. 215.—ANTERIOR CILIARY ARTERIES AND VEINS.
(*From Poirier after Panas.*)

The Conjunctival Veins accompany but are much more numerous than the corresponding arteries. For the most part, i.e. from the tarsal conjunctiva, from the fornix, and the major portion of the bulbar conjunctiva, they drain into the palpebral veins.

Corresponding to the peripheral arterial arcade of the upper lid, there is an important and well-marked venous plexus, which, placed between the tendons of the levator, sends its blood back to the veins of the levator and superior rectus, which again drain into the ophthalmic.

In the circumcorneal zone supplied by the anterior ciliaries the corresponding veins are less conspicuous than the arteries. They form a network some 5 to 6 mm wide, which drains into the muscular veins. It becomes apparent in hyperæmia.

Lymphatics.—The conjunctival lymphatics are arranged in two plexuses. A superficial, composed of small vessels, placed just beneath the vascular capillaries; and a deep, consisting of larger vessels situated in the fibrous layer of the conjunctiva, and receiving the lymph from the superficial plexus.

They drain towards the commissures, where they join the lymphatics of the lids: those from the lateral side go to the parotid nodes, and those from the medial to the submandibular lymph glands.

Nerves.—The nerve-supply of the conjunctiva is derived from the same source as that of the lids generally, but the long ciliaries supply the cornea and circumcorneal zone of the conjunctiva and the lacrimal and infratrochlear supply a much larger area of conjunctiva than of skin.

Nerve endings in the conjunctiva may be considered under two headings: simple, naked, or "free" endings, and "compact", specialised endings, such as the "end bulbs" of Krause.

(a) *Free Endings.*—The nerves having lost their myelin sheath, form a *sub-epithelial* plexus in the superficial part of the substantia propria. From this fibres pass to form an intra-epithelial plexus around the bases of the epithelial cells and send free nerve fibrils between these cells. Many fibres pass to blood vessels.

(b) *The End Bulbs of Krause* (Fig. 216) are round bodies from 0·02 mm to 0·1 mm in length. Each is surrounded by a connective tissue envelope, continuous with the nerve sheath and lined by endothelial cells. In this is found a twisted mass of fibrils. One or two nerves enter the envelope, lose their myelin sheath, and join the central mass.

The classical papers of Weddell, Sinclair and others (1941, 1955, 1967) on the sensibility of skin and cornea have modified considerably views on nerve endings and their functioning in the conjunctiva. According to these observers the so-called end-bulb of Krause is but a stage in the cycle of growth and decay of such specialised organs. Moreover, these special endings are comparatively rare and variable in distribution in the human conjunctiva, "free" endings being much more numerous and widespread.

THE CARUNCLE (Figs. 18 and 217)

The caruncle (diminutive of Latin, *caro*, flesh) is a small, soft, pink ovoid body some 5 mm in height and 3 mm broad, situated in the lacus lacrimalis to the medial side of the plica semilunaris. It is attached to the plica, and fibres of the medial rectus sheath enter its deep surface. Thus it is most prominent when the eye looks laterally, being pulled on by the plica, and becomes deeply recessed when the eye looks medially *and sometimes following tenotomy of the medial rectus.*

It is really a piece of modified skin, so is covered by modified stratified squamous epithelium, and is supplied with hairs, sebaceous and sweat glands. It differs from the skin in containing glands like those of Krause. In the depths of the caruncle the abundant connective tissue is in contact with the septum orbitale and the medial check ligament. *The epithelium* resembles that of the lid margin, but the superficial layer is not keratinised. Also towards the conjunctiva, goblet cells are found. These may occur singly or in groups, forming a kind of acinus.

The Sebaceous Glands resemble those of the eyelids. They produce the characteristic white secretion not infrequently found at the medial canthus.

The Modified Lacrimal Glands are often conspicuous structures. They do not represent the gland of Harder, which is absent in the human. They are placed in the centre of the caruncle, have a typical tubuloacinous structure, and open by a sinuous duct near the plica semilunaris. Around the lacrimal gland tissue there is usually a thin layer of fat.

The Hairs, some fifteen in number, are fine, colourless, and directed towards the nose.

Blood-supply.—The superior medial palpebral arteries. The branches, to reach the caruncle, have to pass through dense connective tissue. This keeps them patent when cut and results in free bleeding, as does a similar arrangement in the scalp.

Lymphatics.—These drain into the submandibular lymph glands.

Nerve-supply.—The infratrochlear nerve.

THE PLICA SEMILUNARIS

The plica semilunaris is a narrow crescentic fold of conjunctiva placed vertically with its concavity facing laterally and lying lateral to and partly under cover of the caruncle. Its lower horn reaches to the middle of the lower fornix, while the upper does not pass up so far. The lateral border is free and separated from the bulbar conjunctiva by a small cul-de-sac some 2 mm deep, present when the eye looks medially, but almost disappearing when the eye looks laterally. The pink colour of the plica is due to its vascularity (Fig. 217) and contrasts with the white of the sclera. In structure it is like that of the rest of the bulbar conjunctiva, but the epithelium instead of six layers consists of eight to ten, and the deepest layer, instead of being cubical, is cylindrical, and contains a lobule of fat and some nonstriated muscle supplied by the sympathetic. Goblet cells are particularly numerous (Fig. 217).

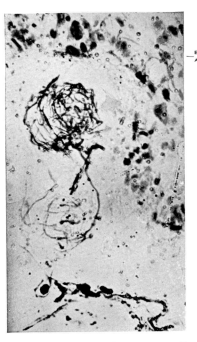

EPITHELIUM
AT LIMBUS

FIG. 216.—FLAT SECTION AT LIMBUS TO SHOW END BULB OF KRAUSE (STAINED BIELCHOWSKY).

The goblet cells may be superficial or grouped and then open on the surface by a narrow duct (intra-epithelial gland of Tourneux) (Fig. 218). Melanophores called cells of Langerhans are always present. They may be non-pigmented in fair people but can always be demonstrated by the Dopa reaction and in other ways.

The connective tissue stroma of the plica is loose and contains numerous vessels and sometimes a nodule of fibro-cartilage. At the base of the plica there is a lobule of fat and sometimes some nonstriated muscle fibres.

Similar structures are found in the caruncle and come from the medial rectus and more especially from the medial capsulopalpebral muscle of Hesser. The plica may represent the third eyelid or nictitating membrane of the lower animals, but see Stibbe (1928).

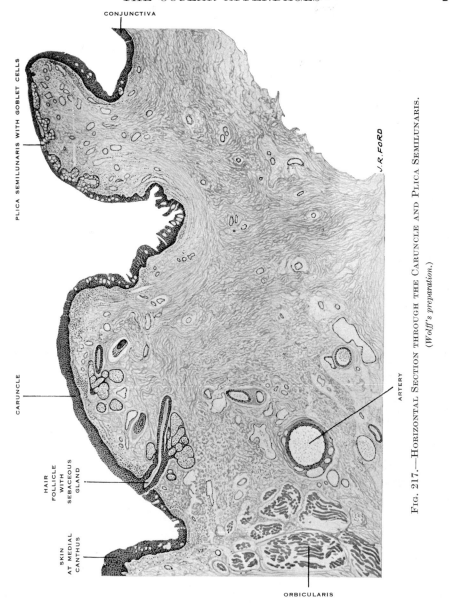

CONJUNCTIVA

PLICA SEMILUNARIS WITH GOBLET CELLS

CARUNCLE

HAIR FOLLICLE WITH SEBACEOUS GLAND

SKIN AT MEDIAL CANTHUS

ARTERY

ORBICULARIS

J.R.FORD

FIG. 217.—HORIZONTAL SECTION THROUGH THE CARUNCLE AND PLICA SEMILUNARIS. (*Wolff's preparation.*)

A still simpler view of the plica semilunaris is that it is an inevitable formation. The conjunctival area here must be generous enough to allow full lateral movement of the eyeball. Thus there is slack to be taken up when the eye looks forwards or medially; hence the fold. No such arrangement exists laterally, for here the fornix is very deep. The absence of a deep medial fornix is a functional necessity to enable the puncta to dip into *superficial* strips of tear fluid (p. 235).

The Lacrimal Apparatus

The lacrimal gland, sited above and anterolateral to the globe of the eye, secretes the tears and pours them through a series of ducts into the conjunctival sac at the upper fornix. The lacrimal gland and its tears are only present in those animals which live in air. In fishes, for instance, there is no lacrimal gland, the water in which they live acting in place of tears. The tears moisten the front of the eye, lubricate it, prevent friction between globe and lids, and also desiccation of the corneal epithelium (see p. 236). The lubricative function is obvious, but it is not usually appreciated with sufficient emphasis that the corneal epithelium provides the basic refractive mechanism of the eye. To provide continuous regeneration and a transparent medium these cells must be alive and wet. The tear fluid is hence primarily of optical importance.

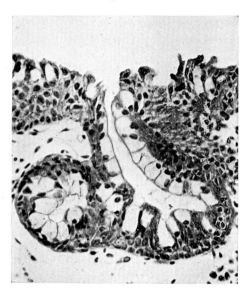

FIG. 218.—SECTION OF PORTION OF PLICA SEMI-LUNARIS TO SHOW GLAND OF TOURNEUX.

Some of the tears evaporate, but the rest make their way medially to the puncta situated in the margin of the lids. From here they are conducted by the lacrimal canaliculi to the lacrimal sac, and then pass into the nasolacrimal duct, which opens into the inferior meatus of the nose.

Under normal conditions almost no tears pass down the nasolacrimal duct; just enough tears are produced to replace evaporation from the cornea and exposed conjunctiva. Thus removal of the lacrimal sac, with consequent obliteration of the drainage channels, is little embarrassment to the average individual.

The Lacrimal Gland

The Lacrimal Gland consists of two portions (Figs. 277, 282, and 283):

(i) A large orbital or superior portion;

and (ii) A small palpebral or inferior portion;

which are, however, continuous behind. *The Orbital Portion* is lodged in its fossa on the anterior and lateral part of the roof of the orbit. It is shaped like an almond, and hence we have for examination a superior and inferior surface, an anterior and posterior border, and a medial and a lateral extremity.

The Superior Surface is convex, and lies in the fossa on the frontal bone, with which it is connected by weak trabeculæ.

The Inferior Surface, slightly concave, lies successively on the levator palpebræ, the lateral expansion of its tendon, and the lateral rectus (Figs. 279 and 282).

The Anterior Border is sharp and in contact with the septum orbitale.

Hence, to reach this portion of the lacrimal gland from the front, one has to divide skin, orbicularis, and septum orbitale.

The Posterior Border, more rounded, is in contact with the orbital fat in the same coronal plane as the posterior pole of the eye.

The Medial Extremity rests on the levator—the *lateral* on the lateral rectus.

The Palpebral Portion, also flattened from above down, is about one-third the size of the orbital portion, and placed so that the anterior border lies just above the lateral part of the upper fornix. It can be seen in this situation through the conjunctiva when the upper lid is everted. It lies for the most part on the fornix and palpebral conjunctiva, but partly also on the superior palpebral muscle. It is separated from the superior portion by the expansion of the levator, but behind this its posterior border is continuous with the rest of the gland (Fig. 282).

The Conjunctival Glands of Krause (Fig. 191) are accessory lacrimal glands in the conjunctiva

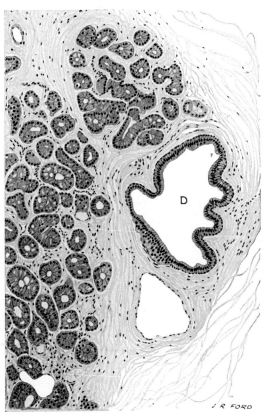

FIG. 219.—SECTION OF THE LACRIMAL GLAND
D = *one* of the ducts.
(*Wolff's preparation.*)

from the fornix to the convex border of the tarsus. They may be regarded as a continuation downwards of the palpebral portion of the lacrimal gland.

Fine ducts pass from both portions of the lacrimal gland to open by ten to twelve small orifices just in front of the lateral part of the superior fornix. One or two also open into the lateral part of the lower fornix.

Structure.—The lacrimal gland is a tubuloracemose gland with short branched gland tubules resembling the parotid in structure (Fig. 219). It consists of masses of lobules, each being about the size of a pin's head. It is not very sharply differentiated from the surrounding adipose tissue, and fat is also found between the lobules.

The acini consist of two layers of cells placed on a thin hyaline basement membrane and surrounding a central canal. The cells of the basal layer are myoepithelial in character and are flat and contractile; the other cells are cylindrical, and form the true secreting cells. At rest these contain granules. After secreting for some time the cells become shorter and the granules disappear. The secretion of the acini passes into very small interlobular ducts, opening into slightly larger ducts which are, however, still intermediary. These finally open into the definitive excretory duct. Mucinogen and zymogen granules occur in the acinar secretory cells. Ultrastructural studies (Scott and Vease, 1959; Ichikawa and Nakajima, 1962) have so far been confined to rodent glands. These studies have shown the basal folding of the secretory cells usually seen in glandular elements, as well as the organelle appearances typical of secretory activity. The former observers recorded the occurrence of naked nerve fibre terminals between the basement membrane and the bases of the cells. They also described several glandular cell types.

The smaller ducts have much the same structure as the acini, but in the large ducts outside the basement membrane is a fibrous coat.

The inter-acinous and inter-lobular connective tissue is hardly present in the young but increases with age. In it are found plasma cells and lymphocytes which may be aggregated into follicles.

The ducts from the orbital portion traverse or are in contact with the palpebral portion. *It thus comes about that removal of the palpebral portion practically does away with the secretion of the whole gland.*

So-called ligaments have been described in connection with the lacrimal gland; none, however, deserve the name.

(a) *Superior* to the lacrimal fossa (= suspensory ligament).

(b) *Inferior*—inferior pole to zygomatic bone.

(c) *Posterior*—where the lacrimal nerve and vessels enter, to the periorbita.

(d) *Internal*—accompanying the ducts.

Vessels.—The lacrimal artery, which enters it on its posterior border, and sometimes a branch of the transverse facial. The corresponding vein joins the ophthalmic.

Lymphatics to the conjunctival lymphatics, and thence to the preauricular glands.

Nerves.—Lacrimal, greater (superficial) petrosal, and cervical sympathetic trunk.

The Fibres of the Greater (Superficial) Petrosal, the "nerve of tear secretion", are the axons of neurons whose somata are in the so-called superior salivatory nucleus (p. 397). They pass out in the nervus intermedius to the geniculate ganglion (but form no synapses there), from which the greater (superficial) petrosal arises. This runs in a groove on the front of the petrous temporal (Fig.

274), then under the trigeminal ganglion to join the deep petrosal (from the sympathetic plexus round the internal carotid artery) to form the nerve of the pterygoid canal in the foramen lacerum (Fig. 289).

The Nerve of the Pterygoid Canal (*Vidian Nerve*), thus composed of parasympathetic (secretomotor) and sympathetic (vasomotor) fibres, joins the pterygopalatine (sphenopalatine, Meckel's) ganglion. Only the parasympathetic fibres

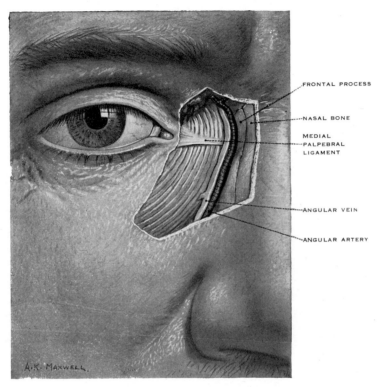

FRONTAL PROCESS

NASAL BONE

MEDIAL PALPEBRAL LIGAMENT

ANGULAR VEIN

ANGULAR ARTERY

FIG. 220.—DISSECTION TO SHOW LACRIMAL APPARATUS. RELATION OF ANGULAR VEIN AND ARTERY TO MEDIAL PALPEBRAL LIGAMENT.

(*Wolff's dissection.*)

relay in the ganglion. The postganglionic secretomotor fibres pass to the zygomatic nerve and reach the lacrimal gland via the connecting branch with the lacrimal nerve. This, the orthodox description, may require some modification. Ruskell (1971) has reviewed the evidence and the observations of his own researches in primates. His own results strongly support a parasympathetic pathway through orbital branches of the pterygopalatine ganglion. These join a "*retro-orbital*" *plexus* (see p. 316), from which *rami lacrimales* carry nonmyelinated postganglionic fibres, both sympathetic and parasympathetic, to the lacrimal gland.

Postganglionic sympathetic fibres may reach the gland by several routes:

(a) along the lacrimal artery (from the internal carotid plexus), (b) through the deep petrosal nerve (and hence also from the same plexus), and (c) through the lacrimal nerve. Ruskell identified sympathetic fibres in the adventitia of the lacrimal artery and (to a very limited extent) in the lacrimal nerve.

The Sensory Fibres are carried by the lacrimal nerve; their cell bodies are in the trigeminal ganglion. (It is important to note that most of the fibres in the lacrimal nerve pass on to innervate palpebral skin.)

THE PUNCTA

Each punctum lacrimale is a small, round, or transversely oval aperture situated on a slight elevation, *the papilla lacrimalis*, at the medial end of the lid

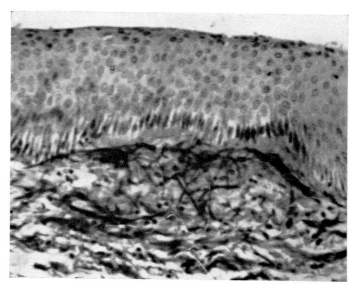

FIG. 221.—PORTION OF WALL OF CANALICULUS.
Note elastic fibres deep to epithelium.

margin at the junction of its ciliary and nearer portions. It is in a line with the openings of the ducts of the tarsal glands, the nearest of which is only 0·5 to 1 mm away. The region of the punctum is relatively avascular, and so is paler than the surrounding area. This pallor is emphasised on drawing the lower lid laterally, *a fact of great value in finding a stenosed punctum.*

The upper punctum is slightly nearer to the nasal side (being 6 mm from the medial canthus) than the lower, which is 6·5 mm from this point. Thus, when the eye is shut the puncta are not in contact, but the upper lies to the medial side of the lower. The upper punctum looks downwards and backwards, and the lower upwards and backwards. *For this reason a normal punctum is only visible if the lid is everted.*

Each punctum, when the eye is opened or shut, glides in the groove between the plica semilunaris and the globe; and is kept patent by a ring of very dense fibrous tissue, continuous with the tarsus which surrounds it. Around this again

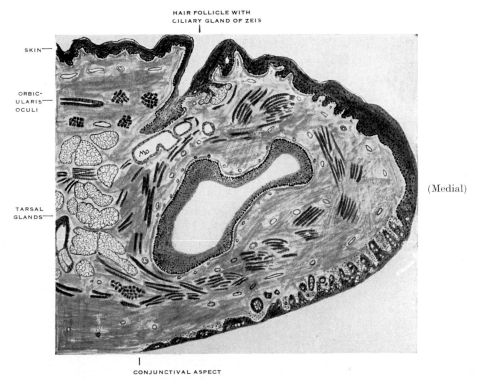

HAIR FOLLICLE WITH
CILIARY GLAND OF ZEIS

SKIN

ORBIC-
ULARIS
OCULI

(Medial)

TARSAL
GLANDS

CONJUNCTIVAL ASPECT

FIG. 222.—HORIZONTAL SECTION OF THE MEDIAL REGION OF THE LOWER EYELID, SHOWING THE LACRIMAL CANALICULUS AT THE JUNCTION OF THE VERTICAL AND HORIZONTAL PORTIONS, SURROUNDED BY FIBRES OF THE ORBICULARIS.

MO = Ciliary gland of Moll. Note goblet cells in conjunctiva.

(Wolff's preparation.)

are fibres of the orbicularis which press the punctum in towards the lacus lacrimalis. Their atrophy in old age makes the papilla lacrimalis more prominent.

THE LACRIMAL CANALICULI

Each canaliculus consists of a vertical and a horizontal portion. *It is, therefore, of great importance in passing a probe to remember that the canaliculus runs at first vertically.*

The vertical portion is about 2 mm long and then bends medially almost at a right angle to become continuous with the horizontal portion. At the junction of the two is a dilatation or *ampulla*. Both horizontal portions slope towards the medial canthus; thus the upper runs downwards as well as medially, while the lower has a slight inclination upwards. Some 8 mm long, the upper being slightly the shorter, they lie in the lid margin.

The canaliculi pierce the lacrimal fascia (i.e. the periorbita covering the lacrimal sac) separately as a rule, then unite to enter a small diverticulum of the sac, the lacrimal sinus of Maier (Fig. 225). The point of entry lies just behind the middle of the lateral surface of the sac about 2·5 mm from its apex.

Structure.—The canaliculi are lined by stratified squamous epithelium (Figs. 221, 222) placed on a corium rich in elastic tissue. The walls are thus so thin and

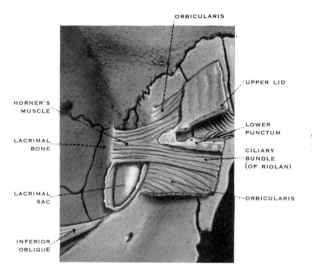

ORBICULARIS

UPPER LID

HORNER'S MUSCLE

LACRIMAL BONE

LOWER PUNCTUM

CILIARY BUNDLE (OF RIOLAN)

LACRIMAL SAC

ORBICULARIS

INFERIOR OBLIQUE

Fig. 223.—The Relations of the Lacrimal Sac and the Pars Lacrimalis (Horner's Muscle).

(*Wolff's dissection.*)

elastic that the canaliculus can be dilated three times its normal diameter, which is 0·5 mm. For the same reason, in pulling the lids laterally and in passing a probe the angle between vertical and horizontal portions can be easily straightened. Also being so close to the edge of the lid and covered by translucent tissue, a coloured fluid injected into the canaliculus can be seen.

Like the punctum the canaliculus is surrounded by fibres of the orbicularis (Fig. 222), which on contraction tend to invert the lower lid and draw the punctum inwards.

The medial third of the canaliculi is covered in front by the two bands which connect the medial palpebral ligament to the tarsi, while behind this is the pars lacrimalis of the orbicularis oculi (Horner's muscle) (Fig. 223).

The Lacrimal Sac

The membranous lacrimal sac is placed in the lacrimal fossa (formed by the lacrimal bone and the frontal process of the maxilla) which lies in the anterior part of the medial wall of the orbit (see also p. 4). The sac is closed above and open below, where it is continuous with the naso-lacrimal duct, a constriction marking the junction between the two. Looked at *from the side* the sac and fossa are seen to slope backwards 15–25°, the line being given by joining the medial canthus to the 1st upper molar of the same side. From the front the sac slopes gently laterally, the duct slightly less so. The two thus make an obtuse angle open inwards (Fig. 225).

The sac is enclosed by a portion of the periorbita which, splitting at the posterior lacrimal crest, encloses the sac to meet again at the anterior lacrimal crest, and thus forms what is called the *lacrimal fascia* (Figs. 223, 224, 225). The lacrimal

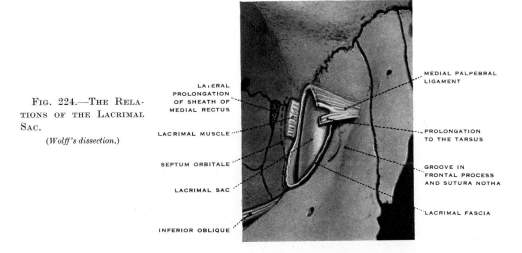

FIG. 224.—THE RELATIONS OF THE LACRIMAL SAC.

(*Wolff's dissection.*)

LATERAL PROLONGATION OF SHEATH OF MEDIAL RECTUS

LACRIMAL MUSCLE

SEPTUM ORBITALE

LACRIMAL SAC

INFERIOR OBLIQUE

MEDIAL PALPEBRAL LIGAMENT

PROLONGATION TO THE TARSUS

GROOVE IN FRONTAL PROCESS AND SUTURA NOTHA

LACRIMAL FASCIA

fascia is separated from the sac by areolar tissue containing a fine plexus of veins continuous with that around the duct, except at the fundus, where it is closely adherent, and, sometimes, on its medial aspect.

Relations.—*Medially* the sac is in relation above with the anterior ethmoidal sinuses (Fig. 3) (which may also at times lie behind and even in front of the sac), below with the middle meatus of the nose. Between bone and sac, however, we always find periorbita.

Laterally are the skin, fibres of the orbicularis and the lacrimal fascia.

For the relation of the medial palpebral ligament to the sac see p. 190.

The inferior oblique arises from the floor of the orbit just lateral to the lacrimal fossa, a few fibres often taking origin from the lacrimal fascia.

The angular vein is the great bugbear in the approach to the lacrimal sac. Lying under the skin it crosses the medial palpebral ligament 8 mm from the medial canthus. Not infrequently a tributary of the angular vein, which can also be seen in the living, crosses the ligament between the medial canthus and parent vein. *It is therefore not safe to make the incision for the removal of the sac more than 2 to 3 mm medial to the medial canthus.*

The lower margin of the medial palpebral ligament is free, but it is continued upwards and laterally as a sheet which blends with the lacrimal fascia covering the fundus of the sac (Fig. 224) (see p. 190).

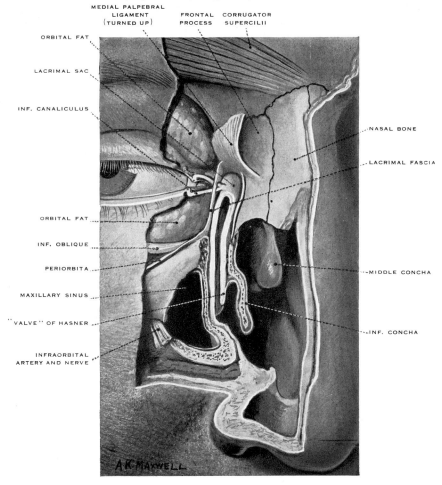

FIG. 225.—DISSECTION TO SHOW THE RELATIONS OF THE LACRIMAL SAC AND THE NASOLACRIMAL DUCT FROM IN FRONT.

(Wolff's preparation.)

As Fisher said (1904), this attachment to the sac may explain how relatively slight blows on the eye (as in boxing) may cause swelling of the lids on blowing the nose. A sudden strain is put on the ligament, which pulls on and tears the sac.

The portion of the sac below the level of the ligament is covered by only a few fibres of the orbicularis, which offer little resistance to distension and swellings of the sac. *It is, therefore, in the area below the ligament that abscesses and fistulæ will open.*

Behind the sac are the lacrimal fascia and muscle; the latter arises from the upper half of the posterior lacrimal crest, runs behind the sac and covers the posterior aspect of the medial third of the canaliculi. Behind this again is the septum orbitale, and then comes the check ligament of the medial rectus (Fig. 197).

The lacrimal sinus (of Maier) is a diverticulum of the upper part of the sac behind the middle of the lateral surface into which the canaliculi open either together or separately.

THE NASOLACRIMAL DUCT

The nasolacrimal duct, the continuation downwards of the lacrimal sac extending from the so-called neck to the inferior meatus of the nose, is only 15 mm in length. It lies in a canal formed mainly by a groove on the maxilla (Figs. 3 and 6) and completed by the lacrimal bone and the lacrimal process of the inferior concha (turbinate bone). It descends posterolaterally, its direction being given in lateral view by a line from the medial angle of the eye to the first upper molar.

The position and shape of the inferior orifice vary greatly. In some cases, where it corresponds to the opening of the bony canal at the highest part of the meatus it tends to be round; in others it runs as a *membranous* tube for some distance under the mucous membrane, and is then found at different points down the lateral wall of the meatus, becoming more slit-like as it descends. It may be very difficult to find.

The nasolacrimal duct lies lateral to the middle meatus (Fig. 225), and laterally makes a ridge in the forepart of the maxillary antrum (Fig. 19), *a relation which explains why epiphora is such a frequent symptom of growths of this sinus.*

The Valves.—Numerous so-called valves have been described in the nasolacrimal duct. They are simply folds of mucous membrane which have no valvular function, since fluids can be blown up the duct to come out at the puncta. The most constant of these folds is the "valve" of Hasner (plica lacrimalis) at the lower end, which represents the remains of the fetal septum (see also Figs. 225, 226). When well-developed (and it usually is) the plica functions adequately in preventing a sudden blast of air (blowing the nose into a handkerchief) from entering the lacrimal sac.

Structure.—The lacrimal sac and duct are lined by two layers of epithelium, the superficial of which is columnar, the deeper flattened. The bases of the columnar cells pass through the deeper layer to reach the basement membrane. The superficial layer is never ciliated, but in it goblet cells occur in variable numbers. Mucous glands have also been described. In the subepithelial layer are lymphocytes, which may be aggregated pathologically into follicles. The actual membranous wall of the sac consists of fibroelastic tissue, the elastic portion being continuous with that around the canaliculi. The nasolacrimal duct is curious in having a rich plexus of vessels around it, forming an erectile tissue resembling in structure that on the inferior concha (turbinate bone). *Engorgement of these vessels is said to be sufficient to obstruct the duct.*

Whilst at its upper part the nasolacrimal duct can easily be separated from the bone, below it is closely adherent, forming a mucoperiosteum, and *thus infection may pass easily from bone to duct or vice versa.*

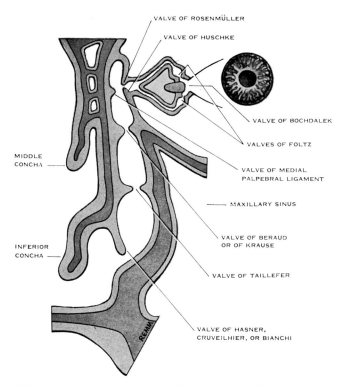

FIG. 226.—SCHEME OF THE SO-CALLED VALVES OF THE NASOLACRIMAL CANAL.

Vessels.—The *arterial* supply comes from the superior and inferior palpebral branches of the ophthalmic (Fig. 277), from the angular artery, from the infraorbital artery and from the nasal branch of the sphenopalatine.

The Veins above drain into the angular and infraorbital veins, while below they run into the nasal veins.

The Lymphatics pass to the submandibular, and deep cervical glands.

The Nerves.—The nerve-supply of sac and duct comes from the infratrochlear and anterior superior alveolar nerves.

There is probably a reflex relation between the nerve-supply of the lacrimal gland and sac, for extirpation of the latter greatly diminishes the tear flow.

THE DISTRIBUTION OF THE LACRIMAL FLUID

At the posterior margin of both upper and lower eyelids there is a collection or strip of tear fluid.

With the naked eye and without the previous instillation of fluorescin these strips of fluid can be made out only with difficulty; but since each acts as a mirror it reflects light strongly so that the brilliant linear reflex that it produces can be seen at some distance. Usually this applies only to the lower strip, since the upper lid margin is normally in shadow.

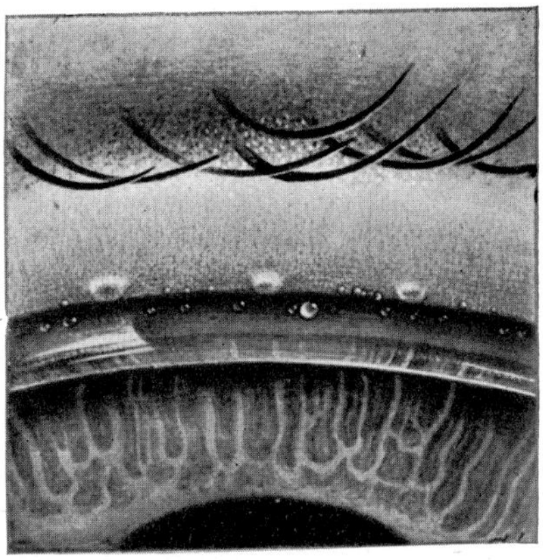

The strips of fluid can be made out better with a loupe and, of course, best of all with the slit-lamp.

With the slit-lamp the strip-like collection of fluid is seen to be between the posterior lid margin of both eyelids and the exposed portion of the globe. That of the lower lid (the inferior marginal strip) runs up on the cornea for a millimetre or so, due to surface tension, and hence

FIG. 227.—THE SUPERIOR MARGINAL STRIP (S).

Note the oil droplets in it, and also some air bubbles.

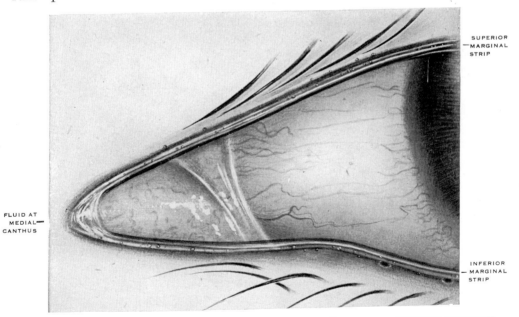

FIG. 228.—WITH THE EYE LOOKING LATERALLY THE MARGINAL STRIPS ARE CONTINUED MEDIALLY BETWEEN THE LID MARGIN ON ONE HAND AND THE PLICA AND CARUNCLE ON THE OTHER. THEY JOIN AT THE MEDIAL CANTHUS.

A.E.—16

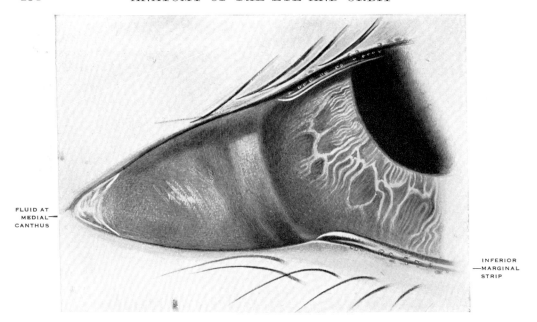

FLUID AT
MEDIAL
CANTHUS

INFERIOR
MARGINAL
STRIP

FIG. 229.—WITH THE EYE LOOKING MEDIALLY A CAVITY APPEARS DEEP TO EACH LACRIMAL PORTION
OF THE LID MARGIN AND THE MARGINAL STRIPS STOP SHORT.

(*Wolff, Trans. O.S.U.K.,* 1946, **66**, 291.)

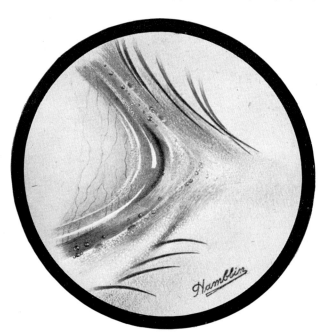

FIG. 230.—THE COLLECTION
OF TEAR FLUID AT THE LATERAL
CANTHUS. IT IS CONTINUOUS
WITH THE FLUID IN THE LATERAL
CUL-DE-SAC.

(*Wolff, Trans. O.S.U.K.,* 1946.)

the tear fluid appears always, that is normally, to be brimming over. It is prevented from actually overflowing, however, by the secretion of the tarsal glands. The anterior limit is at the posterior margin of the openings of the tarsal glands. When the lower lid is drawn away from the eye the tear fluid sinks down into the lower fornix, but immediately returns when the lid is allowed to return to its normal position. In the adult this collection of fluid, where it is in contact with the conjunctiva, contains some folds of this mucous membrane.

The collection of fluid at the posterior margin of the upper lid (the superior marginal strip) runs down on to the cornea for a millimetre or so and ends in a *sharp line*. It is to be emphasized (Wolff, 1946) that there are always droplets of oil, that is of the secretion of the tarsal glands, in these strips of fluid. This may take the form of oil drops or of a film of oil which may at times be seen spreading over the cornea as a typical coloured oil film. The amount of Meibomian secretion on the strips of fluid may be increased, sometimes to a startling extent, by the forceful closure of the eyelids.

When the upper eyelid is lifted away from the globe, the tear fluid runs up towards the upper fornix.

On tracing the strips of fluid at the posterior margin of the eyelids laterally, a veritable tear lake is seen at the lateral canthus. This reservoir contains more obvious fluid than the lacus lacrimalis itself, and is of great importance as it is one of the ways by which lacrimal fluid from the upper lid may reach the lower conjunctival cul-de-sac and the strip of fluid at the lower lid margin. Here, too, the fluid on the side of the skin ends in a sharp line.

The strips of fluid at the lid margins are continued medially between the lacrimal portions of the lid margins on the one hand and the plica and caruncle on the other. The sebaceous secretion of the caruncular gland performs here the same function as do the tarsal glands elsewhere. At least this is true when the eye looks laterally and usually straight ahead. When the eye looks medially a large space appears deep to the lacrimal portion of the lid margins, which now stand right away from the plica and (the lateral part of) the caruncle. The amount of recession of the caruncle varies in different people.

The actual capacity of the lacus lacrimalis is thus greatly increased, but it still contains only a little fluid. This is a thin film covering the plica semilunaris and the slight amount of fluid in the grooves on either side of it and in the little groove to the medial side of the caruncle. One would draw special attention to the fact that it is much more accurate to say that the puncta dip into the strips of fluid at the posterior lid margin than into the lacus lacrimalis. For if it were necessary for them to dip into the tear lake, as universally stated, they could not function in the adducted position of the eye when the puncta are in contact with the cornea, and any person with an internal strabismus would of necessity have a watery eye, which obviously is not the case.

The Conduction of the Lacrimal Fluid

From what has gone before, it becomes clear how one would suggest the tears reach the puncta (Wolff, 1946). Secreted by the lacrimal gland they pass for the most part into the lateral part of the upper fornix, whence they descend to the strip of fluid at the upper lid margin. They reach the upper punctum along this strip or directly under the upper eyelid. The tear fluid reaches the lower lid mainly at the collection of fluid at the lateral canthus and through the lateral conjunctival cul-de-sac. It also communicates at the slight amount of fluid to the medial and lateral side of the caruncle.

Some may also pass from the strip of fluid at the posterior margin of the upper lid to that of the lower at the moment of closure of the lids, and then some ducts of the lacrimal gland actually open into the lower cul-de-sac.

Now the tear fluid is limited by the sebaceous secretion at the mucocutaneous junctions. It will therefore inevitably fill the reservoirs above described. Among these is the inferior marginal strip into which the lower punctum dips. It is in this manner that Wolff suggested the lacrimal secretion reaches its efferent passages.

It will be noted that it has not been necessary to invoke the massage action of the orbicularis, due to its more mobile lateral portion being drawn towards its fixed origin on the medial side, nor to a *flow* of tears over the exposed portion of the globe. It is usually stated that the tears flow over the exposed portion of the globe to reach the lower punctum. But this process has never been observed and many explanations have been offered why it has not been seen. One would say that the reason why no one has seen the tear fluid flow across the eye under normal conditions is that it does not occur. Further, that it is actually prevented from doing so. The main mechanism which stops the tear fluid from flowing down over the cornea is, one would suggest, the oily surface layer of the precorneal film (see p. 240). This is aided by the fact that the upper cul-de-sac acts as a narrow tube, which is closed above.

It seems that if the tears did flow across the eye they could only do so in rivulets, as seen in an exaggerated form in crying, when the above mechanism breaks down with results disastrous for the refraction of the eye.

A thin film of tears is actually *spread* over the cornea by blinking, the upper lid acting in this manner like a swab.

Now we must consider how the tears:

        (a) Get into the lacrimal sac.

        (b) Are discharged into the nose.

The tears get into the canaliculi partly through capillarity, partly through the canaliculi becoming shorter and wider during contraction of the orbicularis.

The orbicularis is attached to the medial palpebral ligament, and this is attached to the sac. Hence, when the orbicularis contracts, the ligament is pulled upon and the lacrimal sac is *dilated* and so sucks in the tears.

Similarly, the lacrimal muscle is attached to the fascia covering the sac posteriorly, and when it contracts will also dilate the sac. We must, however, add here that some hold that this muscle has the opposite action, namely, that it compresses the sac to *expel* the tears.

The tears may be expelled from the sac by its elasticity. Hence, in those pathological cases in which the lacrimal sac has lost its elasticity (atony of the sac), the downward conduction of tears is arrested, although the nasolacrimal duct is quite patent (Fuchs, 1878).

The tears pass into the nasolacrimal duct rather than into the canaliculi, because the former has a wider calibre, and moreover the downward direction is helped by gravity and by any of the "flap-valves" of mucous membrane that may be present (p. 231).

The pumping action of the orbicularis is well seen in the blinking movements that remove excess tears. The one-way flow through the canaliculi and duct causes the lacrimal sac to act like a rubber enema syringe, sucking in fluid at one end (the puncta) and squirting it out at the other end (the inferior meatus).

CHAPTER IV

NORMAL APPEARANCES AS SEEN WITH THE SLIT-LAMP AND CORNEAL MICROSCOPE

THE CONJUNCTIVA

The Bulbar Conjunctiva shows itself as a transparent membrane in which the most striking feature is the vessels.

These form a superficial bright red anastomosing system which is easily distinguished from the more deeply placed reddish-blue episcleral vessels. The superficial vessels move with the conjunctiva, which occurs normally with each blinking movement of the lids. Usually it is impossible to distinguish arteries and veins.

Visible streaming of the blood in the vessels can easily be made out. Usually the blood-current has a somewhat granular appearance. But in the smallest vessels, especially at the loops, the blood-column is not infrequently broken up, and one sees clumps of red cells or even individual cells moving in a somewhat staccato manner.

At the limbus the conjunctiva joins the transparent cornea without a sharp line of demarcation.

The Palpebral Conjunctiva—seen by everting the lids—is smooth and transparent, and the corium presents a rich vascular network, in which one can distinguish a fine subepithelial plexus and larger vessels running at right angles to the lid margin, which are derived from the tarsal arches.

THE CORNEA

When the slit-lamp passes through the cornea it forms a characteristic prism, or more correctly a parallelepiped. In this we recognise four surfaces:

The anterior, corresponding to the epithelium; *the posterior*, corresponding to the endothelium; and the *lateral surfaces*, which form the areas where illuminated and non-illuminated portions of the cornea meet.

With a certain incidence the light may be reflected from the anterior and posterior surfaces of the cornea with mirror-like brightness, and give rise to what are called the anterior and posterior *zones of specular reflection*.

The Anterior Surface appears smooth, translucent, and on it can be seen tears, mucus and oil belonging to the precorneal film (but see p. 242).

The Stroma appears somewhat milky, and has a faintly reticular structure, which Koeppe thinks is due to lymphatics, a view which cannot be upheld.

The Posterior Endothelium can be seen quite clearly (in the posterior zone of specular reflection).

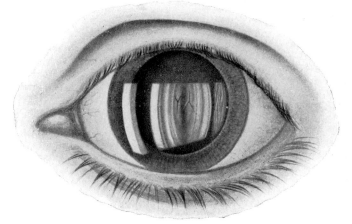

Fig. 231.—Optical Section of the Eye as produced by a Moderate Beam of the Slit-lamp.

The various portions are represented as being in focus simultaneously. To the left is the optical section of the cornea; then comes a dark interval representing the aqueous; next is the optical section of the lens with its bands of discontinuity and Y sutures; behind this the retrolental space is represented dark, while the vitreous is most posterior.

The cells appear slightly yellow in colour. They are mostly hexagonal, sometimes pentagonal, rarely square, and form a mosaic. Sometimes their nuclei may be visible. (Fig. 234.)

Near the limbus dark areas are seen in the mosaic. These are probably due to the (Hassall-Henle) warts on Descemet's membrane. (Fig. 232.)

Bowman's and Descemet's membranes are normally not seen, but become visible when pathologically altered.

The Line of Türck is a vertical line seen in children from 7 to 16 years old, and due to a deposit of leucocytes at the back of the cornea.

The Limbus appears as a transitional zone and has a dentate border. Its limits are not so well defined with the slit-lamp as with the naked eye. Here we find vascular loops placed between the brilliant tongue-shaped prolongations of the sclera. The blood-vessels which come from the conjunctiva and sclera have their connecting loops at the limits of the transparent area. Veins and arteries are distinguished with difficulty. The colour does not help much. Usually one can decide by the direction of the blood-current. But even this may be misleading. For the current

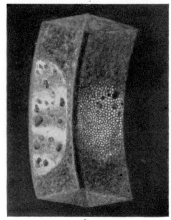

Fig. 232.—The Corneal Prism (Parallelopiped).

The light is coming from the left. In the anterior zone of specular reflection are tears and mucus; in the posterior zone one sees the endothelium and Hassall-Henle bodies (seen as black spots).

(*Modified from Vogt.*)

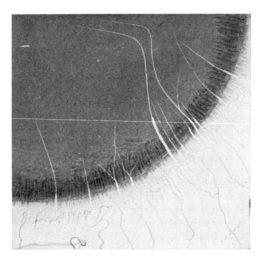

FIG. 233.—SLIT-LAMP PICTURE OF THE NERVES ENTERING THE CORNEA TO SHOW THE CHANGE FROM MEDULLATED TO NON-MEDULLATED PORTIONS.

in a certain vessel may be at times towards the cornea, at others away from it.

Sometimes a *palisade appearance*, which is due to whitish tracts derived from the sclera, is seen at the limbus, more frequently at its upper and lower parts.

The Corneal Nerves are easily seen. They are most numerous in the middle and anterior layers of the cornea. They appear as about thirty whitish filaments, which are better marked near the limbus where they still have their myelin sheath. The myelin always disappears before the first division of the nerve, which is usually dichotomous. The nerves never appear to inosculate. Not infrequently they present small nodosities, usually at a bifurcation (see Mensher, 1974, for a recent survey).

THE PRECORNEAL FILM (WOLFF'S VIEWS)

It is generally emphasised that the precorneal film does not consist of lacrimal fluid alone, but contains also the secretion of the tarsal and conjunctival glands. One would go further and say that although there is probably some slight admixture, each of these three main constituents must be thought of separately; that is, that the oily tarsal secretion, the watery tear fluid and the mucoid secretion of the conjunctival glands have each their special position and function.

As the upper lid moves down in the act of blinking, the marginal strip of tear fluid, with the oil on its surface, is pushed down over the front of the cornea. Above the lid margins is the perfectly smooth (see Cuenod and Nataf) surface of the tarsal conjunctiva, and jutting out from the mouths of the goblet cells are plugs of mucus (Fig. 205). Thus the tarsal conjunctiva, impregnated as it were, with the mucoid conjunctival secretion, forms an ideal polishing cloth for the cornea. As the lid descends, the tarsal conjunctiva

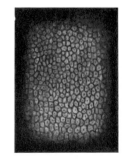

FIG. 234. — THE ENDOTHELIUM AT THE BACK OF THE CORNEA.

(After Vogt.)

passes down in close contact with the corneal epithelium, probably displacing as it does so the watery tear fluid, and then passes up again. In this action the conjunctival secretion is, as it were, rubbed into the corneal epithelium, and forms the deepest layer of the precorneal film. As the lid passes up also, the strip of tear fluid will pass up too, and will form a layer superficial to the mucoid layer. The oily layer remains superficial, floating on the watery tear fluid. It is as if a master artist, with a single down-and-up stroke of his brush, had laid on to the surface of the cornea three perfectly smooth and even coats of paint (Wolff owed this simile to his daughter).

As the lid passes up also, the small particles of the tear film are drawn up by the upper lid as a surface tension phenomenon, and come to rest when the movement of the lid stops.

The relation of the oily, sebaceous secretion to the tear fluid may be fairly accurately represented by placing on a glass microscope slide some water, and on this a minute drop of oil, and then drawing another slide backwards and forwards on these. The drop of oil spreads out into a characteristic colour film floating on the water. It will be seen that the movement of the slide can draw on this film for some distance.

A similar series of events takes place as, in the act of blinking, the lower lid passes up and then down. But these movements are, of course, not so extensive nor so important as those of the upper.

We see then that the precorneal film consists of three parts:

(1) The mucoid layer is deepest. One would suggest that it is this layer which Fischer says remains when closure of the eyelids has been artificially prevented until the cornea has dried. The precorneal film evaporates to a layer 0·05 mm in thickness, which remains constant in spite of further evaporation. Fischer points out that this layer has a composition different from that of the freely moving tears and more like that of the corneal epithelium itself.

(2) The watery lacrimal fluid forms the middle layer. It wets the eye and washes away foreign particles from the front of the eye. It contains most of the bacteriocidal lyzozyme and protein which is organ and animal specific (Ridley).

(3) The oily film is the most superficial. It greatly slows the evaporation of the watery layer deep to it which, owing to its great thinness would, one thinks, otherwise disappear immediately the eye was opened. One would suggest that it is the main mechanism which tends to prevent the tear fluid from flowing down across the cornea. Also the oily surface layer appears to be the fly-paper to which foreign particles adhere. They can thus, as described above, be drawn out of the way by the movement of the upper eyelid without affecting the layers deep to it, and still less the epithelium of the cornea itself.

It is clear that we may say with Treacher Collins and Rollet that the glands of the eyelids are essentially the glands proper to the cornea, which in the interests of vision have been moved out of the way.

CURRENT VIEWS ON THE PRECORNEAL FILM

Wolff's prescience is exemplified in the foregoing account, left *verbatim* from his own writings. Niels Ehlers (1965) has produced a well substantiated modification of Wolff's views, based on biomicroscopical and histochemical observations, and supported by persuasive theoretical considerations. The precorneal film is compressible and elastic. It has clinging properties that preserve its stability, and spreading properties that ensure clear vision immediately after blinking. The film is framed by the watery tears along the lid margins. If the margins are everted (as by an operating speculum) the precorneal film spreads, thins out and evaporates more quickly than normal. Ehlers cannot substantiate the separate layer of mucus that Wolff postulated deepest into the film, on the surface of the corneal

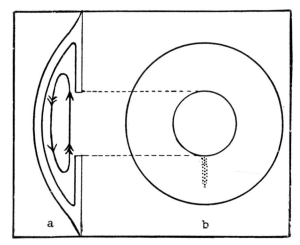

Fig. 235. — Diagram showing the Thermic Circulation of the Aqueous Humour.

On the left (a), sagittal section of the anterior chamber; on the right (b), frontal view. In b is seen the line formed by microscopic deposits on the posterior surface of the cornea.

(From Koby.)

epithelium. The aqueous film is about 10 μm thick and may perhaps contain the mucus dissolved within it. The aqueous film is sandwiched between a lipid surface layer of cholesterol ester and a deep layer of phospholipids which enter also the surface layer of living corneal epithelium. These enclosing lipid layers meet at the limbus; they delay evaporation of the imprisoned water. The two sandwiching lipid layers are derived from the tarsal (Meibomian) glands, and are spread into the precorneal film by the blinking lid margins.

Mishima (1965) is likewise doubtful about the presence of the mucous layer. He concludes that evaporation of the precorneal film produces a hypertonicity that makes water flow from the aqueous through the cornea.

The Anterior Chamber

The anterior chamber is almost, but not quite, optically empty. With the ordinary, broad slit-lamp beam, it appears quite black, but with a very bright, narrow pencil of light, especially if oscillating, a faint relucence along the path of light can be made out (the aqueous flare) (Graves). This is due to the fact that the normal aqueous contains very small particles which are not big enough to be resolved by the magnification used. When larger particles are present they are lit up like dust particles in a beam of sunlight passing across a darkened room.

Convection Currents.—The cornea is cooled by the air. The aqueous, therefore, behind the cornea is cooler than the aqueous in front of the iris. Convection currents are thus set up, the aqueous sinking behind the cornea and rising in front of the iris. Particles in the aqueous will follow these convection currents, which are no doubt responsible for the line of Türck (see Fig. 235).

THE IRIS

Embryologically and for descriptive purposes we may divide the iris into three layers: two anterior, which are mesodermal in origin, and a posterior, the retinal elements which is ectodermal (Fig. 236).

The structure of the iris is seen to differ widely in normal people, and this is essentially dependent on the amount of stroma pigment. The superficial layers of

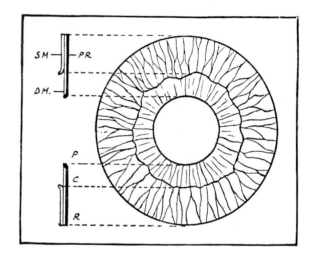

FIG. 236.—DIAGRAM SHOWING THE STRUCTURE OF THE IRIS.

The retinal layer appears at the edge of the pupil, where it forms the pigment border. The mesodermal layer is separable into a deep layer running from the root of the iris to the pupil and a superficial, the axial limit of which forms the collarette. SM = superficial mesodermal layer. DM = deep mesodermal layer. PR = posterior retinal layer. The crypts of the iris situated in the ciliary portion may be considered as openings distributed in the superficial mesodermal layer (anterior). P = pigment border. C = collarette. R = periphery of iris.

(From Koby.)

the blue iris which contains very little stroma pigment appear as a delicate diaphanous tissue, the fibres and trabeculæ of which look like transparent wool (Koby). The dark iris presents a more compact structure on which the vessels are not visible except at the crypts. The surface is smooth, and resembles tinder. Usually clumps of melanocytes producing yellow or brown patches can be seen; but the structure of individual pigment cells cannot be made out with the slit-lamp in the human.

The Superficial Mesodermal Layer is shorter than the deep, and extends from the ciliary border to the *collarette* (circulus minor), which forms a dentate fringe, separated from the underlying middle layer of the iris to a varying degree. It is this superficial layer which gives the ciliary portion of the iris its colour. In it one

finds the iris crypts, and looking through these and the underlying deep mesodermal layer one can, in slightly pigmented irides, see the dark posterior ectodermal layer. This latter becomes more and more difficult to see as the amount of
stroma pigment increases.

The crypts are bounded by the trabeculæ of the collarette, which are the
remains of obliterated vessels that passed to the pupillary membrane during
embryonic life (Lauber and Vogt).

The Deep Mesodermal Layer extends from the ciliary border to the pupillary
edge. In slightly pigmented irides it has a radial fibrillary appearance, and is transparent, so that the deeply pigmented ectodermal layer is visible through it.

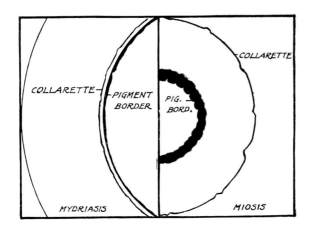

Fig. 237. — Diagram showing
the Relations of the Pigment
Border and Collarette and the
Variations in Thickness of the
former according to the Width
of the Pupil.

To the left, pupil dilated; to the
right, pupil contracted.

(*From Koby.*)

The Collarette (circulus minor) consists of a series of trabeculæ forming a rough
and broken circle, and varies greatly in form. To it are often attached remains of
the pupillary membrane (Fig. 450).

The anterior mesodermal layer is but loosely attached to the deeper one, and
glides freely over it. It does not participate to any marked extent in the movements of the rest of the iris. It thus comes about that, as the pupil dilates, the
pupillary edge approaches nearer and nearer to the collarette—so, when the
pupil is widely dilated, remains of the pupillary membrane may appear to arise
from the edge of the pupil when they are actually attached to the collarette.

There are other changes as the pupil dilates. The pigment ring showing at the
pupillary border is thinned and may disappear. There is a much more decided
step between the collarette, whose angles have straightened out, and the pupillary
margin; the crypts become oblique clefts. The vessels are more tortuous, the
contraction furrows and the peripheral furrows are deeper, and the border zone
disappears.

The vessels of the iris can be made out in non- or very slightly pigmented
irides. The radial vessels can be seen passing to the collarette and then following

one of its trabeculæ. They do *not* form a complete circle. Hence *circulus* iridis minor is not strictly correct.

The Sphincter Iridis can be seen if the iris contains little or a moderate amount of pigment.

The Ectodermal Layer, as pointed out above, can be seen through the crypts in slightly pigmented irides. Its edge is seen at the pupillary border as a fringe of pigment with a crenated margin. This is much better marked when the pupil is small, especially above. The slightest pupillary reaction is made manifest with the slit-lamp.

The dilatator puillæ and the nerves of the iris are invisible.

THE LENS

When the beam of the slit-lamp passes through the lens it is obvious that the portion lit up (the optical section) is not homogeneous. It is divided into a number of bands, some of which are brighter than others. These bands are called by Vogt the zones of discontinuity (Fig. 231). In adults ten bands can usually be made out. Of these, the anterior and posterior bands (of the lens), corresponding to the anterior and posterior surfaces of the lens, are the brightest.

The Fetal Nucleus, which represents the condition at birth, appears as two planoconvex lenses with a central dark interval, which is the most homogeneous portion of the lens and the part which has the least optical density.

In front and behind the fetal nucleus are the *anterior and posterior Y-shaped sutures*. The anterior Y is upright, the posterior is inverted (⅄), contrary to some anatomical descriptions.

The farther we go from the fetal nucleus, the more complicated do the sutures become. Around the fetal

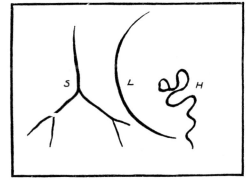

FIG. 238.—DIAGRAM SHOWING THE RELATION OF THE POSTERIOR Y OF THE FŒTAL NUCLEUS (S), OF THE ARCUATE LINE (L), OF THE INSERTION OF THE REMAINS OF THE HYALOID ARTERY (H) IN A RIGHT EYE.

The artery is found on the nasal side, separated from the posterior pole of the lens by the arcuate line, the concavity of which is turned towards the artery.

(*From Koby.*)

nucleus are the *anterior* and *posterior peripheral bands* of the fœtal nucleus. More peripheral still are *the anterior and posterior bands of the adult nucleus*, while beneath the anterior and posterior bands of the lens are the *subcapsular bands* or anterior and posterior bands of disjunction (Vogt).

The Anterior Surface of the lens does not appear homogeneous, but is somewhat irregular, and gives an appearance resembling shagreen (anterior lens shagreen).

At the *Posterior Surface* of the lens, as well as the anterior, there is a zone where the light is reflected vividly (*zones of specular reflection*).

In the posterior zone of specular reflection is seen the *Posterior Lens Shagreen.* It has a slightly yellower tint than the anterior. A marked polychromatic lustre in this posterior region is diagnostic of a complicated cataract.

A corkscrew-like remainder of the *Hyaloid Artery,* which moves with the movements of the eye, is often seen fixed by a whitish dot to the posterior aspect of the lens, just below and medial to its centre and in the concavity of the arcuate line (Fig. 238).

The Arcuate Line is a whitish crescent situated below and medial to the posterior pole of the lens. It is found by tracing the nasal branch of posterior Y till it bifurcates.

The Suspensory Ligament of the lens cannot be seen in the normal eye. When the lens is congenitally dislocated or absent, it may be made out as consisting of cobweb-like strands which are attached in front and behind the equator.

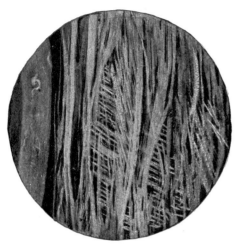

Fig. 239.—The Normal Vitreous Body of a Subject of Twenty Years, the Light coming from the Left.

On the left is seen the posterior band of the lens where the zone of specular reflection has been avoided. On its right the vertical bundles of the vitreous, and a second system of bundles chiefly horizontal and finer. Magnification about × 30. Figure slightly schematic.

(*From Koby.*)

THE REMAINS OF THE PUPILLARY MEMBRANE

1. The commonest form consists of a series of brown dots on the anterior capsule of the lens, usually near the centre, which, when seen with the slit-lamp, have a stellate appearance. These are finer than the remains of posterior synechia, which also when present in any quantity tend to be disposed in a circle.

2. Fine filaments arising from the collarette and branching in the anterior chamber are attached to the front of the lens, where they may end in white tufts or pass across the anterior chamber and be attached to another part of the collarette.

3. Thick cord-like remains which are usually associated with anterior polar cataract.

THE VITREOUS

Only the anterior third of the vitreous can be seen with the slit-lamp as ordinarily used.

Directly behind the posterior band of the lens is the "post-lenticular space", This, with the ordinary broad beam of the slit-lamp, appears optically empty. i.e. quite black (Fig. 231). The less the illumination, the deeper does the space appear. On the other hand, with higher intensities of illumination, faint fibrils can be seen crossing this space.

Comberg believes that the space is capillary only. No hyaloid membrane can be made out with the slit-lamp.

The anterior part of the vitreous appears as wavy milky folds of gossamer-like texture separated by intervals which are optically empty—the whole oscillating with the movements of the eye (p. 176). The folds appear to consist of criss-crossing fibrils. Small nodosities may be seen at the intersection of two fibrillæ.

In old age a powdery appearance in the vitreous is quite common.

BIBLIOGRAPHICAL NOTE

The most complete and classical work on Slit-lamp Microscopy is Vogt's beautiful *Atlas of Slit Lamp Microscopy*: Part I (1930) Cornea and Anterior Chamber, *Berlin*; Part II (1931) Lens and Zonule, *Berlin*; Part III (1942) Iris, Vitreous and Conjunctiva, *Stuttgart*, or (1941), in English, *Zurich*.

In English there are Berliner's Biomicroscopy of the Eye, 1943 and 1949, *New York*, Goulden and Harris's translation of Koby's Microscopie de l'Œil Vivant (Slit-lamp microscopy of the living eye) (in which there is an extensive bibliography), and Harrison Butler's An Illustrated Guide to the Slit-lamp, 1927; also Graves in Recent Advances in Microscopy (Churchill).

Other Standard works by:

Meesman, 1927, *Berlin*.

Lemoine and Valois, 1931. *Paris*.

Koeppe, 1920 and 1922, *Berlin*.

Gallemaerts, 1926, *Paris*.

Busacca, Goldmann and Schiff-Wertheimer (1957): *Biomicroscopie du Corps Vitré et du Fond de l'Œil, Paris*.

CHAPTER V

THE EXTRAOCULAR MUSCLES

THE *extrinsic* muscles of the eye are so called to distinguish them from the muscles inside the globe, the dilatator and sphincter pupillæ and the ciliaris, the intrinsic muscles, composed of nonstriated muscle tissue.

The extrinsic muscles of the eye are six in number: the superior, inferior, medial and lateral recti, and the superior and inferior obliques. In the case of

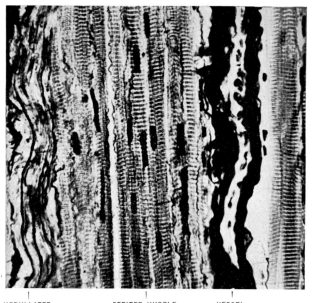

FIG. 240.—STRUCTURE OF HUMAN RECTUS MUSCLE. (STAINED BIELCHOWSKY.)

MEDULLATED
NERVE FIBRES

STRIPED MUSCLE
FIBRES

VESSEL

the superior and lateral recti their posterior ends are U-shaped, while in the inferior and medial they are linear and dentate.

The insertions into the sclera are made by glistening tendons whose fibres run almost entirely parallel to the long axis of the muscle. These fibres consist of collagen supported by thick elastic fibres. Apart from their size they resemble the scleral fibres, being made of the same tissue. But whereas the tendon fibres are practically all longitudinal, the scleral fibres run in many directions (Figs. 40, 63). This results in the tendon having a glistening silky appearance while the sclera is dull white.

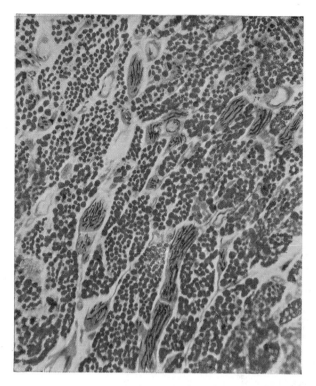

FIG. 241.—TRANSVERSE SECTION OF FIBRES OF A HUMAN RECTUS MUSCLE. (MASSON'S STAIN.)
Note the abundant nerve supply, visible in fascicles between the muscle fibres.

The tendon fibres enter the superficial layers of the sclera, and soon become indistinguishable from it (Fig. 63). Only the cessation of the thick elastic fibres marks the place where one begins and the other ends. Not infrequently one finds slips which leave the main tendon close to its insertion to be attached farther back. These recurrent fibres may be missed in doing a tenotomy (Motais).

Structure of the Extrinsic Muscles.—These muscles, as are those derived from the branchial arches, are more highly differentiated than any other muscles on the body in some respects. Instead of being grouped together in bundles separated by dense connective tissue, the fine fibres are but loosely united and hence easily separated by dissection.

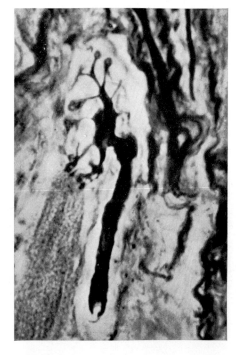

In the intervals between the fibres are unusually numerous nerve fibres (Figs. 240, 241). It must be remembered that each eye muscle receives a nerve which, compared with the size of the muscle it supplies, contains more fibres than other muscular nerves.

Each muscle fibre has a diameter of 9–30 μm, this being less than in other striated muscles. Each fibre is surrounded by a sarcolemma surrounding a granular sarcoplasm in which myofibrils may be seen. This gives the cross-section of the fibril a punctiform appearance. In such a section at least one nucleus is usually visible just internal to the sarcolemma. Each muscle fibre, or cell, is of course a multinucleated structure.

FIG. 242.—MOTOR NERVE ENDING IN HUMAN RECTUS MUSCLE. (STAINED BIELCHOWSKY.)

There are at least two, and perhaps more, types of muscle fibre in the extraocular muscles. Thin fibres (9–11 μm) form a less numerous group chiefly distributed peripherally and sometimes known as "slow fibres". These have grape-like motor nerve terminals. The largest group, the so-called "twitch" fibres, are of the order of 11–15 μm, and these have plaque-like motor nerve endings. There are also a small number of even large fibres, according to some observers, but most current experiment and theory is based on a dual population. The "slow" and "twitch" fibres exhibit considerable ultra-structural details in their endoplastic reticulum and tubule systems and they also differ in pharmacological responses. (Consult Davson and Bach-y-Rita.)

The connective tissue around the fibres constitutes the endomysium and

A.E.—17

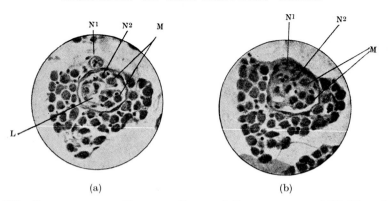

(a)   (b)

FIG. 243.—REPRODUCTION OF FARQUHAR BUZZARD'S ILLUSTRATION OF 1908. The original
description is as follows:

"PHOTOGRAPHS OF THE SAME SPINDLE AT LEVELS A SHORT DISTANCE FROM ONE ANOTHER IN AN OCULAR MUSCLE.
N¹ is an extrafusal nerve bundle which in (b) is being incorporated within the spindle sheath.
N² Intrafusal nerve fibres.
M Intrafusal muscle fibres.
L Lymphatic space.
Note the equality in size between the intra- and extra-fusal muscle fibres, and the thick sheath, with spindle-shaped nuclei."
(By courtesy of the Honorary Editors of the Proceedings of the Royal Society of Medicine.)

contains a large quantity of elastic tissue arranged longitudinally. Similar septa, but surrounding a number of muscle fibres, are called the internal perimysium.

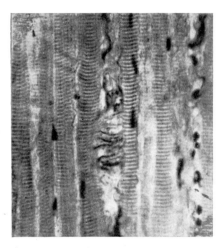

FIG. 244.—SPIRAL NERVE ENDING IN HUMAN RECTUS MUSCLE. (STAINED BIEL-CHOWSKY.)

This contains large elastic fibres, the vessels and nerves, and some connective tissue cells. The internal perimysium is continuous with the external perimysium, or epimysium, which surrounds the muscle.

These muscles are peculiar in the large number of nerve and elastic fibres which they contain. Schifferdecker believes that the elastic tissue helps the muscle in action, and regulates the give of its antagonist. This contributes to the making of the delicacy and smoothness of ocular movements. Apart from these mechanical reasons, however, the rich nerve supply (Fig. 241) is surely the main factor. Each motor neuron supplies relatively few muscle fibres.

The Sheaths of the Muscles.—From the origin for two centimetres the sheath is practically non-existent, being very thin and transparent so that the macro-scopic structure of the muscle is easily visible. From the level of the back of the globe it becomes thicker, opaque and disposed in two layers, the outer or orbital layer with circular fibres and the inner with longitudinal fibres. The inner is continuous with the internal perimysium.

PROPRIOCEPTIVE NERVE ENDINGS

Farquhar Buzzard (1908), described and figured muscle spindles in the eye muscles of man; he knew they were proprioceptive in function. For its historical interest, one of his illustrations is reproduced here (Fig. 243). Yet for many years this was overlooked and the spindles were not seen. For instance Woollard (1931) described fine nonmedullated fibres to the ocular muscles, seen in stained sections,

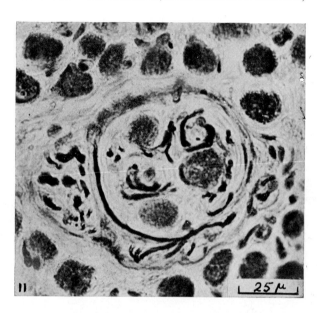

FIG. 245.—TRANSVERSE SECTION OF A MUSCLE SPINDLE IN A HUMAN MEDICAL RECTUS OCULI MUSCLE.

A well-defined capsule is seen with a nerve trunk incorporated in its wall (on the left). Within the capsule there are three intrafusal muscle fibres, capillaries and intricate arrangement of nerve fibres. One nerve fibre partly encircles the spindle, either just inside or within the walls of the capsule. (Paraffin section, Holmes' "silver on the slide" method.)

(*From Cooper and Daniel, 1949.*)

and he wondered if they were sensory—but he failed to see or mention muscle spindles. Daniel (1946), Cooper and Daniel (1949) and Cooper (1951) again described muscle spindles. They are, however, only found in certain regions. Forty-seven have been counted in one inferior rectus muscle. The muscle spindle found in the eye muscles of man is a smaller and more delicate end organ than the comparable structure in the other somatic muscles. Like its larger counterpart, it consists of a group of fine cross-striated muscle fibres with a rich nerve supply enclosed in a torpedo-shaped capsule of fibrous tissue. The capsule is thin, consisting of two or at the most three laminæ of fibrous tissue with characteristic flattened nuclei, and continuous from end to end of the spindle. The muscle fibres within the capsule, the intrafusal fibres, are usually of smaller diameter than the ordinary extrafusal fibres, generally 7 to 20 μm. They may end at the termination of the capsule but most often pass out to become continuous with an extrafusal fibre. The nucleus of the intrafusal muscle fibre is often central instead of being peripheral, as in the extrafusal type (Cooper and Daniel, 1949). Cooper (1951), using goats, recorded *afferent* impulses in the oculomotor nerve. The muscles are exquisitely sensitive, the inferior oblique registering at the order of 1 degree of rotation of the eyeball.

THE ACTIONS OF THE EYE MUSCLES

Movements of the eyeball take place round the centre of movement which corresponds approximately to the centre of the eye. The eyeball as a whole, therefore, is not displaced.

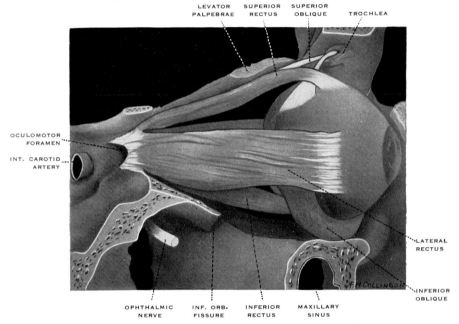

FIG. 246.—DISSECTION TO SHOW THE OCULAR MUSCLES FROM THE LATERAL ASPECT.
Note especially oculomotor foramen.

(From a specimen in the Anatomy Museum of University College.)

The movements may be resolved into those taking place round the three *primary axes* which pass through the centre of the movement, and are at right angles to each other (Fig. 247). These are:

(1) The *vertical* axis, round which the centre of the cornea moves laterally (abduction) or medially (adduction).

(2) The *transverse* axis runs from right to left. Round it the centre of the cornea moves either up (elevation) or down (depression).

(3) The *sagittal* or anteroposterior axis corresponds to the line of vision. Round it the so-called wheel-rotation takes place, better called medial intorsion or lateral extorsion as twelve o'clock on the cornea moves nasally or temporally. It will thus be seen that in naming the movements of the eye about

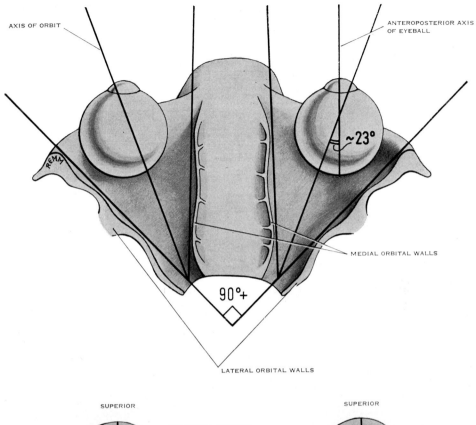

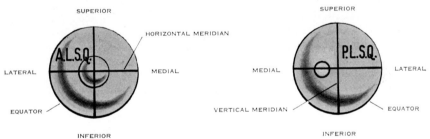

FIG. 247.—THE GEOMETRY OF THE ORBITS AND EYES.

In the upper diagram note the disparity between the orbital axis and the anteroposterior axis of the eyeball. See the text for the significance of this in explaining the actions of individual muscles.

(*Modified from* Gray's Anatomy, *by permission of Churchill-Livingstone and Longmans.*)

the transverse and vertical axes the centre of the cornea (or the pupil) is taken as the moving point, and will indicate in which direction the eye is made to look; while torsion about the anteroposterior axis is qualified from the direction of movement of the upper part of the vertical meridian or, what comes to the same thing, twelve o'clock on the cornea.

This is a necessary convention, for it is obvious that the posterior pole of the eye will go up when the anterior goes down and the lower part of the vertical meridian (or six o'clock on the cornea) will move laterally when the upper moves medially.

Each muscle has *primary, secondary*, and even *tertiary* actions.

The primary action is greatest when the eye is looking in a certain direction, while in this position the subsidiary actions will be least and vice versa.

Thus the primary action of the superior rectus is elevation, and is greatest when the eye is turned out, while the secondary and tertiary actions of adduction and intorsion are increased as the eye turns medially.

Synergic Action.—As elsewhere, extraocular muscles do not work in isolation but in groups of two or more, as synergists. Thus, the visual axis can only be elevated vertically by the synergic action of the superior rectus and inferior oblique, and depression must involve contraction of both the inferior rectus and superior oblique (p. 265).

THE FOUR RECTI

The four recti are attached posteriorly to a short tendinous ring (anulus tendineus communis of Zinn). This is oval on cross-section, and encloses the optic foramen and a part of the medial end of the superior orbital (sphenoidal) fissure, its attachment to the anterior margin of which is marked by the *spina recti lateralis*. The inner surface of the anulus is thickened in its upper and lower parts by two strong bands or *common tendons*.

The Lower Tendon (of Zinn) is attached to the inferior root of the lesser wing of the sphenoid between the optic foramen and the superior orbital fissure. This attachment may be marked by a tubercle (the infraoptic tubercle) (Fig. 1), a roughness, or a small depression. The lower tendon gives origin to part of the medial and lateral recti and the whole of the inferior.

The Upper Tendon (of Lockwood) arises from the body of the sphenoid, and gives origin to part of the medial and lateral recti and the whole of the superior.

Owing to the slope of the orbital roof the origins of the superior and medial recti are on a plane anterior to the others. *Also these muscles are much more closely attached to the dural sheath of the optic nerve* (Fig. 15). It is this attachment of the superior and medial recti to the nerve sheath which is responsible for the characteristic pain which accompanies extreme movements of the globe in retrobulbar neuritis.

With regard to their *length*, which is somewhere about 40 mm, the superior is the longest, then the medial, then the lateral. The inferior is the shortest. The recti extend anteriorly close to the walls of the orbit, and are inserted into the sclera well anterior to the equator by tendons of different widths and at different distances from the cornea. These will be discussed with each muscle, and will be found tabulated below:

	Distance from Cornea	Length of Tendon	Width of Tendon
	mm	mm	mm
Superior rectus . .	7·7	5·8	10·8
Inferior rectus . .	6·5	5·5	9·8
Medial rectus . .	5·5	3·7	10·3
Lateral rectus . .	6·9	8·8	9·2

THE SUPERIOR RECTUS

The superior rectus arises from the upper part of the anulus of Zinn above and to the lateral side of the optic foramen and from the sheath of the optic nerve.

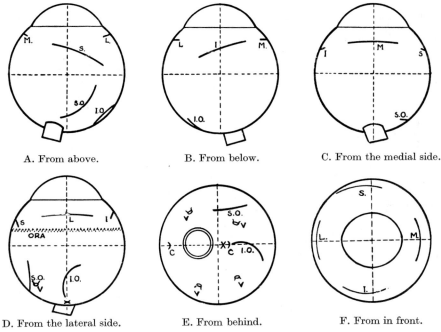

A. From above. B. From below. C. From the medial side.

D. From the lateral side. E. From behind. F. From in front.

FIG. 248.—To SHOW THE INSERTIONS OF THE EYE MUSCLES. (RIGHT EYE.)

X = position of the macula. C = long ciliaries. V = venæ vorticosæ. S.O. = superior oblique. I.O. = inferior oblique. M = medial rectus. L = lateral rectus. I = inferior rectus. S = superior rectus.

Note position of optic nerve. Its centre is just *above* the horizontal meridian. Note also that many authorities place the attachment of the inferior oblique clearly within the posterior inferior lateral quadrant.

This origin lies in the angle formed by the splitting of the dura which lines the optic canal to form the orbital periosteum (periorbita) on the one hand, and the dural covering of the nerve on the other. It is below that of the levator, and is continuous on the medial side with the medial rectus and on the lateral with the lateral rectus.

The muscle passes forwards and laterally beneath the levator, at an angle of 23°–25° with the visual line, pierces Tenon's capsule, and is inserted into the sclera 7·7 mm from the cornea by a tendon 5·8 mm long.

The line of insertion is oblique, 10·8 mm long, and curved so as to be slightly convex forwards. The muscle is about 42 mm in length and 9 mm in width.

Relations.—*Above* the superior rectus are the levator and the frontal nerve, which separate it from the roof of the orbit (Figs. 15, 278, 279).

Below is the optic nerve, but separated by orbital fat, the ophthalmic artery and the nasociliary nerve (Fig. 279). Farther forwards the reflected tendon of the superior oblique passes between it and the globe to reach its insertion (Fig. 246).

Laterally, in the angle between the superior and lateral recti, are found the lacrimal artery and nerve.

Medially, in the angle between the superior rectus on the one hand and the medial rectus and superior oblique on the other, are found the ophthalmic artery and nasociliary nerve (Figs. 279, 280).

RIGHT EYE   LEFT EYE

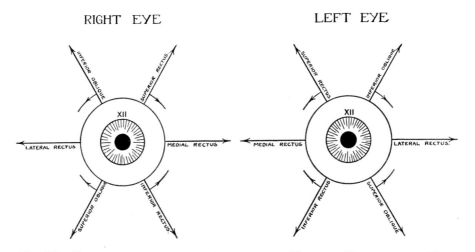

FIG. 249.—DIAGRAM TO EPITOMIZE THE ACTIONS OF THE EXTRINSIC MUSCLES OF THE EYES

The straight arrows show the direction in which the eye is made to look, i.e. towards which the centre of the cornea is moved. The small curved arrows indicate the direction of torsion, i.e. about an anterioposterior axis. Thus the medial and lateral recti make the eye look medially and laterally respectively, while the superior oblique makes the eye look downwards or laterally or causes intorsion (taking XII o'clock as the moving-point).

Note that the diagram only gives the possible actions from the position of rest; thus the superior oblique cannot depress the eye in the abducted position.

Nerve.—The superior rectus is supplied by the superior division of the oculo-motor nerve, which enters the ocular surface of the muscle at the junction of its middle and posterior thirds (Fig. 283).

Blood-supply.—This is from the lateral muscular branch of the ophthalmic artery.

Actions.—The superior rectus, acting alone, would rotate the eye from the primary position of forward gaze in such a way as to turn the visual axis upwards (elevation), and medially (adduction), and to rotate the eye medially around its anteroposterior axis (intorsion). What it accomplishes in reality is dependent upon the actual position of the eyeball and the activity of the other extraocular muscles.

The Primary Action is elevation, which increases as the eye is turned out, and becomes nil when the eye is turned in.

The superior rectus is, in fact, the only elevator in the abducted position of the eye, for the inferior oblique does not elevate the eye in this position. It thus comes about that in a palsy of the right superior rectus, if the patient is asked to look upwards and to the right, he cannot elevate his right eye beyond the middle of the palpebral fissure.

The subsidiary actions are the adduction and intorsion, which increase as the eye is adducted or rotated medially.

THE INFERIOR RECTUS

The inferior rectus is the shortest of the recti. It is attached below the optic foramen and to the middle slip of the lower common tendon.

It passes forwards and somewhat laterally along the floor of the orbit, at an angle of 23°–25° with the visual line, and is inserted into the sclera 6·5 mm from the cornea by a tendon 5·5 mm in length. It is about 40 mm in length and has an average width of about 9 mm.

The line of insertion is 9·8 mm long, markedly convex forwards, always somewhat oblique, so that the nasal end lies nearer the cornea.

The inferior rectus is also attached to the lower lid by means of the fascial expansion of its sheath (Fig. 282).

Relations.—*Above* are the inferior division of the oculomotor nerve and the optic nerve separated by orbital fat, and the globe of the eye (Fig. 282).

Lateral.—The nerve to the inferior oblique runs in front of the lateral border of the inferior rectus or between it and the lateral rectus.

Below is the floor of the orbit, roofing the maxillary sinus. The muscle is in contact with the orbital process of the palatine bone, but more anteriorly it is separated by orbital fat from the orbital plate of the maxilla.

The infraorbital vessels and nerve in their canal also lie below the inferior rectus.

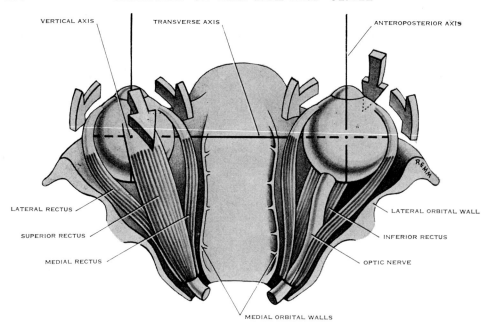

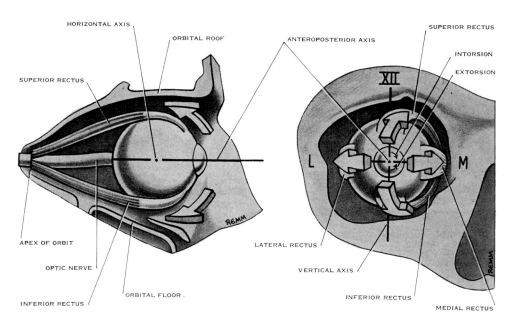

FIG. 250.—DIAGRAMS IN THREE DIMENSIONS TO EXPLAIN THE ACTIONS OF THE RECTI.
See text for details.

(*Modified from* Gray's Anatomy, *by permission of Churchill-Livingstone and Longmans.*)

The inferior oblique crosses below the inferior rectus, the sheaths of the two muscles being united here.

Nerve.—The inferior rectus is supplied by the inferior division of the oculo-motor nerve, which enters it on its ocular surface at about the junction of the middle and posterior thirds (Figs. 282, 283).

Blood-supply.—From the medial muscular branch of the ophthalmic artery.

Actions.—The inferior rectus, acting alone, would depress the visual axis intermedially with a slight degree of extorsion of the axis. By means of its fascial attachment to the tissues of the lower eyelid it also depresses this structure.

The Primary Action is depression, which increases as the eye is abducted and becomes nil when the eye is adducted. The inferior rectus is the only depressor in the abducted position of the eye.

The Subsidiary Actions are the adduction and extorsion, which increase as the eye is turned in.

The Medial Rectus

The medial rectus is in bulk the largest ocular muscle and hence stronger than the lateral. It has a wide origin to the medial side of and below the optic foramen from both parts of the common tendon, and from the sheath of the optic nerve. It is 40 mm in length and is thicker than the other extraocular muscles, though its strap-like belly has a similar width and length.

It passes forwards along the medial wall of the orbit, and is inserted into the sclera 5·5 mm from the cornea by a tendon 3·7 mm in length. The line of insertion is 10·3 mm long, is straight and symmetrical to the horizontal meridian (as a rule).

Relations.—*Above* is the superior oblique, and between the two muscles are the ophthalmic artery and its anterior and posterior ethmoidal branches and the posterior ethmoidal, anterior ethmoidal and infratrochlear nerves (Figs. 280, 283).

Below is the floor of the orbit.

Medially is some peripheral orbital fat, then the orbital plate of the ethmoid, which bounds the ethmoidal sinuses.

Laterally is the central orbital fat.

Nerve.—The inferior division of the oculomotor nerve, which enters it on its lateral surface at about the junction of its middle and posterior thirds.

Blood-supply.—This comes from the medial muscular branch of the ophthalmic artery.

Action.—The medial rectus is a pure adductor. Both muscles act together in convergence. (This statement is only strictly true when the eyeball is in the prim-ary position, i.e. with its geometrical anteroposterior axis in the horizontal plane and directed straight forwards. If the axis is elevated or depressed by the action of other muscles, the medial and lateral recti no longer exert a turning force purely around the vertical axis; they then have in addition a slight elevator or depressor moment, depending upon the position of the eyeball relative to the horizontal plane. Such moments must, however, be small, and their influence of unknown import. To ignore such possibilities, as almost all accounts do, is an over-simplification.)

THE LATERAL RECTUS

The lateral or external rectus arises from both the lower and upper parts of the common tendon from those portions which bridge the superior orbital (sphenoidal) fissure. It is about 48 mm in length, being longer than the lateral rectus; but it has only about two-thirds of the cross-sectional area of the latter.

This origin is continuous, and is strengthened by its attachment to the spina recti lateralis (of Merkel) on the greater wing of the sphenoid. The origin thus takes the form of the letter U (or V), placed so that the opening looks towards the optic foramen, the limbs of the U being referred to as the *upper* and *lower heads* of the muscle (Figs. 246, 263).

The lateral rectus passes forward along the lateral wall of the orbit, at first separated only by a small and variable amount of peripheral fat. More anteriorly, however, it passes inwards towards the globe, pierces Tenon's capsule, and is inserted into the sclera 6·9 mm from the cornea by a tendon 8·8 mm long. The line of insertion is 9·2 mm in length, is vertical or slightly convex forwards, and usually symmetrical.

The lateral rectus can, in the living, often be seen through the conjunctiva and Tenon's capsule (see also paragraph on the expansions of its sheath, p. 269).

Relations.—(a) *At the Apex of the Orbit.*—Between the origin of the lateral rectus and that portion of the lesser wing which separates the optic nerve from the medial portion of the superior orbital (sphenoidal) fissure is a small though very important interval.

The structures which go through it are described as passing between the two heads of the lateral rectus, within the cone of muscles or anulus of Zinn, or the interval is called the *oculomotor* foramen (Fig. 246).

These structures from above downwards are the *upper oculomotor division*, the *nasociliary nerve*, and a branch from the *sympathetic*, then the *lower oculomotor division*, and sometimes the *ophthalmic vein* or veins.

The abducent nerve is in process here of passing from a position below the inferior oculomotor division to one lateral to both and at a level between the two divisions (Fig. 263).

Above the cone of muscles, i.e. above the upper head of the lateral rectus, are the *trochlear, frontal* and *lacrimal nerves, recurrent lacrimal artery,* and the *superior ophthalmic vein*. According to Hovelacque (1927) these structures do not pass through the superolateral part of the superior orbital fissure, as is classically represented, since this is closed by dense fibrous tissue (Figs. 261, 262), and with this the author is in entire agreement. (See also the lacrimal nerve, p. 300.) Below the cone of muscles nothing passes as a rule, sometimes the inferior ophthalmic vein.

(b) *In the Orbit.*—*Above* the lateral rectus are the lacrimal artery and nerve. The lacrimal gland lies anteriorly. The lacrimal nerve runs along the upper border for almost its whole length, the artery only for the anterior two-thirds (Fig. 279).

Below is the floor of the orbit, and anteriorly the tendon of the inferior oblique passes below, then medial to the lateral rectus to gain its insertion (Fig. 246).

Medially, near the apex of the orbit between lateral rectus and optic nerve, are abducent nerve, ciliary ganglion and ophthalmic artery. Between the muscle and the inferior rectus is the nerve to the inferior oblique (Figs. 283, 285).

Laterally, it lies directly against periorbita in its posterior part (Figs. 15, 16), while more anteriorly a slight amount of perimuscular fat intervenes; farther forward still the lacrimal gland lies between it and the bone.

Nerve.—The abducent nerve enters it on its medial aspect, just behind its middle.

Blood-supply.—This is from the lacrimal artery, and from the lateral muscular branch of the ophthalmic artery.

Actions.—The lateral rectus is a pure abductor—that is, makes the eye look directly laterally in the horizontal plane. (See, however, remarks on actions of the medial rectus, p. 259.)

The Superior Oblique

The superior oblique is the longest and thinnest eye muscle. It arises above and medial to the optic foramen by a narrow tendon which partially overlaps the origin of the levator. Its great length is not, however, due to its muscle belly, but to the peculiar length of its deflected tendon.

The fusiform muscle belly, more rounded than that of the other extrinsic muscles, passes forwards between the roof and medial wall of the orbit to the pulley or trochlea of the superior oblique (Figs. 279, 280, 281).

The trochlea consists of a U-shaped piece of fibrocartilage, which is closed above by fibrous tissue, and is attached to the fovea or spina trochlearis on the under-aspect of the frontal bone a few millimetres behind the orbital margin. Through the pulley the tendon is enclosed in a synovial sheath, beyond which a strong fibrous sheath accompanies the tendon to the eyeball.

The muscle, about 1 cm behind the trochlea, gives place to a rounded tendon, which passes through the pulley, then bends downwards, backwards, and laterally at an angle of about 55° (the trochlear angle), pierces Tenon's capsule, passes under the superior rectus, and, spreading out in a fan-shaped manner, is attached obliquely in the posterosuperior quadrant almost or entirely lateral to the mid-vertical plane. The line of insertion is about 10·7 mm long, and is convex backwards and laterally. Its anterior end lies about on the same meridian as the temporal end of the superior rectus (Figs. 246, 248, A).

Actions.—The superior oblique, being attached posteriorly, elevates the back and hence depresses the front of the eyeball. It also would abduct and intort the eyeball if not modified in its activities by those of other muscles.

The Primary Action is the depression, and this increases as the eye is adducted. The superior oblique is the only muscle which can depress in the adducted position. This action is practically nil when the eye is abducted.

The abduction and intorsion are the *subsidiary actions*, and increase as the eye is abducted.

The superior oblique acts with the inferior rectus to make the eye look directly down. The abductor component of the action of the oblique muscles is due to their being attached to posterolateral quadrants of the eyeball with a line of pull posterior to the vertical axis (Fig. 251).

Nerve.—The superior oblique is supplied by the trochlear nerve which, having divided into three or four branches, enters the muscle superiorly and near its lateral border; the most anterior branch at the junction of the posterior and middle thirds, the most posterior about 8 mm from its origin (Fig. 279).

Blood-supply.—This is from the superior muscular branch of the ophthalmic artery.

THE INFERIOR OBLIQUE

The inferior oblique is the only extrinsic muscle to take origin from the front of the orbit; it is also remarkable in having the shortest tendon of insertion (Figs. 277, 282). This is inevitable if it is to have a muscle of sufficient length to match that of the superior oblique. Frequently, the muscle fibres are in part attached directly to the sclera.

It arises by a rounded tendon from a small depression (sometimes a roughness) on the orbital plate of the maxilla a little behind the lower orbital margin and just lateral to the orifice of the nasolacrimal duct. Some of its fibres may, in fact, arise from the fascia covering the lacrimal sac.

It passes laterally backwards, at an angle of about 50° with the visual line (that is, roughly parallel with the tendon of the superior oblique) between the inferior rectus and the floor of the orbit, then near to the lateral rectus to be inserted by a very short tendon (Fig. 84) (often none at all) to the back and lateral portion of the globe, for the most part below the horizontal meridian. The line of insertion is oblique, 9·4 mm long, and is convex upwards. (Different authorities present divergent views of this attachment; in the accompanying illustrations (Fig. 246) it is shown rather higher in the inferolateral posterior quadrant than would be expected if the muscle is to act as a true reciprocal to the superior oblique. See also Fig. 251.)

Its posterior or nasal end is about 5 mm from the optic nerve, *and thus lies practically over the macula* (only 2·2 mm from it (Poirier)) (Fig. 248, E). The anterior, temporal end lies in about the same meridian as the lower end of the insertion of the lateral rectus.

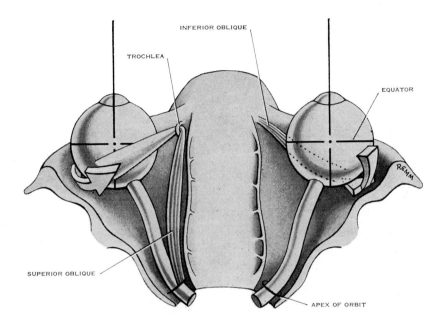

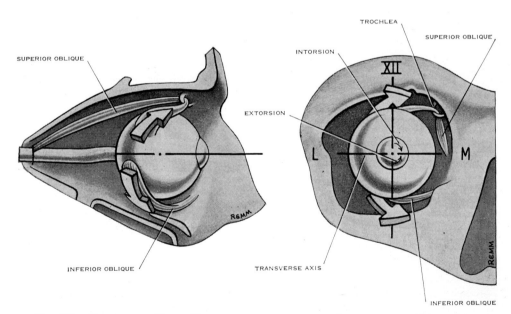

FIG. 251.—DIAGRAMS IN THREE DIMENSIONS TO EXPLAIN THE ACTIONS OF THE OBLIQUE MUSCLES.

(*Modified from* Gray's Anatomy *by permission of Churchill-Livingstone and Longman's.*)

Relations.—Near its origin the lower surface of the muscle is in contact with the periosteum of the floor of the orbit, but farther laterally it is separated from this by fat. Just before the insertion of the muscle, this surface which now faces laterally is covered by the lateral rectus and the capsule of Tenon.

The upper aspect is in contact with fat, then the inferior rectus, then finally spreading out and becoming concave it moulds itself on the globe.

Nerve.—The inferior oblique is supplied by the inferior division of the oculomotor, which crosses above the posterior border about its middle to enter the muscle on its *upper* surface.

The **Blood-supply** comes from the infraorbital artery and the medial muscular branch of the ophthalmic.

Actions.—The inferior oblique is primarily an elevator of the visual axis, for it depresses the *posterior* aspect of the globe. As in the case of the superior oblique, it pulls behind the vertical axis and hence abducts the eye. Because its line of pull is *below* the anteroposterior axis it also acts as an extorter.

The Primary Action is the elevation which increases as the eye is adducted and is nil in abduction. The inferior oblique is the only elevator in the adducted position.

The Subsidiary Actions are the abduction and extorsion, which increase as the eye is abducted and decrease in the reverse movement.

The inferior oblique acts with the superior rectus to rotate the visual axis upwards.

Ocular Movements (Figs. 247, 250, 251).

An extensive literature exists on the topic of ocular movements and the role of individual muscles therein. (Consult, for example, Alpern, Bach-y-Rita, Cogan, Duke-Elder, Davson, Schlossman and Priestley.) An elaborate analysis cannot be undertaken here, but the foregoing basic anatomical facts need adductd pansion.

For all practical purposes movements of the eyeball may be regarded as rotations, the globe being prevented from mere displacement by the resistance of the incompressible soft tissues which surround it and their relative fixity as a mass in the orbit by the multiplicity of connective tissue sheaths, bands, septa, capsules, etc. Each muscle, on its own, would rotate the globe to move its visual axis in the directions shown in Fig. 249. These movements appear complex only because we analyse them into movements around three axes, with corresponding linguistic complication. In reality, of course, no extraocular muscle normally acts alone, nor can it. If we disregard for the moment the integrative movements of two eyes, it is at once apparent that any rotation of an eyeball must alter the distance between the orbital and ocular attachments of all six muscles. Hence, in any movement some will be shortening and some lengthening, and there is abundant evidence (from Sherrington, 1905, to Szentágothai, 1943) to show that such adjustments occur in all six muscles. Such integrations are apparent in the wide-spread concept of "yoking" of muscles, both within one orbit and also in regard to both eyes in binocular coordination. Whatever truth there is in the clinical observations which support such limited views, it appears inescapable that all twelve muscles are exquisitely controlled as a total group in all ocular movements, with the constant feedback of vision to correct any vagaries leading towards diplopia.

If we turn to the actions of individual muscles and consider how they must be modified by each other, a comparatively simple concept of uniocular and binocular activities will emerge.

The medial and lateral recti are natural opponents, whose reciprocal contractions and relaxations swing the visual axis in a horizontal plane. (The visual axis can be displaced through about 45° from the primary "forward gaze" position in any direction. Thus the eye can explore approximately a hemisphere, if we can disregard such natural obstructions as the nose.) But we have already noted that both oblique muscles can act as abductors and the superior and inferior recti as adductors. Moreover, if these two pairs of muscles contract together to an equal extent, their tendencies to elevate or depress the visual axis and to intort or extort it are opposed and hence cancelled out. Thus, the medial, superior and inferior recti act as an adductor group, their abductor opponents being the lateral rectus and both oblique muscles.

Whether in conjugate (parallel) movements of the visual axes (as in scanning relatively distant objects) or in convergent (or divergent) inclination of the two axes to transfer attention from a distant to a proximate focus of regard (or vice versa), the movements of the visual axes are, of course, not necessarily in merely a horizontal plane. Consequently, the changes of tension and length in the pairs of muscles assisting the medial and lateral recti (the superior and inferior recti or the obliques) cannot always be equal, but must be so adjusted by complex neuronal control that the visual axis can, for example, incline smoothly downwards and medially, as in the common movement of transferring the gaze from the distance to objects held or manipulated in the hands. (Head and neck movements are, of course, also commonly involved.) The reverse movement can be carried out with equal nicety in preserving binocular vision. This is a reminder that *divergence* of the visual axes must be carried out with as much skill as *convergence*. Hence, any attempt to assign a particular mystique to the medial recti is misleading. Moreover, convergence movements, when the eyes rotate from the distance to an object to one side or the other, bring one medial rectus and the opposite lateral rectus (with their synergistic partners in each case) into an integrated contraction as precise apparently as in the more usual convergence towards the mid-field carried out by synergy of both medial recti.

With such basic principles in mind the student must thence turn to more detailed monographs for further analysis.

A.E.—18

The Levator Palpebræ Superioris

The levator palpebræ superioris arises from the under-surface of the lesser wing of the sphenoid above and in front of the optic foramen by a short tendon which is blended with the underlying origin of the superior rectus.

The flat ribbon-like muscle belly passes forwards below the roof of the orbit and on the superior rectus to about 1 cm behind the septum orbitale (that is more or less at the upper fornix or a few millimetres in front of the equator of the globe), where it ends in a membranous expansion or *aponeurosis*. This spreads out in a fan-shaped manner, so as to occupy the whole breadth of the orbit and thus gives the whole muscle the form of an isosceles triangle. The fleshy part of the muscle is horizontal, the tendinous part is nearly vertical, moulding itself on the globe of the eye, as indeed does the whole of the upper eyelid. The change of direction takes place above the reflected tendon of the superior oblique.

Attachments.—(*a*) The main insertion of the levator is to the *skin* of the upper lid at and below the upper palpebral sulcus. It reaches this by passing through the fibres of the orbicularis oculi (Fig. 191).

(*b*) *To the Tarsal Plate.*—Some of the fibres of the aponeurosis are attached to the front and lower part of the tarsal plate, forming an identifiable lamina important in surgical exposure of the plate; but the main attachment of the levator here is via the nonstriated *superior palpebral muscle*. This is continuous with the muscular part of the levator, and is attached to the upper border of the tarsus (Figs. 191, 192).

(*c*) The attachment of the levator to the superior fornix of the *conjunctiva* is actually via the fascial sheath of the muscle (see below).

(*d*) The two extremities of the aponeurosis are its *"horns"* (cornua). The *lateral cornu* passes between the orbital and palpebral parts of the lacrimal gland (Fig. 282), which is as it were folded round it, and plays a part in supporting the gland against the orbital roof. The lateral horn is attached to the orbital tubercle and to the upper aspect of the lateral palpebral ligament (Fig. 277).

The *medial cornu* is much weaker than the lateral. It is attached somewhat below the frontolacrimal suture and to the medial palpebral ligament.

The Sheath of the levator has several points of interest. It is attached below to that of the superior rectus (*q.v.*), and it is the tissue between the two muscles which gains attachment to the upper conjunctival fornix (Fig. 214). On the upper aspect of the junction of aponeurosis and muscle the sheath is thickened to form a band (Whitnall), the medial end of which passes up to the trochlea of the superior oblique and to the neighbouring bone and sends a slip to bridge over the supraorbital notch. The lateral end of the band passes above the aponeurosis, and is in part joined to it. Part of it passes into the lacrimal gland and part reaches the lateral orbital wall. Whitnall considers these the true check ligaments of the levator (see, however, Nutt, 1955).

Relations.—*Above* the levator and between it and the roof of the orbit are the trochlear and frontal nerves and the supraorbital vessels. The former crosses the muscle close to its origin from lateral to medial to reach the superior oblique (Figs. 15, 279).

The supraorbital artery is above the muscle in its anterior half only.

The frontal nerve crosses the muscle obliquely from the lateral to the medial side.

Below the levator is the medial part of the superior rectus (which, being the larger muscle, has its lateral edge exposed) and the globe of the eye (Fig. 279).

In front of the tendon at its commencement is the retroseptal mass of fat which is continuous with the upper and medial orbital lobe of fat. Below this the front of the tendon of the levator is in contact with the septum. Behind is the pretarsal space, containing the peripheral palpebral arcade (Fig. 191), and the palpebral portion of the lacrimal gland. The pretarsal space placed behind the tarsal insertion of the tendon is prolonged laterally behind the lateral horn of the levator and contains here the palpebral portion of the lacrimal gland.

Nerves.—(*a*) The *Superior Oculomotor Division*, which reaches the muscle either by piercing the medial edge of the superior rectus (and thus forming another bond between the two muscles) or by winding round its medial border.

(*b*) *Sympathetic Fibres* to the unstriated superior palpebral muscle. These autonomic fibres are probably the axons of neurons whose perikarya are situated in the superior cervical sympathetic ganglia of that side. The axons reach the orbit along the internal carotid artery, pass to the oculomotor nerve in the vicinity of the cavernous sinus (i.e. branch off the cavernous sympathetic plexus), and are distributed to the superior and inferior palpebral muscles along the respective divisions of the oculomotor nerve.

Blood-supply.—This is from the lateral muscular branch of the ophthalmic artery.

Action.—The levator raises the upper eyelid, thus uncovering the cornea and a portion of the sclera, and deepens the superior palpebral fold. Its antagonist is the palpebral portion of the orbicularis.

THE FASCIA BULBI

The fascia bulbi (capsule of Tenon) is a thin, fibrous membrane which envelops the globe from the margin of the cornea to the optic nerve.

Its inner surface is well defined and in close contact with the sclera, to which it is connected by fine trabeculæ. These opposing surfaces were held by Schwalbe to be lined by endothelium, the capsule of Tenon thus forming an articular socket, in which the eyeball moves freely in all directions. The joint cavity, too, was thought by Schwalbe to be a lymph space continuous behind with the lymph space surrounding the external coat of the optic nerve (supravaginal lymph space). But the capsule of Tenon is attached to the globe in front, to the ocular muscles, and to the sclera by the above-mentioned trabeculæ. It is probable, therefore, that while slight movements take place between the globe and the capsule, in more extensive movements the globe and the capsule move together in the surrounding fat.

The posterior surface of the fascia bulbi is in contact with the orbital fat, from which it is separated with difficulty. Anteriorly the fascia bulbi becomes thinner, and merges gradually into the subconjunctival connective tissue. It is separated

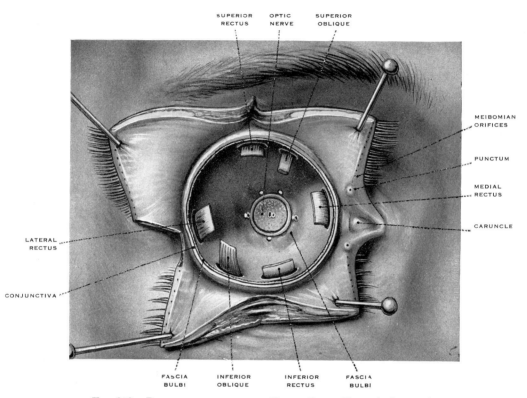

Fig. 252.—Dissection to show the Fascia Bulbi (Tenon's Capsule).
Details visible after removal of the right eyeball.
(*Wolff's dissection.*)

from the conjunctiva by loose connective tissue, and in operations for exposing the ocular muscles can be demonstrated separately from this membrane.

Posteriorly around the optic nerve, where it is pierced by the ciliary vessels and nerves, it becomes very thin, and can be traced only with difficulty to the dural sheath of the optic nerve, with which it is held to be continuous. Schwalbe, however, describes it as being continuous with a membrane which surrounds this sheath to form the supravaginal lymph space—a view which is now held to be very doubtful.

The lower part of the fascia bulbi is thickened to form a sling or hammock, on which the globe rests, and which has received the name of the *suspensory ligament of Lockwood*. That it is effective in supporting the eye is shown by the fact that the globe does not sink down after removal of the maxilla.

The fascia bulbi is pierced posteriorly by the optic nerve (Fig. 252), and around this by the ciliary nerves and arteries; just behind the equator by the venæ vorticosæ, and anteriorly by the six extrinsic muscles of the eye.

Where the fascia bulbi is pierced by the tendons of the extrinsic muscles it sends round each *a tubular reflection* backwards, which clothes it like the fingers of a glove. The reflections differ in the different muscles. In the case of the recti they gradually become continuous with the perimysium, but send important slips or expansions to surrounding structures.

The lateral expansion of the lateral rectus is attached to the orbital tubercle on the zygomatic bone, while that of the medial rectus passes to the lacrimal bone.

These expansions are strong and to some extent limit the action of the muscles. They have therefore received the name of *check ligaments*. (The advent of formalin fixation, which gave a big impetus to the discovery of fascial planes in the body at large, appears to have exerted similar influence in the orbit. "Check" ligaments are legion, and their functional significance is nevertheless generally uncertain and a matter of controversy. For a comparatively recent discourse consult Nutt (1955) for further details.)

The expansion of the superior rectus is attached to the levator palpebræ by a definite band, in which a bursa may be found (Motais). This band is said to ensure the synergic action of the two muscles. Thus, when the superior rectus makes the eye look upwards the upper lid is raised as well.

The expansion from the inferior rectus (Fig. 282) passes from the under-surface of this muscle above the inferior oblique, then deep to the conjunctival cul-de-sac and the palpebral conjunctiva, from which it is separated by the unstriated inferior palpebral muscle (which can sometimes be discerned through the conjunctiva), and then is inserted between the tarsal plate and the orbicularis. By this means the inferior rectus may act on the lower lid as the levator acts on the upper. The lower lid is, in fact, lowered 2 mm and pulled down by its action and the lashes tend to be everted. This movement is, however, aided by the lid being in contact with the globe.

The reflection of the superior oblique passes up to its trochlea, that of the inferior oblique to the lateral part of the floor of the orbit.

From the anterior end of the expansions of all the muscles, fibrous bands pass, to be attached to the conjunctival cul-de-sac. When the muscles act the conjunctiva is pulled back also, and thus is prevented from folding and strangulation, much in fact as the musculus articularis genu pulls the synovial membrane of the knee-joint out of the way in contraction of the quadriceps and prevents it being nipped by the patella.

The Nonstriated Muscles of the Orbit

The capsulopalpebral muscle of Hesser forms the peribulbar portion of the nonstriated muscle of the orbit. It almost completely encircles the eye, but is missing on the lateral side. It consists of superior, inferior and medial palpebral portions. Apart from the muscle of Müller there is no definite origin or insertion to the various portions. Also the fibres of any particular portion may run in various directions. *The Superior Palpebral Portion* consists centrally of the superior palpebral muscle of Müller. This arises from the inferior or bulbar aspect of the levator palpebræ just behind the fornix. Some 15 to 20 mm wide at its origin, it widens a little towards its insertion to the upper edge of the tarsal plate after an almost vertical course of 10 mm (Figs. 191, 253).

It forms a well-defined muscular layer which can be easily dissected, thus differing from other portions of the capsulopalpebral muscle. It lies in connective tissue and fat between the tendon of the levator in front and the palpebral portion of the fascia bulbi and the palpebral conjunctiva behind. It limits the pretarsal space (p. 188).

The Superolateral Portion of the nonstriated musculature extends from the lateral edge of the muscle of Müller to the orbital margin, becoming thinner and less defined. As it does so it divides into two layers which surround the palpebral portion of the lacrimal gland (Fig. 203).

The Superomedial Portion passes to the medial part of the upper border of the tarsal plate. Its fibres are feeble and placed in the fascia bulbi.

The Inferior Palpebral Portion consists centrally of the inferior palpebral muscle of Müller which passes from the ocular surface of the inferior rectus to the lower border of the tarsal plate. For the most part the inferior portion consists of fibres which are dispersed in that portion of the fascia bulbi which separates the inferior rectus from the inferior oblique. Anteriorly the fibres lie between the palpebral conjunctiva and the inferior portion of the septum orbitale in the palpebral extension of the capsule. The inferior portion of the muscle is more or less feeble, especially in its lateral part.

The Medial Portion of the capsulopalpebral muscle is the feeblest. The fibres lie scattered in the fascia bulbi and do not reach the eyelids. They stop about a millimetre from the medial fornix (Fig. 254).

Musculus orbitalis of Müller: for details see p. 22.

Surgical Considerations

From a practical point of view there are four spaces inside the orbit.

(1) Firstly, and most important, is that bounded in great part by the rigid orbital walls, but, anteriorly, by the eye and septum orbitale, including the tarsal plates and tarsal ligaments.

(2) Since the periorbita is for the most part easily detachable there is a potential space between it and the bone.

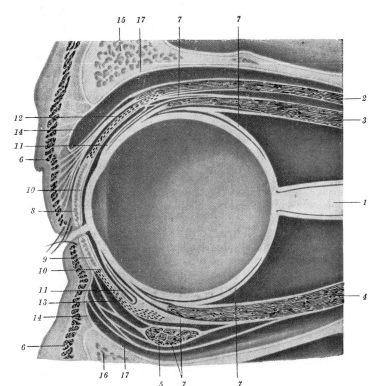

FIG. 253.—SCHEM-
ATIC SAGITTAL SECTION
OF THE EYE AND ITS
SURROUNDINGS.

1. optic nerve.
2. levator.
3. superior rectus.
4. inferior rectus.
5. inferior oblique.
6. orbicularis.
7. fascia bulbi.
8. superior tarsus.
9. inferior tarsus.
10. palpebral conjunc-
tiva.
11. bulbar conjunc-
tiva.
12. superior capsulo-
palpebral muscle.
13. idem, inferior por-
tion.
14. septum orbitale.
15. frontal bone.
16. maxilla.
17. periorbita.

(*From Eisler, after Hesser.*)

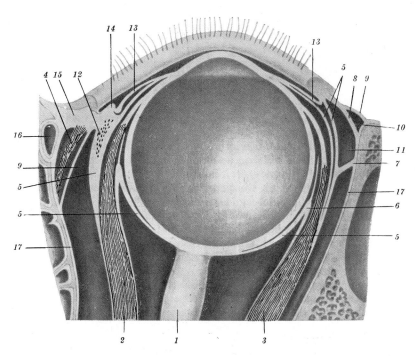

FIG. 254.—SCHEM-
ATIC HORIZONTAL SEC-
TION OF THE EYE AND
ITS SURROUNDINGS.

1. optic nerve.
2. medial rectus.
3. lateral rectus.
4. Horner's muscle.
5. fascia bulbi.
6. fascia bulbi.
7. lateral check liga-
ment.
8. aponeurosis of
levator.
9. septum orbitale.
10. superior recess.
11. recess for lacrimal
gland.
12. medial capsulo-
palpebral muscle.
13. bulbar conjunc-
tival
14. caruncle.
15. medial palpebral
ligament.
16. lacrimal sac.
17. periorbita.

(*From Eisler, after Hesser.*)

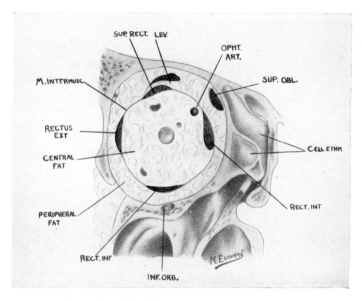

FIG. 255.—THE INTERMUSCULAR MEMBRANE.

Right side, posterior segment. The intermuscular membrane joins the recti and divides the orbital fat into central and peripheral regions. There is a recess containing fat under the levator.

(*From Poirier.*)

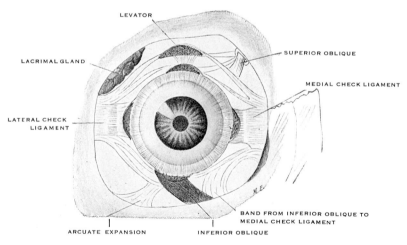

FIG. 256.—ORBITAL EXPANSIONS OF THE OCULAR MUSCLES.

Slightly schematised. The recti sectioned with their sheaths surround the globe and are united by the capsule of Tenon, orbital extensions of levator and superior rectus. Expansion of superior rectus to levator. Arcuate expansion of inferior oblique to floor of orbit. Check ligament from medial and lateral recti, strengthened above and below by superior and inferior expansions.

(*From Poirier.*)

(3) Inside this is the space bounded by the cone of muscles, the intermuscular membrane and the capsule of Tenon.

The intermuscular membrane (Fig. 255) is described by Poirier as follows: "The sheaths of the four recti muscles are joined to each other by an aponeurotic membrane, which becomes thinner as we trace it backwards and anteriorly is continuous with the capsule of Tenon. It is strongest between the superior and lateral recti muscles. In thin and feeble subjects it may be ill-marked, and hence is neither mentioned nor figured by many authors. At the posterior pole of the eye it separates the fat of the orbit into two layers, one central the other peripheral, and controls to a certain extent the progress of infiltrations."

From the above it follows that the muscle cone forms a separate space. Hence an exploration of the orbit outside it can have but little effect on a lesion situated within it. This is illustrated by a case described by Harrison Butler. The orbit was explored several times in a patient with proptosis and rigors and no pus was found. Later, on removal of the eye, the pus was found inside the muscle cone.

(4) The fourth space to be considered is Tenon's capsule, and Harrison Butler and others have recorded cases where a conjunctival incision has been effective in evacuating pus from this space.

The methods, then, that might be employed to relieve tension in the orbit are:

(a) An incision into the orbit outside the muscle cone.

(b) An incision into the orbit with splitting of the lid in a vertical direction and division of one or both tarsal ligaments.

(c) The division of one or other ocular muscle. This not only allows the eye to move farther forwards and so diminishes the pressure behind it, but also opens up the muscle cone and Tenon's capsule, and gives a good view of the back of the eye and anterior part of the optic nerve.

(d) Opening Tenon's capsule by a conjunctival incision.

(e) Temporary resection of part of the orbital wall as in Krönlein's operation.

THE ORBITAL FAT

The orbital fat compactly fills all the space not occupied by the other structures. Indeed, in formalin-hardened specimens it forms so firm a mass that excellent sections of the orbital contents can be cut with a razor by hand.

The orbital fat extends from the optic nerve to the orbital wall and from the apex of the orbit to the septum orbitale. Sometimes the fat pushes the septum in front of it, but never normally passes into the eyelids. The fat varies in its different regions in consistency and in the amount of connective tissue it contains.

The fat consists of lobules of different sizes enclosed in a capsule which is better marked laterally, where it forms a kind of sac for the fat (Charpy). From the capsule septa pass inwards and demarcate the lobules. The interlobular septa are soft, vascular and easily distended with œdema fluid.

The fat is divided by the intermuscular membrane into a *Central* or *intramuscular portion* and a *Peripheral* or *extramuscular portion* (Fig. 255). Posteriorly where there is no intermuscular membrane the two portions run into each other.

The Central Fat around the optic nerve is loose, no doubt to allow for movements of the optic nerve and the ciliary vessels and nerves in excursions of the globe. It is finely lobulated and the septa which surround the lobules are very thin; which make it easy to separate them from each other. In general the lobules are fusiform with the long axis parallel to the optic nerve. At the back of the globe the septa are inserted into Tenon's capsule so that if an attempt be made to separate the fat from the capsule, dentate processes remain attached to the latter. There is thus no space between the fat and the capsule, so that movement of the globe takes place only slightly in the capsule—for in excursions of any extent the fat moves also. Indeed, the capsule of Tenon may in part be regarded as the thickened limiting membrane of the fat.

At the surface of the optic nerve the central fat has a limiting membrane which separates it from the dural covering of the nerve. Between this membrane and the dura is a space traversed by septa which is the supravaginal space of Schwalbe. It is most probably produced by the movements of the fat and optic nerve (Charpy).

The Peripheral Fat is placed between the periorbita and the recti muscles. It is thickest in the region of the insertion of the muscles. It is limited anteriorly by the septum. This fat is covered by a thin transparent membrane which is united to the periorbita by feeble processes easily torn. In spite of its thinness, as long as it is not ruptured, blood passes between it and the periorbita to reach the deep portions of the eyelids, but not the conjunctiva. But if it is ruptured a subconjunctival ecchymosis is produced. Posteriorly the fat covers the recti muscles near their origin. The peripheral fat is situated in the intermuscular spaces and is in the form of four lobes (Winckler). The posterior portion of each lobe passes deeply to become continuous with the central fat, with which indeed it is united by numerous connective tissue septa. Anteriorly its deep surface is in contact with the intermuscular membrane and Tenon's capsule. Superficially each lobe spreads out to cover partially the two muscles between which it lies. The connective tissue membranes which surround the lobes are in contact with the sheaths of muscles and their prolongations, with the periorbita, and with the septum orbitale.

The Superolateral Lobe is placed between the superior and lateral recti. It just covers the edge of the superior rectus and is separated from the superomedial lobe by the frontal nerve. It covers the lateral rectus, especially anteriorly, while the lacrimal gland separates it from the septum.

The Inferolateral Lobe is placed between the lateral and inferior recti. Its lower border lies along the nerve to the inferior oblique. The lobe increases in thickness anteriorly and comes into contact with the inferior oblique muscle. It sends a prolongation to the septum on either side of the arcuate expansion of the inferior oblique.

The Inferomedial Lobe is placed between the inferior and medial recti. It also enlarges anteriorly and sends a prolongation to the septum on either side of the inferior oblique muscle. The remainder of the lobe is placed behind the expansion of the medial rectus to the posterior aspect of the septum, that is, it is posterior to Horner's muscle and the lacrimal sac.

The Superomedial Lobe lies between the superior rectus and levator laterally, and the medial rectus medially. It is partially separated from the periorbita by the superior oblique. Anteriorly this lobe has two prolongations. One passes under the trochlea of the superior oblique and then through the superomedial aperture for hernia of the orbital fat and so reaches the septum. The other passes above the trochlea through the superior aperture. Then it forms a retroseptal roll which lies along the anterior margin of the check ligament of the levator and the lacrimal gland.

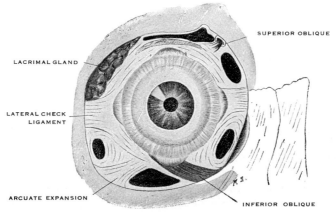

FIG. 257.—THE HERNIAL ORIFICES AT THE BASE OF THE ORBIT.

The eyelids and the septum orbitale have been removed, together with the fat which had herniated through the orifices.

(From Poirier.)

Although the dispositions of orbital fascia and adipose tissue present obvious importance in considerations of the extension of infections and in surgical operations, there is another aspect of these arrangements which is rarely, if ever, alluded to. Collectively these tissues provide a flexible suspension for the orbital structures, and in particular the eyeball. This must preserve an accurate relationsnip to its fellow, if binocular vision is to be maintained.

APERTURES AT THE BASE OF THE ORBIT THROUGH WHICH ORBITAL FAT MAY HERNIATE

If in a dissection of the eyelids the septum orbitale is carefully removed, one sees that the base of the orbit is partially closed by the globe surrounded by its muscles and the fibro-elastic expansions which these send to the walls of the orbit just behind its margins. These expansions and the two oblique muscles bound a series of orifices, five in number, between the orbital margin and the globe (Fig. 257). Through these orifices fat may herniate from the orbit to come into contact with the septum.

The Superior Aperture is in the form of a comma placed on its side. It lies between the roof of the orbit and the upper surface of the levator. The head of the comma, which is medial, is near the pulley and reflected tendon of the superior oblique; the tail reaches the lacrimal gland. Through this aperture fat from the superomedial lobe may herniate and form the retroseptal roll.

The Superomedial Aperture forms an oval with its long axis vertical. It is placed between the reflected tendon of the superior oblique and the medial check ligament. Through it passes that process of the superomedial lobe which is responsible for the common lobulated prominence in old people, which replaces the normal concavity of the region. Through this aperture pass the infratrochlear nerve, the dorsal nasal artery and the angular vein.

The Inferomedial Aperture is also oval. It lies between the medial check ligament, the origin of the inferior oblique, and the lacrimal sac. It is through this aperture that in those animals which have a third eyelid a mass of fat in relation to it passes (Charpy).

The Inferior Aperture is triangular and lies between the inferior oblique, its arcuate expansion, and the floor of the orbit.

The Inferolateral Aperture is small and lies between the arcuate expansion of the inferior oblique and the lateral check ligament.

In general these apertures form a communication between the cavity of the orbit and the deep portions of the eyelids. It is through them that blood and pus pass out of the orbit from the space between the periorbita and the peripheral fat. They reach the septum but are stopped by it (Charpy).

CHAPTER VI

THE ORBITAL NERVES

The Oculomotor or 3rd Cranial Nerve

Superficial Origin.—The oculomotor nerve arises by a series of 10 to 15 rootlets, for the most part from the sulcus oculomotorius, which lies on the medial side of the basis pedunculi. A small lateral component, however, issues from the neigh-

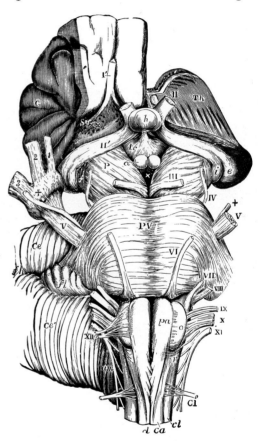

Fig. 258.—Ventral Aspect of the Brain-stem, showing the Attachments of the Cranial Nerves.

The following references apply to the roots of the nerves. I′ = right olfactory tract, divided near its middle. II = left optic nerve springing from the chiasma, which is concealed by the pituitary body. II′ = right optic tract; the left tract is seen passing back into *i* and *e*, the medial and lateral roots. III = left oculomotor nerve. IV = trochlear. V,V = sensory roots of the trigeminal nerves. +, + = motor roots, the + of the right side is placed on the trigeminal ganglion. 1 = ophthalmic, 2 = maxillary, and 3 = mandibular divisions. VI = left abducent nerve. VII = facial. VIII = eighth. IX = glossopharyngeal. X = vagus. XI = accessory. XII = right hypoglossal nerve; at *o*, on the left side, the rootlets are seen cut short. Cl = suboccipital or first cervical nerve.

(*From Quain's "Anatomy".*)

bouring ventral surface of the peduncle. The posterior part of this origin comes close to the upper border of the pons, near the termination of the basilar artery (Figs. 354, 355).

Between the two nerves is the posterior perforated substance.

The posterior cerebral artery runs along the medial side of the origin of the oculomotor nerve, then curls round above the upper rootlets (Figs. 354, 355). It often sends twigs between the rootlets of the nerve. The superior cerebellar artery runs below the origin at the upper border of the pons (Figs. 260, 355).

Course and Relations.—(a) *In the Posterior Cranial Fossa.*—Surrounded by pia and bathed in cerebrospinal fluid, the oculomotor nerve passes downwards and forwards in the cisterna interpeduncularis (Fig. 259), between the posterior

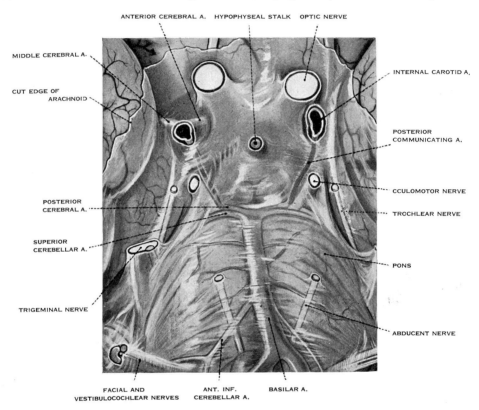

FIG. 259.—THE CISTERNA INTERPEDUNCULARIS AND CISTERNA PONTIS.

A portion of the base of the brain with the arachnoid *in situ* showing the relation of this membrane to the cranial nerves (II to VIII) and to the circle of Willis.

cerebral and superior cerebellar arteries (Figs. 260, 261). The cisterna interpeduncularis is the large subarachnoid space which is formed by the bridging across of the temporal lobes by arachnoid. It contains the cerebral peduncles, the interpeduncular space, and the circle of Willis (Fig. 259).

At first somewhat flattened in form it twists on itself, so that the inferior fibres become superior, and, leaving the arteries, soon becomes a rounded cord. It runs above and medial to the free margin of the tentorium cerebelli and trochlear nerve, and below and lateral to the posterior communicating artery (Fig. 260). It crosses the under-aspect of the optic tract from medial to lateral (Figs. 262, 317). Also above and lateral is the uncus (Fig. 321).

For about 1 cm, i.e. from a point just behind the posterior clinoid process to the point where the nerve pierces the dura, it is in contact with arachnoid.

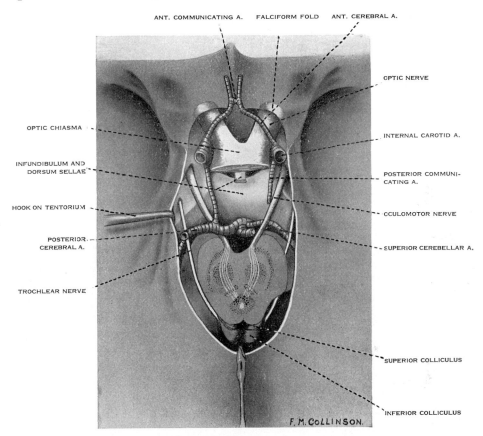

ANT. COMMUNICATING A.   FALCIFORM FOLD   ANT. CEREBRAL A.

OPTIC NERVE

OPTIC CHIASMA

INTERNAL CAROTID A.

INFUNDIBULUM AND DORSUM SELLAE

POSTERIOR COMMUNI-CATING A.

HOOK ON TENTORIUM

OCULOMOTOR NERVE

POSTERIOR CEREBRAL A.

SUPERIOR CEREBELLAR A.

TROCHLEAR NERVE

SUPERIOR COLLICULUS

INFERIOR COLLICULUS

F. M. COLLINSON.

FIG. 260.—THE OCULOMOTOR AND TROCHLEAR NERVES AND THE RELATION OF THE ARTERIAL CIRCLE OF WILLIS TO THE PITUITARY FOSSA.

The mid-brain is divided in the aperture of the tentorium, and the cerebrum removed. On the right side the posterior cerebral and posterior communicating arteries are cut short in order to expose the origin of the oculomotor nerve. On the left side the tentorium and cerebral peduncle are slightly separated so as to show the trochlear nerve more fully.

(From Quain's "Anatomy".)

(b) *In the Middle Cranial Fossa.*—The oculomotor nerve is lateral to the posterior clinoid process and above the attached margin of the tentorium cerebelli. It now lies lateral to the pituitary fossa *above* the cavernous sinus; then, piercing the dura about midway between the anterior and posterior clinoid processes close

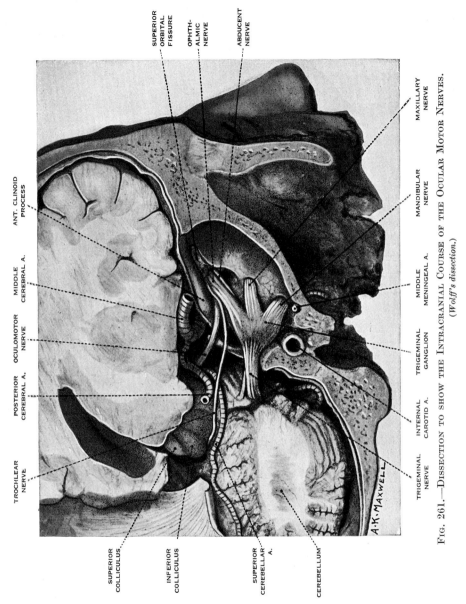

FIG. 261.—DISSECTION TO SHOW THE INTRACRANIAL COURSE OF THE OCULAR MOTOR NERVES.
(*Wolff's dissection.*)

to the prolongation forwards of the free margin of the tentorium cerebelli, it passes through the roof and so comes to lie in the lateral wall of the sinus (Figs. 261, 272, 274).

Here the trochlear and the first and second divisions of the trigeminal nerves are inferolateral to it from above downwards and the abducent nerve, and internal carotid artery actually in the sinus lying below and medial to it (Fig. 368).

In the lateral wall of the sinus the oculomotor nerve receives communications from the first division of the trigeminal and the sympathetic round the carotid artery.

The oculomotor nerve now enters the superior orbital (sphenoidal) fissure, but just before it does so it divides into a small superior and a larger inferior division, and about at this point the trochlear nerve crosses the oculomotor to lie above and then medial to it. The position of this crossing is variable. At the optic foramen the trochlear and trigeminal nerves may be inferolateral to the trigeminal.

At the anterior part of the cavernous sinus, too, the ophthalmic division of the 5th crosses the 3rd from below upwards, and just about this point divides into its three branches (Figs. 261, 284).

(c) *In the Superior Orbital Fissure.*—The two divisions of the oculomotor nerve pass through the fissure within the annular tendon, i.e. between the two heads of the lateral rectus (Fig. 263). They have the nasociliary nerve medial and between them, and the abducent nerve at first below, then lateral. The fourth, frontal and lacrimal nerves pass through the *wide* portion of the fissure above the anulus.

(d) *In the Orbit.*—*The superior division* inclines medially above the optic nerve and just behind the nasociliary to supply the superior rectus on its undersurface at the junction of the middle and posterior thirds (Figs. 280, 282, 283), and the levator palpebræ superioris. The branch to the latter muscle either pierces or curls round the medial border of the superior rectus.

The inferior division, much larger than the superior, immediately divides into three. These are the branches to the medial rectus, the inferior rectus, and the inferior oblique.

The branch to the medial rectus passes under the optic nerve to enter the muscle on its *lateral* or ocular aspect near the junction of its middle and posterior thirds (Fig. 283).

The branch to the inferior rectus pierces the muscle on its upper aspect near the junction of middle and posterior thirds.

The long branch to the inferior oblique runs along the floor of the orbit on the lateral border of the inferior rectus or between this muscle and the lateral rectus. It crosses above the posterior border of the inferior oblique about its middle, and breaks up into two or three branches which enter the *upper* surface of the muscle.

It is this nerve that gives the short stout branch to the ciliary ganglion, for relay to the sphincter pupillæ and the ciliary muscle (Fig. 281).

Communications and Varieties.—For the best accounts of variations in this and other nerves consult Quain (1900) and Hovelacque (1927). Communications between the oculomotor, abducent and trochlear nerves in the cavernous sinus are frequently observed (Sunderland *et al.*, 1946). The superior oculomotor division sometimes communicates with the nasociliary nerve. It may supply (in part) the superior oblique muscle, and it has been described as supplying the lateral rectus when the abducent nerve is absent. Its branch to the ciliary ganglion may be so short that the ganglion is sessile upon the nerve to the inferior oblique muscle.

SUMMARY OF THE OCULOMOTOR NERVE (Fig. 285)

The superior branch supplies:
    Superior rectus.
    Levator palpebræ superioris.

The inferior branch supplies:
    Medial rectus.
    Inferior rectus.
    Inferior oblique.
    Motor root of the ciliary ganglion.

Thus, the oculomotor nerve supplies all the extrinsic muscles of the eye except the lateral rectus and superior oblique, and also innervates the sphincter pupillae and the ciliary muscle.

NUCLEUS AND CONNECTIONS (see also p. 284)

The nuclei of the ocular motor nerves, except the part of the oculomotor which supplies the intrinsic muscles, belong to the somatic efferent nuclear column (Fig. 268) and are composed of rather large multipolar cells like those of the anterior grey column of the spinal cord.

Each oculomotor nucleus forms a small column of multipolar nerve cells some 10 mm long in the floor of the cerebral aqueduct at the level of the superior colliculus. Its superior extremity approaches the floor of the third ventricle, while it ends below on a level with the lower border of the superior colliculus.

Dorsomedial to each oculomotor nucleus is the adjacent central grey zone surrounding the aqueduct; ventrolateral to each is the corresponding medial longitudinal fasciculus (Fig. 263). Inferiorly, or caudally, the oculomotor nucleus is continuous with the trochlear.

Localisation within the Nuclei.—Punctate lesions within these small nuclei are rare; but localised vascular lesions are more common.

Exact localisation within the *human* oculomotor complex of nuclei is uncertain, despite the evidence of partial ophthalmoplegias. However, it is unlikely to be much different from the arrangement in other primates. While the evidence of such experimentation is in some details conflicting, there is nevertheless considerable accord in the results of these studies (see Warwick, 1956, 1964, for discussion). The major twentieth century workers in this field are Abd-el-Malek, (1938), Szentágothai (1942), Bender and Weinstein (1943), Danis (1948) and Warwick (1953); their papers should be consulted for details. For topographical accounts of the primate oculomotor complex of nuclei consult Tsuchida (1905), Le Gros Clark (1926) and Crosby and Woodburne (1943). The formerly accepted scheme of Brouwer (1918) (Fig. 266) has been shown by Warwick (1953) to be very different in the monkey. The formerly accepted scheme is reprinted here for its historical

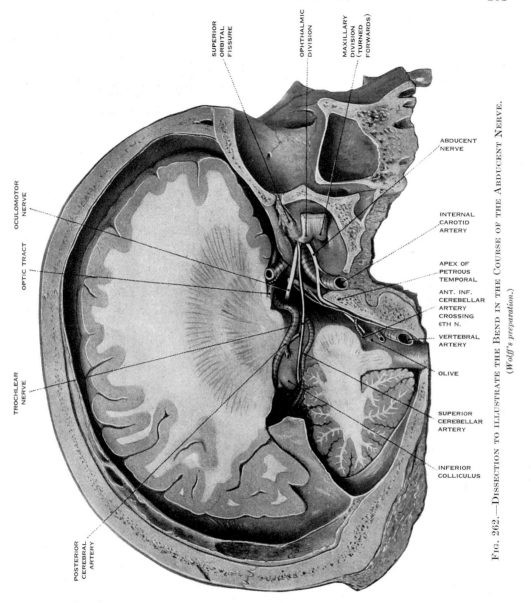

FIG. 262.—DISSECTION TO ILLUSTRATE THE BEND IN THE COURSE OF THE ABDUCENT NERVE.
(*Wolff's preparation.*)

interest only; it cannot be equated with modern work on the mere topography of the human oculomotor complex.

Localization within the Nuclei.—Former Ideas of the Two Nuclei.—The two third nuclei, taken as a whole, consist of five parts: two *main lateral* nuclei; an unpaired central *nucleus of Perlia* which unites the main nuclei and the paired small-celled *nucleus of Edinger-Westphal* situated anteriorly (Fig. 266).

A.E.—19

Modern topographical observations divide the *lateral nucleus* into *ventral* and *dorsal* columns, arranged rostrocaudally in the long axis of the midbrain. The *central nucleus* is absent from some primates, marked in others, variable and unimpressive in mankind. Its degree of development shows no close relation to binocular vision and convergence (Warwick, 1955). The accessory (Edinger-Westphal) nuclei fuse into a median mass at their superior (rostral) extremities, to form the *anteromedian nucleus*. At caudal or inferior levels there is a third midline entity, the *caudal central nucleus*, which is a much better developed mass of neurons than the intermediate median group, Perlia's central nucleus.

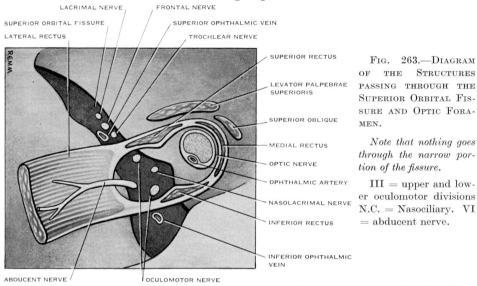

LACRIMAL NERVE
FRONTAL NERVE
SUPERIOR ORBITAL FISSURE
SUPERIOR OPHTHALMIC VEIN
LATERAL RECTUS
TROCHLEAR NERVE
SUPERIOR RECTUS
LEVATOR PALPEBRAE SUPERIORIS
SUPERIOR OBLIQUE
MEDIAL RECTUS
OPTIC NERVE
OPHTHALMIC ARTERY
NASOLACRIMAL NERVE
INFERIOR RECTUS
INFERIOR OPHTHALMIC VEIN
ABDUCENT NERVE
OCULOMOTOR NERVE

FIG. 263.—DIAGRAM OF THE STRUCTURES PASSING THROUGH THE SUPERIOR ORBITAL FISSURE AND OPTIC FORAMEN.

Note that nothing goes through the narrow portion of the fissure.

III = upper and lower oculomotor divisions N.C. = Nasociliary. VI = abducent nerve.

Despite these topographical views, which have been accumulated and refined over many decades, and which are epitomised in Fig. 267, a concept of motor pools (chiefly due to Bernheimer, 1897, and Brouwer, 1918) has been repeated from textbook to textbook (Fig. 266). This diagram, repeated once more here for historical interest, is patently out of accord with the topographical picture and has received little support and much disagreement either from Bernheimer's own contemporary experimenters or those of recent years quoted above. These outdated views may be stated as follows for historical interest only.

The Main Lateral Nuclei contain the centres for the motor nerves to the eye muscles. Each muscle is governed by a well-defined group of cells. These from cranial to caudal are *probably* levator palpebræ, superior rectus, inferior oblique, inferior rectus. The centre for the medial rectus (medial movement) is next to the median nucleus of Perlia.

The Central Nucleus of Perlia is probably concerned with convergence. Thus convergence and medial movement, whose centres lie close together, although often affected together, are not necessarily so.

The Nucleus of Edinger-Westphal probably subserves the pupillary musculature. It is paired and interposed anteriorly between the two lateral nuclei. It is composed of small multipolar cells of the preganglionic autonomic type.

The fibres from the cranial part of the third nucleus are direct, i.e. go to the muscles of the same side; of those from the caudal part some are held to be direct and some crossed.

Modern Views.—The foregoing paragraphs, though curiously vague—particularly as to the central nucleus—are representative of textbook reports until

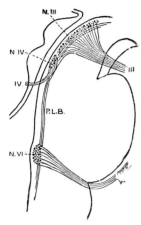

FIG. 264.—OCULOMOTOR, TROCHLEAR
AND ABDUCENT NUCLEI.

Sagittal section showing the nerves (III, IV, and VI) and their nuclei (N.III, N.IV, and N.VI). PLB is the medial longitudinal fasciculus.

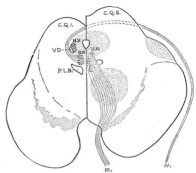

FIG. 265.—OCULOMOTOR AND TROCHLEAR
NUCLEI.

The mid-brain is divided transversely at different levels on the two sides, the section on the right side of the figure passing through the superior, and on the left side through the inferior, colliculus. V.D. = mesencephalic root of the trigeminal nerve. N.V. = its nucleus. C.Q.S. = superior, and C.Q.I. = inferior, colliculus. P.L.B. = medial longitudinal fasciculus. Other abbreviations as in Fig. 262.

comparatively recent years, and it must be noted that they are primarily based upon Bernheimer's experiments on monkeys and Brouwer's speculations upon a median control of convergence. Modern experimenters have substantiated little of these concepts, though their views do differ in some respects. All those quoted above (p. 280) agree that few if any radicular fibres cross before entering the oculomotor nerve. All agree in assigning little importance to the central nucleus. All agree that the accessory nuclei (Edinger-Westphal columns) are the parasympathetic component of the oculomotor complex. A more recent study of these arrangements, studied by retrograde degeneration technique in the cat, has been reported by Tarlov and Tarlov (1971). Their results largely confirm the findings of Warwick (1953), but with interesting differences, which suggest that the dorsoventral arrangement of motor pools may exhibit species peculiarities. These results also differ from the historical diagram of Brouwer and Bernheimer in according with the topography of the oculomotor complex.

Oculomotor Complex of the Monkey.—Warwick (1953) showed that a dorso-ventral rather than a craniocaudal organization exists (Fig. 267). Man has a relatively broader oculomotor complex than the monkey, but it is unlikely that the functional pattern is much different, since the topographical arrangement is basically so similar.

Levator palpebræ superioris is supplied bilaterally from the central caudal nucleus. The superior rectus is supplied from the opposite lateral nucleus (intermediate column). The remaining muscles are supplied ipsilaterally as indicated in Fig. 267.

The anteromedian and Edinger-Westphal nuclei are parasympathetic and supply the sphincter pupillæ and ciliary muscles, but it is still uncertain whether each muscle is supplied by one or both of these nuclei.

Course of the Fibres.—The oculomotor fibres pass with a lateral convexity through the medial longitudinal bundle, the tegmentum, the red nucleus, and the medial margin of substantia nigra, to emerge from the sulcus oculomotorius on the medial aspect of the basis pedunculi (Figs. 260 and 265).

Structure.—Like the abducent and trochlear the oculomotor nerve is large compared with the muscles it supplies. It contains about 24,000 fibres. Most of them are large, but some destined for the ciliary ganglion are small. Most of the fibres are motor and of relatively large diameter, but there are large numbers of fine fibres, some of which may be afferent and possibly trigeminal in the later part of their centripetal courses. Some of the finer fibres have long been considered proprioceptive, and since they were observed to be more prominent in the orbital part of the oculomotor nerve (Tozer and Sherrington, 1910; see p. 285), many subsequent workers have interpreted their experimental results as favouring the view that the proprioceptor fibres of the ocular motor nerves pass to the ophthalmic division of the trigeminal nerve to enter the pons. Boeke (1927) regarded the amyelinate fibres as sympathetic, but they are not affected by cervical sympathectomy (Hines, 1931). Woollard (1931) thought these axons to be proprioceptor. A voluminous and controversial literature has accumulated on this topic. The most recent reviews and experimental studies (unfortunately not easy of access) are the Ph.D. theses of Foster (1973) and Sivanandasingham (1973). The work of Winckler (1937), Cooper and her collaborators (1955), Bach-y-Rita (1964), Manni *et al.* (1967) and Batini and Buisseret (1974) suggests that species differences exist. The most recent studies cited above and those of Bach-y-Rita *et al.* (1964, 1971) indicate that in primates at least some of the ocular proprioceptive fibres enter the brain in the ocular motor nerves (see also p. 292).

The non-medullated fibres in the nerve were regarded by Boeke (1927) as sympathetic, but Woollard (1925) and others hold that they are proprioceptive in function and pass up to the mesencephalic nucleus of the trigeminal nerve.

Cross-sectional Anatomy.—The rootlets of origin of the oculomotor nerve soon join to form a single cord which is surrounded by a thin perineurium and well-marked pial sheath (Fig. 269). On section a few fine interfascicular septa and also a number of small blood-vessels are seen.

Along its course the nerve is intersected by numerous thick irregular septa from the pia, which, however, bear no relation to the future branching. In the cavernous sinus the superior division may at times be seen forming a cap to the nerve; but there is no regular method by which the inferior division separates into its branches (Sunderland and Hughes, 1946).

Fuchs placed the pupillary fibres in the centre of the nerve, drawing attention to the fact that the intrinsic eye muscles often escaped involvement in a fracture of the base of the skull.

Sunderland and Hughes (1946), however, hold that the pupilloconstrictor fibres, which vary in diameter from 3 to 5 μm, are concentrated over the superior arc of the nerve from the cavernous sinus to the mid-brain, and may, therefore, be affected alone in

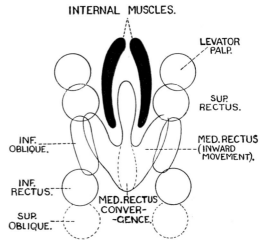

FIG. 266.—VENTRAL (ANTERIOR) VIEW OF THE OCULOMOTOR NUCLEI SHOWING MUSCLE REPRESENTATION. THE ACCESSORY (EDINGER-WESTPHAL) NUCLEI ARE IN SOLID BLOCK.

(After Bernheimer and Brouwer.)

pressure from above. It should, however, be pointed out that fine medullated fibres are scattered through the cross-section of the nerve and that they also occur in the trochlear and abducens.

THE BLOOD-SUPPLY OF THE OCULAR MOTOR NERVES

All nerves are supplied with blood vessels, which are essential for their normal functioning.

The arteries supplying a nerve are derived from adjacent vessels which most often are of small size and only of moderate regularity of position. On reaching the nerve the nutrient artery breaks up into ascending and descending branches which anastomose in the epineurium with similar branches from other nutrient arteries. From such epineural vessels branches penetrate into the perineurium, where further anastomoses occur, and finally small vessels penetrate into the fasciculi and form there a rich longitudinally disposed capillary network which runs up and down the nerve in unbroken continuity. This intra-fascicular network is reinforced along its length by contributions from the various nutrient vessels which reach the epineurium, *but no part of the intra-fascicular plexus may be regarded as being dominated by any one nutrient artery.*

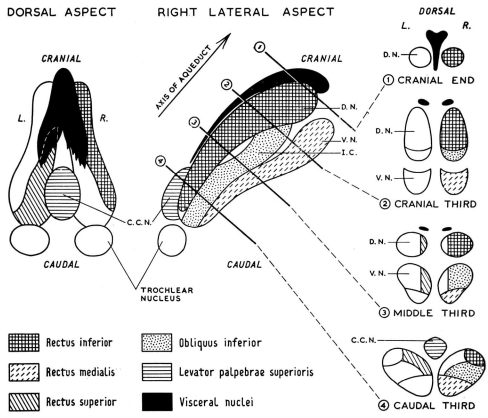

FIG. 267.—LOCALIZATION IN THE OCULOMOTOR NUCLEAR COMPLEX OF THE RHESUS MACAQUE
(AFTER WARWICK, 1953).

The entire complex, including right and left and median somatic nuclei and accessory (autonomic)
nuclei, is shown in dorsal and right lateral views, with representative transverse sections as indicated.
D.N. = Dorsal nucleus, V.N. = Ventral nucleus, I.C. = Intermediate column, C.C.N. = Caudal
central nucleus, L. and R. = Left and Right.

(*By courtesy of C. V. Mosby Company and the artist, Mr. R. E. M. Moore.*)

The blood-supply to the oculomotor, trochlear and abducen nerves is built on the same principle as described above. It is obvious (although not often mentioned as a cause of ocular paralysis) that deprivation of blood-supply to the nerves by spasm, thrombosis, or embolism may produce paralysis or paresis of the muscles supplied.

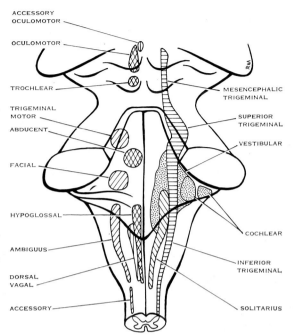

FIG. 268.—DORSAL PROJECTION OF CRANIAL NERVE NUCLEI.

Somatic and branchial motor nuclei are left of the midline, general and special sensory nuclei to the right.

PRACTICAL CONSIDERATIONS

1. **Paralysis** of the oculomotor nerve results in the following:

(*a*) Ptosis from paralysis of the levator.

(*b*) The eye looks laterally, due to overaction of the lateral rectus and superior oblique. Since the eye is in abduction, the depression due to the superior oblique is nil or minimal. There is inability to look upwards, downwards or medially beyond the midline.

(*c*) Intorsion occurs whenever the sufferer is asked to follow the examining finger downwards and laterally (overaction of the superior oblique).

(*d*) The pupil is semi-dilated, from unopposed action of the sympathetic, and does not react to light or accommodation.

(*e*) The patient is unable to accommodate with the affected eye.

2. *The Syndrome of Weber* is oculomotor paralysis on the side of the lesion with a facial paralysis and hemiplegia of the opposite side. The facial paralysis is of upper motor neuron type, the upper part of the face being spared. The syndrome is due to a mid-brain lesion, and involves the facial fibres and those of the trunk and limbs before their crossing.

The Syndrome of Benedikt is like that of Weber, but the hemiplegia is associated with tremors. These may be due to involvement of the red nucleus.

3. It is of interest to note that the oculomotor and trochlear nerves are more commonly affected by pituitary enlargements than the abducent nerve, because the latter is here protected by the internal carotid artery (Fig. 262).

4. The oculomotor nerve may be pressed on by hardening or aneurism of any

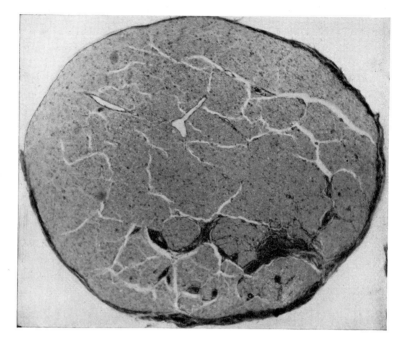

Fig. 269.—Transverse Section of the Oculomotor Nerve near its Emergence.

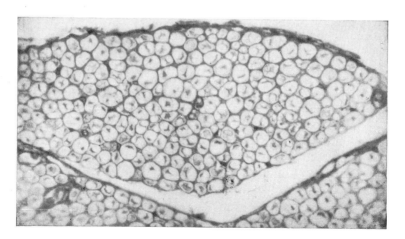

Fig. 270.—Partial Transverse Section of the Oculomotor Nerve.

nearby arteries; namely, the posterior cerebral, superior cerebellar, basilar, posterior communicating, and internal carotid.

THE TROCHLEAR (FOURTH CRANIAL) NERVE

The trochlear is the most slender of the cranial nerves and yet has the longest intracranial course (75 mm).

Superficial Origin (Fig. 271).—After having crossed from the opposite side in the superior medullary velum, which forms part of the roof of the 4th ventricle,

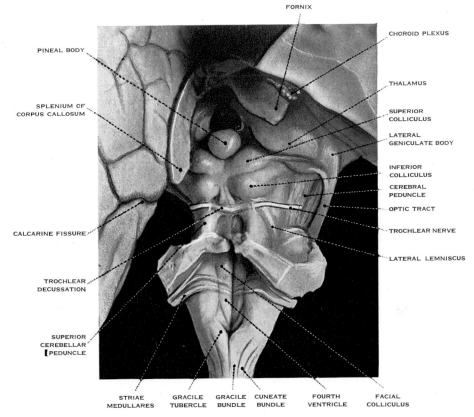

FORNIX

PINEAL BODY

CHOROID PLEXUS

THALAMUS

SPLENIUM OF
CORPUS CALLOSUM

SUPERIOR
COLLICULUS

LATERAL
GENICULATE BODY

INFERIOR
COLLICULUS

CEREBRAL
PEDUNCLE

OPTIC TRACT

CALCARINE FISSURE

TROCHLEAR NERVE

LATERAL LEMNISCUS

TROCHLEAR
DECUSSATION

SUPERIOR
CEREBELLAR
PEDUNCLE

STRIAE
MEDULLARES

GRACILE
TUBERCLE

GRACILE
BUNDLE

CUNEATE
BUNDLE

FOURTH
VENTRICLE

FACIAL
COLLICULUS

FIG. 271.—DISSECTION TO SHOW THE EMERGENCE OF THE TROCHLEAR NERVES.
(*Wolff's preparation.*)

the trochlear nerve leaves the upper part of this membrane by two or three rootlets medial to the superior cerebellar peduncle and just below the inferior colliculus. Its attachment to the velum is very delicate, and the smallest pull will often detach it from its origin. (Nathan and Goldhammer, 1973, have published a special study of the radicles of the trochlear nerve.)

It is the only motor nerve, cranial or spinal, which arises from the dorsal aspect of the central nervous system.

Relations.—(a) *In the Posterior Cranial Fossa.*—Here the nerve is in the subarachnoid space, immersed in cerebrospinal fluid. It is at first posterior to the superior cerebellar peduncle. In this part of its course it is crossed from below upwards by the branch of the superior cerebellar artery to the inferior colliculus. It now runs forwards at the upper border of the pons between and parallel to the posterior cerebral and superior cerebellar arteries (Figs. 261 and 262). It appears on the ventral aspect of the brain, between the temporal lobe and the pons (Fig. 259). At first inferomedial to the margin of the tentorium cerebelli, it soon comes to lie beneath and to be hidden by this membrane (Figs. 260, 318).

The trigeminal nerve, emerging from the lateral aspect of the pons just above its middle, passes forward below and lateral to the trochlear (Fig. 261).

The oculomotor nerve is above and medial, but since its direction is downwards and forwards, and that of the trochlear almost directly forwards, they approach each other as they proceed anteriorly, and as we shall see, eventually cross (Figs. 260, 261, 262).

Just before entering the middle cranial fossa by passing lateral to the dorsum sellæ and while still under cover of the free margin of the tentorium cerebelli the trochlear nerve acquires a very short covering of arachnoid which it loses again where it pierces the dura. In its course through the subarachnoid space it is at first covered by a prolongation of pial tissue, but this quickly yields to an adventitial covering.

(b) *In the Middle Cranial Fossa.*—The trochlear nerve pierces the dura in the lateral angle between the free and attached margins of the tentorium cerebelli, and then lies in the lateral wall of the cavernous sinus above and medial to the trigeminal ganglion and lateral to the pituitary fossa (Figs. 261, 262, 274).

Here the oculomotor nerve is at first above and medial, but just before it enters the superior orbital (sphenoidal) fissure, the trochlear nerve crosses it so as to be at first lateral, then above, then medial.

The first and second divisions of the trigeminal are below and lateral and, in the sinus itself, the abducent nerve and internal carotid artery are below and medial.

(c) *In the Superior Orbital (Sphenoidal) Fissure.*—The trochlear nerve enters the orbit through the *wide* portion of the superior orbital (sphenoidal) fissure close to its upper border above the cone of muscles with the frontal and lacrimal nerves which are lateral to it and the ophthalmic vein which is below it (Figs. 263 and 274).

The oculomotor, nasociliary and the abducent nerves and sometimes the ophthalmic vein pass through the fissure within the common annular tendon (of Zinn).

(d) *In the Orbit*, the trochlear nerve leaves the frontal nerve, which is at first close to it, at an acute angle, and passes medially and forwards beneath the periorbita (periosteum) (Fig. 278) and above the levator and superior rectus (Fig. 279). It divides up in a fan-shaped manner into three or four branches which supply the *superior oblique* on its upper surface near the lateral border, the most anterior branch entering the muscle at the junction of the posterior and middle thirds, and the most posterior some 8 mm beyond its origin.

Nucleus and Connections

The two trochlear nuclei are dorsally situated in the tegmental part of the midbrain, ventrolateral to the cerebral aqueduct (of Sylvius), dorsal to the medial longitudinal bundles (in which they are almost embedded), and on a level corresponding to the superior part of the inferior colliculus (Figs. 264, 265).

Like the oculomotor nucleus, with which each is continuous above, they are the upward continuation of the base of the anterior cornua of the spinal cord.

From each nucleus the nerve fibres run first laterally to reach the medial surface of the mesencephalic root of the trigeminal nerve, then downwards parallel to the aqueduct, then at the lower border of the inferior colliculus they pass medially to decussate completely (or almost so) in the superior medullary velum. The trochlear nerve crosses to the opposite side, and thus each superior oblique is supplied from the contralateral trochlear nucleus. The fibres emerge at the medial aspect of the superior cerebral peduncle.

For central connections see oculomotor nerve (p. 280).

The trochlear neurons are relatively densely staining cells, as showed by basophilic dyes. They are, of course, multipolar, with average dimensions of 40–50 μm. The existence of other nerve cells, possibly interneurons, within or near the trochlear nucleus is a matter of debate. Extrinsic connections are corticobulbar, tectobulbar, and (via the medial longitudinal fasciculus) with various other brainstem nuclei, such as the oculomotor, abducent, vestibular, and possibly others.

There is frequently a small *accessory trochlear nucleus*, caudal (inferior) to the main nucleus.

A proprioceptor component has long been ascribed to the trochlear nerve conducting in pulses from stretch endings in the superior oblique muscle (see Crosby *et al.*, 1962, for discussion of this evidence).

Communications and Varieties

1. While in the lateral wall of the cavernous sinus the trochlear nerve is connected with the sympathetic on the carotid artery, and is joined by a filament possibly containing proprioceptive fibres passing to the ophthalmic division.

2. In one case the trochlear nerve pierced the levator on its way to the superior oblique (Thane).

3. The nerve has been observed in several cases sending a branch forward to the orbicularis oculi, or to join the supratrochlear, the infratrochlear or the nasociliary nerve (Thane).

4. A communication with the frontal nerve is recorded by Berte (Thane).

Consult Quain (1900) and Hovelacque (1927) for further details.

Structure.—The trochlear nerve consists of about 3400 fibres, mostly of large size. (Björkman and Wohlfart, 1936). It also shows close to its origin the vestiges of a degenerated ganglion (Gaskell). See oculomotor nerve (p. 284).

One investigation of human trochlear nerves (Zaki, 1960) showed the nerve to comprise 2400 fibres only, proximal to the cavernous sinus, and 3500 distal to it; this suggests that a large contingent of fibres (observed to be of fairly large diameter), possibly of proprioceptive function, may leave the nerve peripherally perhaps to join the trigemina. Such peripheral communications in the vicinity of the cavernous sinus have, however, been denied by Sunderland and Hughes (1946).

PRACTICAL CONSIDERATIONS

Paralysis of the trochlear nerve produces paralysis of the superior oblique muscle. This results in:

(a) The greatest limitation of movement is seen when, in the adducted position, the patient is asked to look downwards. This is because the superior oblique is only depressor in the adducted position.

(b) The face is turned downwards and towards the sound side.

(c) Diplopia occurs on looking downwards, and is homonymous.

The false image is below, and its upper end is tilted towards the true image, i.e. in the direction of action of the paralysed muscle.

THE ABDUCENT (SIXTH CRANIAL) NERVE

Superficial Origin.—The abducent nerve emerges between the lower border of the pons and the lateral part of the pyramid by seven or eight rootlets, some of which may actually pierce the pons. Unlike the rootlets of the oculomotor and trochlear nerves, which very soon join up to form a common trunk, those of the abducent join up at varying distances from their origin and some may remain separate (Fig. 273) till the nerve pierces the dura.

Course.—It passes upwards, forwards, and slightly laterally in the posterior cranial fossa to pierce the dura lateral to the dorsum sellæ; then runs upwards under this membrane on the back of the petrous temporal near its apex, then forwards through the cavernous sinus. Finally it passes into the orbit through the superior orbital fissure within the annular tendon to supply the lateral rectus muscle. (For variations, consult Nathan et al., 1974.)

Relations.—(a) At its Origin.—The two abducent nerves are about 1 cm apart at their superficial origin, and between them lies the basilar artery at its formation from the two vertebrals. Sometimes an asymmetrical vertebral artery may curve upwards and lie under the nerve. Lateral to it is the origin of the facial nerve to the lateral side of the olive (Figs. 258, 354, 355).

(b) *In the Posterior Cranial Fossa.*—The nerve, at first flat and fasciculated, soon becomes rounded and firmer. Covered by pia it passes upwards, forwards and slightly laterally in the cisterna pontis of the subarachnoid space (Fig. 259) between the pons and the occipital bone (Fig. 261). After a course of 15 mm it pierces the dura at the back of the basilar portion of the occipital bone about

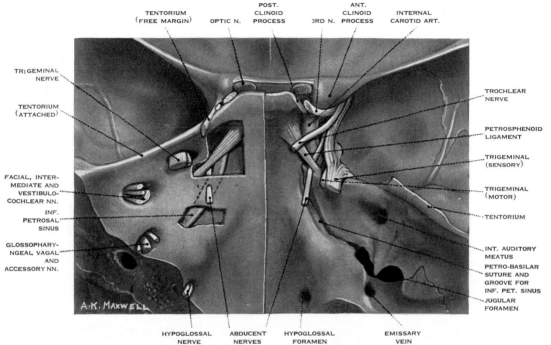

FIG. 272.—DISSECTION TO SHOW RELATIONS OF ABDUCENT NERVE TO THE PETROUS TEMPORAL, INFERIOR PETROSAL SINUS, ETC.

On the right side dura mater has been removed to show osseous relations.

(*Wolff's dissection.*)

2 cm below and slightly to the lateral side of the posterior clinoid process, and just to the medial side of or posterior to the inferior petrosal sinus which lies in the petrobasilar suture (Fig. 272). The sphenobasilar suture is about 1·5 cm from the lip of the dorsum sellæ. Hence the abducent nerve pierces the dura opposite the *occipital* bone.

It is plastered to the pons by the arachnoid (Fig. 259), but does not receive a complete covering of this membrane till a few millimetres from the dural opening.

Just beyond its origin it is crossed by the anterior inferior cerebellar artery (Figs. 262, 273). Usually, i.e. in over four-fifths of the cases, the artery is ventral, but it may be dorsal or pass between the rootlets of the nerve (Stopford, 1916, 1917). The oculomotor, trochlear and trigeminal nerves are above, but are gradu-

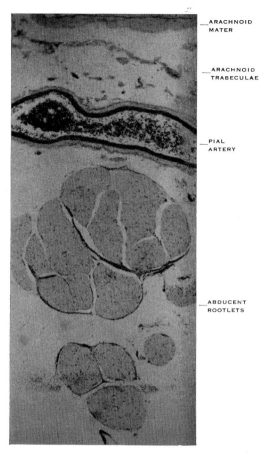

ARACHNOID
MATER

ARACHNOID
TRABECULAE

PIAL
ARTERY

ABDUCENT
ROOTLETS

Fig. 273.—Relation of 6th Nerve to Arachnoid
and Anterior-Inferior Cerebellar Artery.

The abducent rootlets are unlimited here.

ally approaching the abducent as they pass forwards towards the middle cranial fossa.

The abducent nerve passes inferior to the inferior petrosal sinus in an anterolateral direction, and runs almost vertically up the back of the petrous temporal near its apex. It is placed and held here in a groove (Hovelacque, 1927) which has a very variable appearance. Having arrived at the sharp upper border of the bone, it bends forwards practically at a right angle under the petrosphenoidal ligament (of Grüber) and under the superior petrosal sinus to enter the cavernous sinus (Figs. 262, 272). The abducens nerve and the inferior petrosal sinus enter the sinus together by an opening (Fig. 272). Commonly the abducent nerve pierces the inferior petrosal sinus, inside which it then runs to enter the cavernous sinus.

(c) *In the Cavernous Sinus.*—In the sinus the abducent nerve runs almost horizontally forwards. In the posterior part of the sinus the nerve winds round the lateral aspect of the ascending portion of the internal carotid artery, thus making a *second* bend, this time, however, with a lateral convexity (Fig. 272). This second bend varies greatly. It may be very slight, the ascending portion of the internal carotid just pushing the nerve slightly laterally, or it may (as Wolff saw in one case) approach the right angle.

Farther forwards the abducens lies below and lateral to the horizontal portion of the artery (Figs. 262, 368).

The carotid is here surrounded by a sympathetic plexus, which may communicate with the abducent nerve.

In the lateral wall of the sinus from above down are the third, fourth and first, and second divisions of the trigeminal nerves (Fig. 368).

Usually the abducens lies actually in the sinus surrounded by a separate sheath, but it may be adherent to the lateral wall or attached to it by a septum of fibrous dura mater.

Outside the lateral wall of the sinus is the trigeminal ganglion (Figs. 272, 274).

(d) *In the Superior Orbital Fissure.*—The abducent nerve is placed here within the anulus of Zinn, at first below the two divisions of the oculomotor nerve, then lateral and in between the two. The nasociliary is medial (Fig. 263).

(e) *In the Orbit.*—The nerve divides into three or four filaments which enter the ocular surface of the lateral rectus muscle just behind its middle.

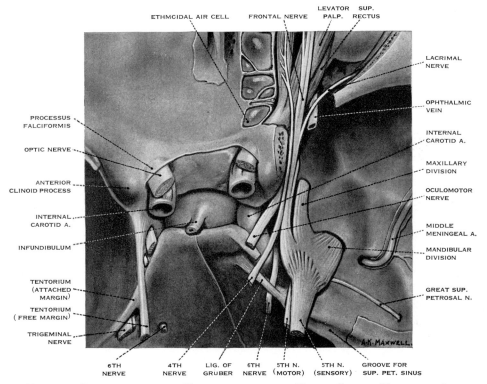

FIG. 274.—Dissection to show Nerves passing from Middle Cranial Fossa into Orbit.
(Wolff's preparation.)

Communications.

From (a) *The Sympathetic* in the cavernous sinus. (b) *From the Ophthalmic* just before entering the orbit.

Variations.

(a) The abducent nerve may arise in two parts, which may remain separate to the superior orbital fissure.

(b) The nerve or part of it may pass above the petroclinoid ligament.

(c) It may give a branch to the ciliary ganglion.

(d) The nasociliary nerve may be a branch of the abducent.

(e) The abducent nerve may be absent, being replaced by the oculomotor.

Nucleus and Central Connections

The abducent nucleus is a small spherical mass consisting of large multipolar cells lying close to the mid-line in the tegmental portion of the pons ventral to the *colliculus facialis*. This is an elevation in the floor of the fourth ventricle, which is produced by the genu of the fibres of the facial nerve (Figs. 271 and 292). The abducent nucleus is separated from the median plane by the medial longitudinal bundle, which is thus ventromedial (while it is ventrolateral to the nucleus of the oculomotor and ventral to that of the trochlear). Partly intermingled with these larger neurons are more numerous small multipolar cells which form the so-called nucleus para-abducens. Since the total number of these two sizes of neuron is about 22,000 (Konigsmark *et al.*, 1969), most cannot be sources of abducent axons (see below). Evidence suggests that some, at least, may ascend through the medial longitudinal fasciculus to the oculomotor complex.

The fibres pass forwards through the whole length of the pons, first medial to the corpus trapezoideum, then lateral to the pyramid, some fibres passing through the latter (Figs. 264, 292).

Connections.—Some axons go from the abducent (and para-abducent) nucleus into the medial longitudinal bundle to the oculomotor, trochlear, and vestibular nuclei; they may be concerned with conjugate movements, one lateral rectus working with the medial rectus of the opposite side. The following is the probable course of the supranuclear fibres for conjugate movement of the globes. Arising from the cortical centres in the frontal lobe the fibres pass in the anterior limb of the internal capsule, and occupy a medial position in the cerebral peduncle. They can be traced as far as upper pontine levels, but probably project to the abducent neurons through unidentified interneurons.

The abducens nucleus is also connected with the visual pathway via the superior colliculus and tectobulbar tract.

Structure.—The nerve contains some 6 to 7 thousand fibres as it leaves the brain stem (Björkman and Wohlfart, 1936). The most recent estimate is 6,600 (Konigsmark *et al.*, 1969).

Some Practical Considerations

1. Division of the abducent nerve results in paralysis of the lateral rectus muscle. There is internal strabismus. The eye *can* move to the middle of the palpebral fissure, but no farther. The diplopia is homonymous, and is worse on looking towards the affected side.

2. Fractures of the base of the skull are very liable to involve the abducent nerve owing to its contact with the basi-occiput and the apex of the petrous temporal bone.

3. Abducent nerve deficit alone has little localising value. The abducens is the most vulnerable of the cranial nerves, and may be affected in almost any type of

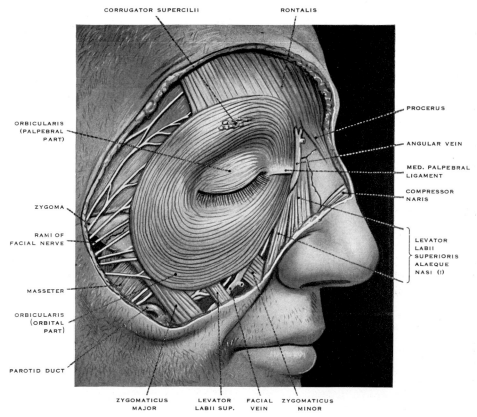

CORRUGATOR SUPERCILII   RONTALIS

PROCERUS

ORBICULARIS
(PALPEBRAL
PART)

ANGULAR VEIN

MED. PALPEBRAL
LIGAMENT

COMPRESSOR
NARIS

ZYGOMA

RAMI OF
FACIAL NERVE

LEVATOR
LABII
SUPERIORIS
ALAEQUE
NASI (?)

MASSETER

ORBICULARIS
(ORBITAL
PART)

PAROTID DUCT

ZYGOMATICUS   LEVATOR   FACIAL   ZYGOMATICUS
MAJOR   LABII SUP.   VEIN   MINOR

FIG. 275.—DISSECTION OF ORBIT FROM IN FRONT.

Stage 1. Orbicularis oculi.

(*Wolff's dissection.*)

cerebral lesion, whether near *or at a distance* from the nerve. Many theories have been evoked to account for this (see Walsh and Hoyt, 1969, Ashworth, 1973).

THE TRIGEMINAL (FIFTH CRANIAL) NERVE

The trigeminal, the largest of the cranial nerves, resembles a typical spinal nerve: it has two roots, sensory and motor, and further, on the sensory root, there is a large ganglion.

Superficial Origin.—The two roots of the trigeminal emerge together, somewhat above the middle of the lateral surface of the pons. The sensory trunk is much larger than the motor, which is placed above and medial to its companion (Figs. 258 and 261).

Course and Relations.—The two parts of the trigeminal pass almost directly forwards, slightly upwards in the pontine cistern of the posterior cranial fossa

A.E.—20

towards a notch at the upper border of the petrous temporal, which they reach after a course of about 1 cm. They are surrounded by separate sheaths of pia, which merge into the connective tissue sheaths of the nerves. Running proximally upon them from the trigeminal cave of dura mater are similar arachnoid sheaths which coalesce a few millimetres posterior to the apex of the petrous part of the temporal bone. The arachnoid and pial sheaths are continuous through "adventitious" connective tissue (Fig. 258).

Inferiorly the facial and vestibulocochlear nerves diverge towards the internal acoustic meatus. *Above* is the cerebellum, the free margin of the tentorium cerebelli, with the trochlear nerve close under it.

The abducent nerve, which is at its origin about 1·5 cm inferomedial to the trigeminal, gradually approaches it, and comes to lie quite close to its medial side at the apex of the petrous temporal (Fig. 272).

The trigeminal nerve pierces the dura under the attached margin of the tentorium cerebelli, which contains the superior petrosal sinus, and, having spread out in a plexiform manner, joins the posterior concave border of the trigeminal (Gasserian) ganglion (Figs. 272, 274). It thus passes through a kind of foramen formed partly by the notch in the sharp upper border of the petrous temporal and partly by the attached margin of the tentorium, which bridges over it (Fig. 272).

The Trigeminal (Gasserian) Ganglion is the sensory ganglion of the trigeminal nerve, corresponding and having a similar structure to the posterior root ganglion of the spinal nerves. (It may harbour herpetic viruses.) It is crescentic or, better, bean-shaped in appearance, the hilum being directed backwards. The ganglion is some 4 cm medial to a point just above the articular tubercle at the root of the zygoma. It lies in a bony fossa on the front of the apex of the petrous temporal, and below this covers that part of the foramen lacerum which overlies the internal carotid artery and greater petrosal nerve.

It is enclosed in a sheath of dura mater prolonged from that of the posterior cranial fossa, which loosely invests the two roots and extends forwards to fuse with the anterior half of the ganglion. This sheath of dura is the cavum trigeminale (Meckel's cave). The dura is lined with arachnoid, so the sensory and motor roots and hence the posterior half of the ganglion is in cerebrospinal fluid. The sheath of dura (i.e. the cave) lies between the fibrous and endosteal layers of the dura mater of the middle cranial fossa.

To its *lateral side* the ganglion has the foramen spinosum, transmitting the middle meningeal artery, which is, therefore, *an obstruction in approaching it by the temporal route*. To its *medial side* is the cavernous sinus, the internal carotid artery, and the ocular motor nerves (Figs. 261 and 262). To the medial side of these again is the hypophysis cerebri (pituitary gland).

Above the ganglion is the uncus and temporal lobe, inferior to it are the greater and lesser (superficial) petrosal nerves, the *motor trigeminal root* and the internal carotid artery.

After extradural approach to the ganglion across the middle fossa there some-times results a *facial* paralysis. This is due to pulling on the greater (superficial) petrosal nerve, producing trauma at the geniculate ganglion. Resultant œdema of the ganglion, or interference with the blood supply, blocks the facial nerve. The palsy is transient and recovery complete.

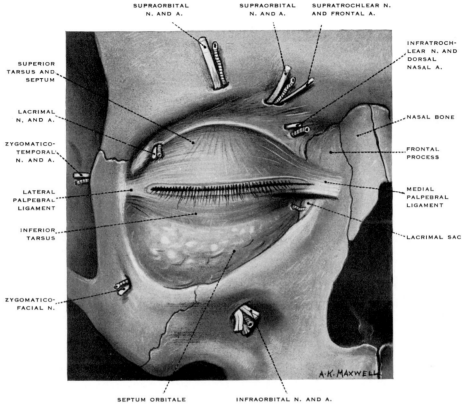

SUPRAORBITAL N. AND A.   SUPRAORBITAL N. AND A.   SUPRATROCHLEAR N. AND FRONTAL A.

INFRATROCH-LEAR N. AND DORSAL NASAL A.

SUPERIOR TARSUS AND SEPTUM

LACRIMAL N. AND A.

ZYGOMATICO-TEMPORAL N. AND A.

LATERAL PALPEBRAL LIGAMENT

INFERIOR TARSUS

ZYGOMATICO-FACIAL N.

NASAL BONE

FRONTAL PROCESS

MEDIAL PALPEBRAL LIGAMENT

LACRIMAL SAC

A·K·MAXWELL

SEPTUM ORBITALE   INFRAORBITAL N. AND A.

FIG. 276.—DISSECTION OF ORBIT FROM IN FRONT.
Stage 2. Obicularis removed to show septum orbitale.
(*Wolff's dissection.*)

The Motor Root of the trigeminal has no connection with the ganglion, but lies on its deep surface, crossing from the medial to the lateral side to join the third division of the trigeminal.

The posterior border of the ganglion is concave, and continuous with the sensory root. From its anterior convex border emerge the three divisions of the nerve, namely the ophthalmic, maxillary and mandibular nerves.

Apart from these branches the ganglion receives communications from the sympathetic round the internal carotid artery and from its posterior part a few filaments pass to the dura.

Small *accessory ganglia* may be found along the concave border of the trigeminal ganglion corresponding to the accessory ganglia found on the posterior root between the posterior root ganglion and the spinal cord.

The trigeminal ganglion contains neurons similar to those in dorsal spinal root ganglia. Most of them are large unipolar neurons, with peripheral processes in the three divisions of the nerve and central axons passing centrally to the nuclei of the trigeminal nerve in the brainstem. Proprioceptor axons pass through the ganglion and have their somata in the mesencephalic trigeminal nucleus. Some degree of functional or somatotopic localisation has been described in the ganglion (Kerr and Lysak, 1964, Lende and Poulos, 1970).

The Ophthalmic Nerve

The Ophthalmic Nerve, the smallest of the three divisions of the trigeminal, enters the medial and upper part of the convex anterior border of the trigeminal ganglion. It extends in the lateral wall of the cavernous sinus enclosed in a separate sheath of dura. Hence it is necessary to incise the dura of the lateral wall of the sinus and *then* the proper sheath of the nerve before it is exposed (Hovelacque, 1927). Superior to it are the oculomotor and trochlear nerves, medially the abducent nerve and internal carotid artery, and inferolaterally the maxillary nerve.

After a course of about 2·5 cm it divides, just posterior to the superior orbital (sphenoidal) fissure into three branches, *lacrimal, frontal* and *nasociliary*, which pass through the fissure to enter the orbit.

In the cavernous sinus it is said to be joined by branches of communication from the ocular motor nerves (probably proprioceptive) and from the sympathetic round the internal carotid artery. The former communications are a matter of controversy (see p. 292). It also sends a *recurrent* branch, the nervus tentorii, to the supratentorial dura mater (Figs. 284, 318). This nerve branches near the origin of the ophthalmic and passes back across the trochlear. It is usually closely adherent to this nerve, and not infrequently passes through it (hence it has been described as a branch of the trochlear) to reach the tentorium.

The Lacrimal Nerve, the smallest of the three terminal branches of the ophthalmic, arises in the anterior part of the middle cranial fossa. It passes through the *wide* portion of the superior orbital (sphenoidal) fissure above the annular tendon lateral to the frontal and trochlear nerves and above and medial to the ophthalmic vein. In the orbit the nerve runs laterally parallel to, and close in front of, the narrow portion of the superior orbital fissure, then forwards along or just lateral to the upper border of the lateral rectus muscle to reach the lacrimal gland. In the distal two-thirds of its course above the lateral rectus, it is accompanied by the lacrimal artery (Fig. 279). Its whole orbital course is sinuous and was described as like a fixed bayonet (Fig. 284) by Hovelacque and Reinhold (1917).

Just before reaching the gland the nerve receives a communication from the

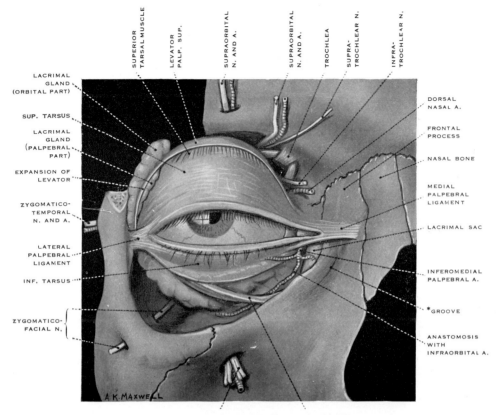

FIG. 277.—DISSECTION OF ORBIT FROM IN FRONT.

Stage 3. Septum removed.

(*Wolff's dissection.*)

* This groove may be mistaken for the lacrimal fossa at operation.

zygomatic nerve (Fig. 283); then, having passed through the gland to which it sends branches, it supplies the conjunctiva and the skin of the lateral part of the upper lid, which it reaches by piercing the septum orbitale. (For the significance of the communication and the autonomic component of the lacrimal nerve, see pp. 225, 316.)

The Frontal Nerve, the largest of the three branches of the ophthalmic, arises in the cavernous sinus just behind the superior orbital fissure through which it enters the orbit.

In the fissure it is placed above the annular tendon between the lacrimal and the trochlear. It runs almost directly forwards under the periosteum (periorbita) and on the levator palpebræ superioris. Towards the front of the orbit it divides into *supratrochlear* and *supraorbital branches.* In the specimen shown in Fig. 279 the division is unusually far back.

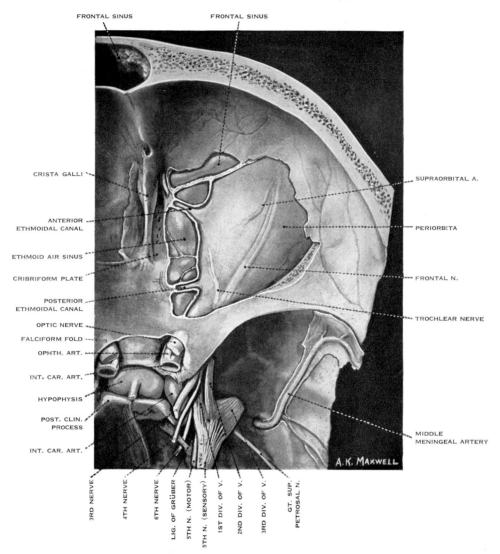

FRONTAL SINUS   FRONTAL SINUS

CRISTA GALLI

ANTERIOR
ETHMOIDAL CANAL

ETHMOID AIR SINUS

CRIBRIFORM PLATE

POSTERIOR
ETHMOIDAL CANAL

OPTIC NERVE

FALCIFORM FOLD

OPHTH. ART.

INT. CAR. ART.

HYPOPHYSIS

POST. CLIN.
PROCESS

INT. CAR. ART.

SUPRAORBITAL A.

PERIORBITA

FRONTAL N.

TROCHLEAR NERVE

MIDDLE
MENINGEAL ARTERY

A.K. MAXWELL

3RD NERVE — 4TH NERVE — 6TH NERVE — LIG. OF GRÜBER — 5TH N. (MOTOR) — 5TH N. (SENSORY) — 1ST DIV. OF V. — 2ND DIV. OF V. — 3RD DIV. OF V. — GT. SUP. PETROSAL N.

FIG. 278.—DISSECTION OF ORBIT FROM ABOVE.

Stage 1. Various structures are visible through the periorbita after removal of the orbital "roof".

(*Wolff's dissection.*)

The Supratrochlear Nerve (Fig. 279), much smaller than the supraorbital, runs forwards to pass above the pulley of the superior oblique near which it sends a twig of communication to the *infratrochlear* branch of the nasociliary.

In company with the supratrochlear artery, and deep to the orbicularis and the corrugator supercilii, the supratrochlear ascends over the orbital margin

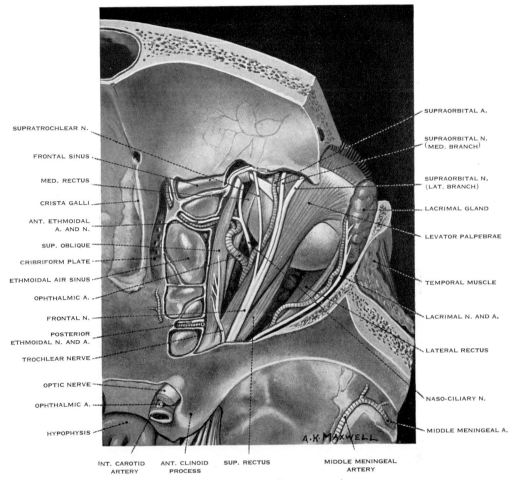

FIG. 279.—DISSECTION OF ORBIT FROM ABOVE.

Stage 2. Periorbita removed.

(*Wolff's dissection.*)

about 1·25 cm from the mid-line. It sends branches of supply to the skin of the forehead and to the upper lid and conjunctiva.

The Supraorbital Nerve, much the larger of the terminal branches of the frontal, continues the direction of the parent nerve. It is above the levator with the supraorbital artery medial to it, and leaves the orbit with this vessel by the supraorbital notch or foramen (Figs. 276, 277).

Occasionally the nerve divides within the orbit into medial and lateral branches (Fig. 279). The lateral branch then occupies the supraorbital notch, and the medial passes out of the orbit about midway between the trochlea of the superior

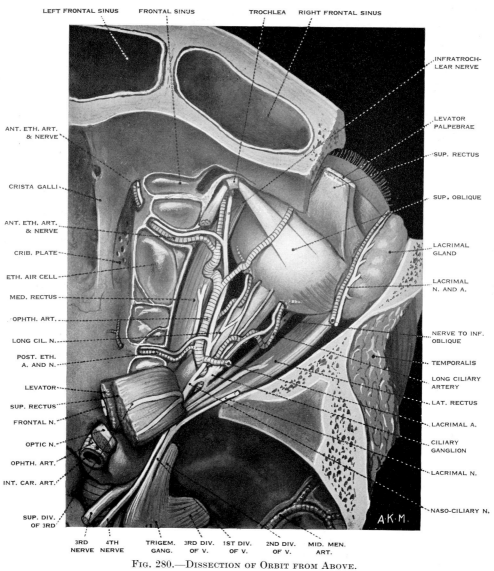

FIG. 280.—DISSECTION OF ORBIT FROM ABOVE.

Stage 3. Levator and superior rectus reflected.

(*Wolff's dissection.*)

oblique and the supraorbital notch. Usually it has a notch (frontal notch of
Henle) or rarely a foramen of its own.

The supraorbital nerve breaks up into branches which reunite with each other
and supply the forehead and scalp to the vertex, and also the upper eyelid, and
the conjunctiva. Those to the scalp are between the periosteum and the orbicu-

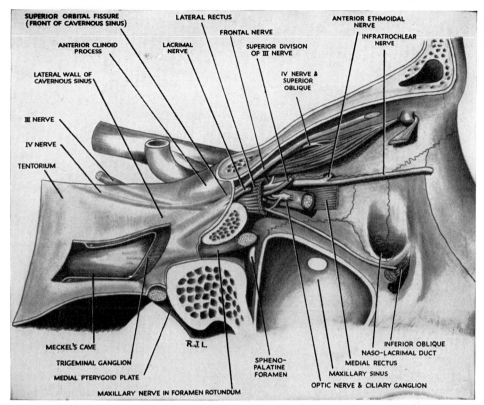

FIG. 281.—A LONGITUDINAL SECTION THROUGH THE RIGHT ORBIT AND MIDDLE CRANIAL FOSSA VIEWED FROM THE LATERAL SIDE. (From Last's "Anatomy, Regional and Applied", by permission of the publishers, Churchill-Livingstone.)

laris and frontalis, which they pierce to reach the skin. They frequently groove the bone, especially in childhood. Rami to the upper lid pass through the orbicularis. The nerve also sends a ramus to the diploë and frontal sinus through a small aperture in the floor of the supraorbital notch.

The Nasociliary Nerve branches from the inferomedial aspect of the ophthalmic, being commonly the first of the three terminal branches to appear. Intermediate in size between the lacrimal and frontal, it lies at first in the lateral wall of the *cavernous sinus*. It passes through the *superior orbital (sphenoidal) fissure* within the annular tendon, between the divisions of the oculomotor nerve close to the *sympathetic root* of the ciliary ganglion, which is below and medial.

In the *orbit* it inclines medially, with the ophthalmic artery above the optic nerve, in front of the superior oculomotor division (Fig. 280), and below the superior rectus muscle. Near the anterior ethmoidal foramen it divides into its two terminal branches, the anterior ethmoidal and infratrochlear.

Branches.—(*a*) *The Long or Sensory Root of the Ciliary Ganglion* is given off in or just in front of the superior orbital (sphenoidal) fissure. It is a slender nerve, usually about 5 to 12 mm long, which passes along the lateral side of the optic nerve to reach the upper and posterior part of the ganglion (Figs. 280, 282).

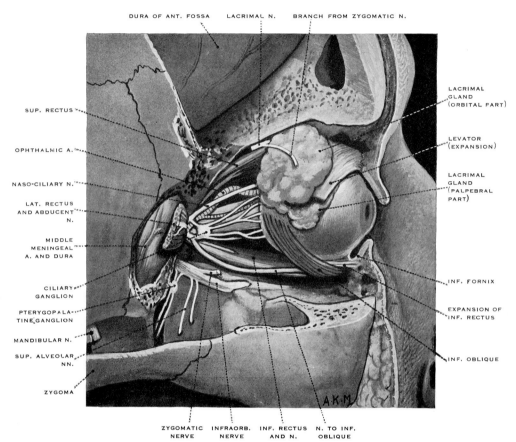

FIG. 282.—DISSECTION OF THE RIGHT ORBIT FROM THE LATERAL SIDE.

(*Wolff's preparation.*)

(*b*) *The Long Ciliary Nerves*, two in number, come off as the nasociliary crosses the optic nerve, to the medial side of which they come to lie. They run with the short ciliaries, pierce the sclera (Fig. 84), and passing between this and the choroid (Fig. 41), supply *sensory* fibres to the *iris, cornea* and *ciliary muscle* and some sympathetic fibres to the dilatator pupillæ (see p. 402).

(*c*) *The Posterior Ethmoidal Nerve* passes between the superior oblique and medial rectus and enters the posterior ethmoidal foramen with its accompanying artery, and supplies the sphenoidal and posterior ethmoidal sinuses.

(d) *The Infratrochlear Nerve* (Figs. 277, 280) is given off as a terminal branch of the nasociliary. It runs forward near the lower border of the superior oblique and passes below the pulley of this muscle, near which it gets a communication from the supratrochlear to appear on the face.

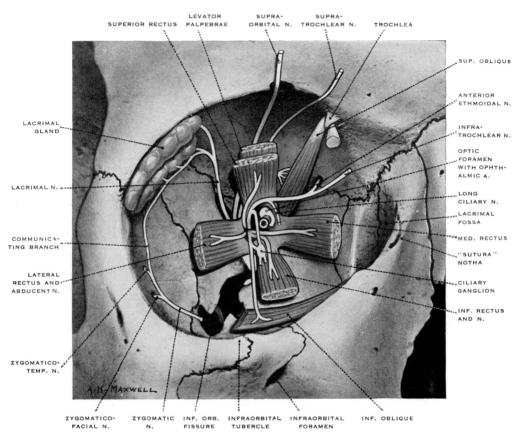

FIG. 283.—DISSECTION TO SHOW ORBITAL NERVES FROM IN FRONT.
(*Based on Wolff's dissections.*)

It breaks up into its branches, which supply the skin and conjunctiva round the medial angle of the eye, the root of the nose, the lacrimal sac and canaliculi and the caruncle. It connects with the supraorbital and infraorbital nerves.

(e) *The Anterior Ethmoidal Nerve* passes between the superior oblique and medial rectus to leave the orbit with the anterior ethmoidal artery by the anterior ethmoidal canal, which lies between the frontal and ethmoid bones. Here it supplies the middle and anterior ethmoidal sinuses and the infundibulum of the frontal sinus. It enters the *anterior cranial fossa* at the side of the cribriform plate of the ethmoid. Inclining medially it passes between the two layers of dura mater to the "nasal slit" in the cribriform plate. In this part of its course it lies partly under or entirely in front of the olfactory bulb (Fig. 287) but separated from it by dura.

Traversing this slit, the nerve reaches the roof of the nose, where it gives *lateral nasal* branches to the upper and anterior quadrant of the lateral wall, and

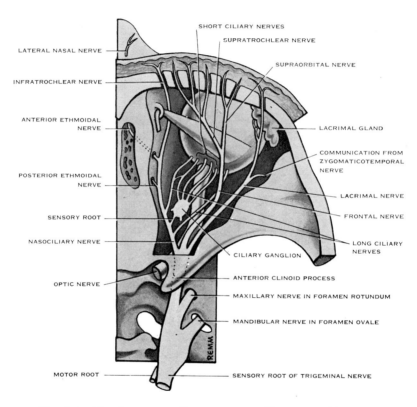

SHORT CILIARY NERVES
SUPRATROCHLEAR NERVE
LATERAL NASAL NERVE
SUPRAORBITAL NERVE
INFRATROCHLEAR NERVE
ANTERIOR ETHMOIDAL NERVE
LACRIMAL GLAND
COMMUNICATION FROM ZYGOMATICOTEMPORAL NERVE
POSTERIOR ETHMOIDAL NERVE
LACRIMAL NERVE
SENSORY ROOT
FRONTAL NERVE
NASOCILIARY NERVE
LONG CILIARY NERVES
CILIARY GANGLION
OPTIC NERVE
ANTERIOR CLINOID PROCESS
MAXILLARY NERVE IN FORAMEN ROTUNDUM
MANDIBULAR NERVE IN FORAMEN OVALE
MOTOR ROOT
SENSORY ROOT OF TRIGEMINAL NERVE

FIG. 284.—THE OPHTHALMIC DIVISION OF THE TRIGEMINAL NERVE.

medial nasal branches to the anterior part of the septum. The nerve next lies in a groove (Figs. 12 and 289) on the posterior surface of the nasal bone, which it notches to appear on the face as the *external nasal nerve*. This supplies the skin over the cartilaginous part of the nose, down to the tip.

Varieties.—Absence of the infratrochlear nerve has been noted, its place being taken by the supratrochlear. Branches have been seen passing from the anterior ethmoidal to the levator; to the oculomotor and abducent nerves; to the mucous membrane of the frontal sinus, as the nerve lies in the anterior ethmoidal canal. For details consult Le Double (1897) and Quain (1900).

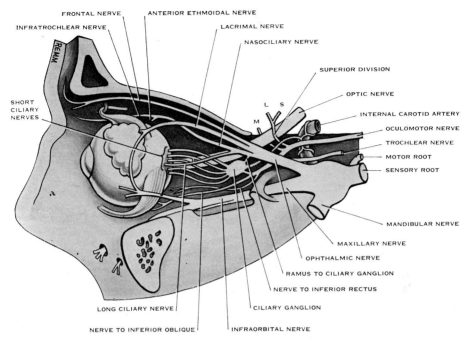

FRONTAL NERVE · ANTERIOR ETHMOIDAL NERVE
INFRATROCHLEAR NERVE · LACRIMAL NERVE
NASOCILIARY NERVE
SUPERIOR DIVISION
OPTIC NERVE
SHORT CILIARY NERVES
INTERNAL CAROTID ARTERY
OCULOMOTOR NERVE
TROCHLEAR NERVE
MOTOR ROOT
SENSORY ROOT
MANDIBULAR NERVE
MAXILLARY NERVE
OPHTHALMIC NERVE
RAMUS TO CILIARY GANGLION
NERVE TO INFERIOR RECTUS
LONG CILIARY NERVE
CILIARY GANGLION
NERVE TO INFERIOR OBLIQUE · INFRAORBITAL NERVE

Fig. 285.—The Ciliary Ganglion and Oculomotor Nerve.

S = nerve to superior rectus. L = nerve to levator. M = nerve to medial rectus. (The sympathetic ramus from the carotid plexus to the ciliary ganglion is not labelled but easy to identify.)

The Ciliary Ganglion

The ciliary ganglion is most easily found by first isolating the nerve to the inferior oblique. This can be done by exposing the inferior oblique from in front; then it is quite easy to see the nerve as it crosses the middle of the posterior border. By pulling gently on the nerve it can readily be identified behind the globe and so leads one to the ciliary ganglion.

The Ciliary Ganglion is a small reddish-grey somewhat polygonal body measuring about 2 mm in anteroposterior and 1 mm in vertical diameter, situated posteriorly in the orbit about 1 cm anterior to the optic foramen between the optic nerve and the lateral rectus muscle. It is in close contact with the nerve, but separated from the muscle by some loose fat. Usually also it is close to the ophthalmic artery (Figs. 280, 281).

It receives posteriorly three so-called roots or rami (Fig. 285):

(1) The long or sensory root;

(2) The short or parasympathetic root;

(3) The sympathetic root.

It is important to appreciate immediately that the sensory and sympathetic fibres pass through the ganglion without interruption. In some vertebrates such fibres by-pass the ganglion, whose only essential "root" is the parasympathetic. (For comparative anatomy see Grimes and Sallmann, 1960.)

(1) *The Long or Sensory Root* comes from the nasociliary, and is given off just after that nerve has entered the orbit. It is a slender nerve about 6 to 12 mm long, which passes along the lateral side of the optic nerve to reach the upper and

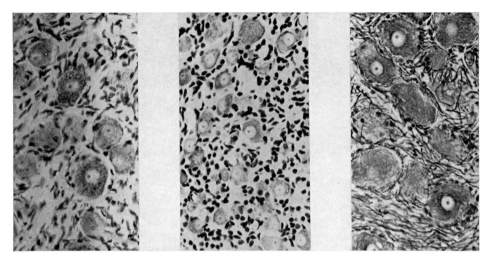

Fig. 286.—Photomicrographs of Ciliary Ganglion Neurons (right and left) and Superior Cervical Sympathetic Ganglion Neurons (centre).

All at the same magnification. Stained by cresyl violet (left and central) and Romanes' technique (right). Contrast size and granule features of the ciliary and sympathetic neurons. The relatively large diameter of ciliary ganglion neurons, both in mammals and birds, has not been widely recognized (Warwick, 1954). They are not typical autonomic neurons.

posterior part of the ganglion. It contains sensory fibres from the *cornea, iris* and *ciliary body*, and possibly (from the sympathetic fibres which often join it) fibres to the dilatator pupillæ.

(2) *The Short or Motor Root* comes from the nerve to the inferior oblique a few millimetres beyond the point where the nerve arises from the inferior division of the oculomotor, much thicker than the sensory root, only about 1 to 2 mm long, and passes upwards and forwards to enter the posteroinferior angle of the ganglion. It carries parasympathetic fibres to the sphincter pupillæ and the ciliary muscle. These synapse in the ganglion.

(3) *The Sympathetic Root* comes from the plexus around the internal carotid artery. It passes through the superior orbital fissure within the annular tendon

inferomedial to the nasociliary. It lies below and close to the long root, with which it may be blended, and enters the posterior border of the ganglion between the other roots. It carries constrictor fibres to the blood-vessels of the eye, and possibly dilator fibres to the pupil.

The blood supply of the ciliary ganglion, despite the voluminous literature on this small structure, has attracted little study. Kuzetsova (1963) recorded observations on the vascularization of the ganglion in human fetal and neonate material; more recently, Eliškova (1969, 1973) has studied India ink preparations

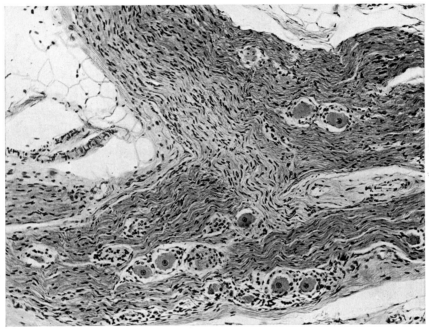

FIG. 287.—SHOWING GANGLION CELLS IN THE SHORT CILIARY NERVES.
(Wolff's preparation.)

(in rhesus and in human fetal and postnatal orbits) and reports the supply to be from the posterior ciliary, muscular, ophthalmic and central retinal arteries.

BRANCHES OF THE GANGLION

The somata of the preganglionic parasympathetic nerve fibres reaching the ciliary ganglion are in the accessory oculomotor nuclei (of Edinger-Westphal) (p. 284). They are, of course, myelinated. They end in the ganglion by forming synapses with the somata and dendrites of the postganglionic neurons. The lightly myelinated axons of these form the short ciliary branches of the ganglion (Fig. 366). These axons are possibly unique, in the myelination, amongst postganglionic nerve fibres. The short ciliary nerves usually contain small groups of displaced ganglion cells (Fig. 287).

The Short Ciliary Nerves, six to ten in number, are delicate filaments which come off in two groups from the anterosuperior and anteroinferior angles of the ganglion respectively. They run sinuously with the short ciliary arteries above and below the optic nerve, the lower group being the larger. As they pass forwards they connect with each other and with the long ciliaries, and having given branches to the optic nerve and ophthalmic artery pierce the sclera around the

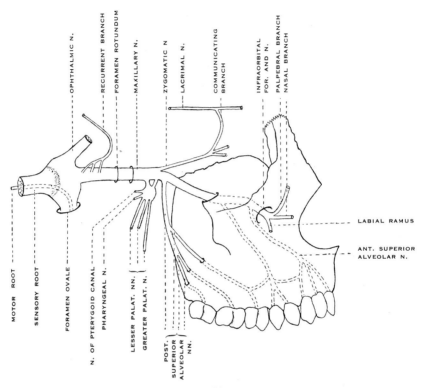

FIG. 288.—DIAGRAM OF THE MANDIBULAR NERVE (L.W.).

optic nerve. They run anteriorly between the choroid and sclera, grooving the latter, to the ciliary muscle, on the surface of which they form a plexus which supplies the iris, ciliary body, and cornea.

Varieties.—The parasympathetic "root" may be so short that the ganglion is virtually sessile on the inferior oblique muscle's branch of the oculomotor. Connections with the trochlear and abducent nerve have been described. For these and other variations consult Quain (1900) and Hovelacque (1927).

The ciliary ganglion contains multipolar neurons, mostly of unusually large size (*c.* 45 μm in diameter) for autonomic postganglion cells. Some observers have claimed to distinguish many classes of cells in the ganglion, but these views have not been sustained. They form a largely uniform population, structurally and functionally (Warwick, 1954). Small numbers of smaller neurons, typical in appearance of the cells in sympathetic ganglia, also occur and may represent either interneurons or aberrant postganglionic sympathetic elements. Experimentally, it is apparent that most of the ganglion cells (c. 97%) innervate the ciliaris muscle, a small number only innervating the sphincter pupillæ (Warwick, 1954). This accords with the great difference in the bulk of these two muscles. It is not certain that the ciliary ganglia provides the *only* source of parasympathetic fibres for the eyeball. The episcleral ganglia of Axenfold (1907) have long been suspected to provide a secondary route. (See Stotler, 1937, and Morgan and Harrigan, 1951, for contrasting views.) A recent study (Phillips, 1972) of episcleral ganglia in primates (including mankind) found them inconstant and insignificant in numbers as a possible route for associated miosis. (For earlier, contrasting opinions, consult Givner, 1939, and Nathan and Turner, 1942.)

THE MAXILLARY NERVE

The Maxillary Nerve, the second trigeminal division, is intermediate in size between the ophthalmic and the mandibular, and issues from the middle of the convex anterior border of the trigeminal ganglion. It runs forwards in the lower angle of the cavernous sinus in a groove (Figs. 261 and 368) on the greater wing of the sphenoid, which leads it to the foramen rotundum.

It passes through this foramen (usually a short canal) into the pterygopalatine fossa. It now turns laterally behind the orbital process of the palatine bone and at the inferior orbital fissure divides into its two terminal branches, the infraorbital and zygomatic nerves.

Relations.—(*a*) *In the Cranial Cavity.*—It lies in the lower angle of the cavernous sinus, in the thickness of the dura mater. Superiorly is the ophthalmic division, while *laterally* is the temporal lobe of the brain.

When the sphenoidal sinus is large it may send a prolongation into the great wing of the sphenoid between the foramen ovale and rotundum, *which may account for the nerve being involved in sinus disease*.

(*b*) *In the Pterygopalatine Fossa.*—Here the nerve is close to the termination of the maxillary artery and a plexus of veins. It is also close to the ethmoidal sinuses in the orbital process of the palatine bone, *and may be involved in ethmoidal disease here*.

Branches.—(*a*) In the cranial cavity a recurrent branch, the so-called *middle meningeal nerve*, supplies the dura mater of the anterior half of the middle cranial fossa.

(*b*) In the pterygopalatine fossa two short branches are attached to the pterygopalatine (sphenopalatine) ganglion, forming its sensory root (p. 315). These are called the **pterygopalatine nerves.**

The **posterior superior alveolar** (dental) **nerves,** usually three in number, branch away just before the maxillary nerve divides in the inferior orbital fissure. They enter canals in the maxilla through small foramina on its infratemporal surface. They supply the molar teeth, the adjoining gingival tissues, their periodontal ligaments, and the mucous membrane of the maxillary sinus.

(c) The **infraorbital nerve** runs forwards from the inferior orbital fissure on the orbital plate of the maxilla. It indents the bone, first into a groove, then into a canal through which it runs with the infraorbital artery to emerge on the face through the infraorbital foramen.

The *middle superior alveolar* (dental) *nerve* is given off in the infraorbital groove and runs down in the lateral wall of the maxilla to supply the upper premolar teeth and the adjoining sinus mucosa. It is variable, occasionally absent, sometimes multiple (Wood Jones, 1939, and Fitzgerald, 1956).

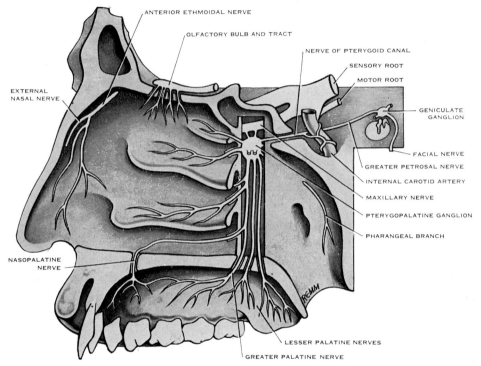

FIG. 289.—NERVES OF THE LATERAL WALL OF THE NOSE.

The *anterior superior alveolar* (dental) *nerve* arises in the infraorbital canal. Passing first *laterally* in the bone, it curves down and medially below the infra-orbital foramen to supply the canine and both incisors, the mucosa of the sinus, and the anterior inferior quadrant of the lateral wall and nearby floor of the nose.

On the face the infraorbital nerve emerges between levator labii superioris and levator anguli oris. It breaks up into a leash of branches, some of which join twigs of the facial nerve. These branches radiate from the overlying cheek downwards, medially and upwards. The *labial branches* supply the skin of the upper lip and the mucous membrane of the vestibule (including the labial gum) from the midline to the second bicuspid tooth. The *nasal branches* supply the lateral side of the lower part of the nose. The *palpebral branches* run up to supply the skin and conjunctiva of the lower lid.

(*d*) The **Zygomatic nerve** inclines laterally from the inferior orbital fissure, and soon divides into zygomaticotemporal and zygomaticofacial branches.

The Zygomaticotemporal Branch ascends in a groove on the *lateral wall* of the orbit, gives a *communicating twig to the lacrimal nerve*, which may carry secretory fibres to the lacrimal gland, and then enters a canal in the zygomatic bone, which leads it to the temporal fossa. It now ascends, pierces the temporal fascia behind the zygomatic tubercle, and having joined with branches of the facial, supplies the skin over the anterior part of the temporal region up to the lateral orbital margin. The lacrimal secretomotor route noted above has been strongly criticised by Ruskell (1971), whose experiments suggest another path (see pp. 301, 398).

The Zygomaticofacial Branch likewise enters a canal in the zygomatic bone, which leads it to the face where, having joined with branches of the facial and pierced the orbicularis, it supplies the skin over the zygomatic bone.

Varieties.—The whole zygomatic nerve may enter one canal and then divide in the bone itself. The lacrimal communication may replace the zygomaticotemporal branch and a twig from the infraorbital take the place of the zygomaticofacial branch. *The Zygomaticofacial Branch* may issue on to the face as two or more branches.

THE PTERYGOPALATINE (SPHENOPALATINE) GANGLION

The pterygopalatine ganglion (of Meckel) is situated in the upper part of the pterygopalatine fossa, just lateral to the sphenopalatine foramen and depends from the maxillary nerve by its pterygopalatine branches (Figs. 282, 288, 289).

ROOTS

Sensory.—The pterygopalatine ganglion receives a contingent of sensory fibres from the maxillary nerve by a posterior ganglionic branch. Most of these fibres leave the ganglion by its various branches to innervate sensitive tissues in the orbit, nose, and pharynx (see below). A few fibres return to the maxillary nerve through an anterior ganglionic connection. None of these fibres are interrupted in the ganglion. They are accidental passengers through a ganglion which is basically autonomic.

Autonomic Motor.—The nerve of the pterygoid canal is formed in the foramen lacerum by the union of the greater petrosal nerve (parasympathetic), from the geniculate ganglion, with the deep petrosal nerve from the sympathetic plexus around the internal carotid artery (Fig. 289). The nerve of the pterygoid canal is thus a mixed autonomic nerve. It passes through the canal in the sphenoid bone and ends in the pterygopalatine fossa, where it joins the ganglion. The deep petrosal nerve comes from neurons in the superior cervical sympathetic ganglion by way of the carotid plexus. Its fibres are post-ganglionic, and traverse the ptery-gopalatine ganglion without relay to enter its branches of distribution. Some fibres return to the maxillary nerve through the anterior ganglionic branch. All the sympathetic fibres thus pass through the ganglion just like the sensory axons. They are mostly vasoconstrictor in function to arterioles in the territory of the maxillary division.

The greater petrosal nerve carries parasympathetic preganglionic fibres, which form synapses with postganglionic neurons in the pterygopalatine ganglion, and which are usually considered to innervate the lacrimal gland, reaching it through the zygomatic nerve and its communication with the lacrimal nerve. (For other views on this secretomotor route see pp. 225, 301.) Other fibres also supply mucous glands in the nose, naso-pharynx, paranasal sinuses and palate. These parasympathetic fibres alone relay in the ganglion; their cell bodies are in the superior salivatory nucleus of the pons, and the fibres leave the brain stem in the nervus intermedius (Fig. 366). The precise identity of this nucleus is not as certain as the term implies; it is probably close to the caudal end of the facial motor nucleus.

The result of stimulation of this pathway is not only lacrimation, but secretion from a wide area of nasal and palatal mucosa—hence the name "ganglion of hay fever" commonly given to this ganglion. To treat intractable hay fever the ganglion is sometimes permanently blocked by alcohol or other injection.

Branches of the Pterygopalatine Ganglion

Each of the branches of the ganglion includes all three components—somatic, sensory, parasympathetic secretomotor and sympathetic vasomotor. *Orbital branches* supply periosteum at the apex of the floor of the orbit. Ruskell (1970, 1971) has drawn attention to experimental evidence indicating that in monkeys these rami provide a route for parasympathetic fibres to the lacrimal gland (see pp. 225, 301, 398).

1. **The Nasopalatine Nerve** (long sphenopalatine nerve) enters the nose by the sphenopalatine foramen, crosses the roof, then descends in a groove on the vomer, giving branches to the mucous membrane all along its course. It passes through the incisive canal to supply the mucoperiosteum behind the two incisor teeth. It is really the largest member of the next group of nerves.

2. **The Posterior Superior Nasal Nerves** (short sphenopalatine nerves) enter the nose through the sphenopalatine foramen, and turn forwards to supply the posterosuperior quadrant of the lateral wall of the nose and part of the septum. (These nerves are hence divisible into lateral and medial groups.)

3. **The Greater Palatine Nerve** descends in a canal which is formed between the maxilla and vertical plate of the palatine bone. Here it gives off multiple twigs that pierce each bone, to supply the mucosa of the maxillary sinus and that of the posteroinferior quadrant of the lateral wall of the nose.

The greater palatine nerve, emerging through the greater palatine foramen, runs forward to supply the mucoperiosteum of all the hard palate up to the incisive canal.

4. **The Lesser Palatine Nerves,** often branches from the greater palatine, pass through the lesser palatine canals and, behind the crest of the palatine bone, pass back to supply the mucous membrane on both surfaces of the soft palate.

5. **The Pharyngeal Branch** passes back through the palatinovaginal canal to supply the mucosa of the nasopharynx.

6. By dissection, microscopy and electron microscopy Ruskell (1973) has recently demonstrated an almost constant branch of the maxillary nerve, just beyond its emergence from the foramen rotundum in the pterygopalatine fossa, which passes into the orbit through the inferior orbital fissure to join the ciliary ganglion. He calls this the *orbitociliary nerve,* and considers that it is probably sensory in function, its fibres passing to the eyeball together with those of the ophthalmic divisions of the trigeminal in the short ciliary nerves. The orbito-ciliary nerve also sends small rami to the retro-orbital plexus (p. 398) described by the same worker.

THE MANDIBULAR NERVE

The mandibular division of the trigeminal nerve is formed by the union of a large sensory branch from the trigeminal ganglion with the motor root of the trigeminal, the whole of which enters this division.

The two nerves pass through the *foramen ovale,* and almost immediately unite into one trunk, which has the tensor palati and auditory tube medial to it and laterally to the lateral pterygoid and middle meningeal artery. (For further details see standard texts, e.g. Gray's Anatomy, ed. Warwick and Williams, 1973.)

NUCLEI AND CENTRAL CONNECTIONS OF THE TRIGEMINAL NERVE

The Sensory Nuclei of the trigeminal nerve extend throughout the brain stem. The mesencephalic part is slender. The pontine and medullary parts together are shaped like a tadpole (Fig. 290). The head is the *principal sensory nucleus* and is situated in the lateral and dorsal part of the pons ventral to the superior cerebellar peduncle. The tail forms the *nucleus of the spinal tract* and becomes continuous with the substantia gelatinosa at the level of the 2nd cervical segment (Fig. 268).

Trigeminal axons from the neurons in the trigeminal ganglion pass dorsally in the pons to synapse with interneurons in the main nucleus; others descend to the spinal nucleus, forming the so-called spinal tract of this nucleus. About 50 per cent of these entering fibres themselves divide into ascending and descending branches; the rest spread out to their destinations without division.

The main sensory nucleus is most probably concerned particularly with fine discriminative touch. The spinal nucleus mediates thermal and tactile sensibility.

Fibres from the ophthalmic division go to the *lowest* part, those from the maxillary division are next, while those from the mandibular division are uppermost.

The mesencephalic nucleus lies in the grey matter lateral to the cerebral aqueduct. It consists of the somata of "primary" sensory neurons, whose axons,

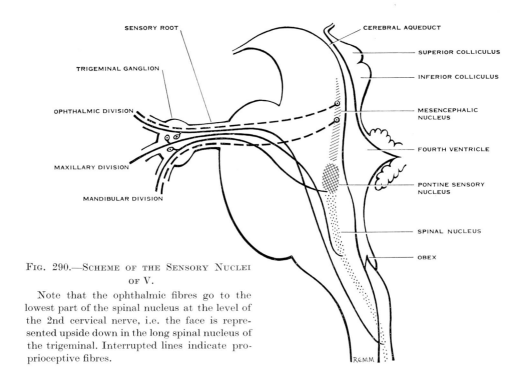

FIG. 290.—SCHEME OF THE SENSORY NUCLEI
OF V.

Note that the ophthalmic fibres go to the lowest part of the spinal nucleus at the level of the 2nd cervical nerve, i.e. the face is represented upside down in the long spinal nucleus of the trigeminal. Interrupted lines indicate proprioceptive fibres.

probably derived from all three divisions of the trigeminal nerve, pass directly through the ganglion (p. 298), a unique arrangement in the central nervous system of mammals (Johnston, 1909).

The Motor Nucleus is in the lateral tegmental region of the pons medial to and nearer the floor of the 4th ventricle than the sensory nucleus. It is in line with the nucleus ambiguus and the facial nucleus (Fig. 268), all three nuclei being branchial or special visceral efferent in morphological terms.

Connections.—Since the trigeminal nerve mediates so much of the head in sensory functions, as well as serving the whole of the masticatory musculature, its central connections with other cranial nerves, especially those of the orbit, tongue, and face, are extensive. The sensory nuclei project to the post central gyrus via the trigeminal lemniscus and the central posterior medial nucleus of the thalamus. There are also extensive projections to the nuclei of motor cranial nerves and tectum, and to the cerebellum, reticular system subthalamic nucleus, etc.

The Facial or Intermediofacial Nerve (7th Cranial Nerve)

The facial nerve is branchial in origin, and hence should contain special visceral efferent (branchiomotor) and afferent (gustatory) nerve fibres, and also perhaps general visceral efferent fibres (parasympathetic). Certain of these components issue as a separate trunk, the nervus intermedius, which is sometimes (as

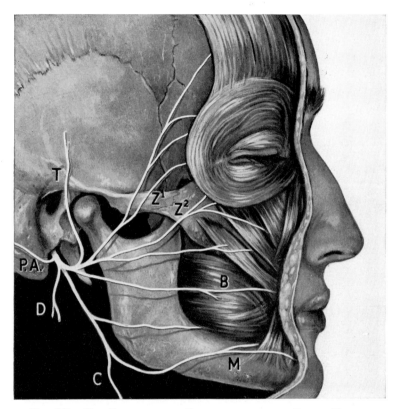

Fig. 291.—The Extracranial Distribution of the Facial Nerve.

P.A. = posterior auricular. D. = branch to posterior belly of digastric and stylohyoid. T. = temporal branch. Z^1. = upper zygomatic branches. Z^2. = lower zygomatic branches. B. = buccal branch. M. = mandibular branch. C. = cervical branch.

in previous editions of this book) considered to be a cranial nerve "in its own right". This is erroneous and misleading. The gustatory and parasympathetic components of the "facial" nerve simply enter or leave the brainstem as a separate trunk. (In a fifth of 73 dissections it was not even a separate nerve—*see* Rhoton *et al.*, 1968.) It is perhaps better to include these two *parts* or *roots* of the nerve under the terms *intermediofacial nerve* or *facial complex*. The usual description of the intermediate nerve or division of the complex as the "sensory root" is also equally misleading, since many of its fibres are efferent parasympathetic, supplying the submandibular and sublingual salivary glands, the lacrimal gland (see p. 225), the palatine and nasal mucosal glands, and to glandular cells in paranasal sinuses.

The facial complex emerges from the brain at the lower border of the pons in the recess between the olive and the inferior cerebellar peduncle (Fig. 352). It is here lateral to the abducent, but medial to the vestibulocochlear, the intermediate part being lateral to the main facial trunk. The two nerves run laterally and forwards in the posterior cranial fossa to the internal acoustic (auditory) meatus. In this part of the course the nervus intermedius is between the facial trunk and the vestibulocochlear, the latter being grooved by it (Fig. 353). Accompanied by the labyrinthine artery these structures enter the meatus, at the bottom

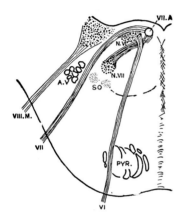

FIG. 292—THE ABDUCENT AND FACIAL NERVES AND THEIR NUCLEI.

The outline represents a transverse section of the lower part of the pons, on to which the course of the facial nerve is projected. VI, N.VI = abducent nerve and nucleus. VII = facial nerve. VII.A = the ascending portion of its root, supposed to be seen in optical section. N.VII = facial nucleus. S.O. = trapezoid body. A.V. = mesencephalic tract of trigeminal nerve. VIII.M. = medial root of vestibulocochlear nerve.

(After Schwalbe, from Quain's "Anatomy".)

of which is the lamina cribrosa, divided into four parts by a horizontal and a less marked vertical partition. The facial, including the nervus intermedius, passes through the anterosuperior quadrant, and enters the facial canal. It now, for a short distance (4 mm), continues laterally more or less in the direction of the internal auditory meatus, then bends backwards over the vestibule to reach the middle ear. The geniculate ganglion is at the bend (geniculum) of the nerve, and here the nervus intermedius fuses with it. Adjacent to the tympanic cavity the nerve is in an osseous *facial canal*, between the roof and medial wall and above the promontory and fenestra vestibuli (ovalis). The bone may be absent in parts, and hence the nerve may more easily be affected in inflammation of the tympanum.

At the junction of the medial and posterior boundaries of the tympanic cavity the facial nerve curves downwards and backwards to issue from the petrous bone by the stylomastoid foramen. The descending portion of this second bend forms a ridge on the medial wall of the aditus, and has above it the bulge formed by the lateral semicircular canal. Having emerged from the skull, the facial nerve gives off two branches (Fig. 291) and then divides into a larger upper and a smaller lower division (temporozygomatic and cervicofacial). These run forwards in the parotid, lying here superficial to the retromandibular (posterior facial) vein and the external carotid artery, and divide in the substance of the gland. These two major divisions of the facial nerve, themselves somewhat variable, subdivide further into temporal, zygomatic, buccal, mandibular and cervical rami, distributed to the facial musculature. (For variations see Hovelacque, 1927.) It is of practical importance to note that in the infant, who has no mastoid process, the facial nerve at its exit from the skull lies more on the lateral than the under aspect of the skull, and if the usual incision behind the ear be made to expose the mastoid antrum it will almost certainly be injured.

BRANCHES

In the temporal bone:
    (a) Major or greater (superficial) petrosal to the pterygopalatine ganglion.
    (b) Branches to the tympanic plexus.
    (c) Nerve to the stapedial muscle.
    (d) Chorda tympani, gustatory to presulcal part of tongue.
At its exit from the stylomastoid foramen:
    Posterior auricular, supplying occipitalis and some auricular muscles.
    Digastric.
    Stylo-hyoid.
On the face:
    Temporal, supplying frontalis, orbicularis, etc.
    Zygomatic, also supplying orbicularis oculi.
    Buccal, to muscles of nose and upper lip.
    Mandibular, to muscles of lower lip.
    Cervical, supplying platysma.

The greater petrosal nerve and the chorda tympani contain fibres which enter or leave the brainstem only in the intermediate nerve; they are gustatory fibres from the tongue and soft palate and parasympathetic secretomotor fibres. The tympanic rami contain fibres which travel in both parts of the facial nerve. All the fibres travelling in the intermediate nerve leave either the geniculate ganglion or the intrapetrous part of the facial nerve, which hence contains no "intermediate" fibres in its extracranial course.

The Greater Petrosal Nerve branches from the geniculate ganglion. It passes through a canal, then runs in a groove on the anterior surface of the petrous temporal (Fig. 274) under the trigeminal ganglion to the foramen lacerum. Here it unites with the deep petrosal, from the sympathetic plexus on the internal carotid artery, to form the nerve of the pterygoid canal, which joins the pterygopalatine ganglion via the pterygoid canal (Fig. 289). The greater petrosal nerve contains taste fibres to the mucous membrane of the soft palate, and also secretory fibres to the palatal, nasal and lacrimal glands (see also p. 225).

The Tympanic Branches join the lesser or minor petrosal nerve as it emerges from the tympanic plexus. These facial fibres thus join glossopharyngeal fibres, and are secretomotor via the lesser petrosal nerve and otic ganglion relay to the parotid gland. Some facial fibres, reaching the tympanic cavity through the tympanic rami, may supply the tympanic membrane and part of the pinna or both aspects. (The secretomotor fibres mentioned above may be derived from the vagus nerve—see Vidić, 1968.) These sensory twigs commonly encroach on the external surface of the tympanic membrane and even on the skin of the external auditory meatus and pinna. Thus is explained the presence here of vesicles in some cases of facial herpes. (For further discussion, see Brodal, 1969.)

The Temporal Branch runs upwards (Fig. 291). It supplies auricularis anterior and superior, and gives a few twigs to frontalis.

The Zygomatic Branches are in two groups. The upper of these (Fig. 291, Z^1) runs subcutaneously across the zygomatic arch to supply frontalis and the muscles of the upper eyelid (orbicularis oculi, corrugator supercilii, procerus) (Fig. 275). Interruption of these nerves prevents full closure of the eyelids, and corneal desiccation and ulceration result. The lower zygomatic branches (Fig. 291, Z^2) cross the zygomatic bone to supply the orbicularis fibres of the lower lid and the upper fibres of the elevators of the upper lip.

The Buccal Branch runs forwards below the parotid duct to supply buccinator and the muscles of the upper lip as far as the midline. These include the zyomaticus major et minor, risorius, levator anguli oris and levator labii superioris alæque nasi.

The Mandibular Branch commonly runs down in the neck and crosses the lower border of the mandible on the facial artery at the anterior border of masseter. Here it is vulnerable to trauma or surgical incisions. It supplies all the muscles of the lower lip depressor anguli oris, depressor labii inferioris, and mentalis.

The Cervical Branch runs down to supply platysma.

Nuclei and Central Connections.—The sensory fibres issuing in the nervus intermedius have their somata in the geniculate ganglion. They are unipolar neurons, whose peripheral processes are distributed as described above. Their central axons reach the cranial levels of the nucleus solitarius, which projects to the ventral nuclei of the dorsal thalamus and thence to the postcentral gyrus. The somatic sensory fibres of the facial (which innervate the tympanic membrane and pinna) have unknown connections.

The motor branchial nucleus of the facial nerve consists of large multipolar neurons like those of the nucleus ambiguus, both being components of the branchial column of the brainstem. The facial nucleus is situated near its point of exit, but the fibres do not pass straight out. They run first backwards and medially through the pons to the floor of the fourth ventricle, where they cross and run upwards medially to the abducent nucleus, forming the colliculus facialis in the floor of the ventricle. The fibres now turn laterally, cross the abducent nucleus again, pass forwards between their own nucleus and the spinal root of the trigeminal nerve, to emerge between the olive and the inferior cerebella peduncle (Figs. 292, 354).

Communications.—Like many other cranial nerves the facial has numerous peripheral connections with others, including the vestibulocochlear, vagal, glossopharyngeal, lesser occipital, trigeminal and transverse cervical cutaneous nerves. It has also been stated to supply the orbicularis oculi via the oculomotor nerve (and other facial muscles via this and other cranial nerves), in an effort to explain the "sparing" of upper facial muscles in supranuclear facial nerve paralysis. These speculations are unfounded, and the explanation is certainly to be found in central connections.

THE VESTIBULOCOCHLEAR (EIGHTH CRANIAL) NERVE

The vestibulocochlear nerve (also known as the stato-acoustic or auditory nerve) is the eighth of the cranial series. It is well-named, because of its two components, vestibular and cochlear, the former serves the phytogenetically older part of the labyrinth, the semicircular canals. The cochlea is less developed in earlier vertebrates. The nerve is continuous with the brainstem immediately inferior to the pons and very close to the facial nerve, the nervus intermedius issuing between them. The inferior cerebellar peduncle is just posterior and the cochlear division of the nerve passes round the lateral side of this to reach the cochlear nuclei, whereas the vestibular division penetrates into the brainstem medial to the peduncle.

The nerve runs laterally and forwards to the internal acoustic (auditory) meatus, its two portions forming a groove in which is the facial, the nervus intermedius lying between them.

Accompanied by the labyrinthine branch of the basilar artery, these structures enter the meatus, at the bottom of which the vestibulocochlear nerve divides into branches which pass through the lamina cribrosa.

The cochlear division passes through the lower and anterior quadrant to reach the cochlea. The branches of the vestibular division pass through the two posterior quadrants. Through the superoposterior quadrant go the nerves to the utricle, superior and lateral semicircular canals. Through the inferoposterior quadrant pass the nerves to the sacculus and posterior semicircular canals. (For recent work on the topography and components of the nerve consult the papers of Bergström, 1973 and the monographs of Rasmussen, 1960, Brodal, 1969, etc.)

Nuclei and Central Connections.—The ganglion of the cochlear division, or ganglion spirale, lies in the cochlear modiolus. Its peripheral fibres come from the spiral organ of Corti.

The ganglion of the vestibular division is in the internal auditory meatus. Its peripheral fibres come from the maculæ and cristæ of the utricle, saccule and semicircular canals. The two nerves are united in the internal auditory meatus, and so run back to enter the brain below the pons lateral to the facial nerve. The cochlear portion now goes to two nuclei, one dorsal and one ventral to the inferior cerebellar peduncle. From the dorsal nucleus fibres pass through the peduncle to join the lateral lemniscus of the opposite side.

The fibres from the ventral nucleus also join the lateral lemniscus, which makes connection with the inferior colliculus for relay of acoustic reflexes. For conscious hearing the lateral lemniscus relays in the medial geniculate bodies, whence fibres traverse the posterior limb of the internal capsule to reach the anterior transverse gyrus of the temporal lobe.

The vestibular fibres are distributed to all the vestibular nuclei (medial, lateral [Deiter's], superior and inferior), which partly correspond to the area acoustica of the fourth ventricle and are partly anterior to the inferior cerebellar peduncle. Some fibres also pass directly into the cerebellum. (For details of the central cochlear and vestibular connections see Rasmussen and Windle, 1960, Crosby et al., 1962, Whitfield, 1967, Brodal, 1969, Williams and Warwick, 1975.)

CHAPTER VII

THE VISUAL PATHWAY

THE visual pathway from the retina may be divided into six levels:
(1) The optic nerve.
(2) The optic chiasma.
(3) The optic tract.
(4) The lateral geniculate nucleus.
(5) The optic radiation.
(6) The cortical areas.

THE OPTIC (SECOND CRANIAL) NERVE

The Optic Nerve, ensheathed in pia, runs as a flattened band from the antero-lateral angle of the somewhat quadrilateral chiasma forwards and laterally and slightly downwards to the optic foramen (Fig. 260). Actually the cross-section behind the optic foramen is pear-shaped, with the rounded end medial. At its entry into the optic canal it receives a covering of arachnoid mater, and since the dura mater is prolonged through the canal as a periosteum, the nerve in fact is from here onwards surrounded by all three meninges, and also, of course, cerebro-spinal fluid (Fig. 259).

Becoming more oval, and acquiring its dural covering, it traverses the optic canal and enters the orbit. As a rounded cord it now runs forwards and slightly laterally and downwards in a somewhat sinuous manner (to allow for ocular move-ments), and is continued into the back of the eyeball. The centre of its cross-section is just *above* and 3 mm medial to the posterior pole (Fig. 248, E).

Its total length is 5 cm, the intracranial portion being about 1 cm, the intra-canalicular 6 mm, the intraorbital 3 cm, and the intraocular 0·7 mm.

Although we speak of the optic *nerve*, it is very important to realise that it is really no nerve at all, but essentially a *fibre tract* joining two portions of the brain. The evidence for this is incontrovertible. Firstly, it is an outgrowth of the brain; secondly, its fibres possess no neurolemmal cells, though other satellite cells occur; thirdly, it is surrounded by the meninges, unlike any peripheral nerve; fourthly (and most cogently), the "primary" and "secondary" sensory neurons of the pathway are both *in the retina*, the ganglion cells corresponding, for example, to those in the gracile or cuneate nuclei in the medulla oblongata.

Relations.—(*a*) *In the Cranial Cavity.*—The nerve lies at first above the dia-phragma sellæ, which covers the pituitary body, then on the anterior portion of the cavernous sinus.

Between the two nerves in front of the chiasma is a triangular space in which is a variable portion of the hypophysis cerebri (pituitary), covered by the diaphragma sellæ (see p. 344).

Above the nerve is the *anterior perforated substance*, the *medial root of the olfactory tract*, and the *anterior cerebral artery*, which crosses superiorly to reach its medial side (Figs. 260, 320, 355).

The Internal Carotid Artery is at first below, then lateral.

The Ophthalmic Artery usually comes off the internal carotid under the middle of the optic nerve (Fig. 280), but since its course here is anteroposterior, and that of the nerve laterally as well as forwards, it may appear at the medial border of the nerve before it eventually passes laterally. At any rate, in this first portion of

OPTIC NERVE COVERED BY FALCIFORM EDGE

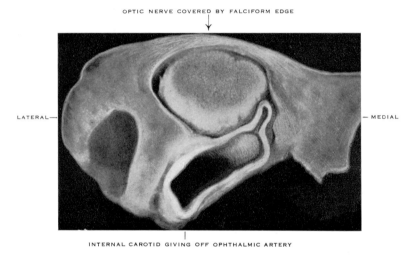

LATERAL —   — MEDIAL

INTERNAL CAROTID GIVING OFF OPHTHALMIC ARTERY

Fig. 293.—Transverse Section of Portion of Sphenoid Bone with Optic Canal at Level of Falciform Edge.

Note ophthalmic artery is medial here.

its course it is nearer the medial border than the lateral (Fig. 293). The nearer the origin of the artery is to the optic foramen, the nearer the *medial* side of the nerve is it placed.

(b) *In the Optic Canal.*—The pia forms a sheath closely adherent to the nerve. The dura constitutes the periosteal lining to the canal and at its orbital end splits to become continuous on the one hand with the periorbita and on the other with the dura of the optic nerve.

Hovelacque (1927) stated the view that a short sleeve only of arachnoid penetrates the cranial end of the canal for 1 to 2 mm, and that the membrane is absent from the remainder of the canal. However, this view is untenable, since cerebrospinal fluid surrounds the nerve as far as the eyeball. Although slight individual variations may occur, the intracranial subarachnoid space always communicates with that around the nerve.

Being in part periosteum, the dura mater is attached to bone. To a variable extent it is also adherent at some point in the canal to the pia mater, giving the optic nerve some degree of fixation in the canal.

But this adhesion varies in its position and in its density. Schwalbe held that it was above, so that only in the lower part did the cranial subarachnoid space

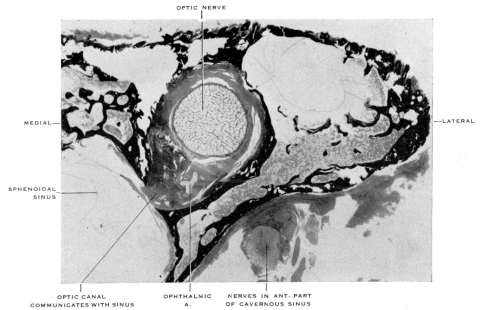

FIG. 294.—TRANSVERSE SECTION OF PORTION OF SPHENOID BONE WITH OPTIC CANAL (BONE DECALCIFIED).

Note dense connective tissue around artery.

communicate with that in the orbit. But Hovelacque (1927), quoting Pfister, stated that the point of adhesion might be anywhere in the circumference of the nerve and indeed most often adjacent to the ophthalmic artery (Fig. 294). There are also here and there weaker trabeculæ which cross from the dura to pia.

The ophthalmic artery crosses below the nerve in the dural sheath to its lateral side. It leaves the dura at or near the anterior end of the canal. Thus the internal carotid artery is to some extent tied to the dural sheath by its ophthalmic branch (Fig. 295); and it is also indirectly attached to the optic nerve by the adherence of the sheaths and by branches to the nerve from the ophthalmic artery.

Medial to the optic nerve is the sphenoidal air sinus (Fig. 294) or a posterior ethmoidal sinus, from which it may be separated by a thin plate of bone only. *This provides the anatomical explanation of a retrobulbar neuritis, following a sinus infection.*

Not infrequently the sphenoidal sinus or a posterior ethmoidal sinus may invade the roots of the lesser wing of the sphenoid, and even the wing itself. The nerve is then surrounded by sinuses.

(c) *In the Orbit* (Figs. 15, 280, 282).—At the optic foramen the nerve is surrounded by the origin of the ocular muscles, that of the superior and medial recti being closely adherent to the dural sheath. *It is this connection which gives rise to the pain (in extreme movements of the globe) so characteristic of retrobulbar neuritis.*

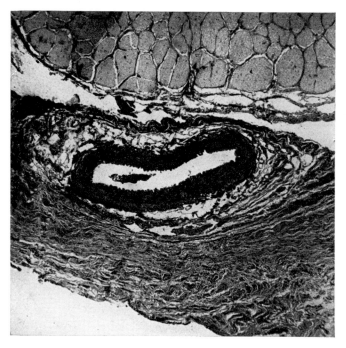

Fig. 295.—Transverse Section of the Sheaths of the Optic Nerve in its Canal.
The ophthalmic artery is here in the dura mater.

Between the optic nerve and the lateral rectus are the divisions of the oculomotor nerve, the nasociliary, sympathetic and abducent nerves and sometimes the ophthalmic vein or veins (Fig. 263).

Farther forwards the muscles are separated from the nerve by orbital fat.

The nasociliary nerve, the ophthalmic artery, and the superior ophthalmic vein cross the nerve superiorly from its lateral to its medial side.

The Ciliary Ganglion is lateral to the nerve, sited between it and the lateral rectus (Figs. 280, 281).

The Long and Short Ciliary Nerves and Arteries gradually surround the nerve as it passes to the back of the eyeball.

The Arteria Centralis Retinæ, a branch of the ophthalmic artery near the optic foramen, runs forwards in or outside the dural sheath of the nerve, then with its accompanying vein *crosses the subarachnoid space* to enter the nerve on its under and medial aspect about 12 mm ($\frac{1}{2}$ in.) behind the eye. At the point of entrance of the vessels the nerve, instead of being round is oval or horseshoe-shaped, and if the vessels enter separately there are two oval regions (Kuhnt, 1890).

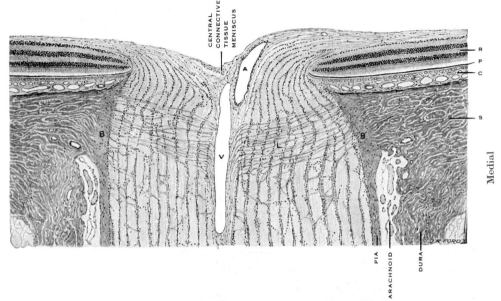

FIG. 296.—HORIZONTAL SECTION OF THE OPTIC NERVE HEAD.

A. = arteria centralis retinæ. V. = vena centralis retinæ. B. = border tissue. L. = lamina cribrosa. R. = retina. P. = pigment epithelium and basal lamina. C. = choroid. S. = sclera.

(d) *The Intraocular Region.*—As the nerve passes into the eye its fibres lose their myelin sheaths, and at the same time there is diminution in the amount of supporting tissue.

This results in the optic nerve being 3 mm in diameter at the back of the globe and only 1·5 mm adjacent to the retina.

The intraocular section of the optic nerve passes through the sclera, the choroid, and finally appears inside the eye as the "papilla" optica, where it becomes continuous with the nerve fibre layer of the retina (Figs. 296 and 301). (It does not, of course, usually project enough to justify the term "papilla".)

We may thus subdivide the ocular fraction of the nerve into *scleral, choroidal,* and *retinal* parts.

The junction between the medullated and non-medullated parts of the nerve is at the back of the lamina cribrosa (Figs. 297, 301)—at the distal end of the subarachnoid space—but this is not a sharp line, for some fibres lose their myelin sheath proximal and some distal to this point.

A.E.—22

The Neighbouring Retina.—The layers of the *retina*, apart from the nerve fibres, end near the borders of the optic nerve, being separated from it, however, by a ring or partial ring of glial tissue called the *intermediary tissue of Kuhnt* (Figs. 298, 301). It is usually stated that the intermediary tissue of Kuhnt can be seen with the ophthalmoscope. This can hardly be true since neuroglia is transparent and also the tissue is covered by the whole thickness of the nerve fibre layer of the retina as it curves round to pass into the optic nerve. In the retinal portion the nerve fibres are in separate bundles, being separated from each other by columns consisting of neuroglial nuclei, fibres and vessels. The individual fibres have extremely fine glial fibres around them.

The boundary of the retina is usually oblique, but more so on the nasal than on the temporal side, where it may be vertical. The inner layers end before the

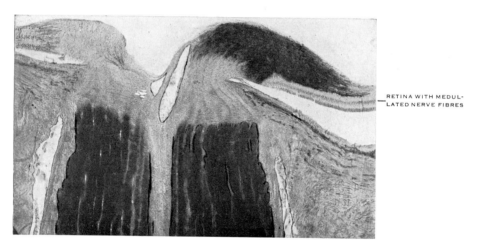

RETINA WITH MEDUL-
LATED NERVE FIBRES

FIG. 297.—SECTION OF THE OPTIC NERVE TO SHOW CONGENITALLY MEDULLATED NERVE FIBRES IN THE RETINA. (WEIGERT'S STAIN.)

Note that the normal medullation stops behind the lamina cribrosa, in which region the fibres are non-medullated.

(From a section kindly supplied by Mr. Percy Flemming.)

outer. The rods and cones become smaller, maybe half their normal size, and cease altogether a little before the pigment epithelium which reaches almost up to the intermediary tissue. The basal lamina may come right up to the nerve fibres but is usually separated by glia.

When the retina ceases a little farther from the periphery of the optic nerve than the choroid, the latter may be visible ophthalmoscopically as a pigmented *choroidal crescent* at the edge of the disc. A localized accumulation of retinal pigment epithelium may cause a similar crescent. Where both choroid and retina fall short of the nerve, a pale *scleral crescent* may be seen.

The Neighbouring Choroid.—The posterior termination of the choroid will

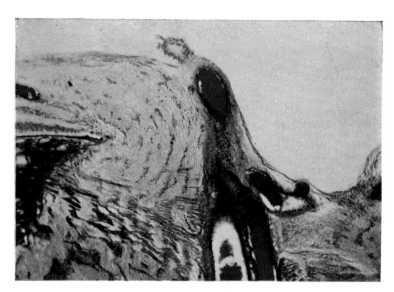

FIG. 299.—SECTION ACROSS OPTIC NERVE HEAD. (MALLORY'S TRIPLE STAIN.)

Red-staining glia covers the physiological cup. Note remains of the hyaloid artery (see Fig. 297).

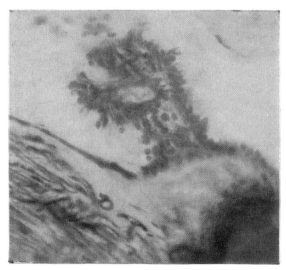

FIG. 300.—DETAILS OF FIGURE 296.

VESTIGES OF THE HYALOID ARTERY, CONSISTING OF GLIAL AND CONNECTIVE TISSUE CELLS (STAINED PINK), OCCUPY THE UPPER HALF OF THE FIELD.

vary greatly as this portion of the scleral canal is widening or narrowing (see types of scleral canal). The boundary may be oblique, pointed, or almost rectangular in sections.

Only the basal lamina, the two layers of which end almost together, reaches the aperture of entry of the nerve. The pigment epithelium continues almost as far as the basal lamina, although the rods and cones have stopped earlier (Fig. 301). The vascular choroidal stroma ends farther from the disc than the basal membrane, the capillaries reaching nearer to it than the smaller vessels (Figs. 298, 301).

The remaining layers of non-vascular stroma form a closely knit tissue containing numerous pigment cells. Pigment cells of different types may thus come

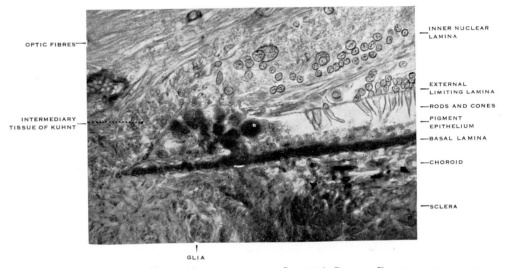

FIG. 298.—EDGE OF OPTIC NERVE (ANTEROPOSTERIOR SECTION). COLLOID BODIES HAVE FORMED ON THE BASAL LAMINA (HYALOID MEMBRANE).

to lie on either side of the basal lamina. The stromal lamellæ of the choroid do not reach right up to the edge of the nerve; they are held away by the border tissue. The laminæ of the suprachoroidea usually have an oblique course between the sclera and the choroid proper, but near the optic nerve they become meridional and run parallel with the sclera. Also pigmentation is dense as we approach the nerve.

The Neighbouring Sclera.—Near the optic nerve the innermost fibres of the sclera are meridional; then meridional and circular, while the most superficial are circular. These outer circular fibres as we approach the optic nerve interlace with the outer longitudinal fibres of the dura in the same manner as they do at the limbus with the cornea. There is a great increase in the number of pigment cells as we approach the optic nerve.

The Marginal (Border) Tissue (of Elschnig) (Figs. 301, 304–306) of the optic nerve is an annular region of neuroglia intervening between the choroid and sclera and the optic nerve fibres. It is basically collagenous tissue, with some admixture of glial cells. It is a scleral derivative, unlike the intermediary tissue of Kuhnt (*vide supra*) and the border tissue of Jacoby, the latter being the backward continuation of Kuhnt's tissue. Both these regions are part of a continuous sleeve of astrocytes around the optic nerve, broken only where the scleral tissue of the lamina cribrosa interlaces with the nerve. (See also p. 334.) With ordinary stains the border tissue differs little from the rest of the sclera, but usually can be distinguished from it. In longitudinal sections it appears as a strip of denser tissue

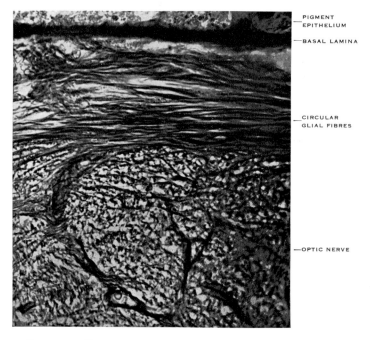

FIG. 304.—TRANSVERSE SECTION OF EDGE OF OPTIC NERVE AT LEVEL OF BASAL LAMINA (HYALOID MEMBRANE). (ZENKER, MALLORY'S TRIPLE STAIN.)

immediately around the optic nerve, and is then continued forwards to delimit the choroid from the nerve fibres. It consists of dense collagenous tissue, in which are also found many glial and elastic fibres and some pigment.

As would be expected, none of the tissues of the eyeball, except the optic fibres, is in direct contact with the optic nerve itself. Even the basal lamina of the choroid is separated from it by the neuroglial tissue (of Kuhnt). See Fig. 301.

The Scleral Canal is the conduit by which the optic nerve penetrates the retina. It is bounded by the border tissue, which separates the nerve fibres from the choroid and anterior third of the sclera proper. It is some 0·5 mm long, and may

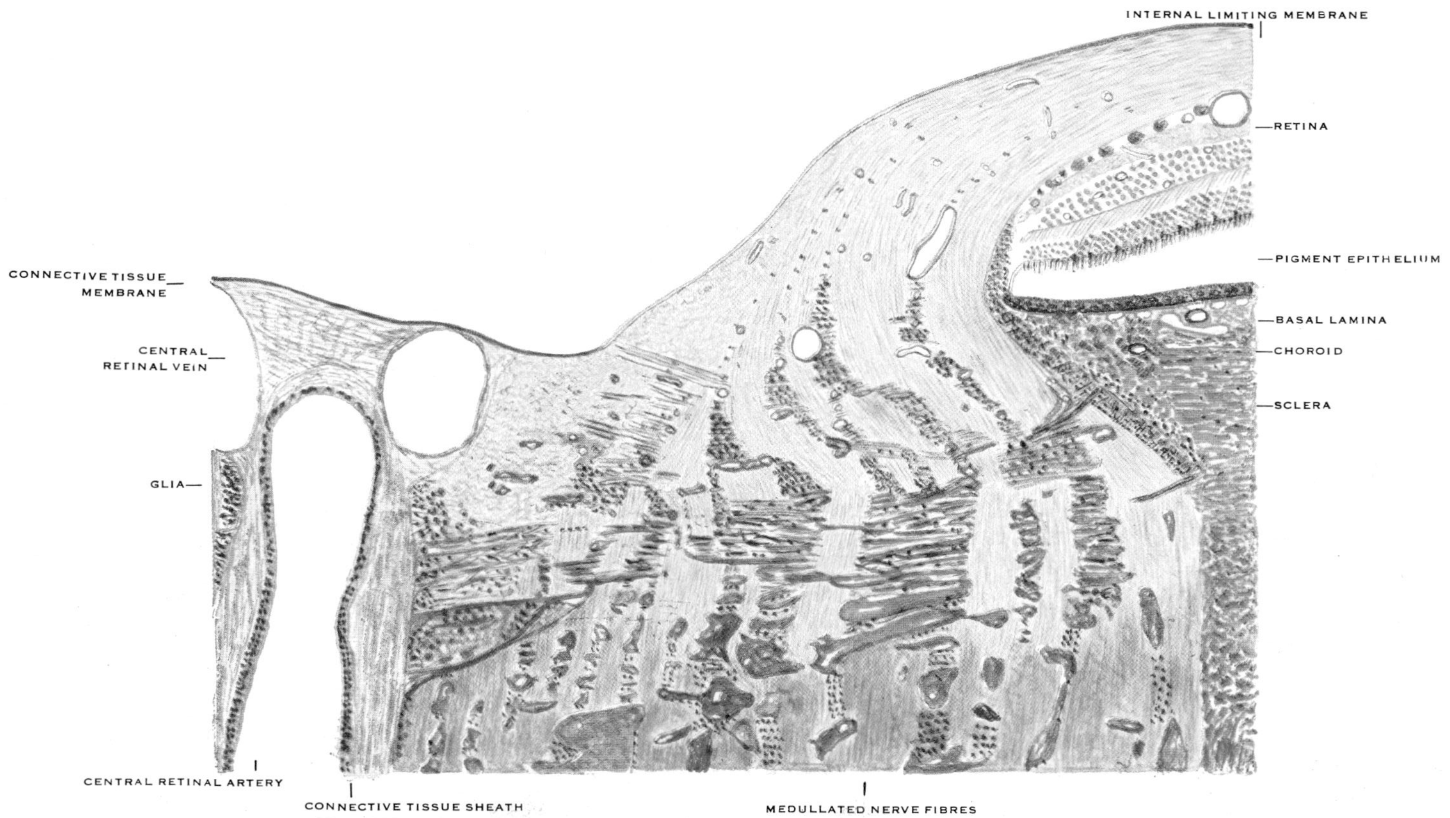

INTERNAL LIMITING MEMBRANE

RETINA

PIGMENT EPITHELIUM

BASAL LAMINA

CHOROID

SCLERA

CONNECTIVE TISSUE SHEATH

MEDULLATED NERVE FIBRES

FIG. 301.—ANTEROPOSTERIOR SECTION OF THE OPTIC NERVE HEAD. (ZENKER. MALLORY'S TRIPLE STAIN.)

CONNECTIVE TISSUE MEMBRANE

CENTRAL RETINAL VEIN

GLIA

CENTRAL RETINAL ARTERY

Connective tissue—blue.

Non-medullated nerve fibres, light red; medullated nerve fibres, darker red: neuroglia, still darker red. Note that the anterior portion of the lamina cribrosa is glial; the posterior consists of alternating layers of glia and connective tissue, but mainly the latter.

Glia separates the anterior portion of the sclera and the whole thickness of choroid from the nerve fibres and is continued anteriorly behind the basal lamina (hyaloid membrane) and pigment epithelium to form the "intermediary tissue" of Kuhnt. This lies in the concavity of the nerve fibres as they sweep into the nerve.

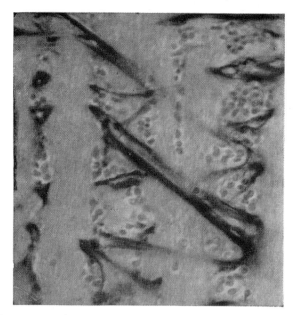

FIG. 302.—LONGITUDINAL SECTION OF OPTIC NERVE. (MALLORY'S TRIPLE STAIN.)
Note columns of glial nuclei and parts of connective tissue septa (stained blue).

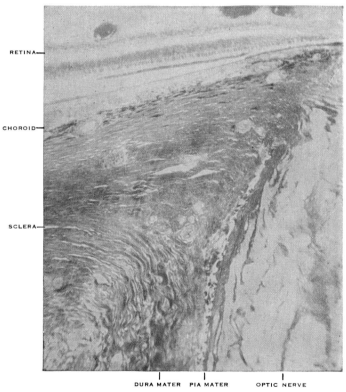

FIG. 303.—SECTION AT THE MARGIN OF THE OPTIC NERVE TO SHOW HOW THE DURA MATER IS
CONTINUOUS WITH THE EXTERNAL STRATA OF THE SCLERA.

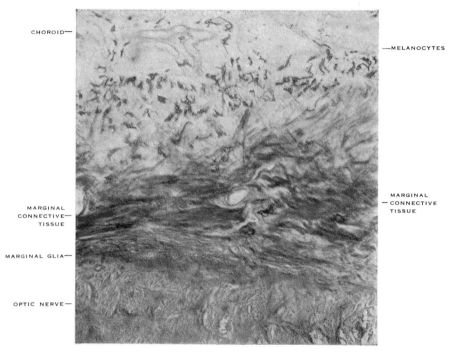

CHOROID—

—MELANOCYTES

MARGINAL
CONNECTIVE—
TISSUE

MARGINAL
—CONNECTIVE
TISSUE

MARGINAL GLIA—

OPTIC NERVE—

Fig. 305.—Transverse Section of Optic Nerve a little posterior to the Basal Lamina and to the section shown in Fig. 302. (Zenker. Mallory's Triple Stain.)

Connective tissue is blue, glia is red.

run straight forward or be directed slightly nasally, temporally, or downwards. For descriptive purposes this *intraocular* part of the optic nerve has been divided by Hayreh and Vrabec (1966) into prelaminar, laminar and postlaminar sections, according to their relationship to the lamina cribrosa. (For detailed differences between these regions consult these workers and also Hogan, Alvarado and Weddell, 1971.)

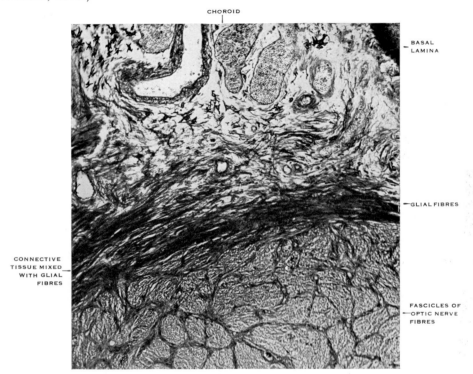

FIG. 306.—TRANSVERSE SECTION OF OPTIC NERVE A LITTLE BEHIND BASAL LAMINA OF THE CHOROID (COMPARE FIG. 304). (ZENKER, MALLORY'S TRIPLE STAIN.)

As regards it shape, there are three types of scleral canal: (*a*) a cone with its narrowest point at the basal lamina; (*b*) the canal narrows to the inner third of the sclera, the portion anterior to this keeping the same diameter; (*c*) the canal narrows to the inner third of the sclera and then widens again, i.e. it is shaped like an hourglass. In (*b*) and (*c*) a scleral ring is present and can be seen with the ophthalmoscope (Kuhnt, 1890).

The Lamina Cribrosa is a sieve-like (cribriform) arrangement of interweaving fascicles of collagen bundles connecting the sclera across the scleral canal. Through its orifices pass fascicles of optic nerve fibres. (Figs. 301, 307, 308.)

In order to understand its structure it is best to consider its development, which in its *posterior portion* is like that of the septa of the optic nerve (see p. 341),

Thus in its scleral portion each trabecula of the lamina cribrosa is essentially the result of the ingrowth of a vessel derived from the vascular circle of Zinn, which is accompanied by connective tissue and glia.

Each trabecula therefore has a vessel in its centre. This is surrounded by collagen bundles and a considerable amount of elastic fibres, external to which are glial cells. The anterior part of the lamina cribrosa has sometimes been said to consist of neuroglial cells, astrocytes; but these merely exist as accumulations,

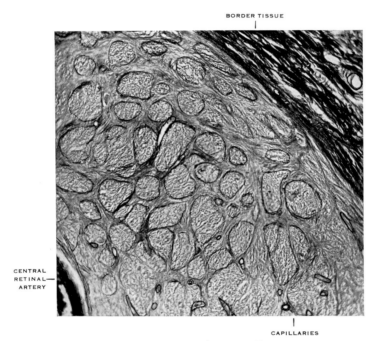

BORDER TISSUE

CENTRAL RETINAL— ARTERY

CAPILLARIES

FIG. 307.—TRANSVERSE SECTION THROUGH THE ANTERIOR PRELAMINAR PART OF THE OPTIC NERVE. (ZENKER, MALLORY'S TRIPLE STAIN.)

Note that the neuroglial tissue between the nerve fibre fascicles corresponds in arrangement with the collagen trabeculæ of the lamina cribrosa (Fig. 308.)

(*Wolff's preparation.*)

between nerve fibre fascicles in the prelaminar part of the nerve, sufficiently to suggest this interpretation in stained sections (Fig. 307).

The amount of elastic tissue in the lamina cribrosa is usually regarded as surprisingly high, considering its relative paucity in the rest of the sclera. It may, however, be much reduced or even absent (Anderson, 1969).

The vessels from the vascular circle of Zinn, as they pass into the nerve, divide and reunite to form a network which fills the interval between the side wall of the scleral canal and the connective tissue around the central vessels.

The form of the lamina cribrosa on transverse section depends on this vascular network. It also forms a net of narrow meshes which are transversely oval (Figs. 307, 308).

In an anteroposterior section it is seen that three to eight dense trabeculæ of hyaline appearance pass out of the side wall of the scleral canal. The most posterior run inwards and backwards (Fig. 301) to reach the central connective tissue a little in front of the outer limit of the sclera and make with the corresponding fibre of the opposite side a letter V with its concavity forwards. The more anterior ones run more directly inwards but are all slightly concave anteriorly. At the posterior boundary of the lamina cribrosa a very thick trabecula often passes out from the sclera (Fig. 301). It contains a correspondingly large artery which has a relatively strong muscularis and well-marked elastica. But in general the limits of the lamina cribrosa are not quite definite, for posteriorly it shades off into the framework of the optic nerve, and indeed some anatomists regard it as simply the continuation forwards of this framework.

THE NEUROGLIA OF THE INTRAOCULAR OPTIC NERVE

Like the rest of the optic nerve, its intraocular part contains much neuroglial, though it is here represented only by astrocytes. This is understandable on developmental grounds, since the optic peduncle is predominantly neuroglial before the optic nerve fibres grow into it (p. 436). Moreover, at a certain stage of development the arteria centralis gives off the hyaloid artery. The origin of this artery is surrounded by a conical bud of neuroglia. Later the artery disappears and all that remains of the bud is a lamella of neuroglia which separates the central portion of the nerve head, including the connective tissue round the central vessels (central connective tissue sheath), from the vitreous (Figs. 299, 300, 301).

This lamella of neuroglia, called the *central connective tissue meniscus* of Kuhnt, replaces the internal limiting membrane, which is absent here, but is continuous with it at the periphery (Fig. 301).

Since there are no connective tissue fibres (except those in the walls of vessels) in the choroidal and retinal portion of the scleral canal, the supporting tissues are all neuroglial. Thus the great majority of cells seen in this region, and forming the "nuclear columns" between the nerve fibre bundles, are glial.

The astrocytes, the only neuroglial elements in this region, are like those elsewhere in the optic nerve. They form continuous sheets as a form of tube around fascicles of optic fibres. Their form is altered by the intrusion of the collagenous element of the lamina cribrosa into the nerve. Their processes are for the most part circumferential with respect to the nerve fibre fascicles. Some of these processes, like those of astrocytes elsewhere, make direct contact with the basement membranes and pericytes of capillaries.

Not infrequently in infants a filamentary remnant of the hyaloid artery may be seen to enter the vitreous for 1–1·5 mm, after a short intrapapillary course.

There are no cells of Müller in the disc and thus no material which binds the nerve fibres together at right angles to their course, as occurs in the retina generally. They can thus be separated much more easily from each other and the tissue distended with œdematous fluid. *This is no doubt the reason why the disc swells so easily in papillœdema while the neighbouring retina remains relatively flat.*

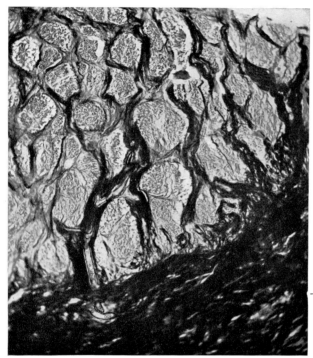

FIG. 308. — TRANSVERSE SECTION THROUGH THE LAMINA CRIBROSA. (ZENKER, MALLORY'S TRIPLE STAIN.)

The elastico-collagenous trabeculae correspond in pattern to the neuroglial arrangement in the prelaminar region. (Compare with Fig. 367.)

(*Wolff's preparation.*)

—SCLERA

Neuroglia also lines the anterior portion of the scleral and the whole of the choroidal portion of the canal of entry of the optic nerve (Fig. 301, 304).

This neuroglia is continued anteriorly beyond the pigment epithelium where it forms the intermediary tissue of Kuhnt. The neuroglia here forms a mass of nuclei and circularly running fibres placed in the concavity of the nerve fibres of the retina as they curve round at the edge of the disc to enter the optic nerve (Figs. 298, 301).

THE SHEATHS OF THE OPTIC NERVE

The optic nerve in the cranial cavity is at first surrounded only by pia, but in the optic canal arachnoid and dura are added.

At the optic foramen the cranial dura splits into two layers. The outer becomes continuous with the periosteum of the orbit (periorbita), the inner forms the dural covering of the optic nerve.

Thus in the canal and in the orbit the nerve is surrounded by three sheaths, namely, **dura, arachnoid** and **pia**.

Between dura and arachnoid is the so-called *subdural space*; between the arachnoid and pia is the *subarachnoid space*. Both these spaces communicate with the corresponding intracranial spaces; thus fluid injected into the subarachnoid space in the cranial cavity easily passes into the subarachnoid space around the optic nerve. The subdural space, as seen in microscopic preparations, is an artefact.

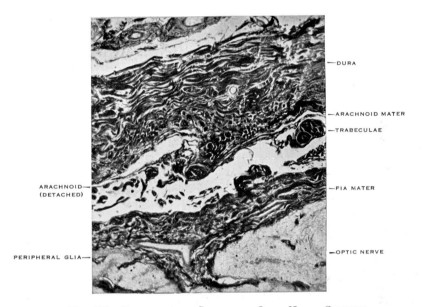

FIG. 309.—LONGITUDINAL SECTION OF OPTIC NERVE SHEATHS.

The "space" is only potential, has no known physiological significance, and only becomes apparent in pathological states. It has received undue attention in normal microanatomy.

The Dura consists of bundles of tough fibrous tissue which are larger than those of the sclera and composed of collagenous fibrillæ, in which are found numerous elastic fibres. The dura varies in thickness from 0·35 to 0·5 mm. It is thickest where it becomes continuous with the sclera.

The central dural fibres run for the most part circularly, the peripheral ones (i.e. those nearest the supravaginal space) tend to run longitudinally with oblique ones interspersed (Figs. 159, 309). Most of the fibres are composed of collagen bundles, but elastic fibres are interspersed between these in small numbers. The collagen fibres have a diameter of 600 to 700 μm, but finer fibres occur.

The outer longitudinal portion (or layer) is loosely made and often divides up into two to five lamellæ. Between the lamellæ are fusiform nuclei which tend to be more numerous in childhood. The nuclei belong to flattened oblong or star-shaped cells which are in close relationship with numerous elastic fibres.

The inner aspect of the dura is covered with a continuous endothelial lining, which very easily becomes detached as an artefact (Fig. 159), and which is then reflected on to the trabeculæ which pass to the arachnoid and pia. Some observers have denied the existence of such a "one-sided" epithelial arrangement. It is difficult to deduce the functional value of such an endothelium.

Where the ciliary vessels and nerves approach the sclera, the lamellæ become condensed, surround these, and eventually blend with the sclera. The ciliary ganglion sends numerous fine nerves with very thick epineurium along the vessels. These form a plexus in which ganglion cells may be present. The vessels have a very thick adventitia and a remarkably thick structureless subendothelial layer.

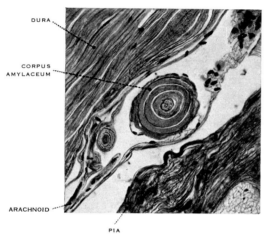

FIG. 310.—CORPORA AMYLACEA IN ARACHNOID.

Around the dura is the so-called supravaginal space, described by Schwalbe (1887) as a lymph space lined by endothelium. It has, however, the structure of loose connective tissue which is easily distensible with fluid (see p. 272).

The Arachnoid is a very thin membrane some 10 μm in thickness, which consists of a central core of largely non-cellular collagenous tissue, covered by flattened fibroblasts on its free surfaces to form a multilaminar membrane in contact with the cerebrospinal fluid. The outer cells of the arachnoid tend to proliferate, even forming endothelial pearls (corpora amylacea) (Fig. 310).

From it numerous trabeculæ pass to the pia, and criss-crossing amongst themselves form a network in the subarachnoid space. Each trabecula consists of a central core of collagenous tissue surrounded by endothelium. Elastin and reticulin fibres also occur amongst the collagen. The continuity of the arachnoid with the pia mater through these trabeculæ has led to the concept of a compound pia-arachnoid meninx, *containing* the cerebrospinal fluid.

The Pia is composed of loose connective tissue, containing collagen, elastin, and reticulin fibres. Its surface presents flattened endothelioid cells like those of the arachnoid. Its deeper layers, next to the optic nerve, may be of neuro-ectodermal origin and it unites with glia elements, leading to the term "pia-glia".

The pia mater sends numerous septa into the optic nerve, which divides its fibres into separate bundles (Figs. 259, 313). Thus the pia is intimately connected with the optic nerve and only separated from it with difficulty. There are numerous vessels in the pia which lie for the most part between the longitudinal and circular fibres. The pia is thus much more vascular than the dura. For ultrastructural details of the meninges around the optic nerve consult Anderson and Hoyt (1969).

The Dura becomes continuous with the outer two-thirds of the sclera, usually without line of demarcation (Fig. 303). The outer fibres pass into the sclera and then bend outwards at an angle of about 110°. They do not run parallel with the scleral fibres, but interlace with them. The inner dural fibres pass in more obliquely.

The Arachnoid ends on a level with the posterior part of the lamina cribrosa by becoming continuous with the sclera (Figs. 296, 303).

The Pia, turning outwards, also becomes continuous for the most part with the sclera, but some fibres run into the choroid and some into the border tissue

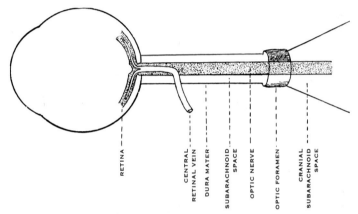

Fig. 311.—Diagram to show the Continuation of the Cranial Subarachnoid Space around the Optic Nerve.

Note how the central vessels cross the space and may be compressed if the intracranial pressure be raised and thus produce papilloedema.

round the optic nerve. The pia increases in thickness as it approaches the bulb by the addition of more circular fibres. Its outer fibres pass outwards into the densely knit meridional fibres of the inner one-fifth or two-fifths of the sclera.

This union of the pia with the inner meridional fibres of the sclera and of the dura with the outer circular fibres gives this transition zone an extremely dense structure which can be made out macroscopically.

The innermost layers of the pia do not end as above described, but pass forwards to the basal lamina between the choroid and the nerve, becoming in fact continuous with the choroid.

Some circular pial fibres insinuate themselves between the fused lamellæ of the suprachoroid lamina, and some run into the border tissue of the nerve. All this tissue has the firm consistency characteristic of the border territories of the sclera.

This dense area of sclera forms a ring which is bounded by a line running from the hyaloid to the outer edge of the dura, and thus gets narrower as we trace it forwards (Fig. 303).

The Subarachnoid Space ends in a cul-de-sac which lies in the sclera and whose

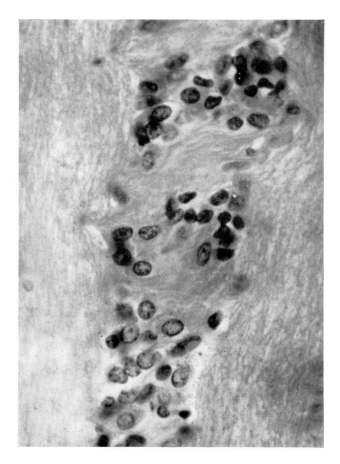

FIG. 312.—NORMAL OPTIC NERVE ($\times$ 220). (MASSON'S STAIN.)
Longitudinal section. Columns of glial nuclei. Note pale and dark types.

anterior extremity reaches the back of the lamina cribrosa (Fig. 296). It is widest anteriorly, where the optic nerve is thinnest, and in a temporally directed scleral canal is wider on the nasal side.

It will thus be seen that for the most part the dura is connected through the arachnoid to the pia by trabeculæ. In most places these tear easily, so that the

---

dura can be made to slide backwards and forwards on the pia. (Normally in the movements of the eye a slight amount of this sliding probably also takes place.)

Close to the eyeball, however, the connection is stronger, and again in the optic canal the relationships of the various sheaths are of special interest.

Here the dura is so firmly united to the optic nerve that it is impossible to separate them (see p. 326). This close union of the dura to the optic nerve is of importance, as the dura is itself firmly united to the bone.

Structure of the Optic Nerve.—The optic nerve is, of course, concerned with *vision*; but although most of its nerve fibres, derived from the ganglion cells of the retina, terminate in the lateral geniculate nucleus, as part of the pathway to the visual cortex, a smaller number establish instead mesencephalic connexions which indicate reflex activity, such as eye movements and pupillary changes. Some optic fibres can therefore be said to be *pupillomotor*, and it is now usually assumed that these may exercise no direct effect on vision. A view still persists that pupillomotor fibres are merely collateral branches of *visual* fibres, but the evidence for this is equivocal. The optic nerve also contains some centrifugal fibres (p. 132), which are motor to blood vessels and perhaps to other retinal elements. The evidence for supposed "trophic" and "retino-retinal" nerve fibres is sparse. If we examine a cross-section of the nerve, we find it is immediately surrounded by the pial sheath, and from this septa pass inwards to divide it into 800–1,200 fascicles (Deyl, 1895). There are about one million fibres in the optic nerve, about 40% of the total afferent fibres in the cranial nerves (Bruesch and Arey, 1942). This makes vision by far the best mediated of the special senses. Polyak (1941) estimated the human optic fibres at 800,000 to 1,000,000; a more recent estimate (Oppel, 1963) being 1,190,000. Kupfer *et al.* (1967) gave a figure of 1·06 to 1·13 million.

The framework of the optic nerve is more obvious its in

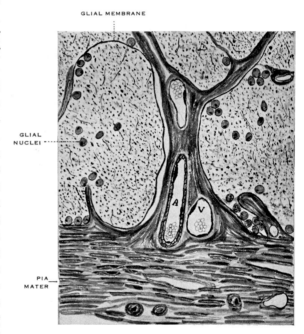

FIG. 313.—TRANSVERSE SECTION OF A SEPTUM OF THE OPTIC NERVE (ZENKER. MALLORY'S TRIPLE STAIN) TO SHOW THAT EACH SEPTUM CONTAINS A VESSEL (OR VESSELS); AROUND THIS IS CONNECTIVE TISSUE AND THEN A GLIAL MEMBRANE.

(Wolff's preparation.)

more vascular part, i.e. distal to the entrance of the central vessels and in the optic canal. Near the chiasma there is a well-marked glial septum which passes obliquely from above downwards and medially to or just beyond the centre of the nerve. This, as well as the trabeculæ, disappears in the chiasma. There are no trabeculæ in the optic tracts.

The Septa.—To understand the structure of the septa it is best to study their development. The developing optic nerve has a glial membrane surrounding it. As the septal vessels, carrying with them connective tissue cells, invade the nerve at about the fourth month of intrauterine life, they invaginate this membrane. Thus each septum has a vessel in its centre; this is surrounded by collagen tissue which in turn is bounded by neuroglia (Fig. 313). The vessels enter the nerve transversely (radially), divide dichotomously repeatedly and, anastomosing with neighbouring vessels, form a vascular net which reaches the centre of the nerve or the central vessels. The septal vessels also send branches anteriorly and posteriorly between the nerve bundles.

The septa pass into the cross-section of the nerve radially. There are some six to nine very thick primary septa which divide the nerve into sectors, and between these a great number of thinner, secondary, septa, 1 mm or less apart. These, as did the blood-vessels, divide repeatedly and dichotomously, and joining with neighbouring septa form meshes which divide the nerve into bundles. The spaces formed by the septa are round or polyhedral, but in man the angles are always rounded in contradistinction to that seen in most animals. There are about 40 septa extending into the whole nerve.

The anteroposterior branches of the septal vessels anastomose with each other and with the transverse branches to form a longitudinal vascular net around each nerve bundle. The septa formed on this scaffolding, therefore, surround the bundles in the form of a tube or cylinder. This tube, however, is not closed, for it is perforated to allow neighbouring nerve bundles to communicate with each other.

It thus comes about that in an anteroposterior section of the optic nerve the longitudinal septa are not continuous. The gaps in each septum correspond to the holes in the cylinder and are normally occupied by columns of glial cells (Fig. 272).

On transverse section also "incomplete" septa are seen. These are so called because they are not completely surrounded by connective (blue-staining) tissue. They are however completed by glia (Fig. 314).

The structure of each trabecula is as follows:

In the centre is a vessel which in the case of the larger septa has a well-marked muscularis and elastica. Around this is a variable amount of loose connective tissue. This in turn is surrounded by dense connective tissue. Around this again are glial fibres and glial nuclei (Fig. 313). Most of the neuroglial cells are astrocytes, but oligodentrocytes and microglial cells have been reported as occurring in small numbers.

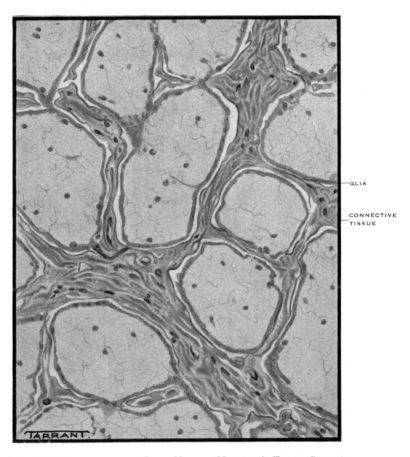

GLIA

CONNECTIVE
TISSUE

Fig. 314.—Section of the Optic Nerve. (Mallory's Triple Stain.)

To show "open" and "closed" compartments. Connective tissue is blue, glia is red. "Closed" means closed by connective tissue *and* glial tissue.

The septa are continuous with the pia and this is the reason why the latter is only separated from the nerve with difficulty.

Lining the pia is the "glial mantle" of Fuchs, which consists of a layer of glial tissue (Fig. 315). This also sends prolongations into the nerve, which not only line the septa but also pass into the nerve bundles themselves. Glial cells lie scattered along the glial prolongations. The glial mantle varies in thickness but is generally

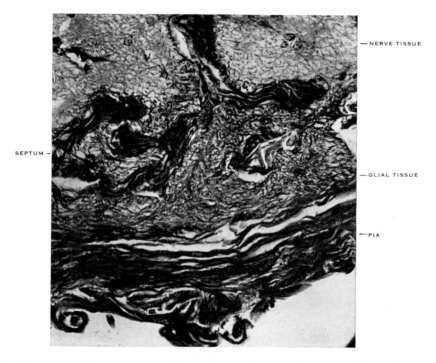

FIG. 315.—TRANSVERSE SECTION OF THE OPTIC NERVE (ZENKER. MALLORY'S TRIPLE STAIN) TO SHOW FUCHS' GLIAL MANTLE.

quite thin. It is greatly thickened, however, in the floor of the third ventricle and, again, just behind the optic canal. This latter thickening lies at the upper and lateral part of the nerve.

From it an important oblique, somewhat triangular, glial (previously described as pial) septum runs from above downwards and medially and backwards, to end in a point a little in front of the chiasma. It sends spidery processes into the nerve which join with the trabeculæ. The septum divides the nerve fibres into a ventro-medial and a dorsolateral portion, the former being the fibres which will cross over to the other side and the latter forming the temporal uncrossed bundle.

The glial septum marks the end of the septal systems of the optic nerve, which are therefore not found in the proximal part of the nerve. The absence of septa accords with the unhindered course of the anterior loops formed by fibres which come from the opposite optic nerve (see p. 377 and Fig. 349).

Also, the end of the glial septum marks the actual beginning of the *physiological chiasma*, i.e. it marks the position where the crossed fibres first separate from the uncrossed, which is there anterior to the *macroscopic chiasma*.

The fibres of the optic nerve vary in diameter from 0·7 to 10 *μ*m; class A sensory fibres (up to 20 *μ*m) are absent. Of these *myelinated* axons about 92 per

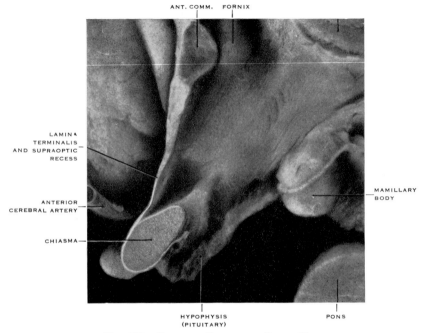

ANT. COMM.   FORNIX

LAMINA
TERMINALIS
AND SUPRAOPTIC
RECESS

MAMILLARY
BODY

ANTERIOR
CEREBRAL ARTERY

CHIASMA

HYPOPHYSIS   PONS
(PITUITARY)

FIG. 316.—SAGITTAL SECTION OF THIRD VENTRICLE.

cent are under 1 *μ*m (Oppel, 1963, Kupfer *et al.*, 1967). Of the larger fibres the majority are less than 2 *μ*m (Chacko, 1948). The smaller fibres appear to be derived from midget ganglion cells (p. 128), the largest axons being concerned with the peripheral retinal area.

Ultrastructural studies of the optic nerve have demonstrated few departures from the characteristics of other nerve fibres (Yamamoto, 1966, Cohen, 1967, Anderson and Hoyt, 1969). It is, of course, possible to distinguish neuroglial processes from nonmyelinated nerve fibres; the latter appear to be concentrated in the peripheral zones of the nerve fascicles. Branching of fibres is described by some observers, denied by others. Yamamoto (1966) suggests that oligodendrocytes are concerned with myelinization and astrocytes with nutrition of the avascular nerve bundles. He finds over 80% of the nerve fibres to be less than 1 *μ*m in diameter.

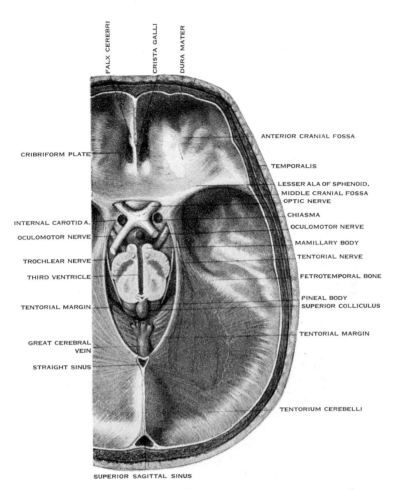

FALX CEREBRI

CRISTA GALLI

DURA MATER

CRIBRIFORM PLATE

INTERNAL CAROTID A.

OCULOMOTOR NERVE

TROCHLEAR NERVE

THIRD VENTRICLE

TENTORIAL MARGIN

GREAT CEREBRAL VEIN

STRAIGHT SINUS

ANTERIOR CRANIAL FOSSA

TEMPORALIS

LESSER ALA OF SPHENOID.

MIDDLE CRANIAL FOSSA

OPTIC NERVE

CHIASMA

OCULOMOTOR NERVE

MAMILLARY BODY

TENTORIAL NERVE

FETROTEMPORAL BONE

PINEAL BODY

SUPERIOR COLLICULUS

TENTORIAL MARGIN

TENTORIUM CEREBELLI

SUPERIOR SAGITTAL SINUS

FIG. 318.—DETAILS OF SUPRATENTORIAL STRUCTURES AFTER REMOVAL OF CEREBRUM.
(*From Hirschfeld and Leveillé.*)

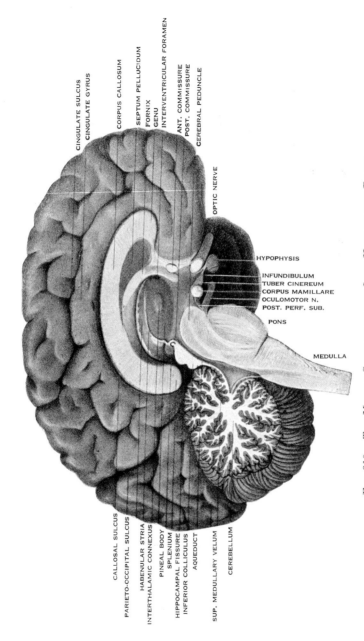

CINGULATE SULCUS
CINGULATE GYRUS
CORPUS CALLOSUM
SEPTUM PELLUCIDUM
FORNIX
GENU
INTERVENTRICULAR FORAMEN
ANT. COMMISSURE
POST. COMMISSURE
CEREBRAL PEDUNCLE

OPTIC NERVE

HYPOPHYSIS

INFUNDIBULUM
TUBER CINEREUM
CORPUS MAMILLARE
OCULOMOTOR N.
POST. PERF. SUB.

PONS

MEDULLA

CALLOSAL SULCUS
PARIETO-OCCIPITAL SULCUS
HABENULAR STRIA
INTERTHALAMIC CONNEXUS
PINEAL BODY
SPLENIUM
HIPPOCAMPAL FISSURE
INFERIOR COLLICULUS
AQUEDUCT
SUP. MEDULLARY VELUM
CEREBELLUM

FIG. 319.—THE MEDIAL SURFACE OF THE LEFT HALF OF THE BRAIN.
(*From Hirschfeld and Leveillé.*)

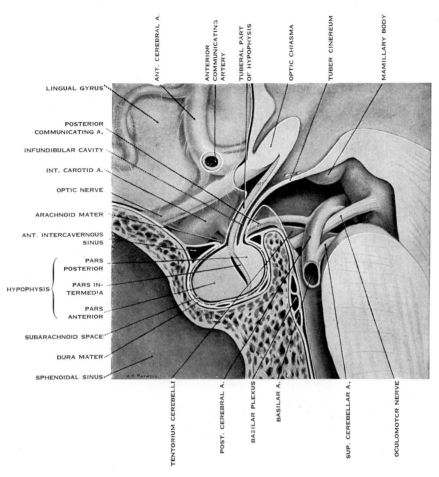

FIG. 317.—DIAGRAMMATIC MEDIAN SECTION OF HYPOPHYSIS (IN SITU).

(The existence of a subarachnoid space around the gland in the pituitary fossa is doubtful.)

(*From Cunningham's "Anatomy".*)

THE OPTIC CHIASMA

The Optic Chiasma is a flattened, oblong band some 12 mm in its transverse diameter and 8 mm from before backwards. It is placed at the junction of anterior wall and floor of the third ventricle, itself forming the floor of the recess which reaches almost to its anterior border (Fig. 316). Clothed in pia it lies obliquely with its posterior border higher than the anterior in the anterior part of the interpeduncular cisterna above the diaphragma sellæ, postero-superior to the the so-called optic groove on the sphenoid (Figs. 260, 317). It is thus suspended in

A.E.—23

and surrounded by cerebrospinal fluid except at its posterior border, which is of course continuous with the brain.

In 80% of causes (de Schweinitz, 1923) part of the hypophysial fossa is anterior to the chiasma; in only 5% is it in the optic groove. In 4% it is posterior to the fossa, and in 12% more of the fossa shows behind the chiasma than in front.

The chiasma is not in contact with the diaphragma sellæ, but is separated

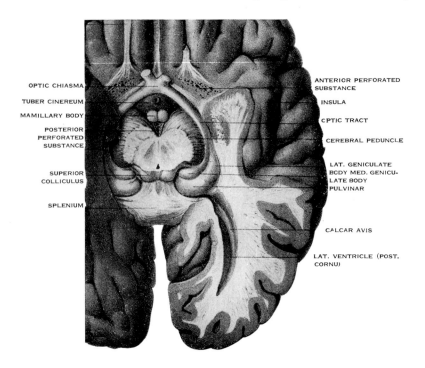

OPTIC CHIASMA

TUBER CINEREUM

MAMILLARY BODY

POSTERIOR
PERFORATED
SUBSTANCE

SUPERIOR
COLLICULUS

SPLENIUM

ANTERIOR PERFORATED
SUBSTANCE

INSULA

OPTIC TRACT

CEREBRAL PEDUNCLE

LAT. GENICULATE
BODY MED. GENICU-
LATE BODY
PULVINAR

CALCAR AVIS

LAT. VENTRICLE (POST.
CORNU)

Fig. 320.—Inferior Aspect of the Brain.
(*From Hirschfeld and Leveillé.*)

from it by 5 to 10 mm. It follows from this that a portion of the cisterna interpeduncularis is inferior to the chiasma (Fig. 317).

Relations.—*Anteriorly* are the anterior cerebral arteries and their anterior communicating branch.

Laterally, the internal carotid artery, as it passes upwards, after having pierced the roof of the cavernous sinus, lies on each side in contact with the chiasma in the angle between optic nerve and tract (Figs. 318, 355). Laterally, too, is the anterior perforated substance (Fig. 320).

Posteriorly is the tuber cinereum—a hollow elevation of grey matter situated between the corpora mamillaria behind and the optic chiasma in front. Laterally it is continuous with the grey matter of the anterior perforated substance and anteriorly with the lamina terminalis. From its inferior aspect the infundibulum (hypophyseal stalk), which is a hollow conical process, passes downwards *and forwards* and through a hole in the posterior part of the diaphragma sellæ to be attached to the posterior lobe of the pituitary gland. The infundibulum is thus in close contact with the postero-inferior part of the chiasma, which it joins at an acute angle (Figs. 260, 317, 355).

Above is the third ventricle, in the floor of which the chiasma makes a prominence which is continuous anteriorly with the lamina terminalis.

The medial root of the olfactory tract lies close above and to the lateral side of the anterior angle of the chiasma (Fig. 320).

Inferior is the hypophysis, and under the lateral edge of the chiasma is the cavernous sinus (with its contents), with the oculomotor nerve the closest relation where it lies on the diaphragma before entering the sinus.

The arachnoid is spread like an apron between the optic nerves. It is attached to the tip of the temporal lobe and internal carotid artery laterally and anteriorly to the frontal lobes (Fig. 259).

(For the arrangement of nerve fibres in the chiasma, see p. 377.)

HYPOPHYSIS CEREBRI (PITUITARY GLAND)

The pituitary gland consists of an anterior lobe derived from the stomatodeum, glandular in structure, and a posterior lobe, formed as an outgrowth from the

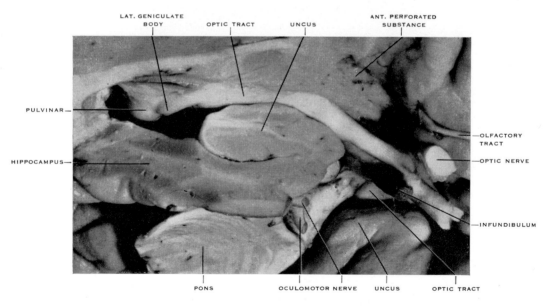

FIG. 321.—RELATIONS OF THE OPTIC TRACT.
The uncus and hippocampus have been divided vertically.

primary brain vesicle, the pars nervosa, having the structure of neuroglia, but containing also fine nonmyelated nerve fibres, and some colloid material coming from the anterior lobe. A cleft separates the anterior lobe from the pars intermedia which, although continuous with the pars nervosa, yet is derived from the anterior lobe.

The hypophysis is a small ovoid body, with maximum and minimum diameters of about 12 and 8 mm. It is situated in the sella turcica (pituitary fossa) on the upper surface of the body of the sphenoid, about midway between the root of the

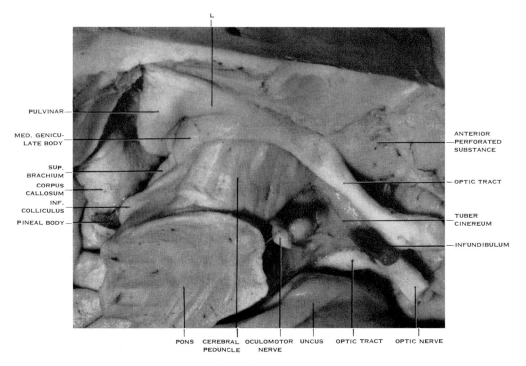

FIG. 322.—RELATIONS OF THE OPTIC TRACT.

A further stage in the dissection of Fig. 321. The uncus and hippocampus have been removed.

nose and the posterior margin of the foramen magnum. In front are the tuberculum sellæ and optic groove; behind, the overhanging dorsum sellæ.

The roof of the pituitary fossa (diaphragma sellæ) is formed by dura mater (Fig. 317), perforated at its centre to allow the pituitary stalk or infundibulum to pass through. This connects the pituitary body with the third ventricle.

On each side the hypophysis is flanked by dura mater, which separates it from the cavernous sinus and the structures within it. In the lateral wall of the sinus from above downwards are the oculomotor, trochlear, ophthalmic and maxillary nerves (Fig. 368). In the sinus itself are the internal carotid artery and lateral to it the abducent nerve.

Fig. 262 shows why the oculomotor and trochlear nerves are more often affected in pituitary tumours than the abducent, which is here protected by the internal carotid artery.

Joining the cavernous sinuses on each side, and situated in the floor of the sella turcica, are the intercavernous sinuses, sometimes regarded as a circular sinus, which is usually represented by a plexus of veins.

In the body of the sphenoid and below the hypophysis cerebri are the two sphenoidal sinuses (see p. 28) separated by a median septum, and having in its lateral wall the carotid buttress, a ledge of bone, which can often be made out in X-rays, and is an important landmark in approaching the gland by the nasal route (see p. 28).

The circulus arteriosus (of Willis) is superior to the hypophysial fossa and an enlarging pituitary tumour may be encircled by it.

The trigeminal ganglion is on the apex of the petrous temporal bone lateral to the cavernous sinus, and above this is the uncus, pressure on which by an enlarging pituitary tumour may evoke olfactory hallucinations.

The meninges blend with the capsule of the hypophysis obliterating the subarachnoid space, and cannot be identified as such (Warwick and Williams, 1973).

The hypophysis receives its blood-supply from the internal carotid by upper and lower hypophysial branches that anastomose with each other. These supply the stalk and posterior lobe, from the capillaries of which a portal system of vessels provides the major supply to the anterior lobe (Xuereb, Prichard and Daniel, 1954). The hypophysial veins drain to the intercavernous plexus and cavernous sinuses (Stanfield, 1960).

THE OPTIC TRACTS

The optic tracts are occasionally described as if they were extracerebral; they are, on the contrary, completely integral with the substance of the inferior aspect of the cerebrum. Moreover, the fibres of the optic nerve, and hence the chiasma and tract, are axons of "secondary" neurons, which are confined to the central nervous system.

Each **optic tract** is a cylindrical band, slightly flattened from above down, which runs laterally and backwards from the postero-lateral angle of the chiasma, between the tuber cinereum and the anterior perforated substance (Fig. 320). It forms the anterolateral boundary of the interpeduncular space.

Becoming more flattened and strap-like, it is united to the upper part of the anterior then lateral surface of the cerebral peduncle, between the internal capsule and the basis pedunculi, i.e. close to the point of disappearance of the peduncle into the cerebral hemisphere (Fig. 322).

Below and parallel to it runs the posterior cerebral artery, but even closer to it is the anterior choroidal. This arises from the internal carotid just beyond (lateral to) the origin of the posterior communicating artery, at the lateral side of the commencement of the optic tract (Figs. 354, 355, 359, 361). It runs backwards and medially, crosses the optic tract on its under surface, and comes to lie on the medial side of this structure. It maintains this relation to the anterior part of the

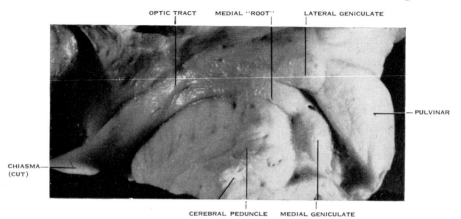

FIG. 323.—THE OPTIC TRACT, ETC., FROM BELOW.

Note two portions of lateral geniculate body with hilum between them. See caption to Fig. 322.

lateral geniculate body. Here it turns abruptly laterally, recrosses the optic tract, and breaks up into a number of branches (see p. 411). The posterior communicating artery may at times cross below the beginning of the optic tract from lateral to medial. The anterior choroidal artery is frequently a branch of the middle cerebral.

Anteriorly the tract has a free surface except for a narrow medial zone, where it is continuous with the outer wall of the third ventricle. As it passes laterally, backwards, and a little upwards round the cerebral peduncle, it rotates outwards slightly on its own axis so that the zone of the brain is at first dorsomedial and finally dorsolateral, the free edge which was at first lateral becoming ventral. The dorsal fasciculi are said to be partially surrounded by the commissures of Meynert and Gudden (see p. 352), while the ventral bundles are free and covered by thin pia mater. The surfaces are at first directed upwards and downwards, but round the cerebral peduncle they face upwards and medially, and downwards and laterally (Fig. 323).

In the first section of its course the optic tract lies superficial on the under aspect of the brain (Fig. 320). It runs above the dorsum sellæ and crosses the third nerve from medial to lateral (Fig. 318). Above is the posterior part of the anterior perforated substance and the floor of the third ventricle, while medially is the tuber cinereum (Fig. 320).

In the middle region of its course the tract lies hidden between the uncus and the cerebral peduncle. It is here also that the flattening commences to conform with the upper aspect of the uncus (Fig. 321). The optic tract here crosses the pyramidal tract which occupies the middle segment of the basis pedunculi. Nearby, just dorsal to the substantia nigra, are the lemnisci carrying sensory fibres. It thus

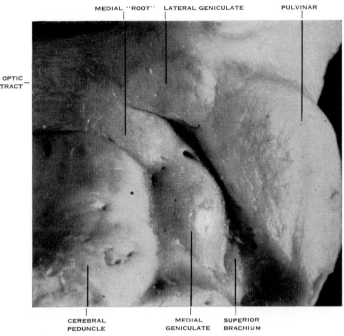

FIG. 324.—ENLARGED VIEW OF A PORTION OF FIG. 321.

The elevation marked as "medial root" is in part due to the medial rim or spur of the lateral geniculate nucleus. The cleft between this and the main lateral geniculate elevation or "body" corresponds approximately to the hilum of the nucleus. See also Fig. 321.

comes about that a single lesion here can affect vision and also the great motor and sensory tracts.

(As will be seen later, the optic radiations also cross and come close to the motor and sensory tracts in the posterior part of the internal capsule, so that here also a single lesion may affect all three.)

In the posterior part of its course the optic tract lies in the depths of the hippocampal sulcus close to the medial part of the roof of the inferior horn of the lateral ventricle. It has the globus pallidus above, the internal capsule medially, and the hippocampus below (Figs. 325, 330). In this part of its course the tract develops a shallow, superficial sulcus, becoming more apparent as it approaches the lateral geniculate elevation. The sulcus marks a division into lateral (geniculate) and medial (collicular) parts or so-called "roots".

The medial root has sometimes been described as being the same as the commissure of Gudden, and is still regarded as a supraoptic pathway (p. 353). It was held to connect the two medial geniculate bodies by passing to the medial side of each optic tract and behind the chiasma, and to be an auditory commissure, a view no longer tenable. The elevation ascribed to the medial "root" is in fact partly

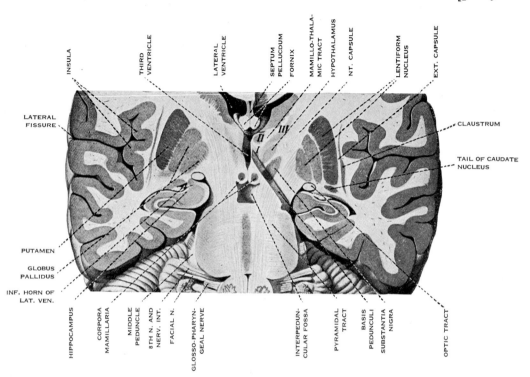

FIG. 325.—A SECTION OF THE BRAIN IN THE PLANE OF THE BRAIN STEM FROM IN FRONT.

On the left the section through the hemisphere is somewhat dorsal to that on the right. I, II and III indicate the anterior, medial and lateral nuclei of the thalamus.

(*From Sabotta.*)

due to the lateral geniculate nucleus, whose medial part is immediately superior (Figs. 328, 329) and may thus augment the elevation (Figs. 323, 324). The nerve fibres in the medial part of the tract therefore pass very close to the lateral geniculate nucleus, but any possible participation of these fibres in visual function is completely obscure in man.

The lateral root spreads over the lateral geniculate body, and for the most part ends in it. The groove between the roots runs into the hilum of the lateral geniculate body, which is usually a definite cleft (Figs. 323, 324).

The fibres of the optic tract, coming from the ganglion cells of the retina, reach three major destinations:

(1) the lateral geniculate nucleus for relay to the visual cortex.

(2) each pretectal nucleus as part of the pupilloconstrictor path.

(3) the superior colliculus for general reflex responses to light.

It should be added at this point that the midbrain connections may also be partly "visual" in function (see p. 513).

The Supraoptic Commissures (of Gudden, Meynert, Ganser, etc.).—It is clear that in many vertebrates, including mammals (and mankind) there are fibres

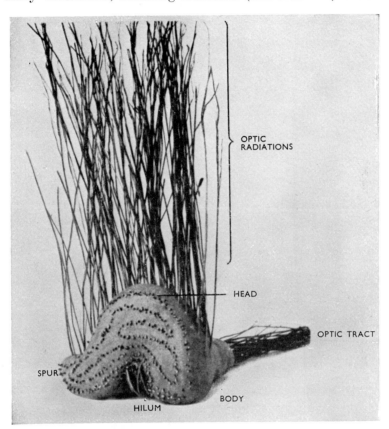

Fig. 326.—Model of Left Lateral Geniculate Body from behind and medial side.
(*After Pfeifer, 1925.*)

other than the retinogeniculate and retinocollicular pathways passing through the optic tracts and chiasma in such a way as to appear commissural. So little is in fact known of the origins and destinations of these groups of fibres that it is impossible to say, even, that they mediate no visual function. Most of such fibres are dorsal to the "visual" fibres, and have been claimed to connect with such structures as the inferior colliculi, periventricular nuclei, midbrain tegmentum, and inevitably, the reticular systems. Most of these arrangements are probably vestigial in higher mammalian brains.

The **Transverse Peduncular Tract** arises from the optic tract, where it enters the midbrain, passes round the ventral aspect of the cerebral peduncle, to enter the brain close to the exit of the oculomotor nerve, with the nuclei of which it is claimed to be connected (Gillilan, 1941) in some mammals. It is said to atrophy when the eye is enucleated, but its visual significance is most equivocal.

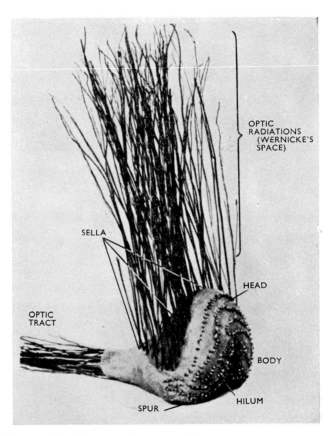

Fig. 327.—Model of Left Lateral Geniculate Body from behind and lateral side.
The origin of the optic radiations from the anterior portion of the saddle (Sella) is seen. This is the stalk of the lateral geniculate body, or Wernicke's field, as it is also called.
(*From Pfeifer, 1925.*)

The **Tract of Darkschewitsch** is another uncertain connection, said to pass from the optic tract to the habenula nucleus (in the wall of the third ventricle, near to the pineal stalk and posterior commissure), and ultimately to the oculomotor nucleus. Little is known of such connections in the human brain. For a discussion of all these obscure projections consult Crosby, Humphrey and Laver (1962).

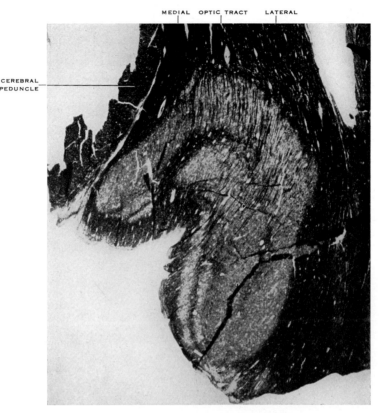

FIG. 328.—HORIZONTAL SECTION OF HUMAN LATERAL GENICULATE BODY WITH TERMINATION OF
OPTIC TRACT. (STAINED WEIGERT-PAL.)

THE LATERAL GENICULATE BODIES

The surface elevation known as the lateral geniculate body is largely produced by the lateral geniculate nucleus, into which the majority of the optic nerve fibres pass. It is the *dorsal* geniculate nucleus of other mammals, there being in many forms a *ventral* nucleus (pregeniculate nucleus), which in man is represented by a few dispersed neurons inferior to, i.e. nearer the surface than, the nucleus itself. The literature on the neurons and connections of this small group of cells is large, but there exist few clear descriptions of its shape and relationship to other adjacent structures, in particular the optic tract. The model by Pfeifer (Fig. 327) corresponds closely with the developmental study of Cooper (1945) and the comparative studies of Chacko (1955). It is an asymmetrical cone, with a rounded apex to its main bulk or body and an incomplete rim, inferiorly. The rim is drawn out laterally as a "peak" or "spur", which is largely responsible for the surface elevation known as the lateral geniculate body. The medial part of the rim is superior to the "medial root" of the optic nerve, and is variably responsible for this surface elevation, which appears to lead dorsally into the medial geniculate body (Figs. 323, 324). The anterior part of the rim is observed by the entry of the optic fibres. Inferiorly the nucleus is hollowed, producing a kind of hilum, which also extends on to the dorsal aspect of the nucleus, which here has no "rim". The hilum may be represented by a superficial cleft or depression (Figs. 323, 324). The close association of the medial part of the nucleus with the medial root of the optic nerve has received little mention in textbooks or papers. (See, however, Wolff, 1953 and Polyak, 1957.)

By far the greater part of the lateral geniculate nucleus lies hidden from a surface view, being enfolded by the pulvinar and only seen in vertical (Fig. 330) and

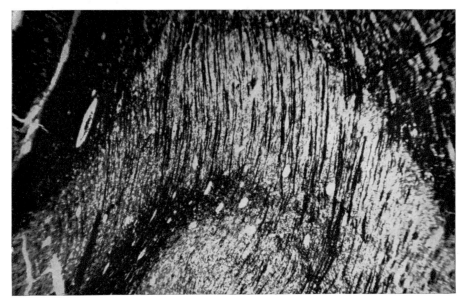

FIG. 329.—As FIG. 326, BUT AT HIGHER MAGNIFICATION.

Note medullated fibres entering lateral geniculate nucleus from the tract. No line of demarcation is visible between medial and lateral portion of the tract.

horizontal sections of the region. On coronal section it appears like a peaked cap, the peak projecting laterally (Fig. 330). On horizontal section it is shown to be related anteriorly with the optic tract which ends therein; laterally with the retrolenticular portion of the internal capsule; medially with the medial geniculate body; posteriorly with the hippocampal convolution, and posterolaterally with the inferior horn of the lateral ventricle. At a higher level the lateral geniculate body is part of the pulvinar which it penetrates (Fig. 330). Here it has anteriorly the pregeniculate grey matter flanked anteriorly by the temporo-pontine fibres of

Türck and the posterior portion of the internal capsule, laterally the area of Wernicke, and medially the medial geniculate body.

On sagittal section it is seen that the fibres of the optic tract divide into two layers (Fig. 330). The inferior of these forms the white layer of the hilum, the superior forms the dorsal portion of the saddle. Between these laminæ which form the capsule of the lateral geniculate body are alternating layers of myelinated fibres and cells which give the body its characteristic appearance (see also p. 380).

From the dorsal portion of the lateral geniculate body pass a mass of fibres

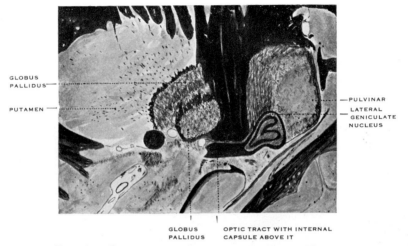

FIG. 330.—PARA-SAGITTAL SECTION OF THE BRAIN (WEIGERT).

Showing optic tract dividing to form capsule to lateral geniculate body; also its relation to the internal capsule.

(*After Lhermitte, slightly modified.*)

(which form its peduncle) into the area of Wernicke. This is a small region of myelinated fibres enclosed by the thalamus medially, the internal capsule laterally, and the lateral geniculate body posteriorly. The main constituents of the area of Wernicke are the fibres of the optic radiation. It also contains the vertical temporothalamic fibres of Arnold.

The lateral geniculate body is connected to the superior colliculus by a slender band called the superior brachium (Figs. 271, 354).

The internal structure of the lateral geniculate nucleus is highly complex. Even macroscopic sections show a laminated pattern (Fig. 352) indicative of a high level of organization. In primates, including man, there are six laminæ of "grey matter" with intervening strata composed largely of neuronal processes, including the terminations of the retinal projection from the ganglion cells. Their precise mode of termination and other connections within the nucleus will be briefly described later (p. 380); but it can be noted here that, just as the responses to light signals excited in the rods and cones undergo a complex shunting or "processing" in the retina, so also is there a further level of interneuronal reaction here, as indeed there occurs a further processing at the cortical level. The geniculate laminæ are like six irregular cones stacked one upon another, and numbered 1 to 6 from the most inferior. They contain the somata of neurons which receive the retinal projection and themselves project to the visual cortex (p. 383). But the connections are not of this simple relay order. The laminæ also contain large numbers of interneurons. (For further details, see p. 380 and consult Minkowski, 1913, Thuma, 1928, Clark, 1941, Glees, 1941, Hubel and Weisel, 1961, Peters and Palay, 1966, Guillery, 1971, 1974, and Szentágothai, 1973.)

THE SUPERIOR COLLICULI

The Superior Colliculi are small rounded elevations situated on the dorsal aspect of the midbrain. They are separated from each other by a vertical median groove, in which depends the pineal body, while a transverse groove separates the superior from the inferior colliculi (Fig. 271). Above each superior colliculus is the thalamus. Superiorly also, in the midline, is the great cerebral vein passing into the straight sinus. Posterosuperior to the whole *tectum*, which comprises all four colliculi, is the cerebellum, both structures covered by pia-arachnoid tissue, between which layers is the cisterna of the great cerebral vein, a local dilatation of the subarachnoid space (Fig. 319).

Afferent Fibres.—(1) From the optic tract via the superior brachium, which runs alongside the lateral geniculate body to the superior colliculus (Fig. 271).

(2) From the occipital cortex via the optic radiations (corticofugal fibres) to the lateral geniculate body, and thence via the superior brachium.

(3) From the spinotectal tract, connecting it with the sensory fibres of the cord and medulla.

Efferent Fibres.—Of the fibres which arise from cells of the grey matter some cross to the superior colliculus of the opposite side, many, after undergoing decussation in the *fountain decussation of Meynert*, make connection with the ocular nuclei, and form the tectospinal tract which connects it with the spinal nerves.

No fibres pass from the superior colliculus to the cortex, i.e. it has no cortical projection.

THE THALAMUS

The thalami are two large ovoid ganglionic masses situated above the cerebral peduncles on each side of the third ventricle and reaching for some distance posterior to the cavity. Its long, anteroposterior axis measures *c.* 4 cm, its maximum width and vertical height being *c.* 2·5 cm.

The anterior extremity of the thalamus is narrow, lies close to the midline, and forms the posterior boundary of the interventricular foramen of Monro (Fig. 317).

The posterior extremity or *pulvinar* is expanded and overlaps the superior colliculus. Medially it presents a well-marked angular prominence, the posterior tubercle, which is continued laterally with but a slight line of demarcation into *the lateral geniculate body.* Inferomedial to the pulvinar, separated by the superior brachium, is *the medial geniculate body* (Fig. 354).

Laterally the thalamus is separated from the *lenticular nucleus* of the *corpus striatum* by the posterior part of the *internal capsule* (Fig. 330).

Each thalamus is an immense collection of neurons of varying size, dendritic fields and interconnections. On the basis of such criteria it has been divided and subdivided into a large series of topographical and, sometimes, functional entities.

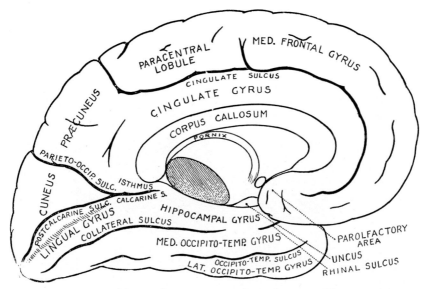

FIG. 331.—THE MEDIAL SURFACE OF THE LEFT CEREBRAL HEMISPHERE.
(From Gray's Anatomy.)

The basic division into *anterior, medial* and *lateral* parts is due to the existence of *laminæ* of myelinated nerve fibres accumulated between these major groups of nuclei. To these may be added the intralaminar, midline (periventricular), and reticular groups. The pulvinar and geniculate bodies belong to the lateral group, the pulvinar (a phylogenetically late development, reaching its zenith in higher mammals) forming almost a quarter of the thalamus at its posterior or caudal end. Since the lateral geniculate body is topographically almost an elevation on the surface of this posterior part of the thalamus, it is tempting to expect some intercommunication between the two, and the existence of this is an old controversy. Minkowski (1913), Brouwer and Zeeman (1926) and others denied any such visual connexions to the pulvinar, whereas Cajal (1909), Elliot Smith (1928),

Le Gros Clark (1932) and Walker (1938) favoured a "tractus geniculothalamicus". The uncertainty persists, and it is noteworthy that the lateral group of thalamic nuclei, to which the pulvinar is ascribed, is primarily concerned with the sensation of pain, according to recent experimenters (e.g. Mountcastle, 1952). Nevertheless, the pulvinar has extensive reciprocal projection relationship with the whole of the

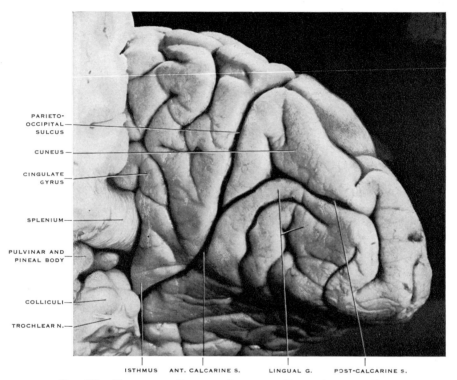

PARIETO-
OCCIPITAL
SULCUS

CUNEUS

CINGULATE
GYRUS

SPLENIUM

PULVINAR AND
PINEAL BODY

COLLICULI

TROCHLEAR N.

ISTHMUS   ANT. CALCARINE S.   LINGUAL G.   POST-CALCARINE S.

FIG. 332.—MEDIAL AND INFERIOR ASPECTS OF RIGHT OCCIPITAL LOBE, ETC.

occipital lobe of the cerebrum, which includes the visual cortex. In summary, geniculopulvinar connections appear to exist in some mammals, but the evidence in human material is at present inadequate. (For details and discussion of these and other thalamic problems, consult Hassler, R., 1955, Crosby *et al.*, 1962, Purpura and Yahr, 1966 and Dewulf, 1971.)

THE OPTIC RADIATIONS

The Optic Radiations (of Gratiolet) or geniculocalcarine pathway, that is the fresh relay of fibres carry the visual impulses to the occipital lobe, arise in the lateral geniculate body (and possibly, as some hold, from the pulvinar of the thalamus as well. This view is, however, dependent upon the existence of a retinopulvinar projection, the evidence for which in man is scanty and negative. The existence of a widespread pulvinocortical projection is not in doubt).

They pass forwards and then laterally through the area of Wernicke (p. 357), as the *optic peduncle*, anterior to the lateral ventricle, and traversing the retro-lenticular part of the internal capsule behind the sensory fibres and medial to the auditory tract. The fibres spread out fanwise to form the medullary optic lamina.

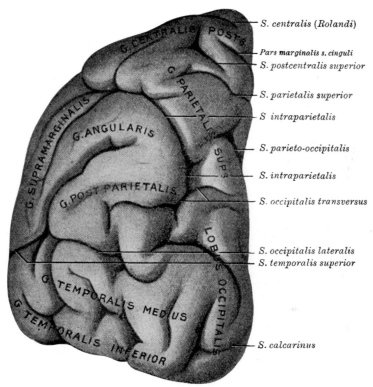

FIG. 333.—LEFT CEREBRAL HEMISPHERE FROM BEHIND. NATURAL SIZE.

G. = Gyrus, S. = Sulcus.

(*From Quain's Anatomy.*)

This is at first vertical but becomes horizontal near the striate cortex. In their course posteriorly the optic radiations lie lateral to the temporal and occipital horns of the lateral ventricle. In this part of their course they are found in the lateral sagittal stratum, which is separated from the cavity of the ventricle by the medial sagittal stratum and the tapetum of the corpus callosum (Fig. 335).

The ventral portion of the optic radiation instead of sweeping straight backwards plunges forwards into the temporal pole before passing backwards as an

A.E.—24

inferior longitudinal fasciculus (Meyer). Interference with this temporal loop of the radiations may cause a superior homonymous quadrantic hemianopia.

The optic radiation as it passes back in the white matter of the cerebral hemisphere lies deep (approximately) to the middle temporal gyrus, so that tumours of this portion of the temporal lobe may give rise to visual defects. The optic radiation ends in the occipital lobe in an extensive area of thin cortex (1·4 mm or less in thickness), in which is the distinctive white stripe or stria first described by Gennari in 1776.

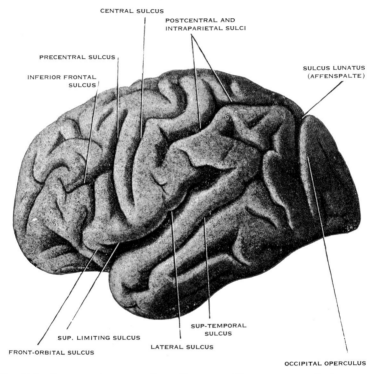

Fig. 334.—Lateral Aspect of Left Cerebral Hemisphere of Chimpanzee.

Note Sulcus Lunatus.

(*From Quain's Anatomy.*)

Apart from these corticopetal fibres the optic radiations also contain fibres that pass from the cortex to the lateral geniculate body and superior colliculus in some animals, including primates, but these have not been substantiated in man. The radiation may also contain descending nerve fibres passing to the nuclei of the ocular motor nerves; but it is likely that this pathway is not direct, but is interrupted at such loci as the para-abducent nucleus, interstitial nucleus, or the posterior commissural nuclear complex (Carpenter and Peter, 1971).

The Calcarine Sulcus

The calcarine sulcus is largely on the medial aspect of the hemisphere. But its anterior end is on the inferior aspect, and posteriorly it may wind round the occipital pole and appear on the lateral surface.

The calcarine is a deep sulcus extending from near the occipital pole, where it usually begins in the centre of the lunate sulcus, the lower limb of which is often grooved by the sagittal sinus (Fig. 331). From here the calcarine sulcus passes forwards, making a bend convex upwards, and ends below the splenium of the corpus callosum. The forked posterior extremity at the occipital pole is sometimes cut off from the rest of the sulcus and then appears as an independent sulcus. Sometimes, as stated above, the sulcus extends round the posterior pole on to the lateral surface, as the lateral calcarine sulcus, and then has the form of a shepherd's crook.

The calcarine sulcus usually runs just above the medial margin of the occipital lobe which is placed at the junction of the falx cerebri and tentorium cerebelli, but may be a varying distance above it.

The parietooccipital sulcus joins the calcarine at an acute angle a little in front of its middle, dividing it into anterior and posterior portions and forming a Y-shaped figure.

If the lips of the parietooccipital and calcarine sulci are widely separated, it will be seen that although on the surface they appear to be continuous they are separated from each other by a small buried vertical *cuneate gyrus*. The gyrus cunei may in fact at times come to the surface when it shuts off the continuity of the two fissures superficially also.

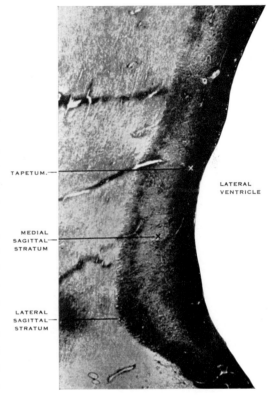

FIG. 335.—STRATA SAGITTALIA.
(*From Brouwer.*)

The posterior part of the calcarine is developed independently of the stem, which is a direct representative of one of the total fissures of the fetal hemisphere, while the posterior part of the calcarine is formed much later by two depressions, which ultimately run together and into the true calcarine. (Sometimes the anterior part of the sulcus is hence called the calcarine *fissure*, distinguishing it from the postcalcarine or, more usually, calcarine *sulcus*, the posterior part of the whole furrow.)

The anterior part of the calcarine sulcus crosses the inferomedial cerebral margin to the inferior surface, where it forms the inferolateral boundary of the isthmus (Fig. 332) which connects the cingulate with the parahippocampal gyrus. Sometimes the calcarine sulcus passes into the hippocampal sulcus as it does constantly in many other primates. As will be seen from Figs. 332 and 336,

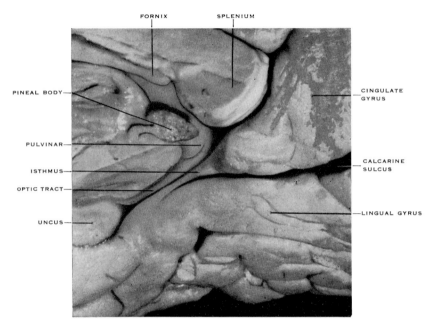

FIG. 336.—THE RELATIONS OF THE ANTERIOR PART OF THE CALCARINE SULCUS.
Further stage in dissection of Fig. 332.

the anterior end of the calcarine sulcus may be fairly close to the colliculi and even to the pulvinar of the thalamus and lateral geniculate body, but its point of termination varies a good deal.

The Sulcus Lunatus is not always present, though it is a constant and marked feature of the lateral aspect of the occipital lobe in apes and monkeys. In man it is small, sometimes continuous with the calcarine sulcus, which it crosses like a T, sometimes separate from it.

The lips of the lunate sulcus, which is a *limiting* sulcus, separate the striate from the peristriate area of the cortex, but the parastriate area is buried within the walls of the sulcus and intervenes between them. The lunate sulcus forms the posterior boundary of the gyrus descendens, which lies posterior to the superior and inferior occipital gyri. Two curved sulci, named the superior and inferior polar sulci, are often discernible near the extremities of the lunate sulcus. The *superior polar sulcus* arches upwards on to the medial aspect of the occipital lobe from the neighbourhood of the upper limit of the lunate sulcus; the *inferior polar sulcus* arches downwards and forwards on to the inferior aspect from the lower limit of

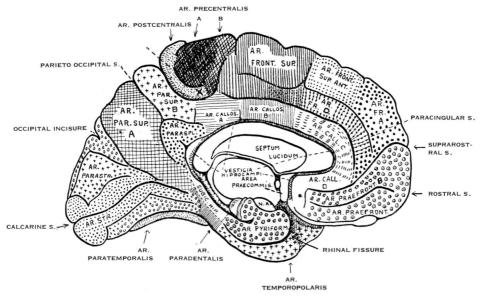

Fig. 337.—Topography of Cortical Areas (Medial Surface).
Note area striata on both sides of the posterior part of the calcarine sulcus, but only inferior to its anterior part. The nomenclature is partly superseded, but is preserved for its historical value.
(AR = Area, S = Sulcus.)
(*Elliot Smith.*)

the same sulcus. These two polar sulci enclose semilunar extensions of the striate area and indicate the expansion of the visual cortex associated with the formation of its large macular area.

The lingual gyrus lies between the calcarine and collateral sulci. Posteriorly it reaches to the occipital pole. Anteriorly it is continuous with the hippocampal gyrus which itself (anteriorly) is lateral to the midbrain (Fig. 331). Anteriorly also the hippocampal gyrus is continuous with the uncus which is recurved and hook-like and forms the posterolateral boundary of the anterior perforated substance. The slit between the uncus and its parent hippocampal gyrus is at the tip of the inferior horn of the lateral ventricle, and here the anterior choroidal artery enters the choroid plexus of the lateral ventricle.

The lateral occipital sulcus runs forward to divide the lateral aspect of occipital lobe into superior and inferior gyri (Fig. 333).

Parietooccipital Sulcus.—The parietooccipital sulcus is best marked on the medial surface of the hemisphere where it appears as a deep cleft extending downwards and a little forwards from the margin of this surface some 5 cm from the occipital pole to near the posterior extremity of the corpus callosum, where it usually joins the calcarine fissure, the two meeting at an angle which encloses a wedge-shaped region of the occipital lobe, the cuneus. On the convex superolateral

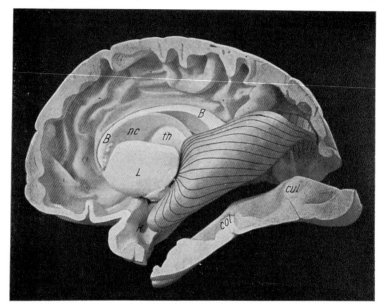

Fig. 338.—The Form and Position of the Geniculostriate Pathway.

K = temporal bend of optic fibres. B = corpus callosum. L = lentiform nucleus. *nc.* = nucleus caudatus. *th.* = thalamus. *col.* = grey matter of collateral sulcus. *cul.* = highest level of grey matter of collateral sulcus.

(From Pfeifer.)

surface the sulcus is continued laterally for a variable distance, generally only a few millimetres (lateral part of the parietooccipital sulcus). This fissure is here taken as the division between the parietal and occipital lobes. In other primates the lateral end of this fissure is in a deep sulcus lunatus (Affenspalte), which intervenes between the parietal and occipital lobes, the cleft tending obliquely backwards, so that the occipital edge somewhat overlaps the parietal (occipital operculum) (Fig. 334) (Quain). The parietooccipital sulcus is about on a level with the lambda or a little in front of the level of that spot: more so in the child than in the adult.

The Striate or Visuosensory Cortex (Primary Visual Area)

The visual cortex is situated for the most part on the medial aspect of the occipital lobe in and near to the calcarine sulcus. A *variable* portion, however, may extend on to the lateral aspect of the occipital pole, and is limited there by a semilunar sulcus, the sulcus lunatus (of Elliot Smith) or *Affenspalte*.

The visual cortex is characterised by the distinguishing *white line* or stria, of Gennari, which is visible to the naked eye, and is best seen on sectioning a fresh brain. Hence the region is called the *area striata*. The stria of Gennari is formed in the fourth layer of the cortex in part by the medullated fibres of the optic radiation but mainly by intra-cortical connecting fibres. The fibres run vertically, transversely and obliquely (Fig. 341).

The calcarine sulcus is divided at the point where the parietooccipital sulcus cuts it into anterior and posterior parts, and while there is visual cortex on *both sides* of the posterior portion (Fig. 339) the stria is found only *below* the anterior (Fig. 337). The approximate limit of the area striata above is the cuneate sulcus in the cuneus or region between the parietooccipital and posterior calcarine sulci. The approximate lower boundary is the collateral sulcus, where this extends posteriorly into the occipital lobe.

If the whole visual cortex be excised and flattened out, it will be found to present the form of an elongated ovoid some 3,000 sq. mm in area. The narrow end of the area lies close

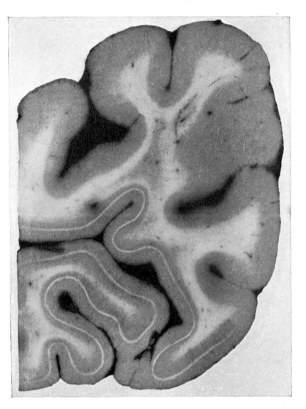

Fig. 339.—Coronal Section of Occipital Lobe to show visual Stria of Gennari in both Walls of Posterior Calcarine Sulcus.

behind and below the splenium of the corpus callosum (see Fig. 337) while the rest of it expands backwards from this point to the occipital pole and beyond it on to its lateral aspect.

At about the sixth month of intrauterine life the area becomes folded along its axis. The fold so formed was called by Huxley the calcarine fissure, because its anterior part produces the prominence of the calcar avis in the interior of the posterior horn of the lateral ventricle. The anterior part of the fissure is much

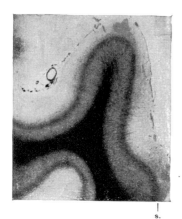

FIG. 340.—VISUAL STRIA (S.).
(WEIGERT'S STAIN.)

Coronal section of posterior calcarine sulcus.

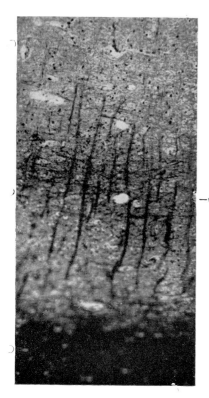

FIG. 341.—VISUAL STRIA (S.)
(Part of Fig. 340 enlarged.)

deeper, more constant in form and position, and earlier in development than the posterior. Phylogenetically, also, it is the older. The calcarine fissure may be continued on to the lateral aspect of the occipital pole as the *sulcus calcarinus lateralis*, and it may reach the lunate sulcus, as already stated above.

The position of the sulcus lunatus is in mankind very variable, and depends on the development of the parietal and temporal association areas. If well developed these may push the sulcus lunatus and thus the visual area on to the medial aspect of the hemisphere, while in some brains it may be a large sulcus well on to the lateral aspect of the brain and resembling that found in apes (the Affenspalte) (Fig. 334). Hence perhaps the variable effects on vision, following localized injuries of the occipital lobe.

Basically the cerebral cortex (except in the allocortex of hippocampal formation, or archipallium, where the pattern is partly of a more simplified form) has a laminar arrangement of the somata or cell bodies of neurons and their processes. This is apparent whether staining techniques show nuclei of cells or their fibres more prominently. Many variant and more complex accounts of this pattern exist (Campbell, A. N., 1905, Cajal, 1911, Brodmann, 1909, Von Economo and Koskinas, 1925, Conel, 1939, Woolsey, 1964, etc.), but in basic details there is much agreement (Billings-Gagliardi *et al.*, 1974). The generalized pattern is as follows:

1. A *plexiform lamina* is most external, and consists of a dense interweaving of neurites (axons and dendrites), or neuropil. The processes include those of intrinsic cortical neurons (mostly stellate cells, see below), the dendrites of pyramidal cells (both situated in deeper layers), and the terminations of afferent fibres reaching the cortex from other parts of

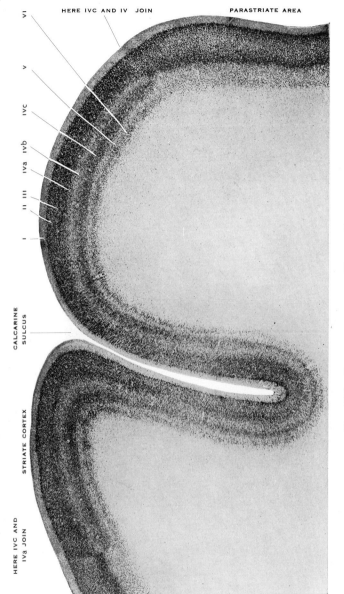

FIG. 342.—LAMINATION OF THE VISUAL CORTEX.

I. *The Plexiform Lamina* is the clear superficial layer. Next comes a thick dark layer which really consists of three portions: layers II, III and IVa.

II. *The External Granular Layer* is the outermost portion of the thick dark layer.

III. *The Pyramidal Lamina* is the middle portion of this layer.

IVa. *The Internal Granular Layer* is the innermost portion of the thick dark layer.

IVb. *The Internal Granular Layer* (the stria of Gennari) is the clear layer that follows.

IVc. *The Internal Granular Layer* is the next dark layer.

V. *The Ganglionic Layer* is the clear layer that follows.

VI. *The Multiform Lamina* is the innermost dark layer.

Note that the stria of Gennari corresponds to IVb and that it is cut off from the parastriate area by the blending of IVa and IVc.

(*After Vogt. Journ. f. Psychologie, 1902–4.*)

the central nervous system, including other parts of the cortex (association fibres). Small neurons with horizontally orientated processes also occur.

2. Internal to this is the *external granular lamina*, so-called from the large number of nuclei of cells visible in it. The layer contains the somata of many kinds of neurons, all influenced in shape by the nature of their dendrites and axons. Thus,

some cells are pyramidal, some stellate (multipolar), and so on. Axons and dendrites from this layer make contacts within it and extend into adjacent layers. Afferent fibres arriving here form innumerable synapses with the local neurons, especially with the apical dendrites of the pyramidal cells.

3. *The pyramidal lamina* is dominated by the familiar "pyramidal" neuron, which has a somewhat conical shape, with apical dendrites, dendrites extending

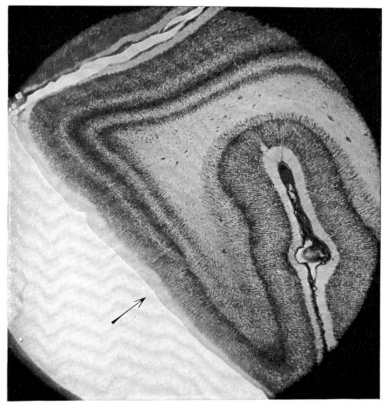

Fig. 343.—Sagittal Section of Neonatal Visual Area—Inferior Margin of Calcarine Sulcus. Note the sudden termination of the stria of Gennari. The area parastriata is to the right.

(*From Pfeifer.*)

from the lower angles, and an axon continuous with its base. This layer also contains many interneurons of stellate type, and these include neurons with processes orientated both vertically (fusiform cells) and horizontally ("basket" cells). Their axons and dendrites extend far beyond their own layer.

4. The *internal granular lamina* is thin and contains largely stellate interneurons and a few pyramidal cells. Although many axons and dendrites are vertically extended, there is a particularly dense aggregation of horizontal processes,

(Fig. 343) forming the so-called external band of Baillarger (Fig. 344). (This is particularly developed in the striate cortex, as already noted above.)

5. The *ganglionic lamina* also contains stellate and pyramidal cells, and in any cortical area the largest pyramidal neurons are in this layer. Like all the laminæ it is, of course, permeated between the actual neuronal somata by a very dense neuropil of dendrites and axons, both local, in passage, and extending to other levels of the cortex.

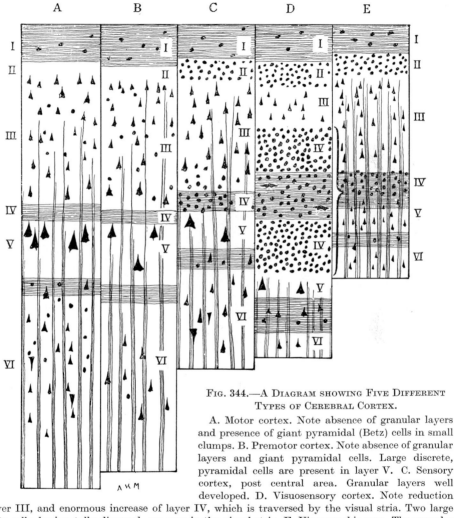

FIG. 344.—A DIAGRAM SHOWING FIVE DIFFERENT
TYPES OF CEREBRAL CORTEX.

A. Motor cortex. Note absence of granular layers and presence of giant pyramidal (Betz) cells in small clumps. B. Premotor cortex. Note absence of granular layers and giant pyramidal cells. Large discrete, pyramidal cells are present in layer V. C. Sensory cortex, post central area. Granular layers well developed. D. Visuosensory cortex. Note reduction of layer III, and enormous increase of layer IV, which is traversed by the visual stria. Two large stellate cells, horizontally disposed, are seen in the visual stria. E. Visuopsychic area. The granular layers are well developed, but large cells are absent from layer five. The relative depths of individual layers, and the relative depths of the whole cortex are approximately accurate.

(From Gray's Anatomy.)

6. The *multiform lamina*, which is nearest to the central "white substance" of the cerebrum, consists of small neurons, most of which are of the "granular" or stellate interneuron type, though a few modified small pyramidal cells also occur. A common form of cell here (the Martinotti neuron) has a long centrifugal axon travelling out to the plexiform layer, and vertically arranged dendritic ramifications in the deeper layers of the cortex.

Much is known of the dendritic and axonal extensions of cortical interneurons and of those cells, chiefly pyramidal neurons, whose axons leave the cortex to

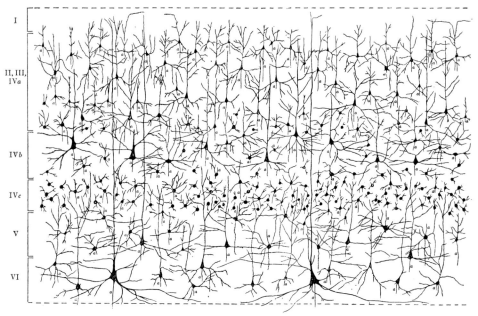

FIG. 345.—COMPOSITE DRAWING OF A SECTION OF THE VISUAL CORTEX OF A MACAQUE MONKEY, MADE FROM GOLGI MATERIAL. TWO MEYNERT CELLS ARE REPRESENTED IN THE MULTIFORM LAMINA. THE APPROXIMATE EXTENTS OF THE CELL LAMINÆ ARE INDICATED ON THE LEFT. THE AXONAL PROCESSES OF THE CELLS ARE MARKED *a*. (LE GROS CLARK, 1942.)

project to the basal ganglia, thalamus, hippocampus, brainstem nuclei and spinal cord. The types of synapses, whether axodendritic, axosomatic, axoaxonal, and so on, or whether excitatory or inhibitor, have been extensively studied in recent decades, and certain repetitive arrangements of neurons into interacting groups have become well established in recent years, both in terms of structure and function (consult Eccles, Ito and Szentágothai, 1964; Szentágothai, 1967). It is clear that in some parts of the cortex those congeries of interacting neurons are set in a columnar manner in the cortex, although it is obvious that complex horizontal interconnection must also exist. The methods of "unit-recording", however, have so far been chiefly instrumental in revealing vertical organization in the cortex, and the striate cortex has been studied with particular attention (see below).

In the proportions of cell types, their actual numbers and in intrinsic and extrinsic connections, the cerebral cortex varies in different areas. Certain major types
of pattern are recognized: one, in which pyramidal cells predominate, is typical of
"motor" areas, whereas another, in which "granular" cells are preponderant, is

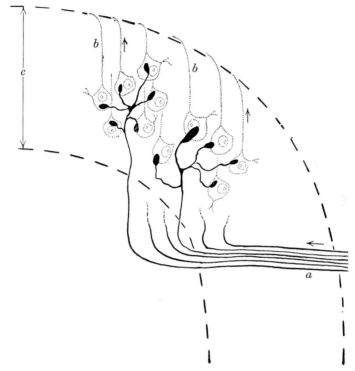

FIG. 346.—DIAGRAM SHOWING THE TERMINATION OF OPTIC FIBRES IN RELATION TO THE CELLS OF
THE LATERAL GENICULATE BODY IN A MONKEY.

A fasciculus of optic fibres (a) is shown entering the geniculate body from the right. From this
fasciculus individual fibres turn out at right angles to enter their appropriate cell lamina (c). Each
fibre ends in a spray of 5–6 branches, and each of these terminates in an end-bulb which lies in
contact with the body of one geniculate cell. The axons of the geniculate cells (b) pass into the fibre
laminæ of the nucleus and run through these to reach the optic radiations. (Glees and Clark, 1941.)

associated with sensory areas. This *granular* type of cortex is most highly developed
in the striate area. Even here, in the 4th cortical layer, there are a few pyramidal
neurons (cells of Meynert), arranged in a single row. Their axons descend through
the optic radiations to reach the superior colliculus and possibly ocular motor
nuclei. The profusion of granular cells in the striate cortex is remarkable; although
it forms a mere 3% of the total cerebral cortex, it is said to contain about 10% of
the total population of cortical neurons. Lamina IV is commonly subdivided
further in the striate cortex (Figs. 342, 345), but such details are beyond this

account. (For a recent description of neuronal organization in this area consult Colonnier, 1969.)

The distinguishing features of the striate cortex are thus as follows:

(1) The visual stria of Gennari distinguishes it from all other cortical areas.

(2) It shares with the other sensory cortical areas a great increase in the number of granular cells. The outer and more especially the inner granular layers consist of a great number of small cells closely packed together. But the whole granular layer (IV) is wider here than in any other cortical area. In fact, the striate area contains approximately one-tenth of the total number of cells in the cerebral cortex.

(3) The basic sexilaminar pattern is complicated by the presence of the visual stria in the internal granula lamina (layer IV), which is considered to consist of two granular sublaminæ, IVA and IVc, with the stria (IVB) between them. The optic radiation and some association fibres terminate in this layer.

(4) The visual stria (IVB) contains a few large cells horizontally placed (Fig. 344), which Cajal thought were the specific cells of vision.

(5) The ganglion layer (V) contains the solitary neurons of Meynert, which are pyramidal in shape, measure about 30 μm, and are arranged in a single row widely spaced. The cells project to the superior colliculus and possibly to ocular motor nuclei.

(6) Their dendritic pattern suggests an integrative function in the cortex (Chan-Palay et al., 1974).

While there is no doubt that the striate or visual cortex (area 17 in Brodmann's terminology) is the main receptor area for the optic radiation from the geniculate body, there are surrounding areas, the peristriate and parastriate zones (areas 18 and 19 of Brodmann) which also receive numbers of such fibres directly, as well as being linked by short association fibres to the striate cortex itself. The main connections of all these areas are summarized below.

Although details are not appropriate to a text of this kind, some reference must be made to the results of electrophysiological study of individual neurons, by the technique of so-called 'unit recording', during recent years. An embarrassingly large volume of work has been recorded, and collectively it has transformed the earlier simple view of the visual pathway as a series of relays, retinal, geniculate or tectal, and cortical, consisting of fairly independent conducting pathways, whose signals are merely transferred en masse to the cortex for decoding.

The disparity in numbers between photoreceptors and ganglion cells in the retina has long provided structural evidence of convergence of pathways, and experimental methods have shown that only some of the macular receptors enjoy individual pathways. Electrophysiological technique has now demolished much of this supposed independence. Collateral synapses between neurons in the retina are responsible for the phenomena of lateral inhibition, inhibitory surround, and the consequential heightening of contrast between stimulated and unstimulated points. A similar but more complex "processing" of coded information in separate conductors occurs in the geniculate nucleus in which a great complexity of interneuronal connections have been shown to exist. Unit recording here also reveals lateral inhibition, and individual neurons can be identified which respond to different kinds of stimulus. There is no clear evidence that geniculate neurons are directly involved in binocular integration; this appears to occur in more complex units of cells, probably arranged in columnar arrays, in the striate cortex. It is not possible to speak dogmatically of the level at which "conscious" vision can be associated with the highly complex neuronal interactions of the visual pathway, though it is tempting to consider the occipital cortex as the locus of this. There is evidence, however, that the information reaching the striate cortex is projected by short association pathways to the peri- and para-striate areas and beyond, and that even more complex integrations of the impulses processed in the striate cortex do occur. The visual pathway thus becomes a most intricate array of interacting conductors, at each level of which a further grade of complex "processing" occurs. How far each level in this neuronal hierarchy can be said to contribute directly to the subjective phenomena which we designate as "seeing" is currently undetermined.

Amongst the plethora of papers in this field it is difficult to select without being invidious. A few representative and recent contributions have been cited which will lead the reader further into the literature. (See Hubel and Wiesel, 1961–72; Glees, 1961; Peters and Palay, 1966; Jones and Powell, 1969–70; Guillery and Colonnier, 1970; Pasik and Pasik, 1971; Rossignol and Colonnier, 1971; Gross *et al.*, 1972.)

Summary of the Connections of the Visual Cortex (Area 17).

(*a*) With the opposite visual cortex by commissural fibres which run in the splenium of the corpus callosum. The striate cortex (area 17) is less profusely connected by such fibres, which are more numerous in the peristriate and para-striate regions (areas 18 and 19).

(*b*) With the frontal eye fields.

(*c*) With parietal "association" areas.

(*d*) With the superior colliculus.

(*e*) With the oculomotor nuclei and other motor nuclei by descending fibres which run in the optic radiations.

The striate visual cortex is directly connected with other parts of the visual cortex and with the frontal, parietal and temporal lobes by abundant association fibres. These are held to integrate the activity of the visual cortex as a whole and to provide an anatomical basis for visuotactile, visuoauditory, and other associative functions including eye movements.

LOCALIZATION IN THE VISUAL PATHS

It is of great clinical importance in the localization of lesions that the fibres in the visual pathways are arranged in a definite orderly manner throughout the visual pathways.

(*a*) **In the Retina.**—The nerve fibres converge towards the disc. On the temporal side is the important papillomacular bundle. There is no overlap between the upper and lower halves of the fibres of the peripheral parts of the retina (Fig.137).

In the retina the line dividing nasal from temporal fibres (in the sense of those that will cross in the chiasma and those that will not) passes through the centre of the fovea. Hence the temporal macular fibres remain on the same side, while the nasal ones cross.

The upper temporal retinal fibres (and some of the nasal portion as well) are separated from the lower by the macular fibres, an arrangement which holds throughout the central visual pathway.

There is still dispute as to how the nerve fibres from the various portions of the retina arrange themselves at the optic nerve head. It is generally held that the fibres from the periphery of the retina pass to the centre of the nerve, while

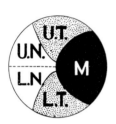 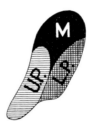 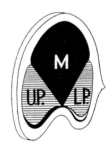

A. In the optic nerve (distal).	B. In the optic nerve (proximal).	C. In the optic tract.	D. In the lateral geniculate nucleus.

The crescents below U.P. and L.P. are the uniocular fibres.

M. = macular. U.T. = upper temporal. L.T. = lower temporal. U.N. = upper nasal. L.N. = lower nasal. U.P. = upper peripheral. L.P. = lower peripheral.

(After Brouwer and Zeeman, 1926.)

Fig. 347.—Distribution of the Visual Fibres.

(Note that in Fig. D, Le Gros Clark and Penman (1934) have shown that only the macular area occupies the posterior two-thirds of the geniculate body.)

those arising close to the disc occupy the periphery of the nerve. But it would now appear that the nerve fibres coming from the periphery of the retina lie deep in the nerve fibre layer and peripheral at the nerve head (see Wolff and Penman, 1950; also Loddoni, 1930) (Fig. 348).

(*b*) **In the Optic Nerve.**—(1) *In the distal region* (Fig. 347, A).—Behind the eye the peripheral fibres are distributed exactly as in the retina; those from the temporal side are lateral in the nerve, those from the nasal side medial. The macular fibres, which constitute almost one-third of the whole nerve (whereas the macular area is only one-twentieth of that of the retina), are laterally placed in the nerve, occupying a wedge-shaped area; but as we approach the chiasma they insinuate themselves among the peripheral fibres, so that (2) *near the chiasma* they are centrally placed (Fig. 347, B).

(c) **In the Chiasma** (Fig. 322).—The *nasal fibres*, constituting about three-quarters of all the fibres, cross over to run in the optic tract of the opposite side. But they do not do this by the shortest route, i.e. along the diagonals.

In the proximal part of the optic nerve the nasal fibres, which hitherto have kept to an orderly arrangement and run parallel with the optic nerve, spread out so that in a horizontal section they occupy the whole width of the nerve and anterior portion of the lateral part of the chiasma (see Williams, 1929).

The most medial of these, representing the fibres from the lower and medial quadrant of the retina, bend medially into the anterior portion of the chiasma and after decussating cross over to the opposite side. The fibres that lie most anterior

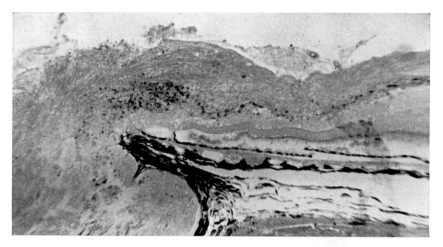

FIG. 348.—MARGIN OF OPTIC DISC AND ADJACENT RETINA OF A RABBIT WITH A PERIPHERAL RETINAL LESION INFLICTED ONE MONTH PREVIOUSLY. (MARCHI.)

Degenerating fibres as shown by the Marchi technique are deep in the nerve-fibre layer and peripheral at the nerve-head.

(*Wolff and Penman, 1950.*)

in the chiasma now form loops convex forwards in the terminal part of the opposite optic nerve, and then having reached the temporal border, pass backwards to the medial and lower part of the tract. *It is because of these anterior loops that a lesion at the termination of the optic nerve may affect both fields.* It is probable that these fibres, i.e. those coming from the lower and medial quadrant of the retina, in crossing over in the chiasma lie next its under-surface, i.e. nearest the pituitary body; for they are first affected in tumours of this body as shown by the early loss of the upper temporal field. The *anterior loops* are crossed at right angles by those fibres in the optic nerve which are still running parallel to its axis, and thus is produced a characteristic basketwork of interlacing fibres (Korbgeflecht of Wilbrand) in the terminal part of the nerve.

A.E.—25

The upper medial fibres coming from the upper and medial quadrant of the retina pass to the lateral side in the terminal portion of the nerve and mingle with the uncrossed bundle. They pass backwards here for varying distances. The most lateral ones actually form loops convex backwards in the beginning of the optic tract before crossing over in the chiasma to the superomedial portion

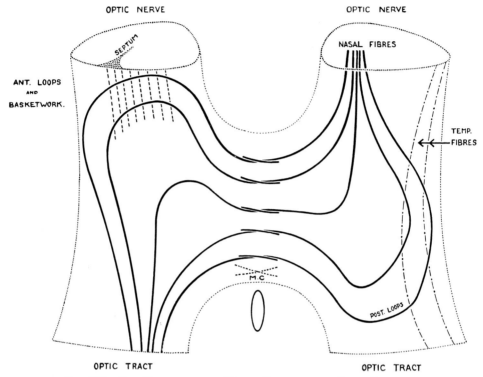

OPTIC NERVE OPTIC NERVE

FIG. 349.—THE DECUSSATION OF NERVE FIBRES IN THE OPTIC CHIASMA.

To avoid confusion only the fibres from one side (except at the actual decussation) are shown.
M.C. = macular crossing.

Note that the most medial of the temporal fibres come much nearer the centre of the chiasma than is shown in the figure. Note also that the macular fibres in fact occupy a much larger part of the chiasma than is shown.

of the tract of the opposite side. The *posterior loops* formed by fibres before their crossing are less prominent than those formed by the crossed medial fibres in the terminal portion of the optic nerve.

The actual decussation takes place in the middle of the chiasma, the anterior fibres crossing each other at more acute angles than the posterior. The fibres cross over not only from left to right but from above downwards as well. For further details on the chiasmal arrangements consult Traquair, 1957; Polyak, 1957; Duke-Elder and Cook, 1963.

The Uncrossed Fibres.—Just anterior to the chiasma the uncrossed bundle forms a compact fasciculus which occupies the whole of the upper and lateral quadrant of the nerve. These temporal fibres run directly backwards in the lateral portion of the chiasma, those coming from the upper part of the retina being above those from the lower. They pass into the tract lying here in the dorsolateral part.

In the chiasma, however, the uncrossed fibres do not form a closed fasciculus, but with them mingle not only the nasal fibres of the same side which have passed laterally before crossing over to the opposite side but also those nasal fibres from the opposite side which form loops in the terminal portion of the optic nerve.

This intermixture of fibres is so marked that in a case of unilateral atrophy of the optic nerve horizontal sections of the chiasma do not reveal the position of the uncrossed bundle. Only in coronal sections can the atrophic area, i.e. the position of the uncrossed bundle, be made out. It then appears in the lateral part of the chiasma as a kidney-shaped area with its hilum medially.

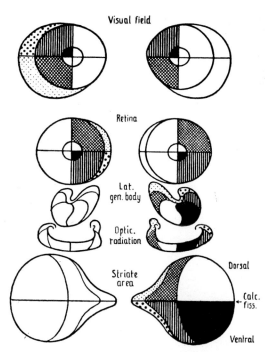

Fig. 350.—Diagram of the Projection of the different parts of the Retina in the Lateral Geniculate Nucleus, the Optic Radiation and the Striate Area.

(*From Brodal, after Polyak, 1933.*)

The Macular Fibres.—In the posterior portion of the intracranial optic nerve the papillomacular bundle is central and keeps this position in the anterior part of the lateral portion of the chiasma. Then the crossed fibres separate from the uncrossed ones and pass as a bundle obliquely backwards and upwards to decussate with the macular fibres of the opposite side somewhat posteriorly in the chiasma. Together with fibres from the central area of the retina the macular axons occupy most of the *central* part of the chiasma, above all other decussating (peripheral) fibres. Lesions here will therefore cause a central temporal hemianopic scotoma.

(*d*) **In the Optic Tract.**—In the chiasma crossed and uncrossed fibres are intermingled, and when they reach the optic tract they are rearranged to correspond with their position in the lateral geniculate body, i.e. the macular fibres (crossed and uncrossed) occupy an area of the cross-section dorsolaterally; the fibres from the lower retinal quadrants are lateral, those from the upper are medial. The fibres from the peripheral portions of the retinæ lie more anteriorly.

(e) **In the Lateral Geniculate Body.**—The fibres from the upper part of the retina go to the medial part of the geniculate body, those from below to the lateral part. The macular area is somewhat cuneiform, involves all the laminæ, and is confined to the posterior two-thirds of the nucleus, broadening towards the caudal pole. It is probable that the peripheral areas farther away from the disc are represented, as in the retina, in the more anterior levels of the geniculate body.

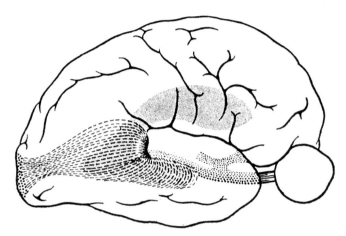

Fig. 351.—Diagrammatic Representation of the course of the Fibres of the Optic Radiation.

The geniculo-cortical fibres from the geniculate nucleus (not visible) curve around the concavity of the lateral ventricle to reach the striate area.

(*From Brodal, after Cushing, 1922.*)

There is a regular "point-to-point" localization of the retina in the lateral geniculate nucleus and there is no bilateral (double) representation of the macula. The body is split up into laminæ, six in number at its centre, which receive fibres alternately from the retina of the same side and the opposite side.

In the human lateral geniculate nucleus, as in that of monkeys and apes, there are six well-defined layers of cells sharply separated throughout most of their extent by medullary laminæ. These layers may be conveniently numbered 1–6 from the hilum of the nucleus (see p. 357). The first two consist of conspicuously large cells, and the remaining four of smaller cells closely packed together. The crossed retinal fibres end in laminæ 1, 4 and 6, while the uncrossed go to 2, 3 and 5 (Fig. 352).

Crossed and uncrossed retinal fibres do not, therefore, end in the same laminæ of the geniculate nucleus, but in such a way that those fibres from corresponding parts of the two retinæ end in neighbouring parts of the adjacent layers. When the fibres enter the lateral geniculate body, crossed and uncrossed fibres are not yet segregated. (For the classical work on this arrangement consult the papers of Minkowski, 1913; Le Gros Clark and Penman, 1934; Glees, 1941; Brouwer and Zeeman, 1942; Polyak, 1957; Meikle and Sprague, 1964.)

Each optic fibre, derived from a retinal ganglion cell, ends within its appropriate laminæ by dividing into five or six terminal branches, and each of these

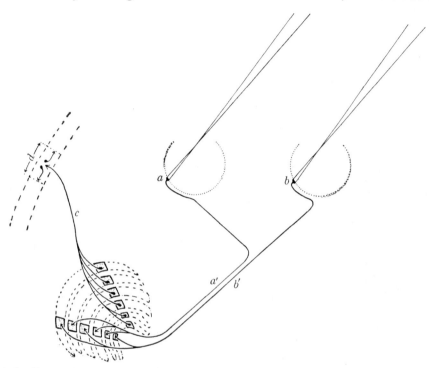

FIG. 352.—DIAGRAM ILLUSTRATING CERTAIN POINTS IN THE CENTRAL REPRESENTATION OF THE RETINA.

Impulses from equivalent spots (a, b) in the two retinæ pass back in the optic tract to the same region of the lateral geniculate body. Crossed impulses (b) terminate in laminæ 1, 4 and 6 and uncrossed impulses (a) in laminæ 2, 3 and 5. Thus the *receptive unit* in the lateral geniculate body with respect to each retina is a band of cells radiating from the hilum of the nucleus, and involving three laminæ. On the other hand, the *projection unit* of the lateral geniculate body on to the visual cortex is a band of cells involving all six laminæ. (Clark (1941), *J. Anat.*, **75**.) It is important to note that while "a" and "b" in this diagram may represent single retinal ganglion cells, the geniculostriate connection, "c", must represent a minimum of six neurons, each with a soma in one lamina alone.

forms a small number of synaptic junctions with the dendrites and soma of a single geniculate neuron. The latter therefore receives impulses from one source only, the retina. This is in great contrast with the motor cells of the spinal cord, which may have as many as a thousand terminal boutons in relation to them, derived from various sources. Glees (1941) found 30–40 terminal boutons related to each geniculate cell. The retinal projection fibres do not necessarily synapse with only one geniculate neuron, and there exists an *intrinsic* population of interneurons, which mediate cross-connections between the pathways passing through the geniculate nucleus. This can no longer be regarded as a simple "relay station", but it is still probable that, despite the complex "processing" of coded information which occurs, the ipsilateral and contralateral streams are predominantly independent; "fusion" does not occur at this level. (For further details of geniculate organization see references on p. 358.)

(The neuronal population of the geniculate body is also influenced, probably in an inhibitory sense, by corticofugal fibres, according to some neurophysiologists. These fibres are reputed to descend from the striate cortex to the geniculate nucleus. If such a cortical "modulating" circuit exists, as seems most probable, it would merely parallel similar projections from other sensory and sensorimotor areas of the cerebral cortex.)

The smallest retinal lesion causes atrophy in all the three layers belonging to that eye; hence, the conducting unit in the optic nerve is a three-fibre unit. The smallest lesion of the visual cortex, on the other hand, causes atrophy in six layers of the lateral geniculate body, and the conducting unit in the optic radiations is probably a six-fibre one. The point-to-point projection of the retina to the lateral geniculate is also carried from the latter to the visual cortex.

(*f*) **In the Optic Radiation.**—The fibres originating in the medial portion of the geniculate body, and representing the upper portions of the retina, form the upper portion of the radiation going to the upper lip of the calcarine fissure; those coming from the lateral portion of geniculate body form the lower portion of the radiation. The macular fibres, as in the geniculate body, continue in the radiation to separate the fibres representing the upper portions of the retina from those representing the lower. This accounts for the fact that one may get a quadrantic visual field defect with a sharp horizontal border.

(*g*) **Localization in the Visual Cortex.**—*It is only in the visual areas that the impulses originating from corresponding parts of the retinæ meet.* Following a lesion of the striate area all laminæ of the lateral geniculate body are affected, which shows that the impulses entering its alternate layers and derived from corresponding parts of the two retinæ pass to the same cortical region. There is a geographical projection or point-to-point localization of the retina in the cortex; that is, each area in the retina is sharply represented in a corresponding area of the striate cortex, and in the adjoining visual areas.

All visual stimuli which impinge upon the corresponding halves of the retinæ (e.g. both right halves) are ultimately transmitted to the lateral geniculate body of the same side, and finally to the ipsilateral striate area (for the most part). Visual stimuli from the left will fall on the right halves of both retinæ, i.e. the temporal half of the right and nasal half of the left. The fibres from the right eye pass without crossing to the right optic tract, those from the left eye cross to continue in the right optic tract. Both sets of fibres reach the right lateral genicu-

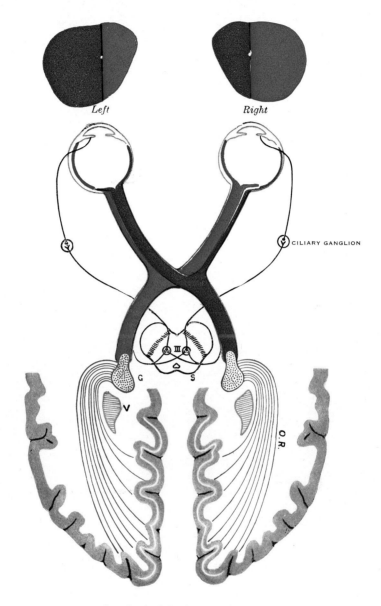

G = Lateral Geniculate Body.
S = Superior Colliculus.
III = Oculomotor Nucleus.
V = Posterior Horn of Lateral Ventricle.
O.R. = Optic Radiations.

Fig. 353.—To show the Course of the Visual and Pupillary Fibres and the Corresponding Fields of Vision.

The cell station in the pretectal nucleus is not shown (see Fig. 362).

late nucleus and the right striate area. Consequently the right striate area is concerned in the perception of objects situated to the left of the vertical median line in the visual fields. This is in line with the fact that the right cerebral hemisphere is concerned in the motor and sensory activities of the left half of the body.

"The retinal projection on the cortex may be represented (approximately—ed.) by picturing one half of the retina spread over the surface of the striate area, the macular region being placed posteriorly, the periphery anteriorly, the upper margin along its upper edge and the lower on its inferior border" (Holmes, 1918).

Thus the upper and lower quadrants of the retina are represented respectively above and below the calcarine sulcus quadrants. The periphery of the retina along the vertical meridian corresponds to the upper and lower limits of the visual area, while the portions which lie next the horizontal meridian are projected in the depth of the calcarine sulcus.

The periphery of the retina along the horizontal meridian is represented in the anterior part of the visual cortex, and as we go centrally in the retina the corresponding area of cortical localisation will be farther back along the calcarine fissure.

The most anterior part of the striate area represents the extreme nasal periphery of the retina which corresponds to the temporal crescent in the visual fields, where vision is monocular.

The maculae are represented posteriorly; but while there is some degree of localization of macular representation in the posterior part of the calcarine fissure and extending on the lateral surface of the occipital pole (Holmes, 1918), it is possible that the macular representation somewhat overlaps that of more peripheral parts of the retina.

The macular area is relatively much later in proportion to the whole striate area than is the macular region in proportion to the whole retina. Because the macula is concerned with the most acute vision and its visual cells are more densely packed than elsewhere, it is more extensively represented in the striate area than the peripheral portion. This apparent disproportion resembles the ratios of representation of the hand, face, and larynx, in the pre- and post-central gyri, as conveyed so forcefully in Cushing's "homunculus". (See Gray's Anatomy, ed. Warwick and Williams, 1973.)

According to Smith (1930): "In a horizontal section through the posterior pole of a human cerebral hemisphere the area striata, distinguished by the presence of the stria of Gennari, is seen to undergo a sudden change in character a short distance behind its midpoint. The thickness of the stria is reduced and the dark band (which is found on its inner side in the part representing the peripheral retina) disappears. The macular cortex begins at this place and extends around the pole on to the lateral surface of the hemisphere to end at the lip of the lunate sulcus. As this lateral part of the area striata is much broader than the medial part, exact measurements reveal the fact that the macular part is at least as extensive as the whole peripheral part. It is possible to identify the macular part of the area striata in many human brains by simple observation of the morphological features of the surface of the cerebral hemisphere. Looking at the posterior aspect of the hemisphere, three semilunar sulci—lunatus, polaris superior, and polaris inferior—may often be seen arranged in a trefoil of shamrock-leaf pattern (grouped around the calcarine sulci in the axis of the area striata). The

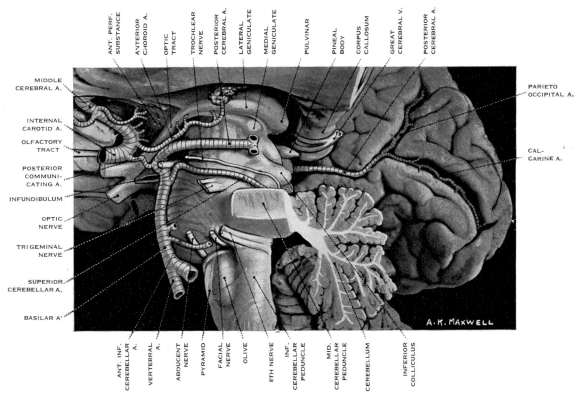

FIG. 354.—DISSECTION TO SHOW THE BLOOD-SUPPLY OF THE VISUAL PATHWAY AND THE RELATIONS OF THE VESSELS TO THE OCULAR NERVES.

(Wolff's preparation.)

rapid expansion of the lateral part of the area striata to afford cortical representation of the macula is responsible for the formation of three opercula bounded by these three semilunar sulci. Hence the presence of this cortical shamrock pattern affords definite evidence of the position and extent of the macular area."

It used to be held that each macula had a double representation, i.e. that each point in the macula was represented in both occipital poles; but most observers now agree with Holmes and Lister (1915) who, from observations on soldiers with gunshot wounds of the occipital region came to the conclusion that each point in each macula had a unilateral representation only. They explain the well-known

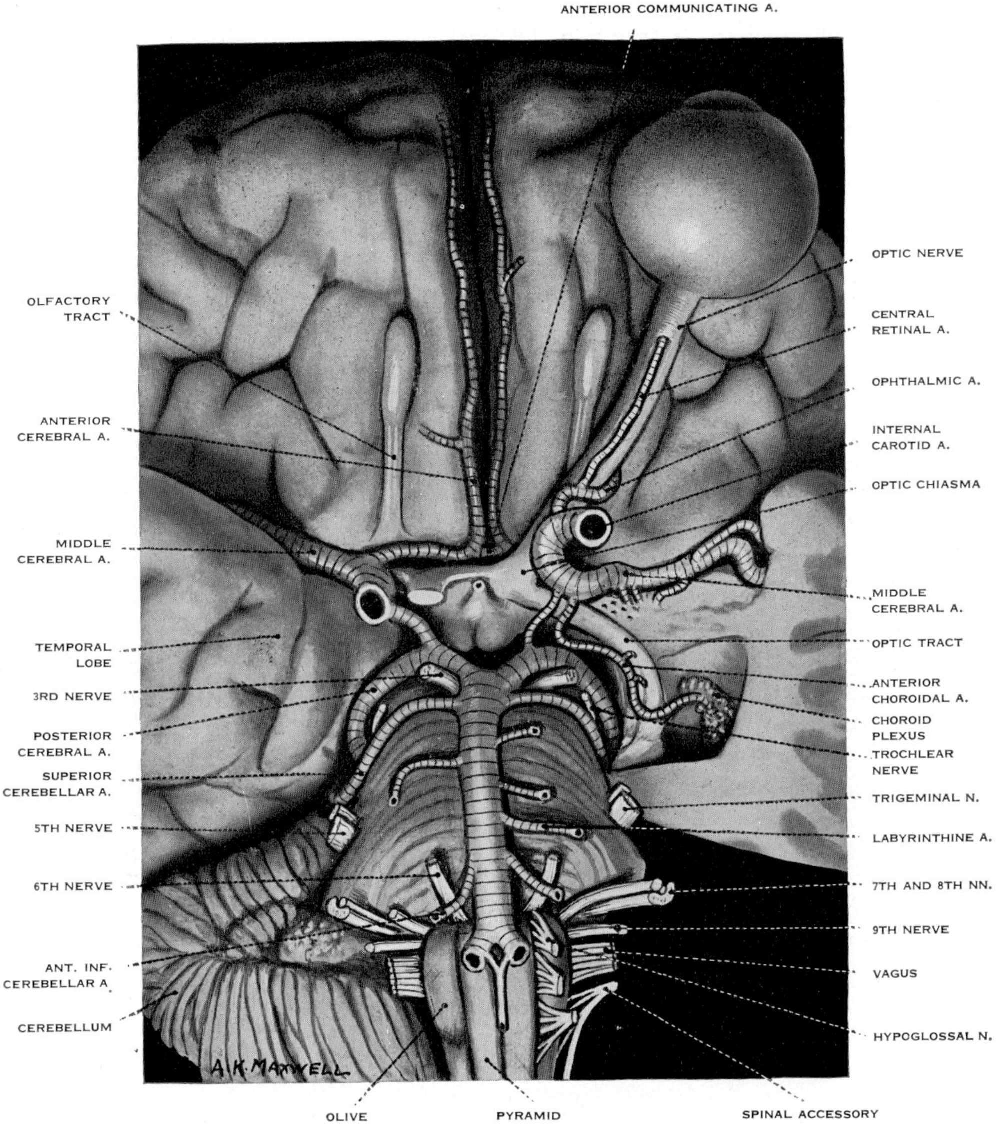

ANTERIOR COMMUNICATING A.

OLFACTORY TRACT

ANTERIOR CEREBRAL A.

MIDDLE CEREBRAL A.

TEMPORAL LOBE

3RD NERVE

POSTERIOR CEREBRAL A.

SUPERIOR CEREBELLAR A.

5TH NERVE

6TH NERVE

ANT. INF. CEREBELLAR A.

CEREBELLUM

A.K.MAXWELL

OLIVE

PYRAMID

OPTIC NERVE

CENTRAL RETINAL A.

OPHTHALMIC A.

INTERNAL CAROTID A.

OPTIC CHIASMA

MIDDLE CEREBRAL A.

OPTIC TRACT

ANTERIOR CHOROIDAL A.

CHOROID PLEXUS

TROCHLEAR NERVE

TRIGEMINAL N.

LABYRINTHINE A.

7TH AND 8TH NN.

9TH NERVE

VAGUS

HYPOGLOSSAL N.

SPINAL ACCESSORY

FIG. 355.—DISSECTION TO SHOW BLOOD-SUPPLY OF OPTIC PATHWAY AND RELATIONS OF VESSELS TO OCULAR NERVES.

Basal aspect.

(*Wolff's preparation.*)

phenomenon that in cases of thrombosis of the posterior cerebral artery the resulting homonymous hemianopia spares the macula (the scotoma falling short of the fixation point by 10°) by the fact that the occipital pole is the border-line territory between the distribution of the middle and posterior cerebral arteries (Fig. 361) and that the former artery will be able to supply the macular area if the latter is blocked. Polyak (1957) has reviewed the literature on this problem most exhaustively and favours the vascular explanation. See also Brodal (1969), who takes a similar view. However, one recent study, admittedly on cats (Stone and Hansen, 1966), does suggest the possibility of a bilateral macular representation at the geniculate level in this species.

THE UNIOCULAR VISUAL FIELDS

The fibres which subserve the uniocular and binocular visual fields run separately in some levels of the visual pathway. Brouwer and Zeeman (1926) found that in the rabbit the binocular field (in this animal only 20 degrees) occupies a very small area in the lateral geniculate body, while nearly the whole of the remainder is taken by the uniocular. But this animal, with laterally directed orbital axes, is representative of those with well-developed panoramic vision, no true binocular vision, and hence of no significance in connection with the primate arrangement.

The human uniocular field, the part seen by one eye only, is represented by the extreme temporal field. The retinal fibres involved are the most nasal. They form the nasal half-moon to the medial side of the crossed bundle and then go to a small strip on the ventral part of the lateral geniculate body (Fig. 347, D).

In the visual cortex the uniocular field is localized anteriorly in the lower lip of the calcarine sulcus. The clinical importance of this is that a lesion of the optic radiation, for instance, may affect one field only.

THE CORTICAL OCULOMOTOR AREAS

1. Frontal.
2. Occipital.
3. Angular Gyrus.

1. The frontal oculomotor area or eye field is the posterior part of the middle frontal gyrus. Stimulation of this area results in conjugate deviation of the eyes to the opposite side, stimulation above the centre results in conjugate deviation downwards, and stimulation below in conjugate deviation upwards. Pupillary responses may also be elicited. Both voluntary and reflex ocular movements may be mediated by this area. (For a review of earlier work see Crosby et al., 1962.)

The path of corticofugal fibres to the ocular motor nuclei is not known, but it probably runs with the pyramidal tract. There is a complete decussation of fibres of opposite sides.

2. The occipital centre is probably concerned with the fixation reflex, i.e. with bringing on to the macula the image of an object which has "interested" the

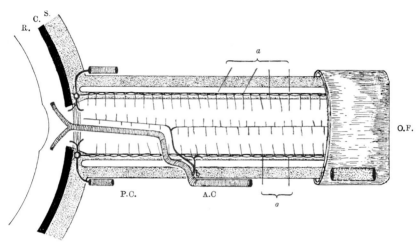

FIG. 356.—SCHEMATIC LONGITUDINAL SECTION OF THE OPTIC NERVE TO SHOW ITS ORBITAL BLOOD-
SUPPLY.

A.C., Arteria centralis; P.C., Posterior ciliary artery; O.F., Optic foramen; R., Retina; C., Choroid;
s., Sclera; a., Group (a) to pial plexus; b., Group (b).

Note that the post-central artery supplies the macular bundle in this part of the optic nerve (p. 389).

periphery of the retina. Stimulation of the visual area causes conjugate deviation of the eyes.

3. Conjugate deviation of the eyes has been produced in animals by stimulation of the angular gyrus, but not in man, in whom operative removal of the area has not resulted in any oculomotor defect.

The blood-supply to these areas is the middle cerebral artery for the frontal and angular gyri and the posterior cerebral for the occipital area.

The Blood-supply of the Visual Pathway

The blood-supply of the *retina* has been considered on p. 145.

The Blood-supply of the Optic Nerve.—The optic nerve, an outgrowth from the brain, has a vascular supply modelled on that organ. The resemblance is great, but not absolute, for here we have no grey matter—no nerve cells. The optic nerve, chiasma, and tracts are covered with pia mater identical with that of the brain. Only those portions of the chiasma and tracts adherent to the base of the brain are bare of pia.

All the arteries which will eventually supply the nerve tissue do so through the pial network of vessels (Figs. 356, 357). This network is rich and fine and extends to the back of the globe. In the intracranial portion of the nerve it is situated on the surface of the pia; in the orbital portion in its thickness, between the longitudinal and circular fibres.

As in the case of the cerebral convolutions there are actually two networks, one inside the other. The outer is the larger and formed of arterioles of fair size; the other, lying within the first, consists of vessels so small that a loupe is necessary to see them. The network is supplied by arteries which probable anastomose slightly in the network, but not before they reach it.

When the vessels pass into the nerve they take with them a coat of pia and also a covering of glia, which constitute the septa. In fact, the distribution of the septa is exactly that of the blood-vessels. Also the thickness of each septum is proportional to the size of the contained vessel. While this is obvious in the orbital portion of the nerve, it is more difficult to make out in the tract and chiasma. In the most posterior portion of the optic nerve (where the septa gradually disappear), in the chiasma, and in the optic tract even the larger vessels are surrounded by only a slight covering of connective tissue which gets less with the smaller vessels and seems to disappear entirely in the capillaries. They are, however, always separated from the nerve tissue by the perivascularis gliæ.

There is a striking contrast between the great vascularity of the pia and the relatively few vessels in the dura mater. The pial network acts as a distributing centre which provides for a regular supply of blood to the nerve. As the vessels pass into the nerve in the septa they divide dichotomously as these do and send branches anteriorly and posteriorly.

The vessels which join it eventually come from the internal carotid and, since the eye has grown out from the brain, its vessels have followed it. This explains why the vessels to the chiasma are short and those to the globe relatively long.

The intracranial part.—The feeders to the pial network are derived from the ophthalmic, superior hypophysial, anterior cerebral and internal carotid arteries.

A cross-section of the nerve shows that the septal network here has a special appearance—whereas in other parts of the nerve the thickness of the septa is fairly constant, in the axial part of the intracranial portion they are not only

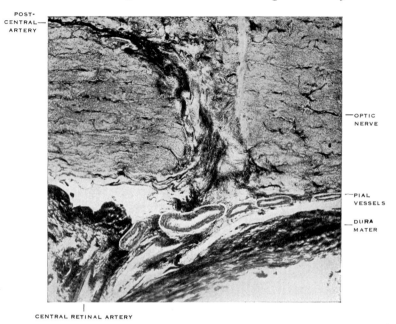

FIG. 357.—LONGITUDINAL SECTION OF THE OPTIC NERVE, SHOWING A LARGE BRANCH FROM THE CENTRAL ARTERY PASSING FORWARDS IN THE SUBARACHNOID SPACE TO THE PIAL PLEXUS; ALSO A POST-CENTRAL ARTERY PASSING BACKWARDS.

(Wolff's preparation.)

thinner but the meshes are wider. Hence smaller vessels supply a large number of nerve fibres. Thus any interference with the blood-supply would, according to Behr (1935), affect first and most markedly the central papillomacular bundle.

The whole of the remaining portion of the nerve and also the whole of the globe is supplied by branches of the ophthalmic artery.

The intracanalicular region is supplied by the ophthalmic, but differs from the orbital part in that the pial network is relatively poor. The branches involved are recurrent rami of the ophthalmic and central retinal arteries and the posterior ciliary arteries.

The orbital part is supplied by two groups of vessels:

(A) Those that pierce the dura behind the entrance of the central vessels.

(B) Those that enter the nerve or join the pial network at the site of entry of the central vessels.

Group A.—In approximately the posterior half of the orbital portion of the optic nerve some six to a dozen small vessels, derived from the ophthalmic and its branches (including the arteria centralis), pierce the dura on various aspects, but mainly above and at the sides. The least pass in from below since this portion is supplied by recurrent branches from Group B.

Having pierced the dura these vessels pass across the subarachnoid space either at right angles or obliquely and, clothed in a portion of dura and arachnoid as is the central artery in like position, reach the pial network.

Group B.—At about the point where the central artery pierces the dura, it gives off one or more branches which diminish its diameter by about one-third. Some of these immediately enter the pia (Figs. 356, 357), dividing into branches which go forwards, backwards, and circularly and, joining the pial network, send branches into the nerve. Others pass into the nerve with the central artery running parallel with it. Although extremely well described by Kuhnt in 1877, these important vessels have often been forgotten in subsequent works and this has led to a great deal of confusion. To emphasize the fact that they do exist one would suggest the name of central collateral arteries (arteriæ collaterales centralis retinæ) (Figs. 161, 356).

A larger vessel of this kind may accompany the central artery to the lamina cribrosa. The collateral vessels send branches into the nerve and hence get narrower as they pass anteriorly. At the point where the central artery bends forwards at the centre of the nerve, a branch of the collateral artery (not of the central retinal artery itself) passes backwards towards the optic foramen (Figs. 356, 357). This branch, the post-central artery, is accompanied by the posterior vein of Kuhnt *and supplies the macular fibres in this portion of their course* (see Magitot, 1908).

While, as we have seen, the collateral arteries get finer as we trace them forwards, the central artery remains much the same size from its point of penetration to its bifurcation. This is due to the fact that, in this portion of its course, the arteria centralis has no branches of any size.

The injections by Beauvieux and Ristitch (1924) of the arteria centralis appear to show that the region of the *lamina cribrosa* is supplied by the arterial circle of Zinn only. A similar view was (ultimately) accepted by Wolff (1961) in the 5th edition of this book. See also Steele and Blunt (1956) and Maysel (1969) and p. 149.

The *nerve head* is supplied by the central artery and the circle of Zinn which also sends branches into the neighbouring retina. The number and size of these branches to the retina are variable, but more evident on the temporal side. Here we find all grades up to what is known as a cilioretinal artery (see p. 148).

The Blood-supply of the Chiasma.—The chiasma is mainly supplied by the anterior cerebral and internal carotid arteries. The small arterial rami from these sources form a network in the pia mater of the chiasma, and this network also receives small "feeders" from the superior hypophysial, anterior and posterior communicating, and even the middle cerebral arteries. It is thus extremely unlikely that a block of any one vessel will have any marked effect on the visual fibres. The anterior cerebrals supply most of the superior aspect while the internal carotids are mainly responsible for the under-surface. The feeding vessels again pass to the pial network and thence into the chiasma.

The Blood-supply of the Optic Tract.—The optic tract is also supplied through the pial network of vessels. This is continuous anteriorly with that of the chiasma.

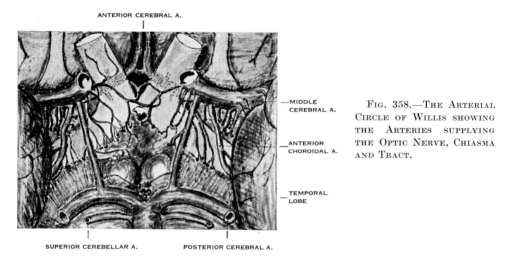

ANTERIOR CEREBRAL A.

MIDDLE CEREBRAL A.

ANTERIOR CHOROIDAL A.

TEMPORAL LOBE

SUPERIOR CEREBELLAR A.   POSTERIOR CEREBRAL A.

Fig. 358.—The Arterial Circle of Willis showing the Arteries supplying the Optic Nerve, Chiasma and Tract.

The feeding vessels come partly from the posterior communicating but mainly from the anterior choroidal artery (Figs. 354, 355, 358, 359, 361). Generally the latter gives several branches to the tract, but the largest of these pass completely through it to enter the base of the brain and supply, among other structures, a portion of the optic radiation.

Shellshear (1927) said that these perforating vessels enter the tract between the crossed (which are the older fibres phylogenetically) and the uncrossed fibres. Sometimes they wind round the tract before entering it. (In this case it is thought that pressure on the tract may disturb nutrition by obstructing the arteries rather than by direct pressure on the nerve fibres themselves.) There is considerable mutual interchange between the anterior choroidal artery and the posterior communicating, and occasionally one or other predominates to the complete exclusion of its fellow (Abbie, 1938).

Injection investigations (François, 1959) have shown the optic tract to be supplied by the anterior choroid artery and by branches of the middle cerebral, overlapping and intermingling, but not anastomozing. That is, each individual

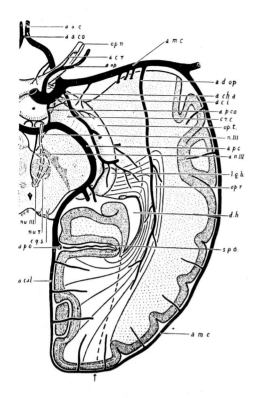

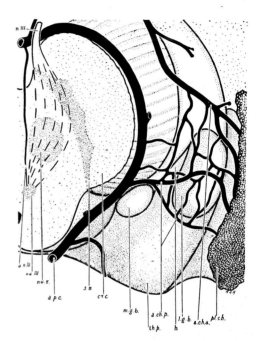

FIG. 359.—TOTAL BLOOD-SUPPLY TO THE VISUAL PATHWAYS, VIEWED FROM THE VENTRAL ASPECT: SEMI-SCHEMATIC (ABBIE).

Note the different sources of supply to the optic radiation. The arrow at the bottom of the figure marks the point of anastomosis between the calcarine and middle cerebral arteries.

FIG. 360.—THE ARTERIAL NETWORK OVER THE LATERAL GENICULATE BODY (SIMPLIFIED) (ABBIE).

Note its derivation from the anterior and posterior choroidal arteries. The specific end-artery from posterior cerebral to the oculo-motor nucleus is indicated.

ABBREVIATIONS EMPLOYED IN THE FIGURES.—a.a.c., anterior cerebral artery; a.a.co., anterior communicating artery; a.b., basilar artery; a.c.i., internal carotid artery; a.c.r., central artery of the retina; a.cal., calcarine artery; a.ch.a., anterior choroidal artery; a.ch.p., posterior choroidal artery; a.d.op., deep optic branch of the middle cerebral artery; a.m.c., middle cerebral artery; a.n.III, artery to oculomotor nucleus; a.op., ophthalmic artery; a.p.c., posterior cerebral artery; a.p.co., posterior communicating artery; a.p.o., parieto-occipital artery; b.ol., olfactory bulb; c.a., anterior commissure; c.c., corpus callosum; c.q.s., superior colliculus; cr.c., cerebral peduncle; f., fornix; h., hilum of lateral geniculate body; h.a., hilar anastomosis; l.g.b., lateral geniculate body; m.g.b., medial geniculate body; n.III, oculomotor nerve; nu.III, oculomotor nucleus; nu.r., red nucleus; op.ch., optic chiasma; op.n., optic nerve; op.r., optic radiation; op.t., optic tract; pl.ch., choroidal plexus; po., pons; s.cal., calcarine sulcus; s.lun., lunate sulcus; s.n. substantia nigra; s.p.cal., posterior calcarine sulcus; s.p.o., parieto-occipital sulcus; t.p., temporal pole; th.p., pulvinar thalami.

artery is a true end-artery, but the amount of overlap explains the absence of hemianopia after occlusion of the anterior choroidal.

The Blood-supply of the Lateral Geniculate Body.—It used to be held that the lateral geniculate body was supplied by the posterior cerebral artery and thus had a different vascular supply from the optic tract. This has been shown by Abbie (1938) and others to be incorrect. In fact, in man, while the main supply, and especially that to the posteromedial aspect, comes from the posterior cerebral, the anterior and lateral aspects are supplied almost entirely by the anterior choroidal artery (Figs. 360, 361). The region of the hilum is supplied through a rich anastomosis from both sources.

The anterior choroidal supplies the fibres coming from the inferior homonymous quadrants of the retinæ, while the posterior cerebral supplies those coming from the superior homonymous quadrants. The intervening region which radiates dorsally from the hilum and contains the macular fibres is supplied by both vessels.

Within the lateral geniculate body the terminal twigs from the penetrating vessels end chiefly in the individual cell laminæ; some pass beyond into the commencement of the optic radiation (Abbie, 1938).

The Optic Radiation.—The blood-supply falls into three parts (Abbie, 1938):

1. While the radiations are passing laterally over the roof of the inferior horn of the lateral ventricle, they are supplied by perforating branches of the anterior choroidal artery.

2. In their posterior course—lateral to the descending horn of the ventricle—they are supplied by the deep optic branch of the middle cerebral artery which enters the brain through the anterior perforated substance with the lateral striate arteries (Figs. 359, 361). (This is a member of the lateral striate group of rami of the middle cerebral artery.)

3. As the radiations spread out to reach the striate cortex, they are supplied by perforating cortical vessels, mainly from the calcarine branch of the posterior cerebral, but also from the middle cerebral artery. It is said that of these perforating vessels those which supply the radiations are independent of those which supply the cortex.

François et al. (1959) put some finishing touches to the above general account. In the first part of the radiation, where the fibres are passing *forwards* from the lateral geniculate body (the *carrefour*), the middle cerebral and even the posterior cerebral overlap the anterior choroid without anastomosis. They confirm the well-known fact that while there are surface anastomoses between the posterior and middle cerebral arteries, all *perforating* branches are end arteries. The optic radiation itself receives few arterioles; these branch on its surface and enter the radiation as non-anastomosing pre-capillaries. The vascular network so formed is completely separate from the vascular network of the cortex.

The Visual Cortex is supplied mainly by the posterior cerebral, especially via its calcarine branch (Figs. 354, 359, 361). The middle cerebral helps at the anterior

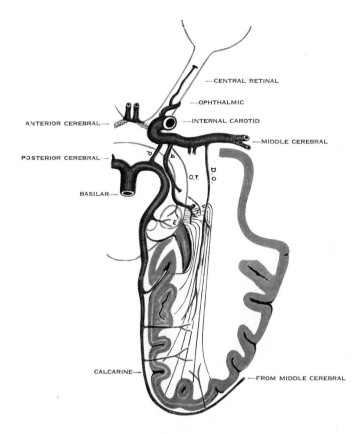

CENTRAL RETINAL

OPHTHALMIC

ANTERIOR CEREBRAL—

—INTERNAL CAROTID

—MIDDLE CEREBRAL

POSTERIOR CEREBRAL—

O.T.

D.O.

BASILAR—

E

CALCARINE—

—FROM MIDDLE CEREBRAL

O.T. = Optic Tract.
E = Lateral Geniculate Body.
A = Anterior Choroidal Artery.
P = Posterior Communicating Artery.
D.O. = Deep Optic Artery (Lateral Striate A.)

FIG. 361.—THE ARTERIES OF THE VISUAL TRACT, INFERIOR VIEW.
(*Modified after Abbie.*)

end of the calcarine sulcus, and on the lateral surface near the posterior pole there is, according to Shellshear (1927), a definite anastomosis between posterior and middle cerebrals, *which may account for the sparing of the macula in cases of thrombosis of the posterior cerebral.* (For an excellent survey of this problem, consult Polyak, 1957.)

Smith and Richardson (1966) give further details of normal variations of vascular pattern, and relate specific arterial branches to their respective areas in the visual fields.

These vessels form a rich network in the pia, from which short branches pass to the grey matter, while larger branches pierce this to reach the white matter. The latter vessels are end arteries, communicating by capillaries only. Thus we may have localised areas of softening in the white matter.

The Blood-supply of the Lower Centres.—The tectum of the midbrain is supplied from a network of vessels coming from the posterior cerebral and superior cerebellar arteries, but the former vessels provide the main supply to the superior colliculi.

According to Alezais and D'Astros (1892), the oculomotor and trochlear nuclei are supplied by specific end-arteries which arise from the posterior cerebral artery and enter the midbrain through the posterior perforated substance (Fig. 358). Stopford, however, stated that these nuclei are supplied from the basilar artery. The abducent nuclei are supplied by a specific end artery which comes from the basilar (Stopford, 1916, 1917). (For further details on the mesencephalic vessels see Lazorthes *et al.*, 1958; Nawab Khan, 1969.)

The Venous Return is partly by the cortical veins and partly by the basal vein which runs close to the posterior cerebral artery. (For the most recent account of the veins draining the brainstem consult the monograph of Duverney, 1975.)

A recent publication by Elišková (1973) describes the blood vessels of the ciliary ganglion in man. The arteries are derived from the lateral posterior ciliary and lateral muscular branches of the ophthalmic artery; the veins, usually four, drain into the inferior ophthalmic vein.

PRACTICAL CONSIDERATIONS

1. Division of one optic nerve results in blindness of that eye and a dilated pupil which does not react to light directly, but does consensually. The vision of the other eye is unaffected; its pupil reacts to light directly, but not consensually. A glance at the diagram (Fig. 364) will make it clear that the reflex can get to the sphincter centre of the affected side, when light is thrown on to the good eye, either through the chiasma or through the posterior crossing in the mid-brain.

The affected pupil will, of course, react to convergence, but does not come under the category of the Argyll Robertson pupil (*q.v.*).

2. Sagittal section of the chiasma results in bitemporal hemianopia (a con-

dition most commonly, but by no means invariably, seen in pituitary tumours). It abolishes neither the direct nor the consensual pupil reactions.

Theoretically, at any rate, a modified Wernicke (see below) ought to be present, i.e. the pupil ought to react when the light falls on the temporal (i.e. seeing) halves of the retina only. Division of the uncrossed fibres of the chiasma leads to binasal hemianopia.

3. Behind the chiasma complete unilateral division of the visual pathway in any part of its course will result in a contralateral hemianopia, e.g. if the left pathway is divided, there results loss of the right halves (temporal of the right side and nasal of the left) of the visual fields.

4. Division of the optic tract produces a contralateral homonymous hemianopia, and, while it abolishes neither the direct nor the consensual pupil reaction, it gives rise to Wernicke's hemiopic pupil reaction, i.e. the pupils do not react when a narrow pencil of light is thrown on the blind halves of the retinæ, but do react if it falls on the seeing portions. It may not be out of place here to state that, owing to the scattering of light by the media of the eye, the test is exceedingly difficult to perform. A lesion of the optic tract may however be distinguished from a lesion of the optic radiation by the following facts. There is often slight ptosis of the same side and inequality of the pupils, the larger one being on the side of the hemianopia. Also the macula is not usually spared and optic atrophy sets in after a time.

5. Since the pupillary and visual fibres part company in the posterior third of the tract, behind this point they are usually affected separately. This accounts for the fact that the Wernicke's hemiopic pupil reaction differentiates a tract lesion from a lesion of the visual pathway behind the point of separation. (See, however, above.)

6. Destruction of the lateral geniculate body gives rise to a contralateral homonymous hemianopia.

While this is the view which is now becoming generally accepted, one must state that some observers hold that the pulvinar of the thalamus must be involved as well to produce it.

7. Destruction of the optic radiation or visual cortex on one side, as occurs in thrombosis of the posterior cerebral artery, gives rise to a contralateral homonymous hemianopia. The pupils are unaffected and the macula is often spared.

If the hemianopia is accompanied by hemiplegia or hemianæsthesia, the lesion is in the posterior limb of the internal capsule behind the lentiform nucleus. Destruction of that portion of the geniculocalcarine fibres, which passes forwards into the temporal lobe, results in a superior quadrantic hemianopia.

8. The visual pathway extends from the eyeball to the occipital pole of the brain. Hence, it may be affected by a great many lesions and thus help in diagnosis.

9. The definite localization throughout the optic system explains the fact that even circumscribed lesions in tract, radiation, or striate area may produce sharply

delimited scotomata in corresponding places in the visual field of the two eyes.

10. In general, a complete hemianopia is much more likely to occur where the visual fibres are tightly packed in a relatively narrow structure such as the optic tract. In the radiations and occipital cortex where the fibres are more widely spread partial defects are more likely developed in the form of a partial homonymous field defects, and quadrantic or smaller scotomata.

The Medial Longitudinal Fasciculus

The Medial Longitudinal Fasciculus is a band of fibres which runs close to the mid-line through the midbrain, pons and medulla. Above, it establishes intricate connections with the region immediately above the mesencephalon, below it is continuous with the fasciculus anterior proprius of the medulla at the decussation of the pyramids. Through this it becomes continuous with the anterior inter-segmental tract of the spinal cord.

In the midbrain it lies ventral to the central grey matter and in the pons it is ventral to the floor of the fourth ventricle. It interconnects the oculomotor, trochlear, abducent and vestibular nuclei (Figs. 260, 264, 265). The nuclei of the oculomotor and trochlear nerves are closely applied to its medial and dorsal aspect, while that of the abducent lies on its lateral side.

The fasciculus has long been known to mediate correlation between the nuclei of the motor nerves of the eye muscles, and between these and all four vestibular nuclei (McMasters, Weiss and Carpenter, 1966). It is one of the most constant features of the vertebrate brainstem, providing an essential "intersegmental" path in the integration of movements associated with vision and hearing. It has extensive connections with the flocculonodular lobe of the cerebellum through the vestibular nuclei (see Brodal, Pompeinano and Walberg, 1962). It is perhaps worth noting that in these highly complex activities at least eight cranial nerves (optic, oculomotor, trochlear, trigeminal, abducent, facial, vestibulocochlear and accessory) are involved, together with many spinal nerves, especially at cervical levels.

CHAPTER VIII

THE ORBITAL AUTONOMIC NERVOUS SYSTEM

THIS consists of two parts, the sympathetic and the parasympathetic systems. Generally the viscera are supplied by each system, and in such cases the sympathetic and parasympathetic systems exercise opposite effects.

The **autonomic nervous system,** like the somatic, has sensory (receptor) connector, and motor (excitor) neurons, but in the former the motor neurons are outside the central nervous system forming various ganglia. The sensory elements, however, are in the same position as those of the somatic system, i.e. in the posterior root ganglia, and connect by means of the sensory root with neurons situated in the spinal cord or brainstem. The axons of connector neurons emerge as white rami communicantes to reach the motor neurons which are either in the ganglia of the sympathetic trunks or in ganglia even more peripherally placed, such as the cœliac ganglia. Hence the motor neurons in these ganglia may be equated with the motor nerve cells in the ventral grey column. In the lateral grey column are the somata of the connector or intercalated neurons of the sympathetic system.

The axons of the cells in the autonomic ganglia are almost always non-medullated. The preganglionic axons which synapse with them are medullated. Usually, many postganglionic neurons are activated by a single preganglionic neuron, producing mass actions or widely disseminated responses. (For general descriptions of the autonomic nervous system, consult the monographs of White, 1952; Mitchell, 1953; Kuntz, 1953; Pick, 1970; Gray's Anatomy, 1973.)

Summary.

Somatic System.—*Sensory (receptor)* neurons, both spinal and cranial, their cell bodies in the posterior root ganglion or its homologue (e.g. trigeminal ganglion).

Motor (effector).—Neurons whose cell bodies are in the central nervous system.

Connector (intercalated).—Neurons also in the central nervous system.

Sympathetic System.—Sensory neuron, cell body in the posterior root ganglion.

The motor (effector) neuron, cell body in the lateral chain ganglia, or in the peripheral ganglion.

The connector neuron starts in the lateral horn of the thoracic region, and leaves the cord by the white rami communicantes.

They are thus *medullated* pre-ganglionic fibres. The post-ganglionic fibres are non-medullated.

The **parasympathetic system** has two outflows, cranial and sacral. It is similarly arranged. The *connector neuron* is in the nucleus of a cranial nerve or lateral grey column of the sacral spinal cord (segments 2, 3 and sometimes 4). The *effector neuron*, however, is in the wall of the viscus innervates. There is an exception to this in the case of part of the cranial outflow, where ganglia are established for relay of the connector neuron on to the effector cell body. These ganglia are the ciliary, pterygo- (spheno-) palatine, submandibular and otic. Only parasympathetic relay occurs here. All four ganglia transmit both sensory and sympathetic fibres

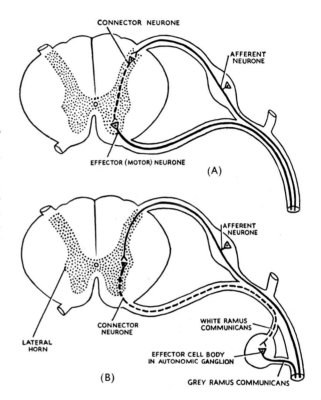

FIG. 362.—(A). A HYPOTHETICAL SOMATIC REFLEX PATHWAY.

(B). AN AUTONOMIC REFLEX PATHWAY.

Note general similarity but differences in the sites of the connector and effector cells. (In fact, reflex pathways are more complex than this. The somatic "connector" is rarely if ever a single neuron.)

(*From Last's "Anatomy: Regional and Applied", by permission. J. & A. Churchill Ltd.*)

to share in the peripheral distribution of the branches, but none of these fibres relay in the ganglia (Fig. 366).

There are thus three outflows of fine medullated nerves to peripheral motor ganglion cells.

    1. Brainstem ·   ·   ·   ·   ·   · cranial parasympathetic.

    2. Thoraco-lumbar ·   ·   ·   ·   · sympathetic system.

    3. Sacral (splanchnic nerves) ·   ·   · sacral parasympathetic.

    1. **The Midbrain Outflow** of preganglionic nerve fibres belong to neurons in the accessory oculomotor nuclei, pass out with the nerve to the ciliary ganglion, where they synapse with motor cells. From here postganglionic *medullated* fibres pass in the ciliary nerves to the sphincter pupillæ and ciliary muscles. This medullation of

postganglionic axons is exceptional. It may be associated with speed of conduction, and in this regard it is interesting to note that the muscles so innervated are necessarily rapid-acting, and hence striated, in the avian eye. The pathway is also largely concerned with accommodation, which is in some characteristics more *somatic* than *visceral* in its activities.

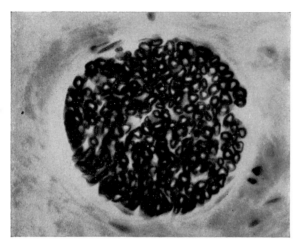

FIG. 363.—SECTION OF POSTERIOR CILIARY NERVE OF RHESUS MONKEY JUST BEHIND THE GLOBE TO SHOW MEDULLATED FIBRES. (WEIGERT'S STAIN.)

There is reciprocal innervation of antagonists. Thus oculomotor stimulation contracts the sphincter and inhibits the dilatator, and likewise the sympathetic is motor to the dilatator and inhibitor to the sphincter.

2. **The Bulbar Outflow** of connector fibres (corresponding to the white rami of the thoracic region) are the axons of small neurons in the so-called *salivatory nucleus*, the identity of which is not entirely certain. (See, however, Lewis and Shute, 1959.) The neurons in question appear to be situated in or near the cranial extremity of the dorsal vagal nucleus. It is customary to divide the nucleus into superior and inferior parts, but the evidence for this is unsatisfactory.

The following are the cranial nerves which contain fibres corresponding to white rami and belonging to the bulbar outflow:

(1) **Superior salivatory nucleus,** secretomotor fibres leave in nervus intermedius for two destinations: (*a*) via greater (superficial) petrosal nerve to relay in pterygopalatine (sphenopalatine) ganglion for lacrimal gland and glands of nose, paranasal sinuses and palate, (*b*) chorda tympani to submandibular ganglion for relay to sublingual, anterior lingual and submandibular salivary glands. (For further details on the routes of parasympathetic fibres to the lacrimal gland and their distribution therein, consult the papers of Ruskell, 1968, 1970, 1971, 1973.)

(2) **Inferior salivatory nucleus,** secretomotor fibres leave in 9th nerve, and by local relay in mucous membrane supply glands of oropharynx. In tympanic branch of 9th secretomotor fibres run in lesser (superficial) petrosal nerve, for relay in otic ganglion to supply parotid gland.

(3) Dorsal nucleus of vagus, motor fibres destined to relay in wall of viscus concerned (heart, lung, intestine).

The **Sympathetic Fibres** which pass to the eye are discussed on p. 402.

THE PATH OF THE LIGHT REFLEX

Two main views have been expressed with regard to the sensors of the light reflex, and are quoted here for their historical interest.

1. Hess (1908 and 1922), in his experiments with diurnal birds which have yellow oil globules between the inner and outer portions of the rods, and nocturnal birds which have none, showed that visual and pupillary reactions to light stimuli of varying intensity and under different conditions of adaptation ran parallel, and came to the conclusion that the outer portion of the rods and cones are the receptor organs—both for vision and for the light reflex. This is the view most widely accepted.

2. Schirmer (1894) believed that the light reflex started in the inner nuclear layer, especially in the amacrine cells. For in diseases of the outer retinal layers, sight is affected much more than the pupil reflex. Von Hippel (1899) pointed out that these cells are absent just in the macular area where the light reflex is most easily obtained.

It is probable that the light reflex can be obtained from any region of the retina up to the ora serrata, and not as Hess thought from the macular area only. But it is certainly much more easily elicited when light falls on the central area; while strong illumination is necessary to produce it from the peripheral retina.

This and other old and heated controversies regarding the pupillary reflex pathway have been admirably reviewed by Lowenfeld (1966) and Lowenstein and Lowenfeld (1969). These workers, whose papers provide the most compendious surveys of the literature on pupillary activity currently available, point out the experimental difficulties involved in evoking and observing pupillary responses from small areas of the retina. In summary, they favour the view that any rod or cone photoreceptors may serve the reflex pathway; and they regard it as improbable that there exist special "pupillary" receptors or receptors other than rods and cones.

The Afferent Tract.—Here again two views are expressed as to whether the visual and pupillary fibres are different or identical. Müller's law of specificity of nerve conduction has even been invoked to support the view that a dual function is involved and hence separate "pupillary" and "visual" fibres must exist. There is no adequate evidence in favour of either view; in particular, the clinical deductions favouring a duality of receptor, ganglion cell and further pathway ignores the improbability of disease selecting one set of fibres rather than the other. There can be no doubt that the axons subserving the sensation of vision and those concerned with the pupillary reflexes have different pathways and connections. Whether the pupillary pathway is formed of branches or collaterals of the retinogeniculate axons or not is still quite uncertain. (See Ranson and Magoun, 1933, and Lowenstein and Lowenfeld, 1969.) The assumptions that axons of small diameter are "pupillary" and the larger ones "visual" or *vice versa* are both poorly supported by evidence.

The pupillary fibres run in the optic nerve; for its division abolishes the direct but not the consensual light reflex. *The pupillary fibres partially cross in the chiasma, as do the visual, a portion going over to the opposite side, while the remainder pass on in the optic tract of the same side.* We know that the pupillary fibres cross in the chiasma, because division of one optic tract abolishes neither the direct nor the consensual pupil reaction. Experimental division of the chiasma abolishes neither the direct nor the consensual light reflex. *Hence there must be a posterior crossing as well.*

The pupillary fibres do not pass from the chiasma to the floor of the third ventricle, for experimental separation of the chiasma (Bumke and Trendelenburg, 1911) from this structure has no effect on the light reflex. *The pupillary fibres run in the optic tract*, division of which causes Wernicke's hemiopic pupil reaction.

They leave the visual fibres at the posterior part of the tract, do not form a cell station at the lateral geniculate body, but run superficially in the superior brachium conjunctivum to the lateral side of the superior colliculus. Division of both superior brachia abolishes the pupil reactions to light on both sides (Karplus and Kreidl, 1913). Even here there is disagreement, for some workers (e.g. Szentágothai, 1942) consider that the pupillary fibres form synapses with neurons in the pre-geniculate nucleus (an almost vestigial group of cells in man, close to the geniculate nucleus), the axons of these cells then passing on to the tectal region. A recent study by Pierson and Carpenter (1974) does not support this view; these workers consider that a retino-pretectal pathway is the principal pupillomotor afferent route.

The fibres which enter the superior colliculus are not concerned with the pupillary reflex; destruction of this body down to the aqueduct has no effect on the pupillary reflex.

The pupillary fibres pass into the midbrain to the lateral side of the superior colliculus to reach the pretectal nucleus (which is an ill-defined collection of small cells anterior to the lateral margin of the superior colliculus), where they have their terminations. The new relay of fibres partially crosses in the posterior commissure and also ventral to the aqueduct, and thus reaches the sphincter centre of the same and opposite side via the medial longitudinal bundle. In man the numbers of axons which cross approximately equals those which do not. The "sphincter centre" is formed by the accessory oculomotor nuclei of Edinger and Westphal.

The literature upon the parasympathetic pupillomotor status of the accessory oculomotor nuclei is immense (see Warwick, 1954), and despite some influential disbelievers the anatomical and physiological evidence is now undeniable. Many of the cells—if not most—in this small-celled component of the oculomotor complex are concerned with accommodation. Attempts to distinguish between the two types of neuron and thus to identify pupillomotor and accommodation "centres" have been few and unconvincing. A recent study (Sillito and Zbrozyna, 1970), using stimulation technique in cats suggests that the classical Edinger-

Westphal columns (p. 283) are concerned with pupilloconstriction, whereas the majority of the anteriomedian nucleus is not.

Summary.

The probable course of the afferent pupillary fibres is as follows (Figs. 364, 365):

They start in the rods and cones—pass through the retina to reach the optic nerve; partially cross in the chiasma like the visual fibres; accompany the visual fibres in the tract to its posterior third, where they leave the tract as a separate bundle of fibres to enter the superior brachium conjunctivum; pass into the midbrain lateral to the superior colliculus to reach the pretectal nucleus; partially

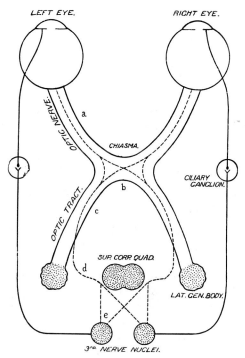

Fig. 364.—Scheme of the Pupillary Path (Interrupted Lines).

Section at (a), i.e. of the left optic nerve, causes blindness of the left eye, abolition of the direct reaction to light of the left eye with retention of the consensual, and abolition of the consensual reaction of the right eye with retention of the direct.

At (b), i.e. of the chiasma, causes bitemporal hemianopia; abolishes neither the direct nor the consensual pupil reaction.

At (c), i.e. of left optic tract, causes contralateral (i.e. right) homonymous hemianopia; Wernicke's hemiopic pupil reaction.

At (d), i.e. of the superior brachium on *both* sides, causes Argyll Robertson pupils.

At (e), i.e. both afferent fibres coming to left nucleus; unilateral (left) Argyll Robertson pupil.

At (e), on both sides causes bilateral Argyll Robertson pupils.

N.B.—*The cell station in the pretectal nucleus (see Fig. 365) is not shown.*

cross to reach the accessory oculomotor nucleus (Edinger-Westphal) of the same and opposite side via the medial longitudinal bundle.

We see therefore that there is a double crossing—namely, in the chiasma and in the midbrain.

The Efferent Path.—The axons of the accessory oculomotor neurons (p. 283) extend into the oculomotor nerve, which they leave in its branch to the inferior oblique muscle. From this a small ramus conducts these preganglionic, parasympathetic, myelinated fibres to the ciliary ganglia, where they terminate in axosomatic and axodendritic synapses with the ganglionic neurons. The latter project *myelinated* postganglionic fibres which reach the eyeball through the short ciliary nerves to innervate the sphincter pupillæ. It is important to note that the majority (95–97% according to Warwick, 1954) of the fibres in this efferent pathway are concerned with the ciliary muscle. The time-hallowed expression—"the light reflex pathway"—is thus something of a misnomer.

The Pupillodilator Fibres.—The so-called dilator centre (of Budge and Waller, 1851) lies in the lateral column of the spinal cord at the junction of its thoracic and cervical regions. The dilator fibres leave the cord via the white rami communicantes of the upper four thoracic nerves. They pass up the cervical sympathetic trunk to reach the superior cervical ganglion, where they form synapses. From here the *postganglionic* fibres run upwards with the sympathetic plexus around the internal carotid artery, which they leave to join the trigeminal ganglion. They pass into the orbit via the nasociliary nerve and enter the eye via the long ciliary nerves and so reach the dilatator muscle. Sympathetic ganglion cells have been found in the internal carotid plexus. These should not be forgotten when considering the effects of extirpation of the superior cervical ganglion (Sunderland and Hughes, 1946). The preganglionic neurons in the spinal cord are thus clearly a kind of motor pool (albeit rather scattered) and not an integrative "centre". Dilatation of the pupil can be evoked by stimulation of the frontal eye field (Crosby, 1953) and by other cortical areas. Although this suggests that the cortex may be involved in reflex pupillo-dilatation, little is known of the connections of such areas to subcortical or brainstem nuclei, and there is no identifiable "higher centre" for this function at the cortical level.

Not all the sympathetic fibres entering the eyeball are concerned with the dilatator pupillæ. A supply to the ciliary muscle has sometimes been suggested; for recent work and a discussion of this controversial subject *see* Génis-Gálvez (1957). A similar controversy surrounds a possible sympathetic vasomotor supply in the retina. (Consult Laties, 1967; Fukuda, 1970.) The most recent study of this topic by Ruskell (1973) was on primates and provided little evidence of such a supply. The same worker (1970, 1971) adduced experimental evidence of a parasympathetic supply to the eyeball, via the facial nerve and pteryopalatine ganglion, which may influence the retinal or choroidal circulation since damage to this pathway lowers intraocular pressure in monkeys.

The Path of the Accommodation Reflex

The accommodation reflex is concerned in the effort to obtain clear images of objects. It is usually accompanied by fixation, which consists essentially of a converging movement of the eyeballs, and by diminution in the size of the pupils. It is, nevertheless, equally possible to alter focus with one eye, in which case the synergic convergence is absent. The afferent path of the whole reflex must be along the visual pathway to the occipital cortex.

Some, however, believe that the *convergence part* of the reflex has a different path and does not involve the occipital cortex. It is held to start in proprioceptive

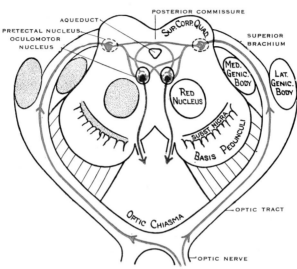

FIG. 365.—DIAGRAM OF SECTION THROUGH MID-BRAIN AND OPTIC CHIASMA TO SHOW PATH OF PUPIL-
LARY CONSTRICTOR FIBRES.

Note especially the pretectal nucleus.

(*From Cunningham's Anatomy, after Ranson and Magoun.*)

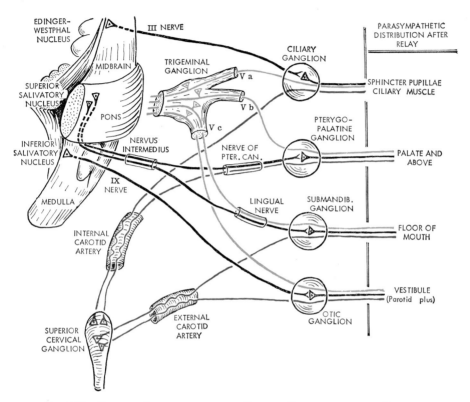

FIG. 366.—PLAN OF CONNEXIONS OF THE CRANIAL PARASYMPATHETIC GANGLIA.

The otic ganglion lies high up near the skull base but by its connexions and branches it is actually the most caudal of the four.

1. Only the parasympathetic roots (black) *relay* in the ganglia. They come from three nuclei, one each in midbrain, pons and medulla. The pontine nucleus (superior salivatory nucleus) relays in the middle two ganglia.

2. The sensory roots (blue) come from the trigeminal ganglion, where their cell bodies lie. The third division (V c) sends branches through the last two ganglia.

3. The sympathetic roots (red) come from cell bodies in the superior cervical ganglion and travel along the internal and external carotid arteries, two on each, to reach their respective ganglia.

(Recent experimental studies suggesting some additions to the above diagram are noted in the text.)

(*From Last's "Anatomy: Regional and Applied", by permission, J. & A. Churchill.*)

impulses in the medial recti. Hence, via the oculomotor nerve or 1st division of the trigeminal to the mesencephalic nucleus of the trigeminal. From here to the constrictor centre of the oculomotor nerve nucleus. Hence, via the oculomotor nerve for an unknown distance. Then leaving the oculomotor nerve it misses the ciliary canglion and makes a cell station in a accessory ganglion (see p. 313), whence it passes to the sphincter pupillæ.

PRACTICAL CONSIDERATIONS

1. The results on the pupillary reactions of division of the optic nerve, the optic chiasma, the optic tract, and the visual pathways behind the point of separation of the pupillary fibres have been discussed on p. 393.

2. Division of both brachia conjunctiva results in loss of the light reflex with retention of the reaction to convergence (Argyll Robertson pupil).

3. For the relation of the superior colliculus to the light reflex, see p. 399.

4. Division of all the pupillary fibres in the midbrain before they reach the oculomotor complex results in bilateral loss of light reflex with retention of the reaction to convergence (Argyll Robertson pupils).

5. If direct and crossed fibres to one accessory oculomotor nucleus only are divided a unilateral Argyll Robertson results. The pupil does not react directly or consensually. The reason for this is easily seen from the diagram, for the sphincter centre of the affected side cannot be reached from either eye. The pupil on the sound side reacts directly and consensually (Fig. 365).

6. Total pupillary paralysis, that is, failure to react to light and convergence, may be due to: (a) a supra-(extra)nuclear lesion; (b) a nuclear lesion; (c) an oculomotor lesion; (d) a lesion of the ciliary ganglion; (e) a lesion of the short ciliary nerves.

7. *The Anatomy of the Argyll Robertson Pupil.*—In trying to fix a site for the lesion, it is very important to remember that in the unilateral Argyll Robertson pupil, the pupil on the affected side does *not* react to light directly or consensually, while the pupil on the sound side reacts to light both ways. There are three main possibilities for the site of the lesion:

(a) That it is on the afferent side of the reflex arc just before the pupillary fibres reach the oculomotor nucleus. This is probably the most generally accepted view. The difficulty about accepting this, and indeed all the other theories, is that it is based on practically no pathological evidence. Current views incline strongly to the belief that the lesion is in the pretectal nucleus (Adler, 1965).

(b) That it is on the afferent side, the lesion being in the superior brachium conjunctivum. Ingvar (1923) and Lenz (1924) believe that the pupillary fibres run superficially in the optic nerve and superior brachium. They hold that the spiro-chætal (or other) toxin is in the cerebrospinal fluid, and will therefore affect the fibres nearest to the subarachnoid space, i.e. pupillary fibres. It will be remembered that Karplus and Kreidl produced the Argyll Robertson pupil by dividing the superior brachia.

(c) That it is on the *efferent* side in the ciliary ganglion (Marina, 1901). While the pupillary fibres are certainly more vulnerable than those which have to do with convergence, it is difficult to see how, if the lesion were in so small a body as the ciliary ganglion, the Argyll Robertson pupil may be present for years and the reaction to convergence not be diminished but actually increased. Cameron (1959) answers this objection by suggesting that only the light-reflex fibres, and not the near-vision fibres, of the third nerve synapse in the ciliary ganglion. This view is untenable on the evidence of experimental iridectomy (Warwick, 1954), but the existence of episcleral ganglion cells should be recalled in this connection.

Argyll Robertson's (1869) original hypothesis, that the lesion is in the cervical spinal cord, affecting "ciliospinal" connections, is now only of historical interest. For a full discussion of these various speculations consult Walsh and Hoyt (1969) and Lowenstein and Lowenfeld (1969). Lowenfeld is of the opinion that the most likely site is just cranial to the accessory nuclei of Edinger and Westphal, which could interrupt not only pretectal connections but also descending inhibitor fibres, rendering the parasympathetic neurons supersensitive to cholinergic influences.

8. *The Sympathetic Pathway.*

Division of the cervical sympathetic results in Horner's syndrome or Horner's triad: ptosis, small pupil and enophthalmos.

The affected pupil does not dilate in the dark or after the instillation of cocaine or after pinching the neck (ciliospinal reflex). In bright light both pupils contract and their inequality disappears.

The affected side of the face does not flush or sweat, and the ear feels colder than on the normal side. The area of absence of sweating includes the whole of the upper limb.

Injury to the cervical sympathetic may result from wounds, accidental or operative, and involvement in growths, etc. The pupillary fibres may also be affected in the lower arm type of brachial birth palsy (Klumpke's paralysis), and in injuries to the spinal cord.

Stimulation of the cervical sympathetic results in exophthalmus, widening of the palpebral fissure, dilatation of the pupil, and often flushing and sweating. It results from pressure by aneurysms, tumours, apical tuberculosis, etc.

THE ROLE OF THE SUPERIOR COLLICULUS

Receiving direct or collateral fibres from the optic tract, the cell bodies of the superior colliculus are connected by tectobulbar and tectospinal tracts with the motor nuclei of the ocular, neck, trunk and limb muscles. Thus may be mediated reflex effects of light—eyeball movements, face (e.g. screwing up the eyes), trunk and limbs (e.g. turning the neck and body, throwing up the hands, jumping, etc.).

Although experiments on various animals, including primates, have shown a retinal projection to the superior colliculus, the number of fibres involved is relatively small in primates, and presumably so in man. (In fact, the region appears to receive other afferents in greater abundance, including axons mediating tactile, thermal pain and auditory modalities of sensation.) Undeniably, also, stimulation of this part of the tectum elicits visual movements (of the eyes, neck and possibly trunk). But these are not necessarily of a reflex character. The superior colliculus projects via the pulvinar of the thalamus to the peristriate cortex, and it receives a projection from peristriate and striate parts of the cortex. It is hence improbable that the long established view of the mesencephalic visual connections as being of a purely reflex nature, with no involvement in the processes of actual vision, is completely valid. Both in birds and mammals there has been a rapid accumulation of experimental and anatomical evidence over the last decade which suggests the existence of alternative visual pathways. (Consult Ingle and Schneider, 1969.) A concept of a "duality" in the mammalian visual pathway has been developed: the mesencephalic route is held to be more concerned with noticing and fixating a visual target, the geniculate pathway with examining and evaluating it. Rapid fixational and slow saccadic movements have been associated respectively with the "two" systems. (See Weiskrantz, 1972; Goldberg and Wurtz, 1972; Sanders, 1974; and Jones, 1974, for references to the extensive literature.) It is probable in man that such alternative systems exist, but they may prove to be the two extremes of altogether more complex arrangements.

CHAPTER IX

THE ORBITAL VESSELS

THE OPHTHALMIC ARTERY

THE ophthalmic artery arises as a vertical branch (Fig. 293), from the medial side of the convexity of the fifth bend of the internal carotid, just after this vessel has left the cavernous sinus by piercing the dura forming its roof. At its origin (Figs. 278, 279, 293), the ophthalmic artery is medial to the anterior clinoid process and inferior to the optic nerve. After a very short course upwards (Fig. 293) it bends forwards at a right angle. It runs directly forwards for a few millimetres under the *medial* side of the nerve, then bends laterally. Usually the origin of the artery lies under the middle of the nerve, but since its course here is anteroposterior and that of the nerve laterally as well as forwards, it may appear at the *medial* border of the nerve before eventually passing laterally (Figs. 274, 355). The nearer the origin of the artery is to the optic foramen, the nearer the medial side of the nerve is it placed, and vice versa.

It passes through the optic canal within the dural sheath of the nerve, at first inferior to the nerve; then, passing to its lateral side, it pierces the sheath near its entrance into the orbit. It will be seen that the internal carotid artery is anchored to the dural sheath by its ophthalmic branch; and it is also indirectly attached to the optic nerve by the adherence of the sheaths and by branches to the nerve from the ophthalmic artery (see p. 325). (Figs. 294, 295.)

In the posterior part of the orbit it lies in the cone of muscles, with the ciliary ganglion and the lateral rectus to its lateral side and the optic nerve medial (Figs. 280, 282).

The artery ascends, crosses between the nerve and the superior rectus to reach the medial wall of the orbit in company with its satellite nasociliary nerve (Fig. 280). It passes forwards between the medial rectus and superior oblique towards the maxillary process of the frontal bone, behind which it divides into dorsal nasal and supratrochlear branches.

The ophthalmic artery and its branches are markedly tortuous.

Summary of Distribution.—The ophthalmic artery supplies the orbit and scalp. One branch transcends all the others in importance—the central artery of the retina. This is an end-artery and its loss (e.g. from embolism) results in complete and irrevocable blindness. Beyond the orbit the ophthalmic artery supplies the forehead to the vertex, and the lateral wall of the nose. Here, especially in the scalp, exists a field of anastomosis between external and internal carotid arteries.

Branches.—Convention dictates that these should be named, but great variation exists and some of the smaller branches are commonly difficult to demonstrate in a dissection of the orbit. The significant branches of the ophthalmic artery are as follows:

1. The central artery of the retina.
2. Long and short posterior ciliary arteries.
3. The lacrimal artery.
4. Lateral palpebral arteries.
5. Recurrent meningeal artery.
6. Muscular branches.
7. Anterior ciliary arteries.
8. Supraorbital artery.
9. Medial palpebral arteries.
10. Posterior ethmoidal artery.
11. Anterior ethmoidal artery.
12. Dorsal nasal artery ⎫
13. Supratrochlear artery ⎬ terminal.
14. Episcleral and conjunctival arteries.

1. **The Central Retinal Artery.**—Its terminal branches anastomose to a limited extent the arterial circle of Zinn around the entrance of the nerve into the eye (see p. 148).

2. **The Posterior Ciliary Arteries** come off as two trunks, while the ophthalmic artery is still below the optic nerve. These divide into some 10 to 20 branches which, running forwards, surround the nerve and pierce the eyeball close to it. The majority, called the *short ciliary arteries*, enter the choroid coat of the eye. Two branches—*the long posterior arteries*—pierce the sclera to the medial and lateral sides of the nerve respectively (Fig. 280). They run forwards between the sclera and choroid to supply the ciliary body, and then, anastomosing with the *anterior ciliary* arteries to form the *circulus arteriosus iridis major* (see p. 94), supply the iris.

3 and 4. **The Lacrimal Artery** arises from the ophthalmic lateral to the optic nerve. It runs forwards at the upper border of the lateral rectus muscle in company with the lacrimal nerve (*q.v.*) to the lacrimal gland, which it supplies. Having passed through or to the lateral side of the gland, it supplies the conjunctiva and eyelids through its *lateral palpebral branches*, which form superior and inferior arcades on the eyelids by anastomosing with the medial palpebral arteries (Figs. 279, 280).

5. **The Recurrent Meningeal Artery** passes backwards through the superior orbital fissure or through a small foramen in the greater wing of the sphenoid to anastomose with the middle meningeal artery, a branch of the maxillary, which in turn comes off the external carotid. This anastomosis is therefore one between

the internal and external carotids, i.e. between the primitive dorsal and ventral aortæ. At times it may be quite large and replace the ophthalmic or middle meningeal in part.

6. **The Muscular Branches** are usually given off as two main branches, *lateral* and *medial*, with a varying number of smaller twigs. These latter come from the main artery and also from the lacrimal and supraorbital. The lateral branch supplies the lateral and superior recti, the levator and superior oblique. The medial branch is the larger of the two, and supplies the inferior and medial recti and the inferior oblique.

7. **The Anterior Ciliary Arteries** (p. 91) are branches of the muscular arteries. They reach the eyeball along the tendons of the muscles, piercing the sclera to anastomose with the posterior ciliary arteries. Before this they form a circumcorneal subconjunctival network (p. 215).

8. **The Supraorbital Artery** (Figs. 276, 280) comes off where the ophthalmic lies above the optic nerve. It lies at first medial to the superior rectus and levator, and then above the latter muscle and under the roof of the orbit. It meets the nerve of the same name at the junction of the posterior and middle thirds of the orbit, and then accompanies it through the supraorbital notch or foramen, and with it crosses the areolar tissue deep to the frontalis (the danger area), and so reaches the scalp, where it anastomoses with the superficial temporal and supratrochlear arteries. It supplies the upper eyelid, the scalp, and also sends twigs to the levator, the periorbita and the diploë of the frontal bone.

9. **The Medial Palpebral Arteries** are derived either directly from the ophthalmic artery or its dorsal nasal branch. There are usually two, one for each eyelid, in which they form arcades with the lateral palpebral arteries (see above). There are usually two (superior and inferior) arcades in each lid (p. 198).

10. **The Posterior Ethmoidal Artery** (Fig. 280) is a small vessel which enters the posterior ethmoidal canal in company with the posterior ethmoidal nerve (nerve of Luschka) when this is present. It supplies the mucous membrane of the posterior ethmoidal air sinuses and upper part of the nasal mucosa.

11. **The Anterior Ethmoidal Artery** (Figs. 279, 280) is larger than the preceding. It comes off where the ophthalmic lies between the superior oblique and medial rectus. It accompanies the anterior ethmoidal nerve through the anterior ethmoidal canal to appear in the anterior cranial fossa. It enters the nose by a slit in the anterior part of the cribriform plate, occupies the groove on the deep surface of the nasal bone, and eventually appears on the face between the lateral nasal cartilage and the nasal bone.

It gives an *anterior meningeal branch* to the dura mater of the anterior fossa; and it also supplies the mucous membrane of the front part of the nasal cavity, the anterior ethmoidal air sinuses, and the skin of the nose.

12. **The Dorsalis Nasal Artery** traverses the septum orbitale above the medial palpebral ligament to supply the skin of the root of the nose and the lacrimal sac.

It anastomozes with the angular and nasal branches of the facial artery. It often supplies the medial palpebral arteries.

13. **The Supratrochlear Artery** (Figs. 213, 276) pierces the septum orbitale with the supratrochlear nerve which it accompanies. It passes upwards, round the medial end of the supraorbital margin about 1·25 cm from the mid-line, and supplies the skin, muscles, and periosteum of the medial part of the forehead. It anastomozes with the supraorbital and with its fellow of the opposite side.

14. **Episcleral and Conjunctival Arteries,** and other small branches, are derived from the larger rami mentioned above. For example, small *temporal* and *zygomatic* arteries, branches of the lacrimal artery, pass into the canals containing the corresponding branches of the zygomatic ramus of the trigeminal nerve.

Variations in the Ophthalmic Artery

1. The ophthalmic artery in 15% of cases crosses beneath instead of over the optic nerve.

2. It may enter the orbit through the superior orbital fissure.

3. The lacrimal often, and the ophthalmic rarely, may arise from the middle meningeal— by an enlargement of the recurrent lacrimal artery which joins the lacrimal to the middle meningeal (that is, marks a union between primitive ventral and dorsal aortæ).

4. The lacrimal may be reinforced by the anterior deep temporal.

5. The branches of the ophthalmic artery show great variation. The supraorbital and posterior ethmoidal are both inconsistent, and there are often accessory ciliary trunks. The dorsal nasal branch may replace the facial in part.

For further information consult Meyer (1887); Quain (1898); Whitnall (1932).

The Cerebral Arteries (Figs. 354 and 355)

The Anterior Cerebral Artery arises from the internal carotid close to the anterior perforated substance, crosses above the optic nerve, and approaching its fellow of the opposite side is joined to it by *the anterior communicating* vessel, which is, as a rule, about 4 mm long. It then curls round the front or *genu* of the corpus callosum, on the upper aspect of which it runs to the splenium, where it anastomoses with the posterior cerebral.

It supplies the front of the caudate nucleus by branches which enter the anterior perforated substance; the corpus callosum; the medial aspect of the hemisphere as far back as the parietooccipital sulcus; a small strip on the upper part of the lateral surface, and the medial portion of the under-surface of the frontal lobe.

So far as vision is concerned the anterior cerebral artery supplies the upper aspects of the chiasma and intracranial portion of the optic nerve.

The Middle Cerebral Artery is the largest branch of the internal carotid, of which it appears to be the direct continuation. It runs laterally into the lateral sulcus, and breaks up into branches on the insula, which supply the lateral aspect of the hemisphere, except for a strip near its upper border (anterior cerebral), and a strip along the lower border (posterior cerebral).

Its **medial** and **lateral striate branches** enter the brain by the anterior perforated substance.

The *medial striate arteries* pass through the medial part of the lentiform nucleus, which they supply, and also send branches to the caudate nucleus and internal capsule.

The *lateral striate arteries* pass between the lentiform nucleus and the external capsule. The largest was called by Charcot the "artery of cerebral hæmorrhage". Abbie (1933–4), however, emphasises the fact that all branches of the middle cerebral artery have become crowded into a small space at the base of the external capsule in the human brain; this is the anatomical basis for the clinical observation that this situation is the commonest site of origin for cerebral hæmorrhage.

So far as vision is concerned the middle cerebral supplies rami to the inferolateral aspects of the chiasma and anterior portion of the optic tract. Via the deep optic branch it supplies the optic radiations, while its terminal branches anastomose with the calcarine branch of the posterior cerebral to supply a small portion of the striate cortex, probably contributing to the macular area (see p. 393).

The Deep Optic Artery (Abbie, 1933), is really a medium-sized member of the lateral striate rami of the middle cerebral artery which turns posteriorly, passing partly through the substance of the putamen, to reach the fibres from the infralenticular and retrolenticular parts of the internal capsule, thus supplying the auditory *and optic radiations immediately after they leave the capsule.* (Figs. 359, 361.)

The Posterior Communicating Artery arises from the internal carotid close to where it becomes the middle cerebral. It is usually a small vessel, but may be so large that its continuation appears to be the posterior cerebral artery. It may even be absent, and the right and left arteries are frequently unequal in size.

It passes horizontally backwards and a little medially to join the posterior cerebral, which is a branch of the basilar, at the superior border of the cerebral peduncle.

It is thus an anastomosis between the internal carotid and vertebral system of vessels.

In its course posteriorly it crosses the under-surface of the posterolateral angle of the chiasma or the beginning of the optic tract from lateral to medial (Figs. 354, 355, 358). Near the cerebral peduncle it crosses above the oculomotor nerve from medial to lateral (Fig. 260).

The posterior communicating supplies the genu and about the anterior third of the posterior limb of the internal capsule. It also sends branches to the globus pallidus and thalamus.

So far as vision is concerned it sends twigs to the under-surface of the chiasma and supplies the anterior third of the optic tract.

There is considerable mutual interchange between the anterior choroidal and posterior communicating (in fact between most of the vessels of the interpeduncular space).

Thus occasionally one or other predominates to the almost complete exclusion of its fellow, and rarely either of these vessels may usurp the stem of the posterior cerebral artery which then arises from the internal carotid and takes over the whole of the supply to the posterior cerebral field (Abbie). (See also Gillilan, 1959, and Alpers *et al.*, 1959).

The Anterior Choroidal Artery arises from the internal carotid just beyond (lateral to) the origin of the posterior communicating at the lateral side of the commencement of the optic tract (Figs 354, 355, 359, 360). (See Abbie, 1934, Carpenter *et al.*, 1954, and Herman, 1966.)

It runs backwards and medially, crosses the optic tract on its under-surface and comes to lie on the medial side of this structure. It maintains this relation to the anterior part of the lateral geniculate body. Here it turns abruptly laterally, recrosses the optic tract and breaks up into a number of branches, which enter the inferior horn of the lateral ventricle to reach the anteroinferior part of the choroid plexus. During its passage backwards the anterior choroidal gives off branches which either pierce the tract or wrap themselves round either its medial or its lateral aspect.

Next to the internal carotid the anterior choroidal artery, by means of these branches, is the most important source of blood to the internal capsule, of which it supplies rather more than the posterior two-thirds of the posterior limb. It supplies in addition the whole of the infralenticular and retrolenticular portions of the internal capsule containing the auditory and optic radiations. The anterior choroid also gives branches to the middle third (pyramidal portion) of the cerebral peduncle, to the tail of the caudate nucleus, to the thalamus and the globus pallidus.

So far as vision is concerned it gives twigs to the pial network supplying the chiasma and is the main source of supply to the optic tract (posterior two-thirds); it also supplies the anterior and lateral aspect of the lateral geniculate body, and by means of branches which pierce the tract, the commencement of the optic radiations (Fig. 361). The supply to the tract is mainly via the pial plexus (p. 387).

The Arterial Circle (of Willis) (Figs. 260, 355, 358) is the anastomosis of the two internal carotids with the basilar. *It is the most important reason why ligature of one or other common or internal carotid does not always produce cerebral softening.* It lies in the subarachnoid space, and surrounds the structures in the interpeduncular cistern.

It is formed as follows: behind, the basilar divides into the two posterior cerebrals; these are united to the internal carotids by the posterior communicatings. From the internal carotid, running forwards and medially, are the anterior cerebrals, and uniting these is the anterior communicating. (For further details and variations, see Fawcett and Blachford, 1906; Watts, 1934; Paget, 1945; Kuhn, 1961; Gillilan, 1962.)

The Basilar Artery is formed by the union of the two vertebral arteries ventral to the pons. It runs upwards near the median groove of the pons on the base of the skull, and at its upper border bifurcates into the two posterior cerebral arteries.

BRANCHES (BILATERAL)

Pontine.—Several on each side to the pons.

Labyrinthine (Internal Auditory) accompanies the facial nervus intermedius, vestibulo-cochlear complex into the internal acoustic meatus, and is distributed to the labyrinth or internal ear.

The Posterior Cerebral Artery.—Each posterior cerebral artery is formed by the bifurcation of the basilar at the upper border of the pons, and winds round the inferior border of the cerebral peduncle of its own side (Figs. 354, 355, 358, 359, 360). It runs below and parallel to the optic tract which is at the upper border of the brain stem. Also above it are the uncus and hippocampal gyrus.

Below and parallel to the posterior cerebral is the superior cerebellar artery, and between the two are the oculomotor and trochlear nerves. The artery passes anterior to or through the radicles of origin of the oculomotor while it is alongside the trochlear at the side of the midbrain (Figs. 354, 355).

The posterior cerebral, continuing backwards above the free margin of the tentorium cerebelli, passes under the splenium of the corpus callosum and enters the anterior part of the calcarine sulcus. Here it divides into branches which run in the parieto-occipital and posterior part of the calcarine sulci respectively. It is important to note that the intracerebral or central branches of these superficial "feeders" do not anastomose with each other. (See Gillilan, 1959 and 1962.)

The *calcarine branch* of the posterior cerebral runs posteriorly in the depths of the calcarine sulcus (Fig. 354). Then it turns around the occipital pole, in the lateral calcarine sulcus if one is present, to reach the lateral surface of the hemisphere. Arterial twigs emerge between the lips of the sulcus and extend above and below to the limits of the striate area. On the lateral surface of the hemisphere the calcarine artery supplies all the striate cortex except the peripheral fringe, where the supply is taken over by small anastomosing twigs from the middle cerebral (Shellshear, 1927; Abbie, 1933).

The calcarine artery also sends perforating branches, the *posterolateral central arteries*, to the posterior portion of the optic radiation as this spreads out to reach the cortex.

In the part of its course near to the lateral geniculate body the posterior cerebral artery gives off a small group of *posterior choroidal arteries* (Abbie, 1933). The ophthalmological interest of these lies in the fact that one of them commonly ramifies on the geniculate body and helps to supply it.

The posterior cerebral thus supplies: (*a*) the medial surface and the posterior part of the lateral surface of the occipital lobe; (*b*) the posterior portion of the optic radiation; (*c*) the whole of the tentorial surface of the hemisphere except the anterior part of the temporal lobe; and also (*d*) central branches to the thalamus, internal capsule, red nucleus, geniculate bodies, tela choroidea and choroid plexus of the lateral ventricle.

So far as vision is concerned the posterior cerebral supplies the posteromedial aspect of the lateral geniculate body, almost the whole of the visual cortex, and is the main supply to the posterior region of the optic radiation.

A block of the right posterior cerebral artery causes:

(*a*) *Destruction of the visual fibres from the right side of each retina, that is, from the left fields—and hence produces a left homonymous hemianopia.*

(*b*) *Sensory aphasia.*

(*c*) *Sometimes hemianæsthesia from involvement of the posterior part of the internal capsule.*

THE VEINS

The orbit is drained by the superior and inferior ophthalmic veins. They and their tributaries, like most head veins, have no valves, are markedly tortuous and display many plexiform anastomoses. They communicate, moreover, with the veins of the face, with the pterygoid plexus, and with the veins of the nose. They drain into the cavernous sinus.

THE SUPERIOR OPHTHALMIC VEIN

The Superior Ophthalmic Vein is formed near the root of the nose by a communication from the angular vein soon after it has been joined by the supra-orbital. It passes into the orbit above the medial palpebral ligament, and then accompanies the ophthalmic artery across the optic nerve and under the superior rectus to the superior orbital fissure, by which having, as a rule, been joined by the inferior ophthalmic vein, it leaves the orbit to enter the fore-part of the cavernous sinus. Its position in the superior orbital fissure is usually above the

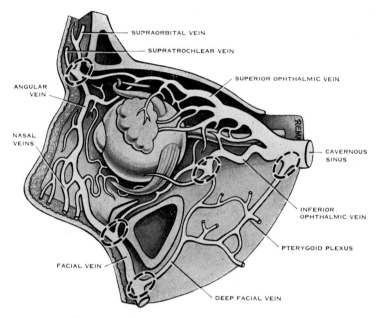

FIG. 367.—SCHEME OF THE VEINS OF THE ORBIT.

cone of muscles, but it may pass between the two heads of the lateral rectus, or occupy the lowest compartment of the fissure.

Tributaries

(a) The inferior ophthalmic vein usually (*vide infra*).

(b) Anterior ethmoidal
(c) Posterior ethmoidal
(d) Muscular
(e) Lacrimal
(f) Central vein of retina

} correspond to the arteries of the same name.

(g) Anterior ciliary.

(h) Two of the venæ vorticosæ or posterior ciliary veins.

The Central Vein of the Retina leaves the optic nerve close to the central artery, but usually nearer the eyeball. As a rule it opens directly into the cavernous sinus, but may end in the superior ophthalmic vein, to which it always gives a well-marked anastomotic branch (Sesemann, 1869). This is of some practical importance.

Graefe thought that papillœdema was due to venous stasis produced by pressure on the cavernous sinus and then back along the vena centralis. Sesemann's observa-tion negatived this theory.

The Anterior Ciliary Veins accompany the arteries of the same name. They pierce the sclera near the cornea, and then, having received some branches from the conjunctiva, join the muscular veins (see also p. 92).

The Inferior Ophthalmic Vein commences as a plexus near the front of the floor of the orbit. It runs backwards on the inferior rectus to enter the cavernous sinus either after having joined the superior ophthalmic vein or separately.

In the latter case, it passes through the superior orbital fissure either between the two heads of the lateral rectus or occupies the lowest compartment.

The inferior ophthalmic vein communicates with the pterygoid plexus through the inferior orbital (sphenomaxillary) fissure; with the anterior facial vein over the inferior orbital margin and with the superior ophthalmic vein. It also gets tributaries from the lower and lateral ocular muscles, the conjunctiva and lacrimal sac, and receives the two inferior vorticose veins.

The Angular Vein

The angular vein is situated at the junction of the veins of the forehead, orbit, and face. It is formed by the union of the supraorbital and supratrochlear veins, and runs down at the side of the nose lateral to the angular artery, across the nasal edge of the medial palpebral ligament some 8 mm from the medial canthus (Fig. 220). It is subcutaneous, and often visible (as a blue ridge) through the skin here, and above and below this point till it pierces the orbicularis. The angular vein (or one of its palpebral branches) is one of the bugbears in approaching the lacrimal sac from the front. It communicates freely with the beginning of the *superior ophthalmic vein*, and is continuous below with the *facial vein*.

Tributaries.—(*a*) **The Supraorbital Vein** runs transversely along the orbital margin deep to the orbicularis, which it pierces under the medial end of the eye-brow to join the supratrochlear and form the angular vein. It communicates with the superior ophthalmic vein through the supraorbital notch, at which point it receives a vein from the frontal sinus and the diploë.

(*b*) **The Supratrochlear Vein** runs down the forehead, accompanying the supratrochlear artery.

(*c*) **The Superior and Inferior Superficial Palpebral Veins.** *One of the upper veins not infrequently crosses the medial palpebral ligament between the angular vein and the medial canthus, where it, too, can be made out through the skin.*

(*d*) **Superficial Nasal Branches**—from the skin of the nose.

The Facial Vein runs obliquely downwards and backwards across the face. It is lateral to and more superficial than its accompanying artery. It crosses the mandible, and joins the retromandibular (posterior facial) vein to form the common facial vein, which opens into the internal jugular.

The (anterior) facial vein communicates with the pterygoid plexus of veins

(Fig. 340), and thus establishes a second communication with the cavernous sinus (q.v.), the first being via the angular and superior ophthalmic veins.

The flow of blood from the frontal region is naturally into the angular and facial veins. But in such a low pressure system it is easy to occlude the facial vein (e.g. lying face down on even a soft pillow) and then blood from the forehead flows via the angular vein into the ophthalmic veins. Hence the danger of septic spots on the forehead and face, which may result in cavernous sinus thrombosis.

THE CAVERNOUS SINUSES

Like the other intracranial venous sinuses, the cavernous sinuses are venous channels formed by the splitting of the dura mater (Fig. 368). They are, of course, lined by endothelium. They extend on each side of the hypophysis and body of the sphenoid from the medial end of the superior orbital (sphenoidal) fissure to the apex of the petrous part of the temporal bone. They are traversed by numerous fibrous trabeculæ, which give them on section the appearance of cavernous tissue, and from this fact they derive their name.

In each sinus is the internal carotid artery, and laterally the abducent nerve. Both these structures receive an investment from the endothelium lining the sinus. The internal carotid artery enters the sinus by passing upwards from the termination of the carotid canal at the medial end of the foramen lacerum, between the lingula and the petrosal process of the sphenoid (Figs. 10, 262). It then runs forwards in its groove on the body of the sphenoid (q.v.) to the medial side of the anterior clinoid process, where it turns upwards and pierces the roof of the sinus between the optic and oculomotor nerves (Fig. 260). While in the sinus it is surrounded by sympathetic filaments.

It is the presence of the artery in the sinus which explains how arteriovenous aneurisms may arise in fracture of the base of the skull.

In the *lateral wall* of the sinus from above down are the oculomotor, trochlear, ophthalmic and maxillary nerves. They are passing forwards to the superior orbital fissure and foramen rotundum respectively. At the anterior end of the sinus the trochlear nerve is above the oculomotor (see p. 290).

To the lateral side of these again, and in contact with the lateral wall of the sinus, are the trigeminal ganglion (Fig. 274) and the temporal lobe of the brain.

Tributaries.—*Anterior*, the ophthalmic veins and the sphenoparietal sinus, which lies along the lesser wing of the sphenoid. *Superior*, the superficial middle cerebral vein.

Drainage.—The superior and inferior petrosal sinuses, and emissary veins through the foramen ovale and the foramen of Vesalius.

Communicating Veins.—The intercavernous plexuses.

The Ophthalmic Veins communicate with the angular vein on the face. *Thus a focus of infection in the upper part of the face may produce thrombosis of the cavernous sinus.*

The sphenoparietal sinus drains from the side wall and vault of the skull.

The Superficial Middle Cerebral Vein drains the cortex alongside the lateral sulcus. Retrograde thrombosis from the cavernous sinus may involve this vein.

The Superior Petrosal Sinus runs along the upper border of the petrous temporal in the attached margin of the tentorum cerebelli. It crosses above the trigeminal and abducent nerves and drains from the cavernous sinus into the transverse. It is usually small.

The Inferior Petrosal Sinus is placed in the groove between the petrous temporal and basi-occipital (Fig. 272). It is often penetrated by the abducent nerve

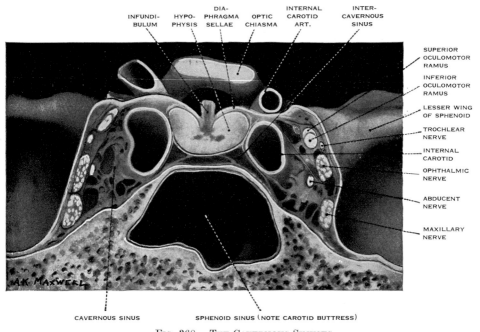

FIG. 368.—THE CAVERNOUS SINUSES.

(After Elliot Smith. Dissection in the Moorfields Hospital Pathological Museum.)

and receives veins from the internal ear. It drains the cavernous sinus into the beginning of the internal jugular vein below the base of the skull.

The petrosal sinuses *explain how thrombosis in the cavernous sinus may spread to the transverse, and finally also produce a swelling behind the ear through the mastoid emissary vein.* This passes through a foramen in the mastoid part of the temporal bone, and unites the sigmoid sinus with the posterior auricular vein. The fact that the auditory veins open into the inferior petrosal sinus marks the route *by which infection of the labyrinth may produce cavernous sinus thrombosis.*

The Emissary Vein which passes through the foramen of Vesalius drains into the pterygoid plexus; so also do the veins that pass through the foramen ovale and foramen lacerum. Moreover, there are indirect communications with the pterygoid plexus via the deep facial vein which unite it to the anterior facial vein, the continuation of the angular, and via the branch which the inferior ophthalmic vein sends to the plexus, through the inferior orbital (sphenomaxillary) fissure (Fig. 367).

The pterygoid plexus of veins corresponds to the second and third parts of the maxillary artery and covers both surfaces of the lateral pterygoid muscle and also the deep surface of the medial pterygoid.

Thus we have an anatomical explanation of how a thrombosis of the cavernous sinus may spread to the pterygoid plexus and produce an abscess so often found post-mortem in this condition in the tonsillar region.

The Intercavernous Plexus connects the two cavernous sinuses across both the roof and the floor of the pituitary fossa. This explains *how thrombosis of the cavernous sinus in the majority of cases becomes bilateral.*

N.B. The "cavernous" nature of the sinuses so designated has been much criticized by Parkinson who has shown, both in corrosion casts and in terms of surgical anatomy, that these sinuses are more usually plexiform like their inter-cavernous connexions. These findings also accord with the embryonic development of these structures. [Consult, Parkinson, D. (1965) *J. Neurosurg.*, **23**, 474 and (1973) *J. Neurosurg.*, **38**, 99.]

LYMPHATICS OF THE ORBIT

The orbit itself contains no clearly demonstrated lymphatic capillaries or lymphoid tissue. That some mechanism for the return of tissue fluids to the venous system must exist seems highly probable, but its nature has not yet been established. The tissues of the lids and conjunctival sac drain to the superficial and deep parotid lymph nodes, and thence to the deep cervical chain of nodes. The medial parts of the lids, especially the lower, also drain to the submandibular lymph nodes, and thence again to the deep cervical. Small lymphoid nodules have been described in the palpebral connective tissue.

CHAPTER X

THE DEVELOPMENT OF THE EYE

THE central nervous system is derived from a thickening in the ectoderm, called the *neural* or *medullary plate*. This is converted into a groove and then into a canal which becomes separated from the surface ectoderm and is called the *neural tube*. The ectodermal cells lining the neural tube are known as neural ectoderm. The cranial end of the neural tube expands to form the three primary brain vesicles.

The eye is partly mesodermal, partly ectodermal in origin. The ectodermal portion is derived from that region of the neural tube (neural ectoderm) which goes to form the forebrain and also from the ectoderm of the surface of the body. The *neural ectoderm* gives rise to all the layers of the retina, to the fibres of the optic nerve, and to the smooth muscle of the iris. *The surface ectoderm* provides the lens and the corneal and conjunctival epithelium, with the lacrimal and tarsal glands. *Mesoderm* provides the remaining structures: cornea and sclera, choroid, iris and ciliary muscle, the vitreous and the "endothelial" cells lining the anterior chamber (p. 457).

There are three stages in the early development of the *retina* and *optic nerve*:

1. The optic groove.
2. The primary optic vesicle.
3. The secondary optic vesicle or optic cup.

The optic grooves appear on each side of the mid-line in the cranial end of the neural plate at a time when the neural plate at this end of the embryo has been converted into a groove, but before its closure to form

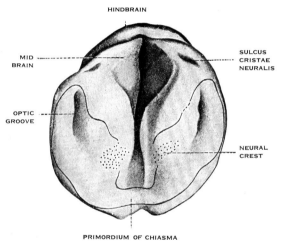

HINDBRAIN

MID BRAIN

SULCUS CRISTAE NEURALIS

OPTIC GROOVE

NEURAL CREST

PRIMORDIUM OF CHIASMA

FIG. 369.—MODEL OF CRANIAL END OF A HUMAN EMBRYO OF TWELVE SOMITES. × 75.

The eye primordium is surrounded by a black line. Laterally it is continuous with the surface ectoderm; to the medial side is the anterior end of the neural crest centrally the areas; of opposite sides are joined by a narrow zone—the foremost part of the primitive brain—which later becomes the chiasma.

(*Fischel, 1929.*)

a canal (the anterior neuropore). The primordium of the retina, in other words, appears very early; in fact, it is already seen in a 2·2 mm embryo.

The areas of opposite sides are joined by a narrow zone which later becomes the chiasma (Fig. 369).

On the closure of the neural tube the optic grooves deepen and appear as hollow symmetrical, hemispherical outgrowths at the side of what is now the forebrain vesicle. The growth is affected by cell division, the mitoses taking place almost entirely on the inner aspect next the cavity of the primary optic vesicle

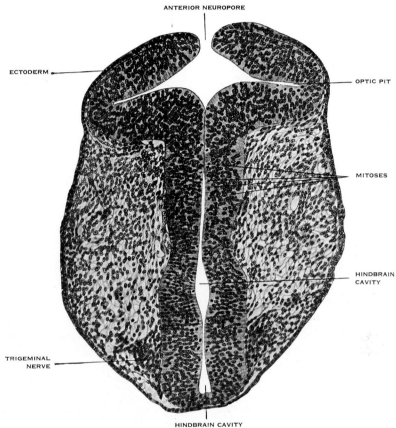

FIG. 370.—HORIZONTAL SECTION THROUGH THE FORE AND HINDBRAINS OF A HUMAN EMBRYO OF EIGHTEEN SOMITES. × 133.

Note that the ocular outgrowth lies lateral to the anterior neuropore.

(*Fischel.*)

(ventricular mitoses). The epithelium of the optic vesicle is high columnar. At first the nuclei are arranged in many layers; later there are many layers of cells.

The cavity of the hollow outgrowth or primary optic vesicle naturally communicates with that of the forebrain vesicle (Fig. 371). The outgrowths are relatively large, and since the optic vesicle is an evagination of the brain itself, it has been described as an "ophthalmencephalon", its cavity as the optic ventricle (Fischel, 1929). As development proceeds, the breadth of the head increases and so does the distance between the brain and the surface ectoderm, with which the optic vesicle remains in contact. As a result of this, the optic vesicle becomes separated from the forebrain by a constriction, its pedicle or stalk, which is best

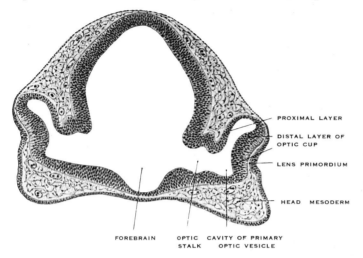

Fig. 371.—Transverse Section through the Forebrain of a 5-mm Human Embryo.

(*From Seefelder, 1930.*)

PROXIMAL LAYER

DISTAL LAYER OF OPTIC CUP

LENS PRIMORDIUM

HEAD MESODERM

FOREBRAIN   OPTIC   CAVITY OF PRIMARY
             STALK   OPTIC VESICLE

marked dorsally (Fig. 371). Meanwhile, the forebrain has developed into the telencephalon (cerebral hemispheres) and diencephalon, and the optic stalk arises from the lower portion of the side wall of the latter. The cavity of the diencephalon, i.e. the future third ventricle, is continued into the cavity of the optic stalk at the recessus opticus. The optic stalk is directed mainly laterally with a slight inclina-tion cranially and dorsally. In the 4 mm embryo the optic vesicle presses on the ecto-derm causing an elevation of the surface which is thus placed laterally (Fig. 377).

The optic vesicles thus, unlike the condition in the adult, lie laterally, being separated from each other by the broad frontonasal process (Fig. 407). In a 19-mm embryo the direction of growth makes an angle of 65° with the mid-sagittal plane, whereas in the adult the corresponding angle made by the optic nerves is 40°.

Opposite the distal end of the primary optic vesicle, but separated from this by a reticulum of protoplasmic fibrils, there is a thickening of the surface ectoderm, which represents the first stage of the development

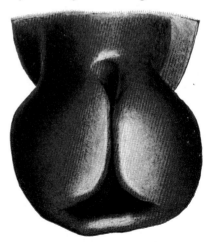

Fig. 372.—Optic Cup of 7-mm Human Embryo. Ventral View (× 100).

(*From Seefelder, 1930.*)

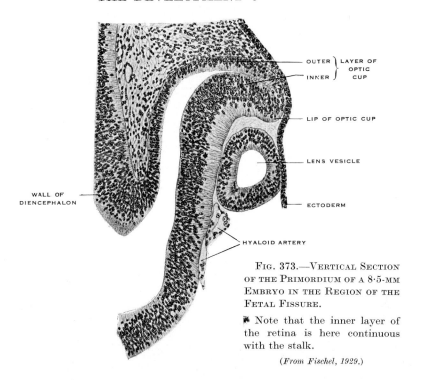

OUTER } LAYER OF
INNER } OPTIC CUP

LIP OF OPTIC CUP

LENS VESICLE

WALL OF
DIENCEPHALON

ECTODERM

HYALOID ARTERY

FIG. 373.—VERTICAL SECTION
OF THE PRIMORDIUM OF A 8·5-MM
EMBRYO IN THE REGION OF THE
FETAL FISSURE.

❧ Note that the inner layer of
the retina is here continuous
with the stalk.

(*From Fischel, 1929.*)

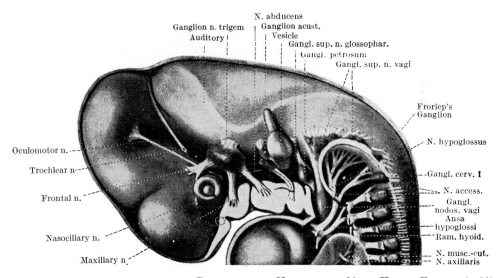

N. abducens
Ganglion n. trigem   Ganglion acust.
Auditory   Vesicle
                     Gangl. sup. n. glossophar.
                     Gangl. petrosum
                     Gangl. sup. n. vagi

Froriep's
Ganglion

Oculomotor n.

N. hypoglossus

Trochlear n.

Gangl. cerv. I

Frontal n.

N. access.
Gangl.
nodos. vagi
Ansa
hypoglossi
Ram. hyoid.

Nasociliary n.

N. musc.-cut.
N. axillaris

Maxillary n.

FIG. 374.—RECONSTRUCTION OF THE CEREBROSPINAL NERVES OF A 10-MM HUMAN EMBRYO (×10).
Note the close relation of the nasociliary nerve to the eye.

(*From Fischel, after Streeter.*)

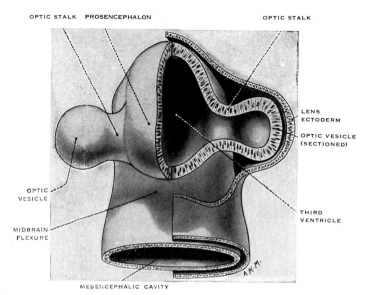

FIG. 375.—SCHEMATIC REPRESENTATION OF THE CRANIAL ASPECT OF THE FOREBRAIN (PROSEN-CEPHALIC) AND OPTIC VESICLES IN A 4-MM HUMAN EMBRYO.

(From Hamilton, Boyd, and Mossman, after Mann.)

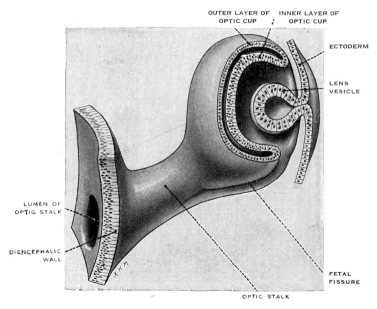

FIG. 376.—SCHEMATIC REPRESENTATION OF THE OPTIC CUP AND STALK IN A 7·5-MM HUMAN EMBRYO.

(From Hamilton, Boyd, and Mossmann, after Mann.)

of the lens (Fig. 369). Similar tissue will be seen to exist later between the lens and the inner layer of the optic cup and there form what is known as the primary vitreous (see p. 451). At this stage it is known as the embryonic supporting tissue of von Szily. With the conversion of this thickening first into a groove and then into the lens vesicle, the primary optic vesicle is first flattened, and then as it were "invaginated" from its distal aspect and below. Thus the two-layered optic cup is produced.

In the mechanism of production of the optic cup it used to be taught that the lens actually pushed in the distal wall of the primary optic vesicle, as one might push in the wall of a toy balloon with one's fist. Its formation is, however, due to

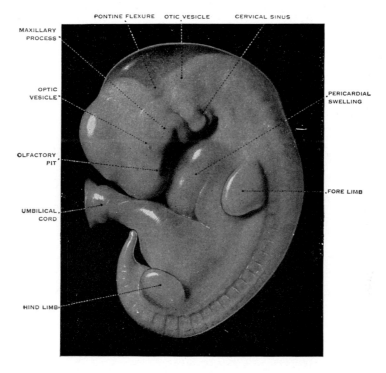

Fig. 377.—The Left Side of a 6·2-mm Crown-rump Length Human Embryo.
(Estimated age, 36 days.)

(From Hamilton, Boyd, and Mossman's.)

the fact that the distal and ventral portions of the vesicle stop growing, while the margins of these areas continue to develop. Thus the lips of the vesicle grow round the developing lens at the sides and dorsally, but not ventrally.

Since the apex of the vesicle, which was originally convex, stops growing, and as it is in contact with the lens, it first appears flattened and then becomes concave. Thus the lumen of the vesicle is reduced to a slit (Fig. 376). Since growth stops below, this area remains depressed, while its margins continue developing and thus is formed the **fetal, ocular or choroidal fissure.**

The function of the fetal fissure, apart from allowing the entrance of mesoderm into the eye, is to provide the shortest route by which the nerve fibres from the ganglion cells can reach the optic stalk and brain. Otherwise, with the formation of the optic cup, they would have to travel round the edge of the cup. For the optic stalk is at first directly continuous with the outer or pigment layer. The direct

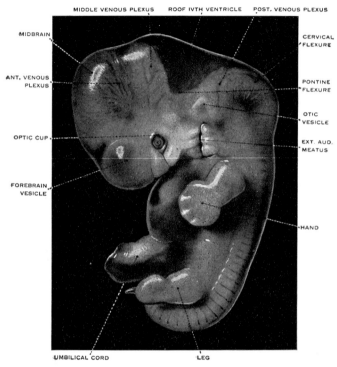

FIG. 378.—THE LEFT SIDE OF A 12·2-MM CROWN-RUMP LENGTH HUMAN EMBRYO.
(Estimated age, 43 days.)
(*From Hamilton, Boyd, and Mossmann.*)

continuity of the inner or nervous layer with the optic stalk is only made possible at the floor of the fetal fissure where it becomes continuous with the floor of the fissure on the stalk (Fig. 372).

In early embryos, between 7·7 and 17·1 mm, the rim of the optic cup may present small *accessory notches*. Their significance is doubtful. Possibly they are made by vessels.

Hence it comes about that as the lens pit is converted into a little pouch or sac, the optic cup also deepens and surrounds it more and more. Also the opening of the cup is gradually differentiated into a laterally directed rounded portion, the primitive pupil, and a ventrally directed part, the fetal fissure (Fig. 372). The fetal fissure extends back along the optic stalk. As soon as it is formed, the fissure becomes filled with embryonic connective tissue which contains the hyaloid artery (future arteria centralis). With the pigmentation of the outer layer of the cup the cleft also is visible through the surface ectoderm.

The optic cup is thus composed of two layers which are continuous with each other at the margin of the cup and at the fetal fissure. The inner layer is much thicker than the outer, and will form the neural portion of the retina, while the

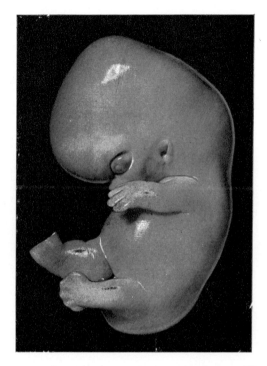

Fig. 379.—The Left Side of a 17-mm Crown-rump Length Human Embryo.
(Estimated age, 47 days.)
(From Hamilton, Boyd, and Mossmann.)

outer layer gives rise to the pigment epithelium only. The neural portion of the retina consists of the pars optica and the pars cæca, which in turn is made up of the pars ciliaris retinæ and the pars iridica retinæ.

The cavity of the primary optic vesicle is potential only, but pathologically can be reconstituted into a real cavity. This happens in detachment of the retina, when fluid collects between the pigment layer (which remains adherent to the choroid) and the rods and cones.

Similarly in the separation of posterior synechiæ the posterior of the two layers of the ectodermal part of the iris becomes separated from the anterior and remains adherent to the lens. This separation re-forms the anterior part of the cavity of the

A.M.—28

primary optic vesicle or ring sinus of von Szily, which indeed may also take place as a senile change.

The fetal fissure closes by its lateral walls growing towards each o ther and eventually fusing. This fusion begins at the centre at the fifth week (15-mm stage) and extends forwards and backwards, to be completed at about the 17-mm stage.

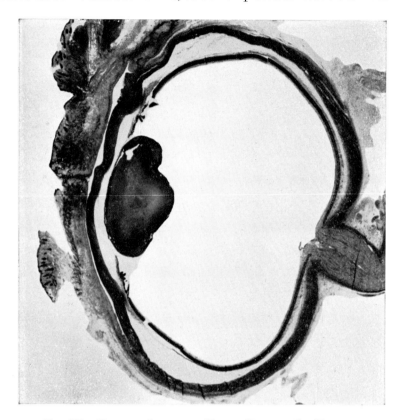

FIG. 380.—VERTICAL SECTION OF EYE OF FETUS OF SIX MONTHS.

The "cavity" between the two layers of the optic cup does, in a sense, persist as the space between the outer segments of the rod and cone processes and the microvilli of the adjoining apical surfaces of the pigmented epithelial cells. The close apposition of these two elements, both of which can be traced embryologically back to the primitive *ciliated* ependyma lining the ventricular system of the fore-brain reflects in a most interesting way upon the origin of the microvilli and photoreceptor segments. As early as 1898 Studrička proposed that photoreceptor cells may have been ciliated or flagellate.

Distally a small notch remains before the fusion completes the primitive pupil, making it round. At the proximal end of the fissure the fusion is complicated by the fact that the inner layer of the cup grows more rapidly than the outer. It thus comes about that there is a slight eversion of the inner layer (Fig. 381), which prevents the pigmented layer from fusing and results in a pale area below the disc. In man, however, this pale area soon becomes pigmented, and usually no trace is left of the fissure except at its extreme posterior end, which remains as the site of entry of the central vessels.

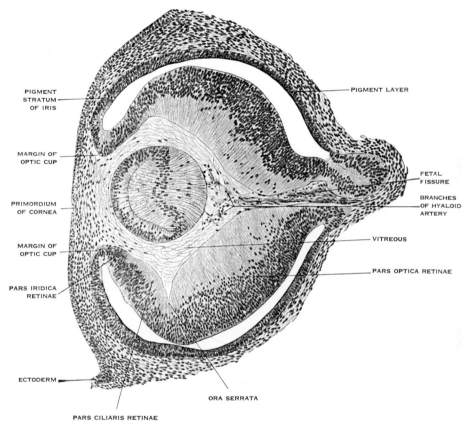

FIG. 381.—SECTION THROUGH THE EYE AND FETAL FISSURE OF A 13·5-MM HUMAN EMBRYO.
× 157.
Note the eversion of the inner layer of the optic cup at the posterior (proximal) end of the fetal fissure.
(*From Fischel, 1929.*)

Non-closure of the cleft results in colobomata (see Mann, 1957).

With the closure of the cleft the portion of the mesoderm which has made its way into the eye through the cleft is cut off from the surrounding mesoderm, and gives rise to the hyaloid system of vessels.

While these changes are taking place, the lens has developed and the meso-

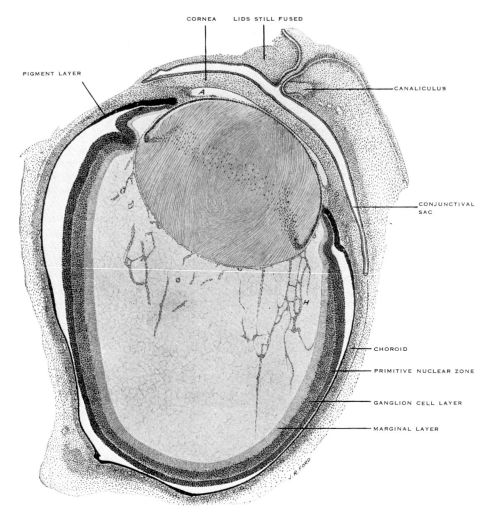

FIG. 382.—VERTICAL SECTION OF THE EYE OF AN EMBRYO OF $2\frac{3}{4}$ MONTHS (38 MM).

A = anterior chamber (possibly an artefact—see p. 442). H = hyaloid vessels.

(Wolff's preparation from a specimen supplied by Dr. A. G. Gilchrist.)

derm around the eye forms the primordium of the choroid and sclera. Thus with the closure of the fetal fissure the eye possesses all its essential parts and forms what may be termed the "embryonic eye".

It is apposite to note here the classical work of Spemann over the three decades, 1900–1930 (see Spemann, 1938). His studies on the amphibian optic outgrowth introduced the concepts of induction in embryonic tissues and of organisers, thus initiating a great train of subsequent workers up to the present day.

The Development of the Retina

Retinal development may be divided for convenience into three stages, which are, however, not sharply separated:

1. The epithelial stage.
2. The stage of differentiation.
3. The stage of growth.

The primordium of the nervous portion of the retina is the distal wall of the primary optic vesicle, and consists at first of a single layer of cylindrical epi-

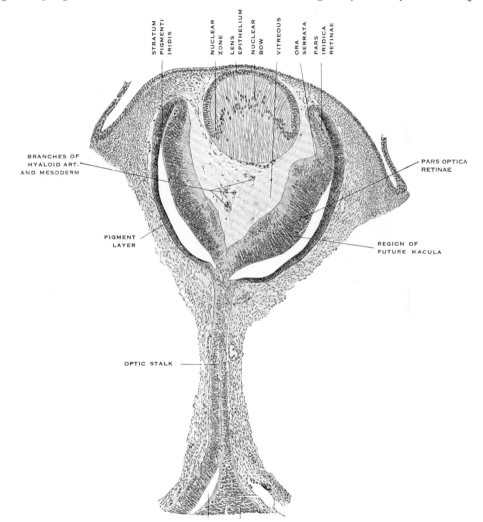

FIG. 383.—LONGITUDINAL SECTION THROUGH THE EYE AND OPTIC STALK OF A 17-MM HUMAN EMBRYO
(× 76).
(*From Fischel.*)

thelium. The nuclei soon divide and become arranged in several layers. Later there are several layers of cells. These cells are at first all alike. The mitoses take place at the side next the future pigment layer (ventricular mitoses), so that the oldest cells get pushed towards and lie nearest the future vitreous (Fig. 384).

By differentiation is meant the different changes which, in view of their different future functions, the various regions of the retina and their contained cells undergo. This stage may also, therefore, be called the stage of specialisation.

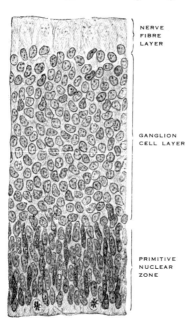

NERVE FIBRE LAYER

GANGLION CELL LAYER

PRIMITIVE NUCLEAR ZONE

FIG. 384.—SECTION OF THE RETINA (NEAR THE POSTERIOR POLE) OF A 31-MM HUMAN EMBRYO.

(*From Seefelder, 1930.*)

The earliest sign of differentiation of the retina is the appearance, at first in the macular region towards the side of the future vitreous, of a clear, almost a nuclear zone as in the central nervous system. This change later affects the more peripheral portions of the retina and also the pars cæca up to the pupillary margin, although here the clear zone is narrower. Thus as the retina rapidly increases in thickness it becomes divided into a **nuclear zone** and a zone containing at first no nuclei—the **marginal layer of His** (Figs. 382, 383). This is formed by anastomotic protoplasmic processes of the retinal cells, and is the primordium of the supporting tissue of the retina—namely, the neuroglia. At the time of the formation of the optic cup the marginal layer is well developed, as are also the internal and external limiting membranes. The retina remains in this primitive condition until the closure of the fetal fissure (17-mm stage).

The Ganglion Cells and the Nerve Fibre Layer.—The ganglion cells are formed from the innermost cells of the *nuclear zone* which invade the *marginal zone* at about the fifth week (in embryos of 11·3 to 13 mm). This latter takes place first in the region of the future macula. These young neuroblasts have a small round nucleus and practically no protoplasm. Later the nuclei grow larger, stain less deeply, and are then easily distinguished from the deeper staining nuclear zone (Fig. 384). No sooner have the ganglion cells invaded the marginal zone than the nerve fibres grow out from them, run parallel to the surface of the retina to find the shortest way to the optic stalk, and thence to the brain. (See Vrabec, 1966.)

The differentiation of the retina proceeds from the posterior portion of the eye anteriorly.

With the formation of dendritic processes from the outer aspect of the ganglion cells, a clear non-nuclear zone is produced between these and the remaining cells, and thus is formed the beginning of the *inner plexiform layer*. Later are added the branching processes of the inner horizontal and bipolar cells.

The Nuclear Layers and Outer Plexiform Layer.—The separation of the two nuclear layers also takes place first in the central area and about the same time as the formation of the inner plexiform layer, while from the primitive nuclear zone a single layer of the outermost cells separates to form the future cones and rods (Fig. 385). Between these cone cells and the remaining cells is a clear zone containing Müller's fibres only.

The outer plexiform (molecular) layer is developed about the end of the fifth month at first by processes of the middle cell layer. In the inner nuclear layer

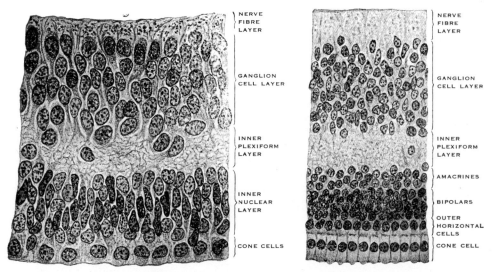

FIG. 385.—MACULAR REGION OF A 65 MM·
HUMAN EMBRYO.

(*From Seefelder, 1930.*)

FIG. 386.—THE MACULAR REGION IN
A FETUS OF FIVE MONTHS.

(*From Seefelder, 1930.*)

Müller's fibres are first developed, then the bipolar cells, then the inner horizontal, amacrine neurons and lastly the outer horizontal cells. Probably no new retinal cells are produced after the sixth month. Thus the relative size of the pars optica of the retina to the whole bulb is much greater in the embryo, since it reaches to the limbus, than in the adult, where it ends at the equator.

Thus mitoses cease first in the central area, so that growth goes on longer at the periphery of the retina. Then new cells are found only in the pars cæca, and finally only at the pupillary margin.

The Rods and Cones.—Up to the middle of the second month, the outer aspect of the inner layer of the optic cup presents only a border made up of tiny cilia which are little apparent and often stuck together. This border is like the surface of the cerebral ventricles and the ependyma of the canal of the spinal cord, whose cavity is homologous with the interparietal cavity of the retina: it is the ciliated border of the ependymal epithelium. Many embryologists have held that it is these cilia which form the outer members of the rods and cones.

The rods and cones are developed from a single row of cells which separate from the primitive nuclear zone (Fig. 385). The diplosomes which lie in the outer side of these primitive cells play an important part in their development (Fig. 388).

The young cone cells have a small round deeply staining nucleus and a fair amount of protoplasm which lies next the outer limiting membrane. Later the

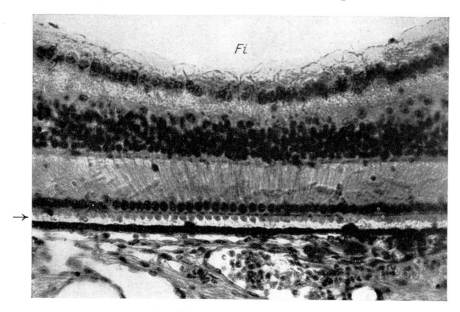

FIG. 387.—FOVEA OF THE NEWBORN.

Extensive foveal depression Fi. The transitory layer of Chievitz has disappeared, the outer nuclear layer is thinned and the ganglion cells reduced to a single row. The cones are still very immature (arrow) (this applies only to the foveal cones) while at the periphery the stumpy form has long since changed.

(*From Pfeifer, after Wolfrum.*)

protoplasm and the diplosomes break through this, and the cone cells become cylindrical and more like epithelial cells. Threads pass outwards from the diplosomes which, becoming surrounded by a soft protoplasmic material, form the outer portion of the cones. The rods are developed in a similar way.

The Macular Area and Fovea Centralis.—In the third month a marked thinning is seen in the retina of the posterolateral quadrant. All layers are affected. *This, however, does not constitute the macula.* The appearance of the macular area is shown by a thickening of the ganglion cell layer at about the fifth month (fetus of 122 mm according to Seefelder, 1930) between the above area and the papilla.

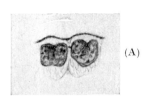

(A)

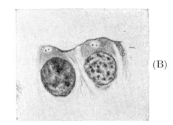

(B)

Cone Cells from the Central Area of a 65-mm Fetus.

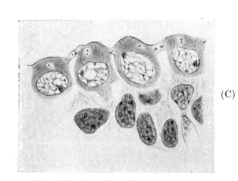

(C)

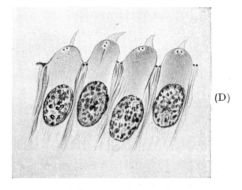

(D)

Cone Cells from the Central Area
of a 80-mm Fetus.

Cones from Para-central Area of
345-mm Fetus.

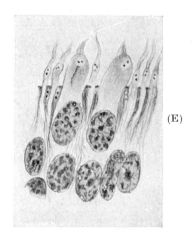

(E)

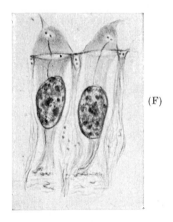

(F)

Rods and Cones from the
Para-central Area of a
345-mm Fetus.

Central Cones of a
420-mm Fetus.

Fig. 388.—Stages in the Development of the Rods and Cones.

(From Bach and Seefelder, 1912.)

In the fifth month there is developed in the central area an additional fibre layer, namely the transitory layer of Chievitz, which disappears only after birth. Its significance has not yet been decided. It is formed through the separation of the amacrine neurons from the remainder of the inner nuclear layer (Fig. 381).

The development of the fovea commences at the end of the sixth month by a thinning of the ganglion cells, which move away to leave a central shallow depression. This is deepened by a thinning of the outer layers, except of course the outer nuclear layer, which remains as before, one layer thick. Up to the time of the formation of the fovea the development of the macula precedes the remainder of the retina, but after this it falls behind, especially with regard to the neuro-epithelium. Thus in the macular region the cones appear later than in the remaining portions of the retina and at birth the foveal cones are still very plump

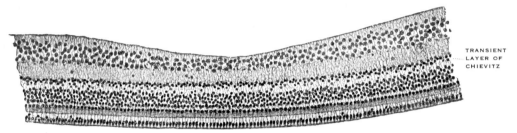

TRANSIENT LAYER OF CHIEVITZ

FIG. 390.—THE FOVEA CENTRALIS OF A FETUS AT THE END OF THE SIXTH MONTH.
(*From Seefelder, 1930.*)

structures (Fig. 387), about 5 μm in diameter and only 8 μm in height, and it is only when the child is several months old that the cone gets its definitive form, and only then can the central area show its superiority over the remainder of the retina. Hence also the reason for the absence of central fixation at birth. It is remarkable that the fovea centralis is as far away from the nerve head at its formation as in the adult.

The thickening of the outer cell layer in the region of the fovea arises after birth, and results from the fact, according to Drault (1912), that as the limbs of the cones get thinner they are more crowded together and therefore also their nuclei.

Some degree of macular differentiation occurs after birth, particularly in an increased density of retinal pigment cells (Streeten, 1967).

THE OUTER RETINAL LAYER (PIGMENT EPITHELIUM)

With the invagination of the primary optic vesicle, the two layers of the secondary optic vesicle which have at first the same epithelial structure start differentiating. The cells of the outer layer are at first high cylindrical, occupy its whole thickness, and have their nuclei arranged in two or three rows.

Pigmentation of the cells starts in embryos of from 6 to 7 mm at about three weeks and these appear before any other pigment in the body. Yellowish granules

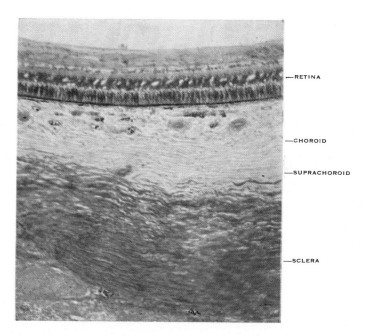

—RETINA

—CHOROID

—SUPRACHOROID

—SCLERA

Fig. 389.—Coats of Eye of Fetus of Six Months.

The choroid appears as a reticulum in which the vessels are enmeshed.

appear which rapidly become darker and eventually appear black. They are formed for the most part in that portion of the cell nearest the retina. The anterior portion is pigmented first and then the process passes backwards. This pigmentation makes the vesicle visible through the surface ectoderm.

By the time the embryo has reached 10 mm the whole of the outer layer is pigmented. As development proceeds the pigment cells become flatter, i.e.

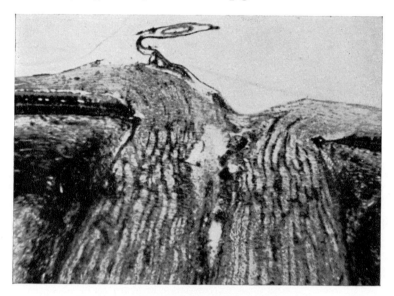

FIG. 391.—OPTIC DISC OF FETUS OF SIX MONTHS.
Note hyaloid artery.

cubical with the nuclei arranged in a single row, probably because they have to line a larger area.

The pigment is formed in the cell itself (Miescher, 1923). Probably there is a colourless precursor of the melanin pigment, of the nature of dioxyphenylalanine (dopa) which is converted to melanin by a peroxidase enzyme. The continuation forwards of the pigment epithelium of the retina forms the stratum pigmenti ciliaris and the stratum pigmenti iridis.

For the most detailed overall accounts of retinal development the reader should consult Seefelder, 1930 and Mann, 1964. See also Duke-Elder and Cook, 1963 for extensive bibliographies and an excellent general survey.

THE OPTIC NERVE

The optic nerve is developed from the optic *stalk* or *pedicle*. Its cavity communicates on the one hand with the cavity of the diencephalon, and on the other with the primary optic vesicle (Fig. 370).

After the formation of the optic cup the fetal fissure extends back on the optic stalk, which also becomes "invaginated" from ventrally. Hence a transverse section of the optic stalk resembles that of the optic vesicle, with a thick inner wall and a thinner outer one (Fig. 392).

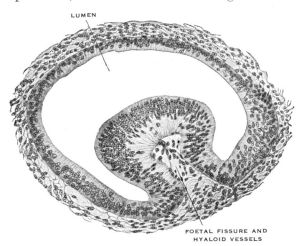

LUMEN

FOETAL FISSURE AND
HYALOID VESSELS

FIG. 392.—TRANSVERSE SECTION OF THE OPTIC STALK OF A 9-MM HUMAN EMBRYO. DISTAL PORTION.
(*From Fischel, 1929.*)

As development proceeds the distance between the diencephalon and the surface ectoderm increases more and more, and this necessitates a lengthening of the optic stalk which is at first short, broad and wide. A new piece is drawn out of the side wall of the diencephalon. The optic stalk thus comes to consist of a distal primitive portion which is grooved by the fetal fissure and a proximal portion, added later, which is not (Figs. 372, 375).

The closure of the continuation backwards of the fetal fissure converts the optic stalk into a rounded cord. The cavity of the stalk is closed by the development of the nerve fibres which grow towards the brain from the ganglion cells.

Nerve fibres first appear in the ventral and lateral portions of the stalk, so the cavity becomes semilunar (Fig. 394), and at first displaced dorsally; later when the dorsal fibres grow it is displaced ventrally and disappears about the third fœtal month.

The epithelial cells forming the walls of the stalk develop into the glial system of the nerve. At the third month the glial cells become arranged in rows parallel to the long axis of the optic nerve and between these the nerve fibres run. Glial tissue also develops round the hyaloid artery and around the periphery of the nerve. The glial tissue or glial mantle around the hyaloid artery at its entrance into the vitreous forms a protruding mass (glial cushion or Bergmeister's papilla), which not only clothes the artery

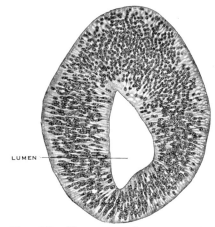

LUMEN

FIG. 393.—TRANSVERSE SECTION OF THE OPTIC STALK OF A 9-MM HUMAN EMBRYO. PROXIMAL PORTION.

(*Fischel, 1929.*)

and some of its branches, but fills the physiological excavation of the optic nervehead as well (Figs. 415, 416). With the regression of the hyaloid artery this glial mantle disappears also.

Bergmeister's Papilla.—As the optic nerve fibres pass from the ganglion cells to the optic stalk they have to traverse the remainder of the retina. As they do this they cut off a cone-shaped mass of glial cells at the centre of the disc, which is known as Bergmeister's primitive epithelial papilla. This becomes vascularised by the hyaloid artery, and supplies this vessel and its branches with their sheaths (Seefelder, 1910; von Szily, 1921–2). Later, with the disappearance of the hyaloid system the papilla also atrophies, the amount of atrophy determining the depth of the physiological cup.

Remains of the papilla are always found in the glial sheaths of the vessels and the glial tissue which separates the optic cup from the vitreous (the central connective tissue meniscus of Kuhnt). (Figs. 300, 301.)

The fibrous (mesodermal) septa of the optic nerve are developed from the mesoderm of the vessels which invade the nerve at the middle of the third fetal month, and which have the form and position of the future septa (see p. 342). The mesodermal lamina cribrosa is only formed in the last fetal months, and then has not the strength of the previously existing glial lamina.

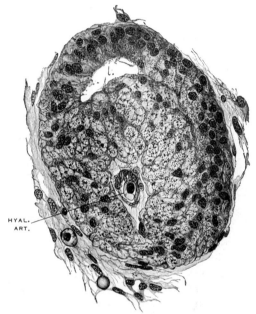

FIG. 394.—TRANSVERSE SECTION OF THE OCULAR END OF THE OPTIC NERVE OF A 19-MM HUMAN EMBRYO.

(From Seefelder, 1930.)

The nerve sheaths are derived from the head mesoderm, and develop concurrently with the posterior part of the sclera. At the fifth month dura, arachnoid, and pia can be distinguished from each other.

Myelination of the nerve fibres takes place from the brain distally, and reaches the lamina cribrosa just before birth. The so-called "congenital" nerve fibres, seen not infrequently near the disc (Fig. 297), are therefore not really congenital at all, since they are medullated after birth. At six weeks the optic fibres penetrate the under-surface of the forebrain; at about seven and a half weeks the chiasma has been formed by partial decussation of the fibres and at nine and a half weeks the optic tract is plainly present.

By the fifth month of gestation the vascular patterns of the nerve are well established, including the arterial circle of Zinn. The nerve is now about 1·2 mm in diameter and 7–9 mm long; these dimensions increase to 2·7 mm and 25 mm during the ninth month. Thus its growth in length is almost complete, but myelination is not. The process has reached the disc, but the actual amount of myelin is less.

The Development of the Lens

Stages:

    (*a*) Lens placode or plate.
    (*b*) Lens recess or pit.
    (*c*) Lens pouch or sac.
    (*d*) Lens vesicle.

At the 4·5-mm stage the surface ectoderm opposite the distal part of the primary optic vesicle is thickened by the cells assuming a high columnar form, and their nuclei, many in mitosis, are usually arranged in a single layer (Rabl, 1903). This thickening is called the *lens placode* (Fig. 371). A groove or pit appears in this. The pit deepens into a pouch which closes and forms a *vesicle* at about four and a half weeks. The *lens vesicle* moves away slightly from the surface ectoderm, being connected to it, however, by a protoplasmic reticulum, the embryonic supporting tissue of von Szily (p. 426).

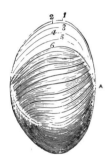

With the formation of the lens vesicle the primary optic vesicle is invaginated to form the optic cup. At this stage the optic cup is almost completely filled by the lens (Fig. 373). During the invagination of the lens rudiment the cells in its anterior part, which will form the lens epithelium, are inverted, so that their basement membrane faces anteriorly.

Fig. 395.—To illustrate the Course of the Fibres in the Fetal Crystalline Lens.

A = anterior pole.
P = posterior pole.

(*After Allen Thomson, rom Quain's Anatomy.*)

The mitoses subserving the growth of the lens occur posteriorly, in the cells towards the free surface of the placode and later towards the cavity of the vesicle. The proliferation of cells (in the human) is so rapid that some cells are thrown off into the lens pit and into the vesicle. They mix with the fluid in the vesicle and soon degenerate, but some have believed that they later form the thin layer of amorphous substance beneath the anterior epithelium. While the vascular capsule is present the lens grows very quickly. Hence it is almost full-grown in foetal life.

The cells of the posterior part of the vesicle become columnar and eventually elongate to fill the lens vesicle. These primitive lens fibres run from the front to the back of the lens; *later none do*. The lengthening of the cells first takes place in the centre of the posterior wall, which therefore bulges convex forwards into the cavity of the vesicle. This lengthening is the first sign of transformation of the cells into lens fibres and is associated with the loss of power of multiplication which stops when the cells are about 0·18 mm long (Fischel, 1929). The vesicle is completely obliterated in this manner by the 16 mm stage.

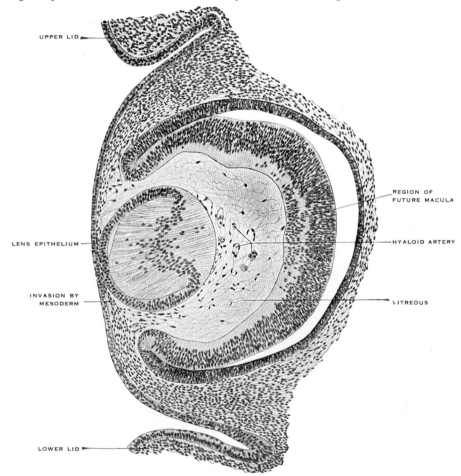

UPPER LID

REGION OF FUTURE MACULA

LENS EPITHELIUM

HYALOID ARTERY

INVASION BY MESODERM

VITREOUS

LOWER LID

FIG. 396.—SECTION THROUGH THE EYE OF 17-MM HUMAN EMBRYO (× 148).
(*From Fischel, 1929.*)

The nuclei of the lens fibres pass anteriorly, and at the equator form a line convex forwards (the nuclear bow) (Fig. 382), which is continuous laterally with the equatorial nuclei of the cells of the anterior epithelium which will form all except the first fibres.

The rest of the lens fibres, and all those formed subsequently and throughout life, are formed from cells at the equator of the *anterior* layer of the lens vesicle. These cells continue to proliferate throughout life, forming the anterior epithelium of the lens.

The new lens fibres formed from the equatorial cells are laid down concentrically round the filled-in lens vesicle, and thus the lens gets its laminated structure. Also the new fibres are laid on tangential to the equator; hence on equatorial section the lens shows radial lamellæ. At three months there are 1474 radial lamellæ and 2250 in the adult, numbers characteristic for the human (Fischel).

As pointed out above, none of the fibres run completely from the front to the back of the lens. At the two surfaces of the lens mass the thicker ends of the fibres end in sutures, later to become the so-called lens stars. Thus the earliest fibres are anteroposteriorly diametric, whereas all later ones are circumferential.

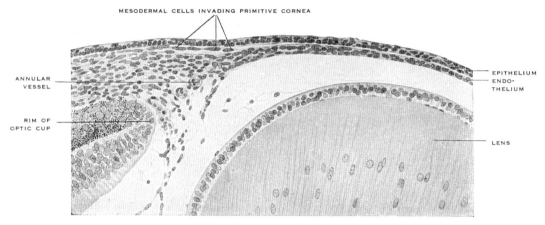

MESODERMAL CELLS INVADING PRIMITIVE CORNEA

ANNULAR VESSEL

RIM OF OPTIC CUP

EPITHELIUM
ENDO-
THELIUM

LENS

FIG. 397.—ANTEROPOSTERIOR SECTION OF A 23-MM HUMAN EMBRYO.
(*From Seefelder, 1930.*)

The first indication of the sutures is seen in the second month, but only becomes really plain in the fourth month. Their formation comes about from the fact that as the new-formed lens fibres pass in a bow round the primitive ones, and being of equal length, the nearer the axis they end anteriorly the farther away they end posteriorly, and vice versa (Fig. 395). At first the lens fibres end in a vertical suture anteriorly and a horizontal one posteriorly (Fischel). Later these become Y-shaped, vertical anteriorly, inverted posteriorly (Fig. 231). The fibres formed later, for instance the superficial ones of the adult lens, start and finish in the more complicated stellate figures, conforming, however, to the above rule (see also p. 166).

Within the lens vesicle and later in the lens itself, there is not inconsiderable tension which plays an important part in the regular growth of the lens fibres. The lens grows very rapidly so long as it is supplied by its vascular capsule. It thus comes about that at birth it has already acquired its definitive anteroposterior diameter and two-thirds of the equatorial. It is more or less spherical at birth. The anteroposterior flattening of the adult is brought about by the method of laying on of the lens fibres and the pull of the suspensory ligament.

The Lens Capsule.—At the 13-mm stage the lens epithelium secretes its hyaline capsule. It is primarily an ectodermal basement membrane, which becomes thicker as the lenticular vesicle is formed.

For modern accounts of lenticular development see Barber (1955); Vrabec (1955); O'Rahilly and Meyer (1960); and Mann (1964).

THE CORNEA

After the formation of the lens vesicle mesoderm cells grow into the protoplasmic fibrillæ (the so-called anterior vitreous) between the lens and the surface ectoderm. They become arranged in a single row parallel to the surface and go to form the posterior limiting lamina, Descemet's endothelium (Fig. 397). Many years ago Kölliker (1861) noted that in birds at a very early period a thin structureless ectodermal membrane is laid down, which apparently formed the scaffolding on which the cornea is built. Hagedoorn (1928) holds that such a directing membrane ("Richtungshäutchen") exists in the anterior vitreous of all vertebrates. Mesoderm grows in firstly as the endothelium behind this membrane and secretes Descemet's membrane, and secondly as a wedge-shaped mass which forms the substantia propria between the epithelium and the primary cornea. See also Mann, 1931.

Into the space between Descemet's endothelium and the surface ectoderm there grow more mesodermal cells from the region of the edge of the optic cup. These form the substantia propria of the cornea. The differentiation of these cells into the corneal fibrillæ takes place from behind forwards. The surface ectoderm forms the epithelium of the cornea. The substantia propria may be formed by a second mesodermal invasion (Hogan *et al.*, 1971). Collagen fibrils are identifiable at about the 25-mm stage (end of 7th week). They attain their final width by the 85-mm stage (Schwarz, 1961).

The posterior membrane is formed in the fourth month by a secretion from the endothelial cells, whereas the anterior limiting lamina (Bowman's membrane) is simply a condensation of the anterior corneal fibrillæ.

As development proceeds the cell content of the cornea diminishes. Wandering cells appear about the fourth month.

The cornea is transparent from the first as is all early embryonic tissue.

THE SCLERA

The sclera arises through a condensation of the mesoderm round the optic cup. The anterior portion is formed first—no doubt associated with the insertion of the eye muscles. The limbus is at first much farther back, lying over the ciliary body, but gradually shifts forwards. The definition of the whole sclera extends from about the 20 mm to the 35-mm stage. Its differentiation beyond this lies largely in the development and condensation of collagen bundles, from the third

A.E.—29

month onwards. As its collagenous nature becomes more defined it is more clearly distinguished from the stroma of the choroid.

The *fascia bulbi* (Tenon's capsule) is developed in the same way as the sclera, but somewhat later, and again the anterior portion is differentiated before the posterior.

THE PUPILLARY MEMBRANE

Of the mesoderm which invades the anterior vitreous, i.e. the protoplasmic reticulum between the surface ectoderm and the lens, the anterior zone is non-vascular, and, as we have seen, forms the main substance of the cornea. The posterior and major zone, in which vessels develop, becomes the iridopupillary lamina (Figs. 402, 404, 452).

The peripheral region of this unites with the rim of the optic cup to form the iris, while the central region is the pupillary membrane (Figs. 400, 404).

The pupillary membrane is thus developed in the mesoderm posterior to the posterior limiting lamina (Descemet). It consists of numerous anastomosing vessels and a fibrillary tissue between them. It forms, in fact, the anterior part of the tunica vasculosa lentis, with the remainder of which it is continuous under the rim of the optic cup. As the edge of the pupil grows forwards, however, this continuity is broken. The pupillary membrane is nourished, as is the iris, by the long posterior ciliary arteries, and is thus entirely independent of the hyaloid system and continues to develop when the latter is regressing.

The pupillary membrane is at first attached to the edge of the pupil, but later comes to arise from the front of the iris. This is due to a split in the mesoderm between the sphincteric portion of the iris and the pupillary membrane. After the eighth month the pupillary membrane begins to disappear. Remains of it may, however, frequently be seen in the new-born baby and sometimes persist throughout life (Fig. 452). They arise from the *anterior* aspect of the iris in the region of the circulus iridis minor (collarette) (see p. 247).

THE ANTERIOR CHAMBER

The Anterior Chamber commences peripherally as a slit in the mesoderm between the cornea and iris, which gradually travels centrally. The appearance of this cleft is probably due to the disappearance of the mesoderm between the developing iris and cornea at about the 30–40-mm stage. Some observers have, however, considered that it appears much later, and that such early appearances are due to sectioning artefacts (see Fig. 382).

The anterior chamber is soon separated from the lens by the pupillary membrane. It is always shallow and is still so at birth.

The region of the future angle is at first filled with loose mesodermal tissue (uveal framework of H. Virchow), which later disappears, except for the portion at the extreme periphery. The sinus venosus scleræ is present at three months,

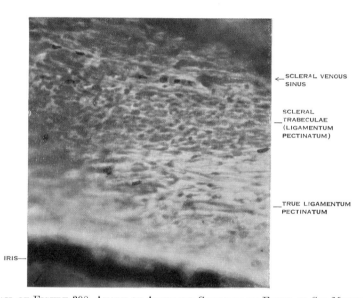

← SCLERAL VENOUS
   SINUS

__ SCLERAL
   TRABECULAE
   (LIGAMENTUM
   PECTINATUM)

__ TRUE LIGAMENTUM
   PECTINATUM

IRIS—

FIG. 399.—DETAIL OF FIGURE 398. ANGLE OF ANTERIOR CHAMBER OF FETUS OF SIX MONTHS.
The Scleral Venous Sinus (Canal of Schlemm) contains blood.

and from the first carries blood corpuscles (Seefelder, 1930) (Fig. 399). For other views on this topic, see Allen *et al.*, 1955.

THE UVEAL TRACT

The choroid, ciliary body and iris are partly mesodermal, partly ectodermal in origin. They are formed from the neurectoderm of the optic cup and the mesodermal and vascular covering of the whole cup.

The mesodermal moiety of the uveal tract probably depends for its development on the optic cup, especially on its pigment layer. Normally, it covers the optic cup from the stalk to the pupillary margin, and should any region of the cup be missing the mesoderm does not develop and a coloboma results.

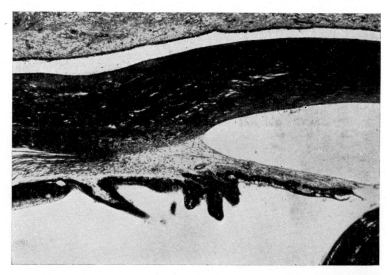

FIG. 398.—CILIARY REGION OF EYE OF FETUS OF SIX MONTHS.

Note how the true ligamentum pectinatum iridis which is present in the human at this stage fills the future angle of the anterior chamber. It passes forwards to the end of Descemet's membrane.

As soon as the lens vesicle has become detached from the surface ectoderm, mesoderm grows between the lens and the optic vesicle on the one hand and the surface ectoderm on the other. Thus the optic cup and lens become embedded in a common mass of mesoderm which is pierced by the optic nerve. From this mesoderm is developed the choroid, the ciliary body, the stroma of the iris, as also the sclera and non-epithelial laminæ of the cornea. Peripherally this mesoderm is continuous with the general adjacent mesoderm mass, from which are derived the fascia bulbi, the episcleral tissue, and the orbital fat; anteriorly it becomes continuous with the mesoderm of the skin, i.e. of the future eyelids. The septum orbitale is also genetically the boundary between the connective tissue of the skin and that around the optic vesicle. All this connective tissue is originally quite homogeneous. But soon it divides into two regions which are differentiated by the relative density of their packing and the shape of the cells. The mesoderm adjacent to the differentiating pars optica of the retina becomes vascularised.

The epithelium of the pars cæca is at first high columnar with the nuclei arranged in several layers. Later there are several layers of cells. A small clear marginal zone which reaches to the pupillary margin forms as in the pars optica. With the general increase in size of the eye and the formation and forward growth of the iris, these cells are converted into a single layer of cubical cells which become lower as we go towards the pupillary margin.

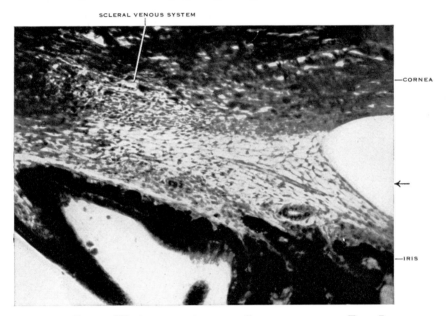

FIG. 400.—DETAIL OF FIGURE 399. ANGLE OF ANTERIOR CHAMBER FILLED BY TRUE LIGAMENTUM PECTINATUM AS OCCURS IN LOWER ANIMALS. (COMPARE FIG. 48.)

Between the scleral venous sinus and the ciliary region is the primordium of the definitive scleral trabeculæ (ligamentum pectinatum), as indicated by the arrow.

The iris is in part neurectodermal, derived from the marginal region of the cystic cup; the tissues from this origin are the sphincter and dilatator pupillæ and both layers of the epithelium on the posterior aspect of the iris. The mesodermal invasion is responsible for the stroma and vessels of the region.

Up to the end of the third month of embryonic life there is no true iris, and the margin of the optic cup extends but a little way beyond the equator of the lens (Fig. 382). The retinal and mesodermal portions are continuous with those of the ciliary body without line of demarcation, and, moreover, the mesodermal tissue is not delimited from the pupillary membrane. The development of the iris as such commences about the middle of the fourth month by a forward growth of the rim of the optic cup with its overlying mesoderm. It is preceded by a spur-like process of mesoderm which is continuous with the pupillary membrane. The iris thus becomes more or less differentiated from the ciliary body and pupillary membrane.

At this period a space, *the marginal ring sinus*, is present between the two layers of ectoderm forming the rim of the optic cup. It is at first small, but increases in size up to about five months, when it gets smaller, to disappear at seven months. It represents the last trace of the cavity of the primary optic vesicle. It is interesting to note that at this point the cells of the vesicle which form its two layers come into contiguity at the *apical* aspects, or luminal surfaces.

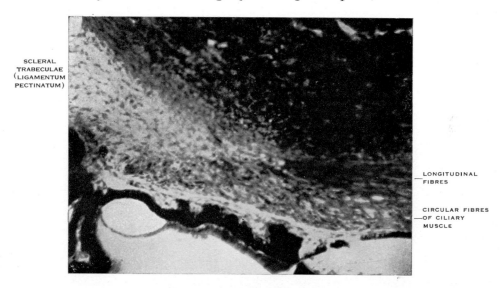

SCLERAL
TRABECULAE
(LIGAMENTUM
PECTINATUM)

LONGITUDINAL
FIBRES

CIRCULAR FIBRES
OF CILIARY
MUSCLE

Fig. 401.—Detail of Figure 380.

Note how far back true ligamentum pectinatum passes at this stage. Circular fibres of ciliary muscle can be readily distinguished.

The epithelium of the cavity which they originally lined is a continuation of the brain cavity. Thus they are potentially ependymal cells, which are frequently ciliated. The occurrence of occasional ciliated cells in the iridial epithelium is therefore not surprising.

The sphincter pupillæ is developed at this period from the pigment epithelium of the rim of the optic cup. The peculiarity of this derivation of the iridial muscles from ectoderm is well-known. At the 10-mm stage there is a proliferation of the cells of the stratum pigmenti iridis at the pupillary margin and a mass of cells grows backwards towards the ciliary border. The slight amount of contained pigment disappears and the cells are differentiated in plain muscle cells. These cells become limited peripherally by a ridge of pigment known as Michel's spur. At about the sixth month the sphincter begins to separate from the cells that gave it origin, passes into the mesodermal portion of the iris and is invaded by vessels. Numerous connections with the pigment epithelium, however, always persist, and Michel's spur represents the most peripheral of these. Pigment cells, derived from the anterior portion of the optic cup, pass through the sphincter and into the iris stroma to form *the clump cells* (Figs. 25, 76, 77). At birth the sphincter pupillæ is still closely adherent to the epithelial cells of the pupillary border. The dilatator pupillæ is also derived from the same ectodermal cells at the end of the sixth month. The nuclei of the cells of the stratum pigmentum, first in the ciliary

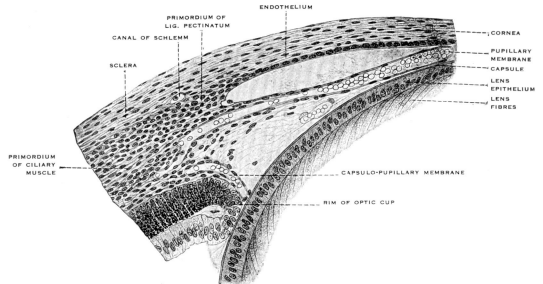

FIG. 402.—REGION OF THE ANGLE OF THE ANTERIOR CHAMBER IN AN 88-MM HUMAN EMBRYO.
(*From Seefelder, 1930.*)

zone, wander from their anterior to their posterior portions in which also the pigment collects. The anuclear portions become drawn out and arrange themselves radially to the pupil; then muscle fibrillæ form in them and thus the dilatator is formed. Thus whereas a whole cell of the anterior layer goes to form a muscle fibre of the sphincter pupillæ, only part of it forms a fibre of the dilatator. The anterior epithelium already contains pigment when the iris commences to form. Pigmentation of the posterior epithelium commences at the pupillary margin, and reaches its base at about the sixth month. The iris develops in width more slowly than the rest of the eye; so the pupil gets wider up to the beginning of the seventh month. At five months the iris is hidden by the limbus and resembles the condition of aniridia.

After the eighth month the pupil becomes smaller, due to the development of the sphincteric portion of the iris. With the disappearance of the pupillary membrane changes take place in the front of the iris with the formation of iris crypts. At about this time the *anterior border or limiting layer* can be recognised. It is formed by several rows of star-shaped cells which anastomose with each other and which may at times contain pigment cells at birth. The pigmentation of the stroma usually takes place in the first years after birth, and appears to be under the control of the sympathetic system. Also the pattern of the anterior

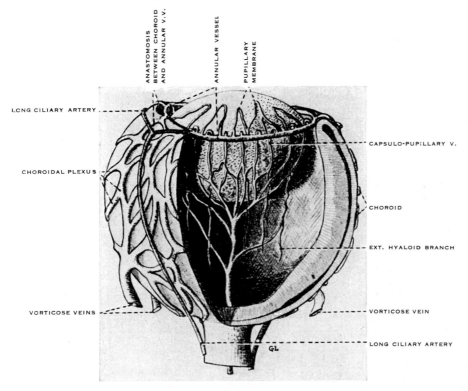

FIG. 403.—SCHEME OF THE VESSELS OF THE EMBRYONIC EYE.
(*Leplat and Dejean, 1939.*)

surface of the iris is produced during the first year, and generally the iris is not fully formed till twelve months after birth.

The Ciliary Body.—The neural ectoderm of the optic cup forms both layers of the epithelium of the ciliary body, while the mesoderm is responsible for the stroma, the ciliary muscle and the vessels.

The junction of the pars optica and parts cæca retinæ, i.e. the future ora serrata, can be made out quite early owing to the sudden diminution of thickness at this point (Fig. 381). But the ciliary epithelium is also demarcated from the retina proper by the formation of the ciliary folds early in the third month. Vessels sink into these folds and form what is for the most part a venous net. At the sixth month the ciliary arteries have formed the circulus iridis major and given off branches to the pupillary membrane, the stroma of the iris and the ciliary region.

During fetal life the most anterior of the ciliary folds lie behind the peripheral portion of the iris and then gradually move backwards. The longitudinal portion of the ciliary muscle is formed from the mesoderm next the sclera at the fourth month, while the circular portion develops at the end of the sixth month. The anterior portion of the ciliary muscle and the ligamentum pectinatum are developed from a continuous mass of mesodermal cells in the neighbourhood of the future angle of the anterior chamber (Fig. 402).

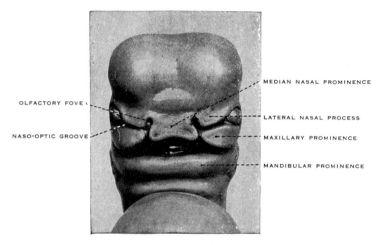

FIG. 407.—MODEL OF THE FACE OF AN EMBRYO (RECONSTRUCTION BY HIS) TO SHOW THE PROMINENCES WHICH FORM IT. THE MANDIBULAR PROMINENCES HAVE FUSED AT THIS STAGE. (The clefts between the maxillary and nasal prominences are diagrammatic—no actual clefts exist, but merely surface grooves.)

(*From Whitnall, 1932.*)

By the fourth or fifth month of intra-uterine life the tendinous fibres of the ciliary muscle are well differentiated, and can be followed directly into the fibres of the ligamentum. The essentially circular fibres of the scleral spur condense round some of the tendinous fibres, leaving a variable number to continue beyond the tip of the spur directly into the ligament. Thus the adult relationships are established.

At first only the corona ciliaris is present. The orbiculus ciliaris is formed at the fifth month by the limit of the true retina, i.e. of the pars optica moving backwards towards the equator. By this, too, the original small teeth of the ora serrata are lengthened.

The Choroid.—The primitive choroid is developed in the mesoderm round the primary optic vesicle, which it clothes as a vascular venous net. It is thus a very early formation (Figs. 382, 403). It is at first very cellular but gets less so as time

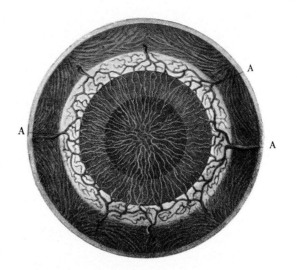

FIG. 404.—THE PUPILLARY MEMBRANE OF A FETUS OF ABOUT 3½ MONTHS.
The ciliary arteries (A) have been injected.
(*From Hirschfeld and Leveillé.*)

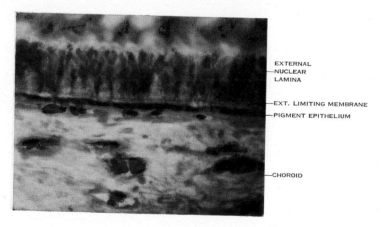

FIG. 405.—DETAIL OF FIGURE 389.

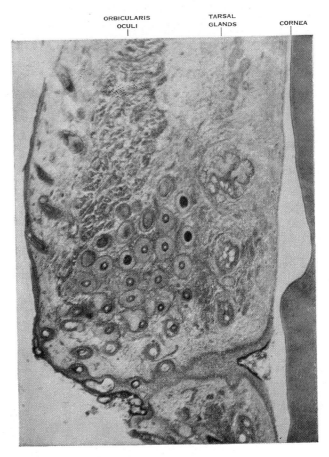

ORBICULARIS
OCULI

TARSAL
GLANDS

CORNEA

FIG. 406.—VERTICAL SECTION OF FUSED EYELIDS IN A FETUS OF SIX MONTHS.
Note tarsal glands, hair follicles, and ciliary muscle are easily distinguishable.

goes on. It gradually divides into two and then more layers of vessels. By the fifth month all the layers of the choroid can be recognised, including, last of all, the elastic lamina. The time of pigmentation of the choroid varies. The pigment is developed in the melanoblasts or fixed cells of the choroid usually during the fifth month, and first in the neighbourhood of the posterior ciliary arteries.

The final anatomical relationships between the three tunics of the eye are determined by function rather than by embryonic origin.

Thus the corneo-sclera and the uveal tract derived from the same mass of mesoderm are separated from each other in the adult eye anteriorly by the anterior chamber and posteriorly by the suprachoroidal space. They are only attached where the ciliary muscle arises from the scleral spur and at the optic nerve. On the other hand, the uveal tract is closely connected with the inner coat. Thus the pigment layer of the retina derived from the outer layer of the optic cup rarely separates in the living from the choroid and never from the ciliary body. Thus also the anterior layer of the pars iridica retinæ is inseparably connected with the iris, as are also the sphincter and dilatator pupillæ which are derived from it.

THE LIDS

The embryonic eye occupies a lateral position in the head covered only by a thin layer of ectoderm. At the beginning of the second month a circular fold

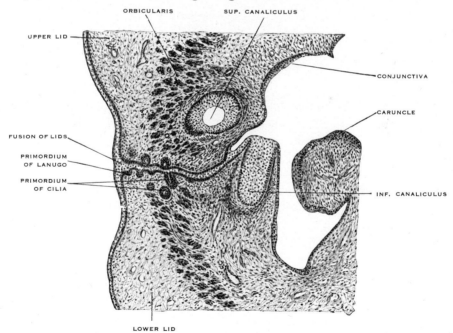

FIG. 408.—SECTION OF THE FUSED LIDS OF AN EMBRYO OF 14 CM ($\times$ 45).

(After Fischel, 1929.)

forms around and at some distance from the eye. The palpebral fissure is therefore at first round with no angles and relatively wide. The upper and lower regions of the fold grow towards each other and so angles are formed and the upper and lower eyelids demarcated from each other. The eyelids meet and unite loosely at two and a half months (Figs. 382, 408), union taking place from the edge towards the middle. At about the fifth month they start separating again through keratinization of the cells of the united edges, separation being completed at the seventh or eighth month.

The Tarsal Glands are developed about the end of the tenth week by the ingrowth of a regular row of solid columns of ectodermal cells from the lid margins directly behind the posterior row of cilia. These later acquire a lumen and begin

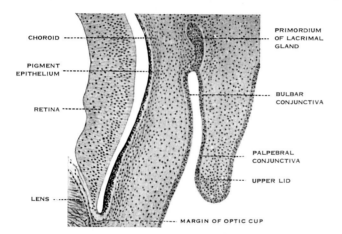

CHOROID

PIGMENT
EPITHELIUM

RETINA

LENS

MARGIN OF OPTIC CUP

PRIMORDIUM
OF LACRIMAL
GLAND

BULBAR
CONJUNCTIVA

PALPEBRAL
CONJUNCTIVA

UPPER LID

Fig. 409. — Sagittal Section of the Lateral Portion of the Upper Lid of an Embryo of 34 mm.

(*From Poirier, after Cirincione, 1908.*)

secreting at the end of the fifth month. The ciliary glands (of Moll and Zeis) are outgrowths from the ciliary follicles.

The Tarsus is formed as a condensation of the mesoderm around the tarsal and Zeis's glands.

The first hairs of the eyebrows make their appearance when the lids unite. They are said to be the first hairs of the embryo.

The Cilia appear a little later, first in the upper lid and then in the lower. They develop as epithelial buds from the lid margins soon after their union. Two or three rows, one behind the other, are formed. As the follicles of the cilia and the tarsal glands grow into the embryonic connective tissue, they split the ciliary muscle (of Riolan) from the remainder of the orbicularis.

The Lacrimal Gland is developed by about eight cuneiform epithelial buds which grow towards the end of the second month from the superolateral side of the conjunctival sac (Fig. 409) and repeatedly divide. With the development of the levator and the fascia bulbi, the gland is divided into orbital and palpebral portions. The full histological differentiation does not, however, take place till after birth, so that tears are not produced till about the beginning of the third month.

The Conjunctival glands (of Krause) are developed as growths of the basal cells of the upper conjunctival fornix and to a slight extent from the lower fornix at about six months.

The Lacrimal Sac.—The primordium of the lacrimal sac forms in a solid column of cells which, derived from the surface ectoderm, sinks into the furrow between the lateral nasal and maxillary prominences at about the 10-mm stage. At the 15-mm stage it is free from the ectoderm and grows upwards into the lids to form the canaliculi and downwards into the nose to form the nasolacrimal duct. The lower canaliculus is the thinner of the two and grows farther laterally than the upper. Hence the lower punctum is lateral to the upper.

Errors in development, such as multiplication of the canaliculi or puncta and abnormal diverticula, arise from abnormal division or outgrowths of the primitive solid column of cells.

Canalisation of the solid cellular columns takes place by a degeneration and shedding of the central cells (Fig. 409), first in the region of the lacrimal sac, at about the third month. It reaches the nose at six months and the puncta at seven months. The debris of these cells may cause blocking of the nasal duct, *and give rise to a mucocele, not uncommon in the first few weeks of life.* (Consult Cassidy, 1952.)

The Conjunctiva is developed from the ectoderm lining the lids and that covering the globe (Figs. 382, 409).

The Lacrimal Caruncle.—According to Ask (1907), the caruncle develops by cutting off a portion of the lower lid with its contained cilia, sebaceous and sweat glands, by the ingrowth of the inferior calculus.

The Semilunar Plica develops from the conjunctiva at about five and a half weeks.

THE DEVELOPMENT OF THE VITREOUS

The primordium of the vitreous is present at the earliest stage of the primary optic vesicle, between this vesicle and the surface ectoderm (Fig. 410), but its actual origin is still uncertain. At an early stage the optic cup is filled with an almost featureless mesenchyme, from which the first vitreous tissue (the *primary vitreous*) is probably derived. The fibrils and protoplasmic processes of these cells show some continuity with the tissues of the lens and retina, and this has led to a concept of partial retinal origin of the vitreous. Bach and Seefelder (1911) have, however, claimed that no such processes can be seen within the optic cup prior to the entry of mesodermal cells. However, the appearance of fibrils in fixed material may be due to artefact. Thus has developed a highly controversial situation, dominated more by the statement of "views" than the illuminative effect of valid observations.

As the lens separates from the retina the mesenchymal tissue extends and forms a network which fills the space between them. It will be noted that the reticulum stains the same way as the basement membranes.

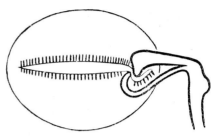

FIG. 410.—DEVELOPMENT OF THE LACRIMAL CARUNCLE
(EMBRYO OF 170 MM).

Note how the lower canaliculus cuts off a piece of the lid margin which forms the caruncle. Actually the eyelids are fused at this stage, but are drawn separated to show the developing tarsal glands (vertical lines).

(*From Ask, 1907.*)

The primitive vitreous is vascular, the vessels being formed in the first place by vaso-formative cells which are present from the earliest stages. Then it is invaded by the hyaloid artery and its branches.

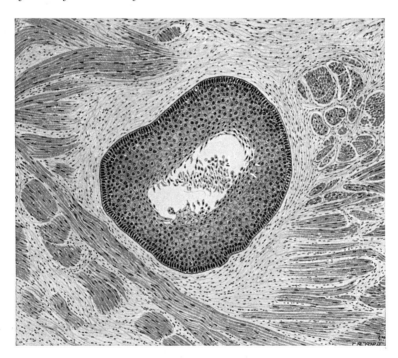

FIG. 411.—TO SHOW THE FORMATION OF THE LUMEN IN THE LACRIMAL CANALICULUS OF A FETUS
OF ABOUT EIGHT MONTHS.

The debris of the central cells may at times cause the mucocele not uncommon in the first weeks of life. Around are fibres of the orbicularis.

(*Wolff's preparation.*)

Formation of the Definitive Vitreous.—When the primitive vitreous with its vessels fills the whole vitreous cavity there appears on the surface of the retina a

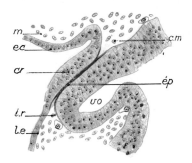

FIG. 412.—SECTION OF THE EYE OF A SHEEP EMBRYO OF 7·5 MM AT THE STAGE OF THE
PRIMARY OPTIC VESICLE. (STAINED PICRO-BLACK-NAPHTHOL.)

e.c. = head ectoderm; m. = mesoderm; v.o. = optic vesicle; c.r. = lens thickening; l.e. =
basement membrane of ectoderm; l.r. = basement membrane or limitans of optic vesicle; e.p. =
their thickening forming the retino-lenticular material of union; c.m. = wedge of mesoderm.

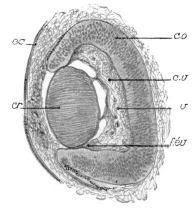

FIG. 413.—SECTION OF THE EYE OF A SHEEP EMBRYO OF 20 MM.

c.o. = optic cup; e.c. = head ectoderm; c.r. = lens; c.v. = primitive vitreous; v. = its vessels
f.é.v. = fan-like fibres or faisceau isthmique.

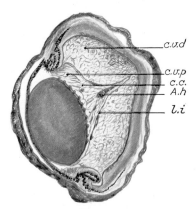

FIG. 414.—SECTION OF THE EYE OF A SHEEP EMBRYO OF 90 MM.

c.v.d. = definitive vitreous; c.v.p. = primitive vitreous filling hyaloid canal of Cloquet; l.i. =
intervitreous condensation; A.h. = hyaloid artery; c.c. = primitive vitreous.

(From Dejean in the Traité d'Ophthalmologie, 1939.)

A.E.—452]

dense layer. This forms the definitive or secondary vitreous arising like the primitive from the basement membrane of the retina (but not from the optic disc). It
enlarges rapidly, pushing the primitive vitreous and its vessels before it. It is at
first homogeneous but soon becomes lamellar. It is characterized by being avascular and fine-meshed.

The primitive vitreous is then pushed behind the lens, into the ciliary region
and to the central axis, where it surrounds the trunk of the hyaloid artery.

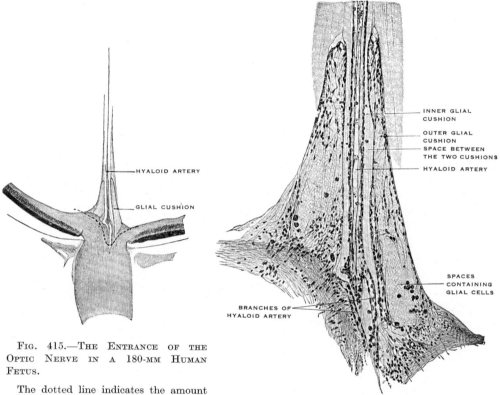

FIG. 415.—THE ENTRANCE OF THE
OPTIC NERVE IN A 180-MM HUMAN
FETUS.

The dotted line indicates the amount
of atrophy to form the normal physiological cup.

(*From Seefelder, 1930.*)

FIG. 416.—THE REGION IN FIG. 415 ANTERIOR TO
THE DOTTED LINE, ENLARGED.

(*From Bach and Seefelder, 1930.*)

The Intervitreous Condensation.—This is a lamellar-like condensation between
the primitive and definitive vitreous. It runs forwards from the disc to the back
of the lens, then bends round to reach the ora serrata. It forms the walls of the
hyaloid canal and the anterior limiting layer of the vitreous (Fig. 414).

For a full discussion of the origin of the vitreous consult Duke-Elder (1963) and
Mann (1964). The consensus of opinion is that neural ectoderm (retina), surface
ectoderm, and mesoderm all contribute. The primary vitreous is compressed by

the secondary, and is said to be the only part of the vitreous of mesodermal origin. It corresponds to a small part of the vitreous adjacent to the zonule, behind the lens, and in the vicinity of the hyaloid canal. The main bulk of the vitreous (secondary) and the zonule (tertiary) are in the same view derived from neurectoderm.

The Ciliary Zonule.—The zonule is developed during the third month (60-mm stage) onwards from the so-called *tertiary vitreous*, which itself is thought to be derived from the neurectoderm of the ciliary region (Mann, 1964).

The Internal Limiting Layer of the Retina.—The essential part of what we have called the internal limiting layer of the retina (see p. 133) is derived from the basement membrane of the retina, which, as we have seen, is present from the earliest stages of development. It thus has the same origin as the vitreous and stains the same way. At about the 11-mm stage the feet of the fibres of Müller reach it and form the irregularities on its retinal aspect.

POST-NATAL DEVELOPMENT OF THE VITREOUS

At birth the hyaloid canal extends horizontally backwards from a point a little below and to the nasal side of the posterior pole of the lens.

The extreme anterior end of the main trunk of the hyaloid artery extends horizontally backwards from the lens capsule along the first part of the canal. After birth the remains of the artery curl up like a corkscrew and hang down behind the lens. The walls of the hyaloid canal become very lax and hang down, moving with the movement of the eye and head (Mann, 1964); its attachment to the back of the eye probably remains as the arcuate line.

THE HYALOID SYSTEM OF VESSELS

As the optic cup develops two systems of vessels appear, (*a*) inside it and (*b*) on its exterior (Fig. 403).

(*a*) The hyaloid artery, a branch of the ophthalmic, *enters* the optic cup by the fetal fissure, and drains anteriorly into the annular vessel. It also anastomoses with the vessels of the optic stalk.

(*b*) A second set ramifies *on the surface* of the optic cup and will eventually form the choroid (*q.v.*). The most anterior part of this plexus forms the annular vessel round the rim of the cup. This vessel has been considered by some authorities to be an artery; but although it is impossible at this stage to differentiate arteries and veins structurally, it is most probably a vein since the hyaloid artery drains into it.

The circulus iridis major is later developed in the same position as the annular vessel, but is not derived from it.

The hyaloid artery divides repeatedly, and gradually forms a network of vessels covering the back of the lens (the tunica vasculosa lentis). Other branches of the artery practically fill the vitreous chamber at this stage and reach their greatest development at the middle of the third month (vasa hyaloidea propria) (Fig. 355).

The hyaloid artery at first emerges from the middle of the optic disc (Figs. 415, 416, 417), but later diverges more and more to the nasal side. It at the same time becomes smaller and smaller, while the arteria centralis grows larger. Eventually the hyaloid artery appears to be merely a ramus of the central retinal artery.

The hyaloid system of vessels disappears first at the peripheral parts of the vitreous (about the fifth month), and concurrently with this the point of division of the main hyaloid artery moves further forwards and its attachment to the lens becomes more medial. The venous return of the whole system is via the capsulo-pupillary membrane, which covers the lens from its equator to the edge of the pupil.

Vascularisation of the Optic Nerve and Retina

At first the optic nerve and retina are avascular because the hyaloid system supplies the developing lens and the vitreous only. At two and a half months with

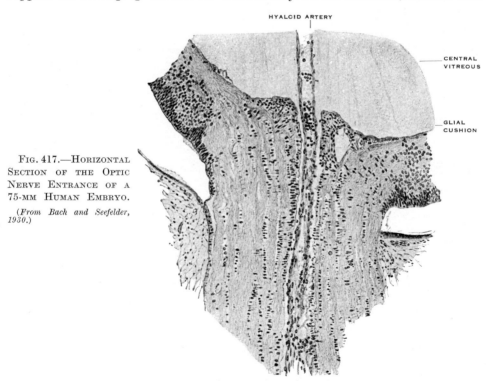

HYALOID ARTERY

CENTRAL VITREOUS

GLIAL CUSHION

Fig. 417.—Horizontal Section of the Optic Nerve Entrance of a 75-mm Human Embryo.

(*From Bach and Seefelder, 1930.*)

the invasion of the septal vessels a plexus of veins forms round the hyaloid artery while it is still in the optic nerve. In this, two vessels can be distinguished early, and these unite near the optic disc to form the vena centralis retinæ. After this, at about three and a half months, the retinal arteries are developed as two buds from the hyaloid artery which grow into the nerve fibre layer of the retina and later become canalised. Similar buds form the retinal veins.

The vessels gradually grow out towards the ora serrata, and at the eighth month the vascular arrangements of the retina are complete.

That portion of the hyaloid artery enclosed in the optic nerve becomes the arteria centralis.

THE ORBITAL SKELETON

The osseous orbit is formed in the circum-ocular mesoderm. This is, however, derived from several sources:

1. Superiorly, from the mesodermal capsule of the forebrain.
2. Inferolaterally, from the maxillary prominence.
3. Medially, from the frontonasal prominence.
4. Posteriorly, from the pre- and orbito-sphenoids.

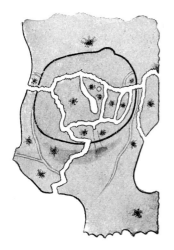

FIG. 418.—DIAGRAM TO SHOW THE APPROXIMATE POSITION AND NUMBER OF CENTRES OF OSSIFICATION IN THE BONES WHICH FORM THE ORBIT.

The centres appear between the sixth and eighth weeks of fetal life, and, except for the sphenoidal, have fused into component bones before birth (6th to 7th month). In very rare cases one of the secondary centres may remain ununited.

(*Whitnall, 1932.*)

The optic vesicle at first lies at the side of the head between the head fold and the maxillary prominence (Fig. 407). As this prominence grows forwards and forms the floor and lateral wall of the orbit, the eye passes forwards too. The frontonasal prominence divides into two lateral and two medial nasal processes.

Each lateral prominence goes to form the medial wall of the orbit (including the frontonasal prominence, the lacrimal and ethmoid bones) of its side and eventually unites with the maxillary prominence.

The roof of the orbit is formed from the capsule of the forebrain.

The optic nerve passes into the eye between the two roots of the orbito-sphenoid, which are attached to the orbitonasal septum. The development of this region and of the optic canal has recently been examined and previous observations reviewed by Kier (1966). He has explained the genesis and true nature of "double" optic foramen.

All the bones of the orbit (including the greater wing of the sphenoid) are membrane bones, but the pre- and orbito-sphenoids belonging to the base of the cranium are developed in cartilage. As it is formed round the eye, the orbit is at first much more of a sphere than in the adult, and also the orbital opening is more circular.

The eye at first grows faster than the orbit, whose margin at six months only reaches to the equator.

THE EXTRINSIC MUSCLES

The most recent and most detailed account of the development of the human extraocular muscles is that of Gilbert (1957). The muscles are developed in three separate, but closely associated, mesenchymal condensations, which correspond to the premandibular, mandibular, and hyoid head cavities of lower vertebrates, and which are from the first associated with the oculomotor, trochlear and abducent nerves. By the 9-mm stage the muscles are individually differentiating, but the levator palpebræ superioris does not delaminate from the superior rectus until the embryo is 55 mm. The three condensations probably correspond to pro-otic myotomes; hence the triple nerve supply. (For an excellent review of these phylogenetic problems see Duke-Elder and Cook, 1963.)

SUMMARY OF THE ORIGIN OF THE VARIOUS TISSUES OF THE EYE (FROM MANN, 1949)

Surface Ectoderm gives rise to:

Lens.

Epithelium of cornea.

Epithelium of conjunctiva (and hence), lacrimal gland.

Epithelium of lids and its derivatives, and cilia, the tarsal glands, and the ciliary and conjunctival glands.

Epithelium lining lacrimal apparatus.

Neural Ectoderm gives rise to:

Retina with its pigment epithelium.

Epithelium covering ciliary processes.

Pigment epithelium covering posterior surface of iris.

Sphincter and dilatator pupillæ muscles.

The optic nerve (neuroglial and nervous elements only).

Associated Paraxial Mesoderm gives rise to:

The blood-vessels, i.e. the choroid, the arteria centralis retinæ, ciliary vessels, and other vessels of the orbit which persist, as well as the hyaloid artery, the vasa hyaloid propria, and the vessels of the vascular capsule of the lens which disappear before birth.

The sclera.

The sheath of the optic nerve.

The ciliary muscle.

A.E.—30

The substantia propria of the cornea, and the endothelium of its posterior surface.
The stroma and anterior epithelium of the iris.
The extrinsic muscles of the eye.
The fat, ligaments, and other connective tissue structures in the orbit.
The upper and medial walls of the orbit.
The connective tissue of the upper lid.

Visceral (Mesoderm of Maxillary Process) below the eye gives rise to:

The lower and lateral walls of the orbit. The The structures lying behind and below
the eye (i.e. the alisphenoid, zygomatic, and orbital plate of maxilla).
The connective tissues of the lower lid.

A list of age-length relationships at representative stages is added for reference (crown-rump length in mm):

4 weeks (28 days) . . . 7·8 mm	11 weeks (77 days) . . . 59·2 mm
5 weeks (35 days) . . . 12·2 mm	12 weeks (84 days) . . . 70·5 mm
6 weeks (42 days) . . . 17·6 mm	18 weeks . . . 130·0 mm
7 weeks (49 days) . . . 24·0 mm	24 weeks . . . 190·0 mm
8 weeks (56 days) . . . 31·3 mm	30 weeks . . . 250·0 mm
9 weeks (63 days) . . . 39·6 mm	36 weeks . . . 310·0 mm
10 weeks (70 days) . . . 49·0 mm	39 weeks . . . 340·0 mm

PRINCIPAL LANDMARKS IN OCULAR GROWTH

The following table from Mann (1957) shows in italics the changes of greatest moment in the production of developmental abnormalities:

Period	Structures undergoing change	Approx. size of embryo at end of period	Approx. age at end of period
	Organogenetic period		
1	*Optic pit changes into optic vesicle.* Lens plate forms	3 mm	3–4 weeks
2	Lens pit and vesicle appear. *Optic vesicle invaginates to form optic cup.* Pigment appears in outer layer of optic cup	7 mm	End of 4th week
3	*Fœtal fissure closes.* Lens separates from surface and *primary lens fibres form.* Retinal differentiation begins. Tunica vasculosa lentis begins	14 mm	6th week
	Neofetal period		
4	Secondary lens fibres begin. Tunica vasculosa lentis fully formed. Lid folds develop. *Ectodermal layers of iris begin*	70 mm	3 months
	Fetal period		
5	The following appear: Arteria centralis retinæ, ciliary muscle, sphincter and dilator of pupil, sclera, ciliary body and outer layer of choroid. *Posterior vascular capsule of lens begins to retrogress*	110 mm	4 months
6	*Pupillary membrane retrogresses.* Pars plana begins. Medullation of optic nerve begins	250 mm	7 months

Period	Structures undergoing change	Approx. size of embryo at end of period	Approx. age at end of period
7	*Hyaloid artery disappears.* Medullation reaches lamina cribrosa	300 mm	9 months

Neonatal period

8	*Macula lutea finally differentiates*	—	4–6 months after birth

Postnatal or adolescent period

	Further formation of *secondary lens fibres.* Growth of whole eye	—	25 years

(For other views on stages of ocular development, *see* O'Rahilly, 1966.)

THE EYE AT BIRTH

The eye at birth is less spherical than in the adult. This is due to the bulge of the postero-lateral quadrants.

Its anteroposterior diameter varies from 12·5 to 15·8 mm, and the vertical diameter from 14·5 to 17 mm. To offset the comparative shortness of the eye which would make it exceedingly hypermetropic, the media are more highly refractive than in the adult, the seat of the excess of refractivity being in the lens. These dimensions are taken from Fuchs (1884). Weiss (1887), however, gives the following measurements for the anteroposterior, vertical, and transverse diameters respectively, 16·4, 15·4 and 16 mm. Sorsby and Sheridan (1960) found natal measurements to be respectively 17·9, 17·3 and 18·4 mm.

The cornea is relatively large, its diameter (10 mm) being three-fifths that of the anteroposterior axis.

It is more curved at the periphery than at its centre, i.e. just the opposite of the condition in the adult.

The medial rectus is very close to the cornea.

The corneal stroma contains more nuclei than in the adult. The lamina cribrosa is not fully consolidated for several months after birth.

The stroma of the uveal tract has no pigment except possibly posteriorly near the optic nerve.

The pigmentation of the anterior border layer of the iris commences in the first few days of life.

The pupil is small and does not dilate fully.

The anterior chamber is shallow and its angle is narrow. It is filled by trabecular tissue.

The ligamentum pectinatum is still somewhat fetal in character, i.e. it still fills the angle to a large extent.

The ciliary processes are still in contact with the iris.

The stroma of the ciliary body is very cellular, but the various types of muscle can be recognised.

The ridges of the ciliary processes are as dark as the valleys between them.

The macula is as far from the disc as in the adult. A depression in it is just visible. The cones are still short and stumpy. Relative to the rest of the retina the macular region is thus markedly retarded.

The teeth of the ora serrata are just visible, and the retina passes much more gradually into the pars ciliaris. The two nuclear layers fuse, and are continued into the ciliary epithelium.

A fold of the retina at the ora serrata is often found, but this must be regarded as an artefact.

The orbicularis ciliaris is very short, so that the retina lies just behind the ciliary muscle.

The nerve fibres behind the lamina cribrosa are still not medullated.

The lens is rounder than in the adult, and on account of its anterior bulging the anterior chamber is shallow.

For details of postnatal dimensions see Duke-Elder and Cook (1963).

Postnatal Growth and Changes in the Eyeball

The eye grows rapidly in the first years of life, the vertical diameter growing faster, so that the eye becomes more nearly spherical. The rate then decreases till puberty, when it again becomes more rapid till the early twenties (Weiss, 1887).

There is a distinct parallel between the growth of the eye and that of the brain. Thus, from birth to adult life, the eye grows 3·25 times and the brain 3·76. The body, on the other hand, increases 21·36 times.

The increase in size during the first years of life affects mainly the anterior segment, i.e. the cornea and the sclera up to the insertions of the muscles. Thus the cornea reaches adult size at about two years or earlier.

The later growth affects mainly the posterior segment, but the distance between the fovea and optic nerve remains the same as at birth.

Myelination of the optic nerve is completed in the first three weeks after birth, and seems to be hastened by exposure to light. Thus a premature baby will have its medullation farther advanced by the time it reaches the ninth month than a newly born full-term child.

The fovea is not properly developed till one month after birth.

There is little difference between the ciliary and pupillary zones of the iris at birth. This can be made out at about six months.

The colour of the iris changes in the first few years of life, depending on the amount of stroma pigment laid down.

The Ciliary Body.—As the retina recedes, so there is an increase in the size of the orbiculus ciliaris. The line of demarcation between the retina and ciliary body is well marked, but does not reach adult relationships till about seven years.

As the ciliary processes are displaced backwards the angle of the anterior chamber widens to adult size between two and four years.

There is no muscle of Müller at birth (Fuchs, 1884). It is only after the fifth year that the ciliary muscle, and thus the whole ciliary body, takes on a triangular form.

The lens grows rapidly in the first years of life and becomes flatter, owing to being pulled on by the ever-widening circle formed by the ciliary body. The lens continues growing throughout life (p. 167).

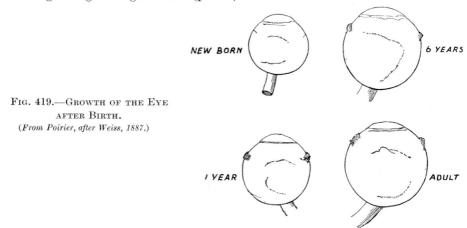

FIG. 419.—GROWTH OF THE EYE
AFTER BIRTH.
(From Poirier, after Weiss, 1887.)

The eye of the new-born child is normally hypermetropic. The increase in axial length would, however, render it myopic were it not for this flattening of the lens.

The eyes get farther apart and the orbits enlarge especially anteriorly, so that their temporal borders are more widely separated. As the eyes separate they also tend to diverge, since the separation makes the lateral rectus act to greater and the medial rectus to less advantage than before.

Signs of Age in the Eyeball

The cornea flattens with age, but more in the vertical than in the horizontal meridian. This gives rise to an astigmatism against the rule. *Hence the onset of astigmatism against the rule in emmetropes after about forty years may be regarded as normal, and, further, for the same reason, astigmatism with the rule tends to lessen and that against the rule tends to increase with age.*

The arcus senilis is a manifestation of the fatty degeneration which tends to take place with age throughout the fibrous tunic of the eye.

It starts above and below as two grey crescents, close to and parallel with the corneal margin. The crescents eventually fuse and become whiter and more opaque. The ring so formed is thicker above than below. There is always a portion of clear cornea between it and the limbus. It is sharply defined peripherally, but fades more gradually into clear cornea centrally.

Fatty degeneration first affects the superficial stroma and the anterior limiting lamina (of Bowman). Peripherally it is limited by a line passing from the end of the anterior lamina obliquely outwards for a varying distance into the sclera.

The sclera becomes thicker and more rigid. There is a tendency for the deposition of fat, which changes the colour from white to yellowish.

In the uveal tract there is a great increase in the amount of connective tissue. The ciliary body, therefore, thickens and the circumlental space is diminished. Senile myosis and rigidity of the sphincter pupillæ are also due to increase in the amount of connective tissue in its neighbourhood.

The various glass-like membranes become thicker, and there is a great tendency to wart formation seen specially at the periphery of the posterior limiting lamina (of Descemet) and in the basal lamina (membrane of Bruch).

The warts on the basal lamina are secreted by the pigment epithelium which covers them, but thins over the summits of the elevations. They, therefore, appear with the ophthalmoscope as yellowish-white spots surrounded by a narrow pigmented border. The spots in Tay's choroiditis are of this nature.

The pigment epithelium tends to show areas of atrophy, especially round the disc.

CHAPTER XI

COMPARATIVE ANATOMY

RESPONSE to the light stimulus does not in itself indicate an organ of vision. We know that many inorganic substances react to light. One of the most remarkable examples of this is seen in the photographic plate. Also, as is well known, a colourless solution of eserine goes pink when exposed to light.

Plants, too, respond to light. Thus the portions above ground as a rule grow towards the light (positive photropism) while the roots grow away from it (negative phototropism). Although the formation of chlorophyll, the hæmoglobin of plants, depends on the presence of light; but we do not postulate an organ of vision.

A

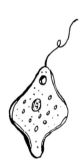

FIG. 420.—EUGLENA VIRIDIS (A FLAGELLATE) WITH ITS "EYE-SPOT".

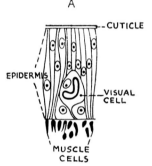

FIG. 421.—VISUAL CELL AND EPIDERMIS OF THE WORM STYLARIA LACUSTRIS.

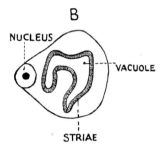

FIG. 422.—THE VISUAL CELL UNDER GREATER MAGNIFICATION.

In the unicellular animals (Amœbæ, Infusoria) the animal usually reacts as a whole in its response to light; thus the amœba crawls away from a beam of light thrown on it. On the other hand, *Paramœcium bursaria*, which contains algæ, swims towards the light which is necessary for its symbiotic chlorophyll-containing partners to build up starch and sugar. But even in the Protozoa there may be some specialisation. Thus it has been found that the anterior region of *Euglena viridis*, an infusorian, is much more sensitive to light than the posterior. In this anterior portion there is an "eye-spot" which at first was thought to be the most primitive eye. But later the area most sensitive to light was shown to be in front of this. In *Stentor*, another protozoon, the anterior end also is especially susceptible. When light falls on this part, the animal turns away and seeks a shady corner.

In the multicellular animals (Metazoa) there is further specialisation. In the earthworm, for instance, there are specialised visual cells first described by Hesse in 1895 and since found in many other animals. Each cell is shorter and wider than the other epithelial cells among which it is placed; also, the protoplasm is clearer and contains vacuoles; at its proximal end it is continued into a filament, probably a nerve fibril (see also p. 472).

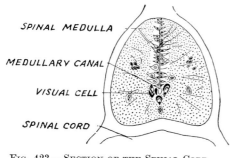

FIG. 423.—SECTION OF THE SPINAL CORD
OF AMPHIOXUS.

(*From Poirier, after Hesse.*)

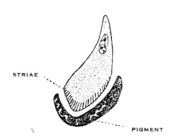

FIG. 424.—VISUAL CELL OF
AMPHIOXUS.

Earthworms are sensitive to bright light and crawl away from it. They come out of their burrows before dawn to feed, but, at break of day, they return. The return to the burrow is an expression of negative phototropism.

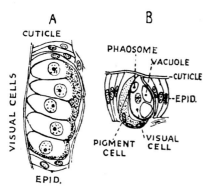

FIG. 425.—THE EYE OF STYLARIA
LACUSTRIS.

A = on transverse section.
B = on horizontal section.

(*From Bütschli, after Hesse.*)

In passing up the animal scale, we find that to arrive at true vision we pass through three stages:

(*a*) **Phototropism.**—The animal as a whole moves either towards or away from the source of light (positive or negative phototropism), as we saw in the *Paramœcium bursaria* and amœba.

(*b*) **Sensation.**—Here the animal receives the light stimulus by a special mechanism, but does not recognise it as light. As an example of this, we saw how the earthworm avoids sunlight. Also the tubeworm rapidly withdraws its feathery tentacles (each of which is possessed by an "eye") when the light falling on it is shaded. This "shading reaction" (an expression of negative phototropism) is present in many sluggish and sessile shore creatures. It is obviously protective. A fish in search of food casts a tell-tale shadow. This shadow will cause barnacles to close, sea squirts to contract up into gelatinous blobs, and burrowing bivalves to withdraw their soft protruding siphons into the sand. On the other hand, a sudden shading of the light will cause the sea urchin to bristle up its spines. Thus, this "shading reaction" enables the invertebrate to hide or arm itself at the approach of its enemies.

(c) **Specific Sensation.**—Here the animal, owing to the development of the central nervous mechanism of vision, recognises the light as light. It is only animals which have the last type of vision which really *see* in the true sense of the word.

(The distinction between (b) and (c) is not a clear one. In both cases "central" nervous systems may be involved, and always are in all higher invertebrates and, of course, all vertebrates. At what level in a nervous system or in evolution "recognition" of light occurs depends essentially upon what is implied by "recognition". The evolution and arena of "consciousness", which is inherent for some in the use of the word "sensation", are equally difficult problems. It is always dangerous to classify in biological fields.)

CLASSIFICATION OF THE TWO BIG GROUPS OF VISUAL ORGANS

A. **The epithelial eye of invertebrates** developed from the skin.
- Simple eye:
  1. Single epithelial cell.
  2. A collection of epithelial cells:
     (a) Flat.
     (b) Cup-shaped.
     (c) Vesicular.
- Compound or faceted eye.

B. **The cerebral eye of vertebrates** developed from the central nervous system.

A. The most rudimentary "eye" is the visual cell. This, as we have seen, is an epithelial cell, but slightly differentiated and well seen in worms.

In the next stage we find a mantle of pigment associated with the cell (Fig. 424). The pigment is there to absorb the light and to convert it into heat and possibly other forms of energy. In *Amphioxus* these visual cells lie deep next the medullary canal (Fig. 423). A further stage is seen in the worm, *Stylaria lacustris*, in which a number of these cells have become grouped together (Fig. 425). Such a rudimentary eye, whether consisting of one or more cells, is called an ocellus (= little eye).

Cup-shaped Eyes.—In these the visual cells of the surface epithelium have sunk in so as to line a fossa or cup. Thus there is a greater crowding together of visual elements and a better orientation of the incident light. They have some directional value.

These eyes, although superior to the flat eyes, and although they have arrived at a certain degree of differentiation, consist almost exclusively of visual cells. They form a simple depression, open widely on the surface (Fig. 426). A further advance is seen where the opening is more or less closed, the "eyes" then opening on the surface by a small hole or "pupil" only (Fig. 429). These latter are formed on

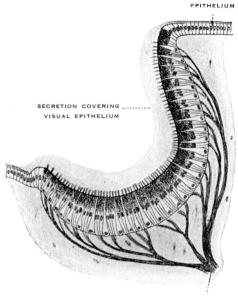

EPITHELIUM

SECRETION COVERING
VISUAL EPITHELIUM

OPTIC NERVE

FIG. 426.—THE EYE OF PATELLA—A MOLLUSC
(STILL WIDE OPEN ON TO THE SURFACE).

The visual epithelium consists of pigmented
visual cells and non-pigmented secretory cells.

(*From Hesse.*)

the principle of the pin-hole camera—i.e. a dark chamber with a small hole leading into it.

A further stage is seen where, apart from the visual cells, a kind of lens formed by the cuticle is present, and between the lens and the retina a transparent substance. This is formed by secretory cells placed among the visual cells (Fig. 431).

Cup-shaped eyes are seen in the arthropods and molluscs.

Vesicular Eyes.—This is a further stage in development. Here, the opening in the depression is closed so that the eye forms a vesicle, which sinks in from the surface and becomes covered over by surface epithelium (Figs. 432, 433).

Such eyes are seen in the ocelli of spiders and scorpions and in cephalopods, or octopuses, with the most advanced invertebrate eye. Nautilus, a cephalopod, however, still has a simple cup-shaped eye which opens on the surface (Fig. 429).

In the *cephalopods* (Fig. 435) the eye is partially contained in a cartilaginous

FIG. 427.—THE EYE OF
THE WORM, PLANARIA
GONOCEPHALA.

The free end of the visual cell bears cilia and passes into the crescent formed by the pigment cells.

(*From Hesse.*)

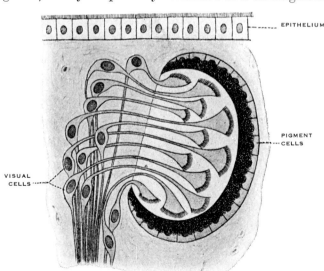

EPITHELIUM

PIGMENT
CELLS

VISUAL
CELLS

orbit. The proximal (deepest) part of the vesicle forms the retina, the distal part is responsible for the posterior portion of the lens. The surface ectoderm becomes thickened to form the anterior portion of the lens (which joins the posterior part), and is so folded that it forms a kind of iris, pupil, cornea and anterior chamber which is open at one point to the surrounding fluid in which the animal lives.

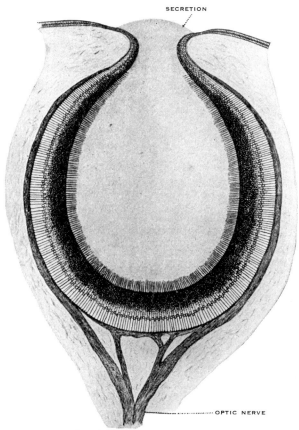

FIG. 428.—THE EYE OF THE SNAIL HALIOTIS.
(The opening is much narrower than in Fig. 426.)
(*From Hesse.*)

The mesoderm between the optic vesicle and the ectoderm forms two laminæ of cartilage (equatorial and iridic), and outside these is formed the silvery membrane or tunic which passes forwards to the pupil. Ciliary and iridic muscles are also found, so that accommodation and pupillary movements are provided.

The Compound or Faceted Eye is found in the arthropods, especially in the crustaceans and insects. It is formed by the union of a number of modified ocelli. Each ocellus, which goes to form an eye, is called an ommatidium (resembling an eye). The number of ommatidia varies from one to many thousands.

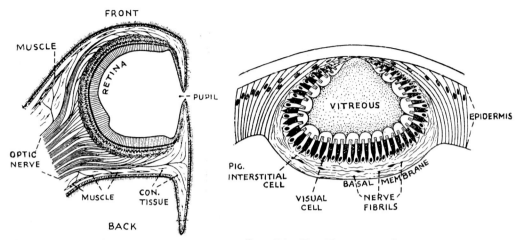

FIG. 429.—THE EYE OF NAUTILUS, A
CEPHALOPOD.
(*From Bütschli.*)

FIG. 430.—THE EYE OF THE CARNIVOROUS WORM,
NEREIS CULTRIFERA.
(*From Bütschli, after Hesse.*)

An ommatidium usually consists of the following: the dioptric apparatus is formed by a corneal facet and a lens cone. Behind this are the retinal cells, usually four to eight to each corneal facet forming a *single* unit, from which a single nerve fibre passes to a collection of nerve cells, the optic ganglion.

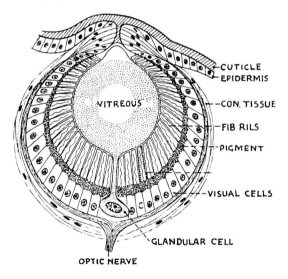

FIG. 431.—THE EYE OF THE WORM,
PHYLLODOCE LAMINOSA.
(*From Bütschli, after Hesse.*)

It is the fact that in the ommatidium a number of retinal elements are structurally and functionally united to form a single unit *the retinule*, which distinguishes it from the ordinary ocellus.

The whole eye usually forms a portion of a sphere and on section is fan-shaped.

The surface, which is formed by the corneal facets united together, appears smooth to the naked eye, but under the loupe or microscope it forms a mosaic. The facets are hexagonal in the insects, quadrilateral in crustaceans, and convex in Lepidoptera.

B. **The Vertebrate or Cerebral Eye.**—Unlike that of the invertebrate, the vertebrate eye is remarkable for the uniformity of its development and general structure.

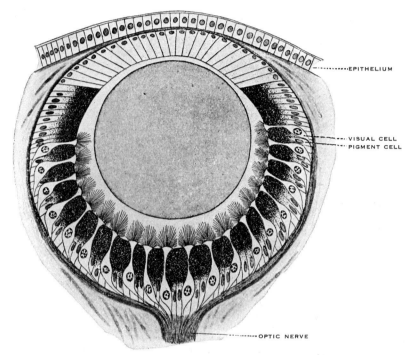

Fig. 432.—The Eye of the Snail, Helix pomatia (completely cut off from the surface).
(From Hesse.)
The visual cells have cilia. The space between the lens and retina is filled with secretion.

(It should be noted here, despite the contrasts drawn above between the eyes of Invertebrates and Vertebrates, that the "cerebral" eye of the latter is also in ultimate origin ectodermal, its lens being directly so derived.)

Generally speaking, the cerebral eye consists of a retina, a dark chamber, and a dioptric apparatus.

There are, however, exceptions, such, for instance, as in the cyclostomes, *Proteus anguineus, Amphioxus, Ascidia*, the mole, and others. In the cyclostomes generally the eye is a simple vesicle under the skin; only in the adult lamprey is it more developed, and one finds traces of a lens, cornea and iris. In the larva of this animal the lens is still a vesicle. Such myxinoids have no lens.

The Proteidæ or amphibian urodeles are cave-dwellers. In them the eye is

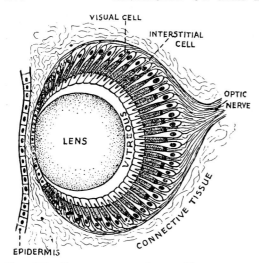

FIG. 433.—SCHEME OF THE CLOSED VESICULAR
EYE OF A GASTROPODE MOLLUSC.
(From Bütschli.)

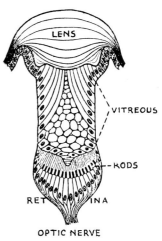

FIG. 434.—SECTION OF THE
OCELLUS OF THE SPIDER, SAL-
TICUS.
(From Bütschli, after Grenacher.)

also a simple vesicle under the skin and does not contain a differentiated refracting
apparatus. The eye has no orbital cavity, being wholly functionless, and is

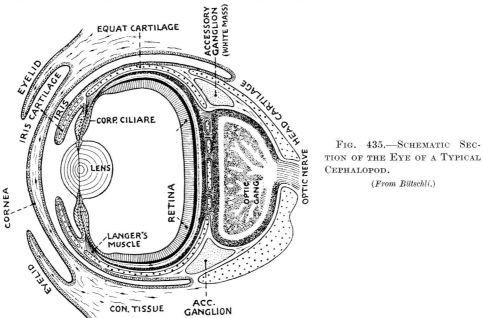

FIG. 435.—SCHEMATIC SEC-
TION OF THE EYE OF A TYPICAL
CEPHALOPOD.
(From Bütschli.)

practically hidden in the masseter muscles. It is very rudimentary, about 0·5 mm
in diameter, and seen with difficulty as a dark shadow under the skin.

In the mole the eye is more differentiated, but is still very small, being about 2 mm in diameter. It is practically covered by the skin, in which there is always, however, a hole (Ciaccio, 1875). This varies from 0·10 to 1·0 mm in the *seeing* mole (*Talpa europa*), to 0·50 to 0·20 mm in the blind mole (*Talpa cæca*). At any rate, in the latter type the hole is too small for vision, and as was already realised by Dante, the mole sees through its skin.

Then there is the *lancelet* (*Amphioxus*), a primitive chordate, which really lies between the invertebrates and vertebrates. Its "eyes" are unicellular ocelli, which are placed next the medullary canal (Figs. 423 and 424)—the central hollow of the creature's dorsal nerve cord—and thus far from the surface. The light can reach the eyes because the animal is small and transparent.

The "eyes" of *Amphioxus*, too, are said to lie between the invertebrate and vertebrate types. Here the eyes have sunk into the depths, but have not grown back to the surface as do vertebrate eyes.

In the larva of *Ascidia*, also, a rudimentary eye is attached to the medullary canal.

Thus in the genesis of the vertebrate eye there are three stages:

(*a*) Development of the eye from the surface ectoderm (epithelial eye of invertebrates).

(*b*) The eye sinks in to lie next the medullary canal (*Amphioxus*, larva of *Ascidia*, the sea-squirts, which are, in the adult, sessile chordates, but free-swimming as larvæ.

(*c*) The eye grows out again to the surface (cerebral eye of vertebrates).

In the epithelial eye of the invertebrates as a rule the light strikes the retinal cells before the nerve and the retina is called a *direct* or converse retina. Exceptions occur in a shellfish, Pecten, and in some spiders (Fig. 440).

In the cerebral eye of vertebrates, the retina being produced from the anterior "invaginated" portion of the optic vesicle, the light strikes the nerve fibres first, and the retina is said to be of the *inverted* type.

The Comparative Anatomy of the Retina

The Retina of the Invertebrates.—The invertebrate retina consists of visual cells and their processes. In the vertebrate retina to these are added the bipolar, the ganglion cells, and supporting fibres.

The photoreceptor cells of the invertebrate are of two main kinds:

(*a*) A cell with a ciliated border or a striated zone ("Stiftchensaum" of Hesse).

(*b*) A rod-like cell.

The latter is the only form that occurs in the vertebrate retina. A third type of photoreceptor is one with a phaosome or phaosphere, i.e. a large vacuole which undergoes changes when exposed to the light (Fig. 425, B). (It has been noted elsewhere that vertebrate photoreceptors are, in fact, potentially ciliated cells, being "ependymal" derivatives.)

(a) Cells with a Striated Zone

The single cell constituting the primitive eye may be ciliated. Often the cells contain large vacuoles round which the striæ are arranged (e.g. in the leech) (Figs. 424, 436).

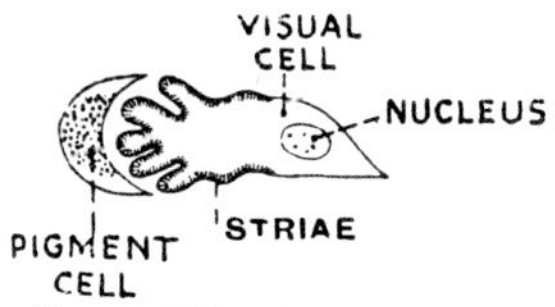

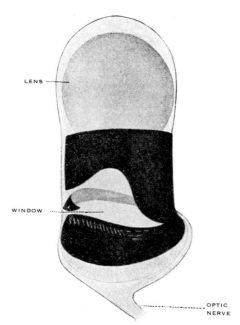

Fig. 436.—Eye of Trematode Worm (Tristomum papillosum).

(*From Bütschli, after Hesse.*)

The striated portion is often enlarged to increase the area of light reception, and, to the same end, the cell may present digitations as in *Tristomum papillosum* (Fig. 436) a trematode worm.

The nerve fibre leaves the cell opposite the striated region and, indeed, according to Hesse, is continuous through the cell with the cilia.

(b) Rod-like Photoreceptors

These are found in many worms, in the ocelli of arthropods and in the eyes of molluscs. Such cells also form the neuro-epithelium of the vertebrate retina and

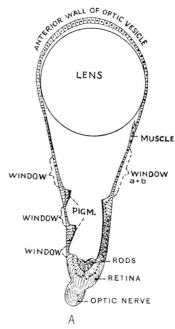

Fig. 437.—The Telescopic Eye of Pterotrachea coronata, a Mollusc.

(*From Hesse.*)

Fig. 438.—Telescopic Eye of Pterotrachea coronata, on Section.

(*From Bütschli, after Hesse.*)

are usually arranged in a single layer. But in the scallop (*Pecten jacobeus*) there are two layers of cells between which are the nerve fibres, and behind the proximal visual cells there is a layer of epithelial cells rich in pigment (Fig. 441). In the cephalopods the visual cells are rod-like and form a single layer resting on the choroidal cartilage.

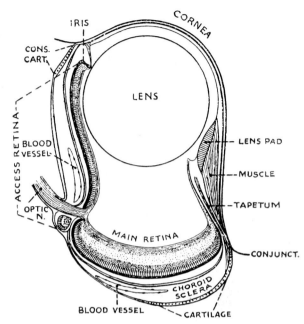

Fig. 439. — The Telescopic Eye of a Deep-sea Bony Fish, Disomma anale.

(*From Bütschli, after Brauer.*)

The nerve fibres leave the eye posteriorly by several holes in the cartilage.

Generally speaking, the nerve fibres pass into a ganglion which may be directly behind the eye or in the central nervous system.

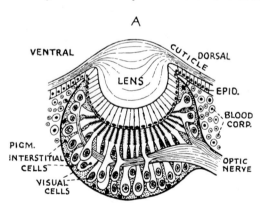

Fig. 440.—The Inverse Eye of a Spider, Tegenaria domestica.

(*From Bütschli, after Widman.*)

The Retina of the Vertebrates is generally more complex than that of the invertebrates. Here we find two tiers of neurons. The photoreceptors are nearest the sclera.

Rods and cones are found in all classes of vertebrates except in certain rudimentary forms. *Amphioxus* is of course an exception, having only unicellular "eyes" (Fig. 423), but it is, of course, a chordate, not an invertebrate. Some have more cones, others more rods.

Ascending the evolutionary scale, we find more rods and cones per sq. mm. Thus Mann (1928) found in a strip of retina 1 mm long and 0·1 mm wide 100 cones in the lamprey, 125 in the frog, 327 in the hen, while at the human macula there were 652.

A.E.—31

The Pigment Epithelium is much the same in all classes of vertebrates, but it may contain, apart from pigment, oil droplets in great variety, and crystals of guanine.

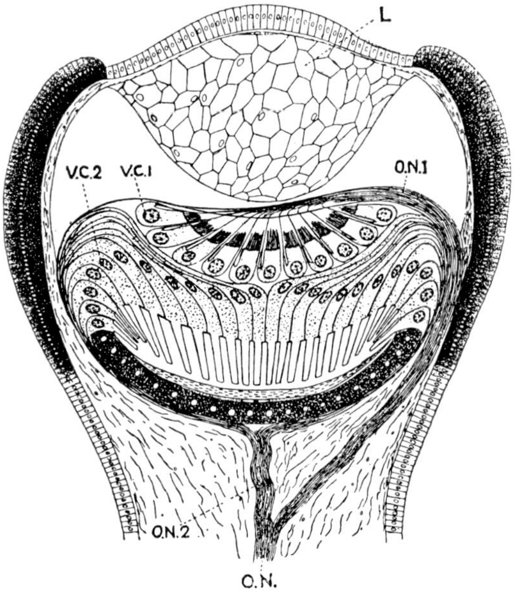

The pigment is morphologically different from that of the choroid. In the choroid it is almost entirely amorphous, in the retina crystalline (Greeff, 1899). The retinal pigment is epithelial in origin, in the choroid mesodermal.

In those animals which have a tapetum the retinal pigment in the region of the tapetum is absent.

In the outer nuclear layer one finds in certain vertebrates the fibres (*massues*) of Landolt. These are filaments ending in knobs towards the outer limiting membrane and probably derived from the bipolar cells (inner nuclear layer).

The Area Centralis.—In all vertebrates there is found an area where the visual cells are narrower and more closely packed—an area of more acute vision than the rest of the fundus. Such an area has even been described in some invertebrates: Hess (1913) found it in some cephalopods, and a trace of it is seen in certain plathelminths (flat worms), and also in many insects. In man and most other

Fig. 441.—The Eye of the Mollusc, Pecten
Jacobeus.
(*From Hesse.*)

L. = lens. V.C.1 = first layer of visual cells. O.N.1 = nerve fibres from this layer. V.C.2 = second layer of visual cells. O.N.2 = nerve fibres from this layer. O.N. = optic nerve.

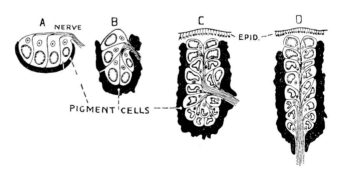

Fig. 442.—Schematic Representation of Stages in the Change from the Inverse Eye of Clespine (A) and Nephelis (B) to the Converse Eye of the Leech (Hirudo) (D).

(*From Bütschli, after Hesse.*)

primates the area is characterised by a yellow pigment, hence the name macula lutea (see p. 141). In the centre of this is the fovea centralis.

The Retina of Fishes is complex, and differs much in the different species. In general, however, it resembles that of the mammals.

The pigment epithelium is often characterised by numerous granules of guanine (Kühne and Sewall, 1880), specially in the gold-fish, perch and bream.

These granules may be brilliant white or reddish yellow in colour. They were first described in 1836 by Della Chaie, who called them ophthalmoliths.

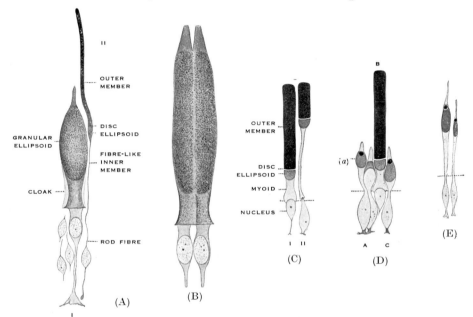

Fig. 443.—(A) Rod (II) and Cone (I) of the Perch. (B) Large Double (or Twin) Cone of the Perch. (C) Red (I) and Green (II) Rods of the Frog. (D) Visual Cells from the Retina of a Frog which has been in Strong Light (A = double cone, one part (a) of which has an oil droplet. B = rod. C = cone with oil droplet). (E) Cones of the Sparrow (note oil droplets).

(After Greeff, 1873.)

They are abundant, especially in the upper part of the eye, and, from the reflex to which they give rise, have been mistaken for a tapetum. (See Walls, 1942.)

The rods and cones are very long, so that, especially in the teleosts, the neuro-epithelium may occupy one-third to one-half the whole thickness of the retina (Schultze, 1873). The rods and cones often resemble each other very closely, and Greeff (1900) and Schultze doubted the existence of the latter in selachians (sharks).

The largest cones are found in the perch, where they are often double (Fig. 443, B). Usually there are no oil droplets, but Schultze found colourless ones in the sturgeon between the outer and inner segments of the cones. A kind of membrane or cloak is often seen round the rods and cones.

The outer nuclear layer has four rows usually, but there are six in the bream and one in the lamprey. Many medullated nerve fibres are found.

Area Centralis.—It used to be believed that there was no area centralis in fishes, but Carrière (1885) showed it in *Hippocampus* and Krause (1886) in *Syngnathus*, belonging to the lophobranchs. Hesse found it in cephalopods, in selachians (*Scyllium*), and in the bony fishes, red mullet and the minnow.

THE RETINA OF AMPHIBIANS

Rods and cones are found, the former being usually more numerous. They are much larger than in the human, the smallest being double the size of mankind's.

The pigment cells are very large, covering eight to fifteen visual cells in the frog. They contain numerous oil droplets. The frog has two kinds of rods:

(*a*) Violet-red, the larger and more numerous.

(*b*) Green.

The intercalated disc which lies between the inner and outer segments of the rods is better marked than in other animals (Fig. 443, C and D). Oil droplets are found between the two segments of the cones. They may be colourless or slightly yellow.

The visual cells all end in a ramifying footpiece. (Generally speaking, the cones end in this way and the rods in a knob.) Cajal (1894) describes double cones and rods.

The fibres of Landolt are more numerous than in any other vertebrates.

The nerve fibres from the right side of the retina go to the left side of the disc and vice versa (corroborated by Wolff's own preparations).

In *Proteus anguineus* and *Axolotl* (cave-dwellers), which belong to the tailed amphibians, the retina is primitive and little differentiated, and fills practically the whole bulb.

THE RETINA OF REPTILES

The retina is generally characterised by the predominance of the cones over the rods. The crocodile and gecko are exceptions.

The pigment epithelium is like that of the vertebrates generally except in the crocodile, where in the upper part of the retina it contains guanine crystals as well as pigment.

The cones often contain oil droplets. They are abundant and coloured in the tortoise, fewer and almost colourless in the lizard.

The outer nuclear layer consists of two rows of large cells like those of the amphibians.

Both the rod and cone fibres end in a ramifying footpiece, and since this is the usual termination of the cone fibres, it was believed that only cones were present. *Rods and cones are, however, best distinguished by their connections rather than by the type of termination.* (Also by their staining reactions, see p. 112.)

The inner nuclear layer is very wide. In the crocodile a horizontally striated area centralis is found. In the reptiles the cells of the pars ciliaris retinæ are very large. (See Mann, 1933.)

THE RETINA OF BIRDS

The retina of diurnal birds contains many cones and few rods. In the fowl and pigeon, however, in a certain area, coloured yellow in the former and red in the latter, the rods are more numerous.

In the nocturnal birds the rods are much more numerous.

The neuro-epithelium is especially distinguished by the *oil droplets*, which are more abundant here than in any other vertebrate. The oil droplets are situated between the inner and outer segments of rods and cones, but more numerous in the latter (Fig. 443, E).

In the diurnal birds the droplets are of varied and bright colours. Most usually they are red, but there are different shades of yellow, green, and blue. In the nocturnal birds the droplets tend to be yellow. The pigments producing these colours were called chromophanes by Kühne and Sewall (1880).

In the posterosuperior quadrant of the retina in fowls the yellow droplets predominate and give this area its yellow colour. The same quadrant in the pigeon is red, giving rise to the red area in these birds. The remaining portion of the fundi appears slightly red in fowls and slightly yellow in the pigeon, owing to predominance of these colours in the oil droplets.

The fibres of Müller are narrower, and in the distal portion of the inner granular layer break up, like those of the reptiles, into a brushwork of fibres.

Area Centralis and Fovea.—Birds have an area centralis, often two. A fovea is often present, and in some, including the pigeon and sparrow, two in each eye according to Müller (1872).

Rochon-Duvigneaud (1943) stated that insect and grain-eating birds, which have their eyes more or less lateral and whose visual axes make an angle of 120° or more with each other, have a single fovea more or less central. The nocturnal birds of prey and the swallow have a double fovea, one central, the other lateral— the latter being placed behind and below the former.

In some birds a band-shaped area of acute vision may be associated with the macula. Where two maculæ occur, they may be joined by such a band (Wood, 1917).

THE RETINA OF MAMMALS

A central area is present in most diurnal mammals, although it is said to be absent in the mouse, rat and sheep. Only man and some other primates have a macula and fovea centralis subserving binocular and stereoscopic vision. However, a fovea occurs, often containing rods only (not cones, as in man) in some representatives of all classes of vertebrates except the Agnatha (lampreys, etc.). (See Prince, 1949; Walls, 1963.)

In tarsius, the sole surviving representative of a group between lemurs and monkeys, there is a great crowding together of the rods in the macular region, but there is no spreading apart of the various layers so that light may fall directly on the neuro-epithelium. This takes place first in the marmoset (Woollard, 1926). A "true" macula shows considerable modification in arrangement of its photo-receptors and neurons, but also an exclusion of blood vessels from the area.

MYELINATED NERVE FIBRES IN THE RETINA

What occurs as a rarity in man is normally present in a number of animals.

The rabbit has a well-marked horizontal band of opaque nerve fibres on either side of the disc (Fig. 455).

Johnson (1901) found myelinated nerve fibres in the retina of *Perameles lagotis* and other marsupials by ophthalmoscopy.

In the dog (Fig. 461) the nerve fibres of and all round the disc are medullated and Kolmer (1936) saw them in *Dentex* and *Lophius*.

THE CHOROID

The choroid occurs only in the vertebrate eye; it is usually about 0·5 mm deep, but in the whale and seal may be thicker than 1·5 mm.

The pigment is most abundant peripherally, that is, in the suprachoroidal lamina, but is absent here in birds and fishes. Thus in the latter the *silvery membrane* (argentea), which is placed between the lamina suprachoroidea and the layer of large vessels, shows through.

The Silvery Membrane (argentea) of the choroid of fishes (especially of the bony fishes) is placed between the suprachoroidea and the large vessels. It extends over the whole choroid and also over the iris.

It is formed of crystals of guanine which give the membrane its brilliant white appearance, and are responsible for the metallic lustre of the iris of fishes and cephalopods.

The Choroidal Gland.—The choroid of fishes is thicker than that of other vertebrates, and has a spongy structure. It is very vascular, especially in its posterior part. The retina thus appears to rest on a vascular cushion. To this posterior thickened portion the name of choroidal gland has been given. It is particularly well developed in certain ganoid fishes such as *Amia*, and in some other teleosts, for instance the angler fish (*Lophius*). The 'gland' is of unknown function, but is usually only present in fish with a special branchial (pseudo-branchial) efferent vessel, which conveys aerated blood direct to the choroid. It is also said to be an arrangement to smooth out vascular pressure in the eye (Walls, 1963).

The Tapetum is seen in most mammals. It is responsible for the green reflex seen in the cat's eye and the emerald green in that of the dog. It is best seen in the carnivore, ruminant, horse, cetacean, seal and dolphin. One also finds it in fishes, but not in rodents, reptiles (except the crocodile), and amphibians.

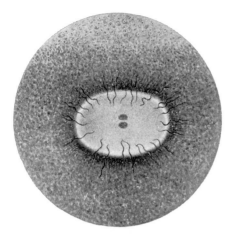

FIG. 444.—THE FUNDUS OF THE HORSE.

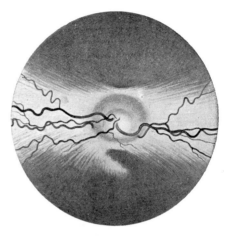

FIG. 445.—THE FUNDUS OF THE RABBIT.

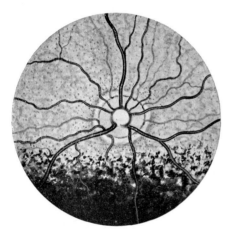

FIG. 446.—THE FUNDUS OF THE DOG.
The pale area above is the tapetum.

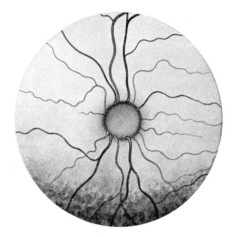

FIG. 447.—THE FUNDUS OF THE CAT.
The pale area above is the tapetum.

The (Choroidal) Tapetum may be cellular or fibrous. It may occupy the whole fundus, but more often only the upper and back portion. It is found in the mammals and in certain cartilaginous fishes (skate, shark).

Among birds, only in a few, such as the ostrich, exhibit the "eyeshine" or reflected light usually associated with a tapetum. No true tapetal structure has been established in any avian eye. The bright reflex from the ostrich eye is (according to Walls) produced by the lamina vitrea on the inner surface of choroid, which is especially thick in this animal.

The tapetum is placed just deep to the choriocapillaris, and is visible because this and the retina are devoid of pigment. Among the carnivores the tapetum is usually cellular, consisting of several layers of flattened cells. Among the herbivores and dolphins the tapetum is fibrous, i.e. composed of fine fibres, also in several layers. The tapetum reflects the light strongly, and on account of its stratified structure diffracts the light and gives rise to the different colours seen in the fundus.

In the horse the tapetum is extensive; in the lamb and ox it extends especially on the temporal side; in the goat it is quadrilateral and symmetrical round the posterior pole. It is triangular in the roebuck, the dog, and the cat.

In the dog it is usually entirely above the disc, in the cat it reaches a little below this area. It is brighter in the carnivores than in the herbivores, and is thickest in the ox.

In some animals there is also what is called a *retinal tapetum*. It is formed of crystals of guanine, and occurs in certain teleosts such as peroids (perch) and cyprinoids (gold-fish). It is typical of the bream, and in the crocodile it is of the same nature. In the crocodile the upper portion of the fundus is brilliantly white but becomes redder in the dark (Abelsdorff, 1905).

We must not forget, however, that in the higher molluscs (cephalopods) and in the bony fishes there is the *argentea* or "silvery membrane" named after the crystals which give it a silvery brightness. But this is not a tapetum, for it is placed outside the layer of large vessels and, being covered by pigment, is not seen from the interior of the eye (Ovio, 1927).

The Fundus

The Colour.—In those animals which have no tapetum the colour of the fundus comes from the blood in the choroid modified by the density of the pigment epithelium. Otherwise, it is the tapetum which is responsible for the colour.

A red colour in the fundus is seen in primates (including man, but excluding some lemurs), and also in some insectivores.

A yellow colour (principally) is seen in the lemuroids, bats, in some cats, elephants and squirrels.

A green colour is the least frequent; it is seen in some carnivora and in the ruminants, except the goat and camel, in which it is red.

In the ox the disc is pink and transversely oval. It has no physiological cup, and often remains of the hyaloid artery are seen on it. The retina is well vascularised. The fundus generally is red, but there is a large blurred green tapetum below the disc. The fundi of the other ruminants are similar, but the disc is round in the goat, semilunar in the sheep, and the tapetum is absent in the pig.

In the horse (Fig. 444) the disc also is transversely oval, and has no physiological cup. From it numerous small vessels run for a short distance only into the fundus (paurangiotic). The tapetum is greenish blue and above the disc. Generally the fundus is reddish grey, but varies with the colour of the animal. Myelinated fibres are often seen.

In the marmot and squirrel the disc forms a longish horizontal band. It is kidney-shaped in the wolf, jackal and fox. It is white in lemurs, bats, rodents, edentates, marsupials, *Echidna*; bright red in the hedgehog and mole; black or green in the galagos and loris. In the carnivores it may be white, grey, brown, maroon or red.

In the guinea-pig the disc is small, round, greyish white and placed in a dark grey retina, which is almost devoid of vessels.

In the rabbit the disc is pale pink, transversely oval, and deeply excavated. It is continued at the sides into bands of medullated nerve fibres, to which the vessels are confined (Fig. 445). There are no retinal vessels on the rest of the fundus, but in the albino rabbit the choroidal vessels show through.

In the dog the disc is round or triangular. It is characterised by a well-marked venous ring (Fig. 446). The arteries are small, cilioretinal, and leave the disc at its periphery. The tapetum is yellowish green, and for the most part in the upper part of the fundus. Remains of the hyaloid artery are not infrequently seen.

In the cat the disc is grey and round, and since the vessels leave it peripherally, it looks something like a glaucoma cup (Fig. 447). The bright reddish-green tapetum surrounds the disc and occupies the upper part of the fundus. Remains of the hyaloid artery are often seen.

In birds the fundus is difficult to see, owing to the fact that the pupil is small and is not dilated by atropin (Ovio, 1927). The disc is hidden by the pecten which is attached to it and its continuation downwards, which is known as the cauda.

In the pigeon the two foveæ are seen as dark spots.

In reptiles the disc is difficult to see owing to the small pupil. The hyaloid circulation is visible. In the crocodile the disc is black (Hirschberg, 1882; Abelsdorf, 1898).

In amphibians the circulation is visible in the hyaloid system owing partly to the great magnification produced by the lens and partly to the large size of the blood corpuscles.

In the frog the disc forms an oblique streak (see Hirschberg, 1882).

In fishes.—In the minnow the entrance of the optic nerve is marked by a round disc not well defined, which has a wing-like prolongation upwards and medially. The vessels converge on the disc and some project into the vitreous.

In the eel a disc is not seen, but the nerve entrance is marked by the point of convergence of the whitish nerve fibre bundles and the retinal vessels.

In the pike there is a worm-like streak provided with pigment, from the middle portion of which the nerve fibres radiate. No retinal vessels are seen.

The selachians have no hyaloid or retinal vessels.

Among the bony fishes many have a hyaloid network which Virchow (1881) divided into three types:

(*a*) The hyaloid artery and vein enter at the ora serrata (ganoids).

(*b*) The artery enters at the disc, and the vein leaves at the ora serrata (gold-fish).

(*c*) Both enter at the disc (eel).

In the cephalopods there are many discs, as the optic nerve enters through a number of holes (Fig. 435).

(For the most voluminous record of ophthalmoscopic examination of the fundus in many mammals, from which much of the above is taken, see Johnson, 1901, and also Prince, 1949.)

THE CILIARY BODY

In the human eye and that of the higher apes we find the ciliary body formed of two main components:

(*a*) Muscular.

(*b*) Ciliary processes (essentially vessels).

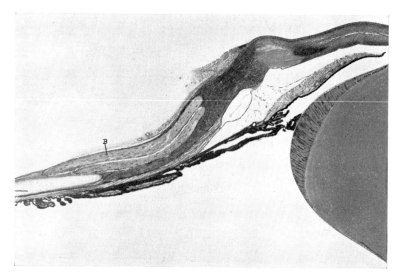

FIG. 448.—NORMAL DOMESTIC FOWL'S EYE. ANTEROPOSTERIOR SECTION.

Note especially the normal adhesion of the ciliary process to the lens pad, which largely takes the place of our suspensory ligament, the large sinus venosus scleræ, and the bone and cartilage in the sclera.

There is an analogous organ in the cephalopods, in which a structure similar to the iris is also seen (Fig. 435), but apart from this a ciliary body is only found in the vertebrates, in which, however, it varies greatly. The muscular element is the more constant.

The Ciliary Processes are absent, or practically so, in fishes and amphibians. In birds their numbers may be 200 as compared with 70 in man. They may be so large as to leave an impression on the lens. In the human the ciliary processes do not touch the lens (0·5 mm away), nor are they in contact with the iris. But in some animals such as the rabbit they are in contact, a condition which obtains in the human embryo up to the last months.

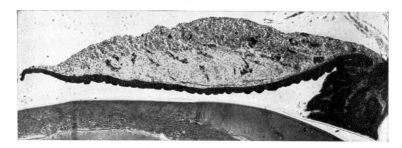

Fig. 449.—Detail of Figure 446. Iris and Lens of Domestic Fowl.

Note sphincter of iris is anterior. Note also adhesion of ciliary process to lens (in place of suspensory ligament). Compare human embryo at three months (Fig. 353).

The Ciliary Muscle.—In mammals there are at least two major components, a peripheral part of meridional fibres (Brücke's muscle), and a more central region of fibres circumferential with respect to the lens (Müller's muscle). There are also oblique fibres, and even more complex arrangements in man (see p. 69). Birds are said to exhibit both these muscles and also, anterior to them (i.e. nearer the limbus) and composed of radial or meridional fibres. However, the homology of the mammalian and avian components is uncertain, and perhaps more interesting and remarkable is that the avian ciliaris, unlike the mammalian, is largely composed of striated muscle tissue—presumably an adaptation to rapid focusing in fast-moving animals (but see below).

This passes from the deepest layers in the cornea to the anterior part of the sclera. The size of the ciliary body depends on the amount of accommodation and not on the amount of intraocular fluid. Thus in man the ciliary muscle is more developed than in other mammals. In the ass the amplitude of accommodation is 16D, in the dog 2·5 to 3·5D, and in the cat only 1D (Hess, 1913). It is feeble in herbivora and rodents, who have little power of accommodation, but well developed in diving birds and those that fly swiftly; for instance, the swallow.

In birds (and reptiles) the contraction of the ciliary and Crampton's muscles raises the pressure in the vitreous. This pushes on the lens, which, being held peripherally by the iris, can only bulge forward axially. In most birds, except the nocturnal species, the power of accommodation is very great. Hess (1913) found 40 to 50D in the cormorant.

In the bony fishes, in which there is only a rudiment of a ciliary body, there is hardly a trace of ciliary muscle. In fact some authors deny the existence of a muscle and describe a ciliary ligament which binds the ciliary body to the corneo-sclera.

Fishes whose eyes are normally fixed for near vision have to accommodate for distance. This is done by the retractor lentis muscle which pulls the whole lens backwards. In some amphibians a high degree of miosis takes the place of accommodation, while in others the lens is pulled forwards by the protractor lentis (Hess, 1913).

The ciliary muscle and that of the iris in birds and reptiles (Sauropsida) are striated, while in mammals they are not.

THE IRIS

Arthropods.—When we speak of the iris of the arthropod we mean the pigment and iridic tapetum. Each facet of the compound eye when looked at with the microscope appears to have a pupil surrounded by pigment.

Cephalopods have a real iris with pigment and a double sphincter and dilator. The pupil in the cephalopods is horseshoe-shaped, and in some species on contracting it forms a straight or curved line, which, however, remains open at the extremities. This type of dumb-bell-like pupil is also seen in the dogfish.

Vertebrates always have an iris. It is, however, rudimentary in some deep-sea fishes with telescopic eyes.

In fishes the iris has a metallic lustre owing to the crystals of guanine in the silvery membrane which extends into the iris. The same applies to the iris of cephalopods. Here the membrane is partially covered by chromatophores which give the iris its special colours.

The amphibians and reptiles have similar reflexes, but it is doubtful whether these are due to crystals of guanine, although they are present in the crocodile and chameleon.

Among birds the iris is brown in the singing varieties, yellow in the birds of prey. The herons, parrots, and pheasants have reddish irides, due to oil droplets of different refractions rather than to micro-crystals. Almost always the iris of birds has a black edge which may make the pupil appear larger than it really is.

The musculature of the iris, like that of the ciliary body, is striped in the sauropsida (birds and reptiles) and smooth in all other vertebrates.

In the fishes, amphibians, and cephalopods the muscles are rich in pigment.

In the lower animals there are no iris crypts, and the anterior epithelium is well marked.

The pupil, when constricted, is not always round; when dilated it is always more or less circular. It is round as in the human in birds, except the owl, in many reptiles and fishes, and even in some amphibians.

The pupil is oval with the long axis horizontal in the horse, ox, goat, kangaroo, and in certain fishes; oval with long axis vertical in the seal and alligator; vertical slit in the cat, fox and owl.

In nocturnal selachians, such as *Scyllium*, *Torpedo*, etc., it is a slit.

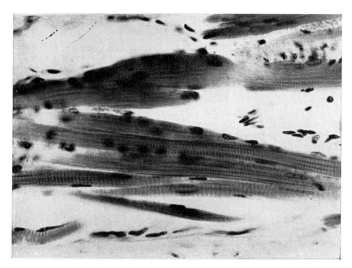

FIG. 450.—STRIPED CILIARY MUSCLE FIBRES OF FOWL.
(McDonagh and Wolff, 1939.)

There is a pupillary operculum in the skate, and in *Pleuronectes* (sole, etc.), which swim on their sides near the bottom of the sea, the pupil not only closes completely, but the upper part hangs over the lower.

In the Sauropsida the pupil is often displaced nasally and downwards (corectopia); in the amphibians downwards, and in the salamander upwards. *Gecko* has a vertical slit with irregular borders.

In some animals the pupil extends beyond the lens so that an aphakic portion is present, as obtains after iridectomy in the human. This is especially seen in some bony fishes.

It would seem that the essential structure of the adult iris in the different species of animals is determined by the embryonic ocular circulation, especially the presence or absence of a pupillary membrane and the number and position of the branches of the hyaloid artery.

The pupillary membrane exists only in mammals, who alone possess the arteriovenous anastomosis of the lesser circle. The vascular pattern of the iris is necessarily different in submammalian species. The degree of pigmentation and the shape of the pupil, however, are at any rate in part determined by function of habitat (see Mann, 1931 and 1957).

The Dioptric Apparatus

In the most primitive eyes, such as those of the worm, *Stylaria lacustris* (Figs. 421, 425), the light acts directly on the epithelial cells of which it is composed, without first passing through a dioptric apparatus.

But soon a rudimentary refractive mechanism appears. It may be a simple transparent mass secreted by the epithelial cells, or it may be the cuticle covering the eye which becomes thick and transparent, or it may be the visual cells themselves which become differentiated into bodies refracting the light so as to focus it on the visual cells proper.

In the cephalopods there is a cornea-lens. This consists of two half-spheres in contact with each other.

A transparent mass, the primitive vitreous, always fills the cavity of the eye. Generally it is secreted by the undifferentiated cells between the visual cells.

In *Phillodoce laminosa*, a worm, there is only one of these secretory cells, but it is very large (Fig. 431).

In the compound or faceted eyes each "eye" has a small transparent cornea behind which is a cone-shaped lens.

The Cornea

Vertebrates.—*The cornea* is constant in vertebrates. It is generally larger in mammals and fishes, and, relative to the bulb, smaller in birds and reptiles, larger in nocturnal than diurnal birds.

In the cat and rabbit it is one-third of the bulb, in the bat and mouse one-half of the bulb.

It is more or less flat in fishes, acuminate in nocturnal birds. In several species of parrot it forms a keratoconus, while it is also prominent in the mole. In the whale and seals there is a high degree of astigmatism. In the horse the cornea is pear-shaped, being larger on the temporal side. Generally the astigmatism is greater in eyes with an oval or slit-like pupil.

The corneal epithelium is very thick in fishes and lies almost loose and not smooth as in the human. In some terrestrial animals the superficial layers are keratinized. *Tetrophthalmus* swims on the surface of the water with half its cornea out of the water and half in. Here only the upper half is keratinized. In man the epithelium has 5 layers (Virchow, 1910) (6 according to Ciaccio, 1881), the horse 20 (Virchow, 1881), amphibians 2–4, the ox 8–10, the rabbit 6.

In the calf, sheep, guinea-pig, chimpanzee, and in many birds and fishes, the corneal epithelium is so pigmented that this can be seen with the naked eye. With the microscope, pigment can be found in most corneæ.

In some cyprinoids (gold-fish) the cornea is vascularized, in others only during embryonic life.

In man the cornea is never vascularized except in disease.

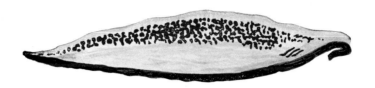

FIG. 451.—IRIS OF DOMESTIC FOWL, STAINED WITH SUDAN III, TO SHOW FAT IN THE SPHINCTER MUSCLE WHICH IS HERE PLACED ANTERIORLY (SEE FIG. 448).

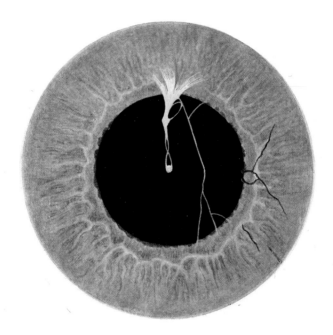

FIG. 452.—PERSISTENT PUPILLARY MEMBRANE AND TWO CAPSULO-PUPILLARY VESSELS.
(*From Mann, 1928, after Silcock.*)

In fishes and aquatic mammals the cornea is many times thicker at the periphery than at the centre.

The substantia propria in the lower vertebrates consists of regular lamellæ throughout. In man and the higher vertebrates this obtains in the central area only. Elsewhere it is broken up by the "fibrous cordage" superficially, and by elastic fibres in the deeper parts. The cornea is a powerful lens, but only in those animals which live in the air. It loses its refractive power in water. The human cornea exerts a dioptric power of over 40 dioptres, the lens only a fraction of this —perhaps 18–20 dioptres at birth, but 10 dioptres or less after 20 years.

THE LENS

Generally speaking, as we pass up the vertebrate scale the lens becomes less and less spherical, but in fishes it is nearly round and often protrudes anteriorly to be almost in contact with the cornea. This is due to the fact that the cornea has no refractive power and the lens has to make up for it. In amphibians it forms a sphere, but is flattened anteriorly. Not infrequently one finds a lenticonus anterior or posterior. This is seen especially in the falcon and finch.

Among mammals the mouse and rat have a spherical lens. In the carnivores the lens is more convex anteriorly; in the herbivores and primates it is the posterior surface which is more convex.

As regards size, the nocturnal animals have a large lens, but in the owl it is small. In some fishes it is very big (moonfish and whiting).

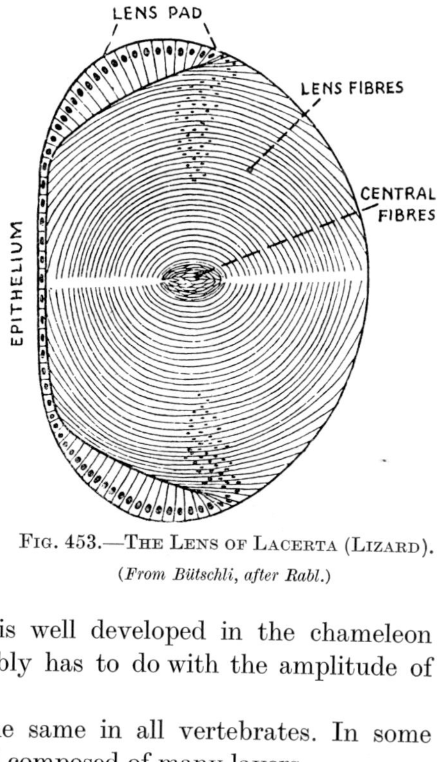

FIG. 453.—THE LENS OF LACERTA (LIZARD).
(*From Bütschli, after Rabl.*)

The nuclear zone in Sauropsida (birds and reptiles) develops in a peculiar way to form the soft lens pad (Fig. 452). This is well developed in the chameleon and lizards and is huge in birds. It probably has to do with the amplitude of accommodation.

The general structure of the lens is the same in all vertebrates. In some animals (horse) the capsule is very thick and composed of many layers.

LENS SUTURES

There are three types of suture (Rochon-Duvegneaud, 1943).

(1) *A Punctiform* central suture like a small, non-recessed umbilicus with irregular borders. It is seen in birds, some bony fishes, and reptiles, and is pro-

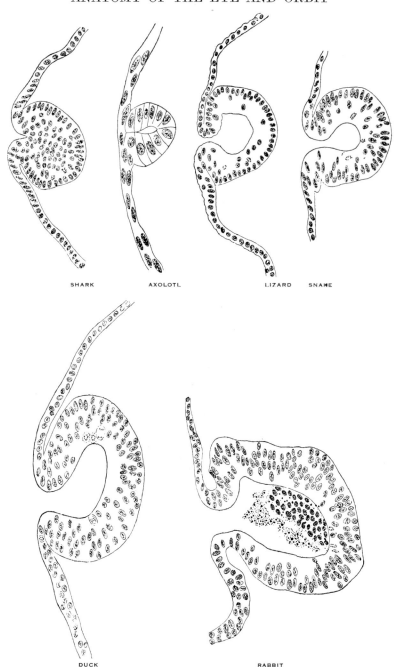

FIG. 454.—THE PRIMORDIUM OF THE LENS AT THE SAME STAGE IN DIFFERENT VERTEBRATES.
Note that the debris of cells inside the saccule occurs only in the mammal.
(*From Rabl.*)

duced by a great tapering of the lens fibres from the equator backwards and forwards so that the ends are so small that they can be accommodated in the small round suture (Fig. 456a).

(2) *A Straight Line*, often quite short. This type of suture is seen in many selachians, bony fishes, and in the rabbit, etc. It is produced by the fact that although they taper somewhat the ends are too large to end in a point suture and so they have to be accommodated on a line (Fig. 456b).

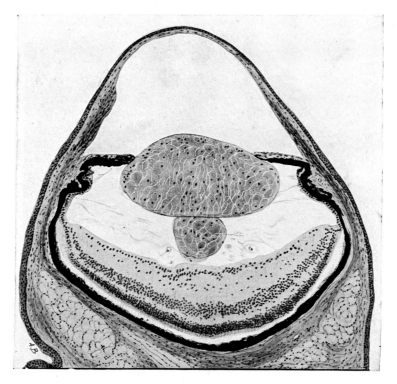

FIG. 455.—THE EYE OF A MOLE.

This presents a conical cornea with thinning of the central region and a very deep anterior chamber. There is a curious posterior extrusion of lens substance which almost touches the retina.

(From Rochon-Duvigneaud.)

(3) *Star-shaped Suture*. This type of suture is seen in mammals and especially in man. Here the ends, although there is *always* some tapering, are wider still and require more room than could be furnished by a straight line, which therefore bifurcates, producing a star with three branches (Fig. 456c). More branches are often necessary.

It will thus be seen that the usual description of the lens fibres as bands with

A.E.—32

parallel borders is incorrect. They must taper in varying degrees from the equator towards the two poles.

The multiplication of sutures—there may be six or even nine in the human—is brought about by a large number of short fibres; these stop short and create a number of secondary sutures which complicate the primary three of the newborn.

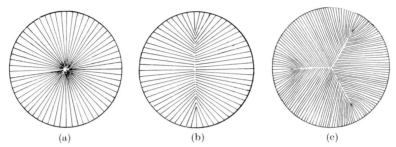

(a)   (b)   (c)

FIG. 456.—DIFFERENT TYPES OF LENS SUTURE.

(a) Lens of a pigeon, showing the sutures terminating anteriorly in a central point.
(b) Lens of a shark with a simple linear suture.
(c) Lens of a guinea pig with a triradiate suture.

(*From Rochon-Duvigneaud, 1943.*)

SUSPENSORY APPARATUS

The lens is held in position by the ciliary zonule of Zinn in all vertebrates. In birds the zonule, although less extensive, is much stronger than in mammals, and much more like a ligament between the lens and the ciliary processes (Figs. 448 and 449). In fishes it is reduced to a triangular band consisting of strong fibres which are attached to the upper pole only of the spherical lens. Fishes and amphibians have muscles in connection with the lens. Fishes have a muscle known as the retractor lentis. It runs from the falciform process, and is attached to the back of the lens below and to the nasal side of its centre. It pulls the lens laterally and backwards and is associated with accommodation. (This muscle is sometimes termed the campanula of Haller.)

In amphibians there is a protractor lentis. In the urodeles it is a filament which runs from the summit of a ciliary process to the corneoscleral junction. It is in relation with the fetal fissure, and appears to be of ectodermal origin. It pulls the lens forwards.

In the frog there are two protractor lentis muscles, one ventral, the other dorsal.

In some fishes, too, a retractor lentis arises from the region of the choroidal fissure.

ANTERIOR CHAMBER

In cephalopods the anterior chamber is very large, reaching to the back of the bulb, and since in these animals the cornea is perforate, it is filled with the fluid in which the animal lives.

But in those whose cornea is not perforate (squid, octopus) it is filled with a fluid analogous to our aqueous.

The anterior chamber is very large in birds and small in fishes. In some birds it may be 8 mm deep.

In the cat it is 2·5 times greater than in man.

THE VITREOUS

The vitreous is not entirely analogous to the primitive vitreous which fills the eye of invertebrates and which is a simple secretion (see p. 486). Little is recorded of its comparative anatomy. (See Walls, 1963.)

ORGANS OF PROTECTION

In fishes the cornea may be considered as such, for, being submerged in water, it takes no part in the refraction of the eye; so also the chitinous cornea of the ocellus and faceted eyes. Primitive eyes are protected by their position because they are covered by the epithelium forming the surface covering of the body. (See below under Eyelids, Lashes, etc.)

ORBIT

The invertebrate eye is more or less buried in ectoderm. Only in the cephalopods is there a rudimentary cartilaginous orbit.

The orbit is constant in vertebrates, but varies in size, in completeness, and in the distance apart. In relation to the size of the bulb the manatee (*Trichechus*) has a large orbit, while in the owl the eyes are, as it were, walled in.

In man and monkeys seven bones form the orbit. The inferior orbital fissure is narrowest in man and monkeys. It is much larger in other vertebrates; so large, in fact, that the lateral wall may be absent and then the orbit opens into the temporal fossa and even, in the case of the amphibia, into the pharynx. In the horse the superior orbital fissure is a long canal (Nussbaum, 1902), and in ruminants, rodents, and some other mammals it is joined to the optic foramen.

In man the lateral wall is shorter than the medial, while in some other mammals this wall, although partly membranous, is the longer.

The two bones always present are frontal and sphenoid. The ethmoid, on the other hand, does not take part in the orbit in the common mammals and often the palatine does not either.

In fishes the orbital cavity, much reduced, has accessory bones. The frontal is often divided into several parts.

In fishes the roof of the orbit is formed by 1 to 6 bones.

In *Pleuronectes* (flat fish) the two orbits are asymmetrical and of different sizes. When young, these fishes resemble ordinary fishes, and have their eyes symmetrically placed. Later, when they come to lie on one or other side at the bottom of the sea, the lower eye, which is the left in the sole and the right in the turbot, makes its way through a hole in the frontal bone to come to lie next its fellow. They thus have what is known as a *migratory eye*.

In the lower vertebrates the lacrimal bone is little developed and really only makes its appearance in reptiles.

In *Ornithorhynchus, Echidna*, the marsupials, and edentates it is a simple plate perforated by the nasal canal. In the primates it is limited to the orbit, and does not reach the surface of the face.

In the bird, lizard, crocodile and tortoise the orbits are close together. In the camel and hare there is one optic foramen for the two orbits. In man, monkeys, and nocturnal birds the orbits are anterior, in the dog and cat they are slightly lateral. In fishes, birds, ruminants, and carnivores they are lateral. In rodents, amphibia, and in some fishes they tend to be above.

The relative sizes of eye and orbit are interesting (Dexler, 1893):

Pig	·	·	·	·	1 : 2·4
Ewe	·	·	·	·	1 : 1·6
Goat	·	·	·	·	1 : 1·8
Horse	·	·	·	·	1 : 3
Ox	·	·	·	·	1 : 6

In the elephant the orbit is very large in relation to the eye (Virchow, 1881).

An Aponeurosis more or less extensive and containing muscle fibres is present in the orbital cavity. These muscle fibres in the frog help to move the bulb and the lower lid, in birds the lower lid only. This musculature is continuous with that of the maxillary region, which is directly continuous with the orbit (Burkard, 1902). In amphibians, reptiles, and birds, the muscle tissue is striped. In the frog, salamander, and lizard it forms individual muscles, which are attached to the globe and more especially the lower lid.

Sharks have a cartilaginous peduncle which passes from the back of the globe to the back of the orbit. It is expanded anteriorly, and prevents the globe from being drawn back too far—a function taken over in the higher mammals by the fascia bulbi (capsule of Tenon) and the orbital fat.

THE SCLERA

In the most rudimentary ocellus the cup of pigment alone forms the outer covering of the eye; but most of the ocelli are surrounded (besides this) by the basement membrane of the sensory epithelium or even by a connective tissue capsule.

A true sclera is present only in the vertebrates. It is fibrous in mammals, partly cartilaginous, partly bony, in the other classes of vertebrates. It is strengthened by a cartilage in birds, reptiles and fishes, and in some amphibia. Traces are also found in some lower mammals (monotremes). The cartilage has the form of a cup perforated by the optic nerve.

In bony fishes and birds (Figs. 448, 459) the sclera is strengthened by cartilage and bone. In fishes there are usually two lateral lamellæ of bone, but these may be joined and form a ring (as in tunny and sword-fish).

In birds there is a posterior bony cup and an anterior intrascleral ring.

Eyelids

Lids are found only in vertebrates. *Fishes*, owing to the fact that they live in water, have no, or only rudimentary, lids, which are in any case immobile. Among the sharks, the lids are more developed. The upper is the larger, while the nictitating membrane does the work of the lower (Harman, 1899). In *reptiles* there are many varieties of lids.

In *chelonians* they are thick and only slightly mobile, in *lizards* thin, and usually only the lower one is mobile. In the chameleon they are well developed, but joined so as only to leave a small circular orifice between them.

In the slow-worm, and other limbless lizards, the lower lid is transparent at the centre, and is the only mobile one.

It is also transparent in the geckos, but here it is adherent to the upper lid, as in serpents.

In the snakes the eye is covered by the lower lid, which is transparent, and forms a "lunette" or window, through which the animal sees. Hence arose the idea that the serpent had no lids, and it is also responsible for the "fixed stare" of these animals.

In *birds* the lower lid is by far the more mobile.

In *amphibians* special glands associated with the upper lid are observable, while the lower lid and nictitating membrane were well developed. Lunettes somewhat like those in snakes are found in certain fishes, such as the eel and lamprey, but here the "lids" are not mobile, being a direct continuation of the skin and adherent to the front of the cornea.

The Tarsus.—In the higher animals the lids are strengthened by a tarsal plate, consisting not of cartilage but of dense connective tissue. Even in the dog it is only slightly marked; in birds and lizards it is formed only in the lower lid, and is entirely absent in the parrot, duck, tortoise, alligator. In the iguana and other lizards traces of hyaline cartilage occur (Cords, 1922).

The Palpebral Opening varies in size and shape. It is generally, relative to the size of the animal, smaller than the human. Only in the elephant is it relatively larger. The smallest (relatively) are found in the camel and seal.

The Tarsal Glands, which are modified sebaceous glands of the skin, are little developed in other mammals other than mankind.

It has been suggested that they represent a row of lashes which have disappeared in man, but may reappear in the condition of distichiasis when the tarsal glands are said to be absent.

Richiardi (1877) considered them absent in camels. They are replaced by the sebaceous glands in the huge caruncle of this animal, which fills the whole of the medial canthus.

In birds, only traces are found and they have the appearance of sebaceous glands of the skin, with the hairs of which they are still often found associated.

EYELASHES

Lashes are well developed, not only in primates, but also in the dog and pig. They are absent in the cat. Traces are found in the ostrich and vulture, where they are formed of rudimentary feathers. In the horse they are absent in the central portion of the upper lid.

Eyebrow.—The eyebrow is found not only in man, but in the higher apes. In the cat it is represented by a few long hairs, and in the camel there is a similar formation below the lower lid.

THE PALPEBRAL MUSCLES

Lid movements are usually accomplished by the orbicularis and levator palpebræ superioris. But in sharks, amphibians and snakes there is no orbicularis. In the elephant there is a depressor palpebræ inferioris (Virchow). In the aquatic mammals there is a muscle in the form of a tube which is distributed all round the lids—in fact, a dilator rimæ palpebrarum (Stannius, 1839; Virchow; 1881).

Nonstriated muscle was found by Müller (1872) in human lids, and above the inferior orbital fissure, here mixed with elastic fibres. In other mammals it is much better developed, forming an orbital muscle which may act as antagonist to the retractor bulbi. All these are supplied by the sympathetic. The orbital muscles are striated in lower animals, nonstriated in mammals, but appear to have a common origin from the periorbital aponeurosis (Groyer, 1903).

The palpebral or tarsal muscles of Müller, nonstriated in man, are striated in aquatic mammals. These arise with the recti, which divide into two—a part going to the eye, the other to the lids. But in most mammals the lid portion is nonstriated.

In mammals also parts of the tarsal muscles enter the nictitating membrane. If nonstriated, they have a sympathetic nerve supply; but when striated, they are innervated by the nerves of the adjacent extraocular muscles.

Lashes, unlike ordinary hairs, have no arrector pili muscles as a rule, but Zietschmann (1904) found traces in the horse and pig.

The orbicularis is considered a cutaneous muscle, but in man it is independent of the other facial muscles, while in lower animals its common origin with these is more evident. In the lower animals the orbicularis hardly extends beyond the orbital margin.

In birds (Riehl, 1908) the orbicularis, levator, and depressor of the lids are nonstriated.

The Conjunctiva

The conjunctiva in fishes is cutaneous. Lymph nodes have been noted in the calf, dog and pig. The horse has many "lymphoid" papillæ.

Sweat glands have been described in the bulbar conjunctiva of the goat, pig, and ox. The utricular glands of Manz at the limbus have been seen in the pig, ox, lamb, and fox, and have also been described in man (Manz, 1859). Recent monographs, such as Walls (1963), ignore these structures.

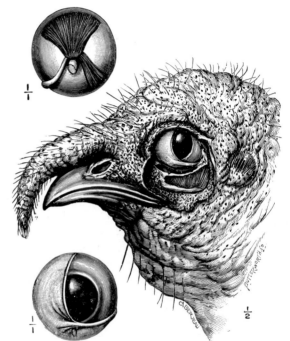

FIG. 457.—Head of Turkey.

The insets show the pyramidalis and quadratus, also the termination of the tendon in the nictitating membrane. The relation of the tendon is also shown in the large figure.

(*From Bland Sutton, 1920.*)

Visible Pigmentation of the conjunctiva near the corneal margin is present in many animals. Müller (1872) found ramifying pigment cells which appeared possessed of remarkable contractile powers.

In the Japanese and Chinese (Steiner, 1923), the bulbar conjunctiva is always more or less pigmented. This pigmentation increases with age and in those who are much exposed to bright sunlight. It is even more marked in negroid peoples.

The Nictitating Membrane, or third eyelid, is conjunctival in origin. It is best marked in mammals, especially the Herbivora, and in Sauropsida, and Amphibia. Generally speaking, one finds this membrane less developed, as the hand is more able to wipe the eye (Ovio, 1927). Thus it is well developed in the ungulates, less so in carnivores. In man and other primates it is absent, but some, for instance the chimpanzee, have one. In man it is represented by the semilunar fold. Usually it is placed at the medial angle of the eye, and extends vertically. It passes laterally somewhat obliquely in front of the eye. In the frog and the shark the nictitating membrane is inferior, and passes upwards in front of the eye, like the curtain of the ancient Greek theatre (Hirschberg, 1882).

In bony fishes the nictitating membrane is on the temporal side.

The nictitating membrane in many animals contains a plate of cartilage, which is especially big in the large Herbivora. Traces of this have been seen in man, more especially in the dark races (Giacomini, 1887).

Elastic fibres are very abundant in the nictitating membrane. The margin is often pigmented, and consists of a special band of elastic tissue, the limbus marginalis, which Kajikawa (1923) believes holds the membrane in place without muscular action when in front of the eye, as obtains in the tendons of the extremities in birds.

In birds and some amphibians such as the frog, the nictitating membrane when stretched becomes transparent in the centre, forming a sort of window through which the animal can see.

In birds and reptiles, but best developed in the former, the nictitating membrane is controlled by two special muscles, the pyramidalis and the quadratus, which, with the retractor bulbi, are supplied by the abducent nerve.

The quadratus arises from the sclera, behind the tendon of the superior rectus, passes downwards, and ends above the optic nerve in a tendinous loop through which the pyramidalis passes.

The pyramidalis, smaller than the quadratus, arises from the sclera below and passes upwards. It ends in a tendon which curves round the lateral side of the optic nerve, then above it, to pass through the tendon of the quadratus. It continues on, and is attached to the nictitating membrane near the medial angle of the eye. The membrane may, in fact, be regarded as the expanded tendon of the pyramidalis. In the tortoise these muscles are present, but much reduced. In the frog, the membrane is drawn up by the retractor bulbi muscle. In mammals, it has no connection with any muscle. Here movement of the membrane is affected by simultaneous retraction of the globe. The cartilage which it contains, and which is prolonged backwards, in the form of a tongue-shaped process, is in contact with a special mass of orbital fat. As the globe passes backwards the membrane is prevented from doing likewise, and so it naturally covers more and more of the eye.

The Lacrimal Caruncle is found in nearly all mammals, but is almost always larger than in man, and especially so in the camel, where it fills the whole of the medial angle of the eye. In the dog, the lacrimal caruncle (as in man) contains many accessory lacrimal glands, and the deeper layers of the epithelium are pigmented.

THE LACRIMAL ORGANS

The Harderian Gland occurs in all vertebrates except primates. It opens by two ducts on the nasal side of the conjunctival sac, and secretes an oily (Cetacea) or a mucous material. It is large in mammals, especially in the Herbivora. It is rudimentary in the lower apes, but is absent in the anthropoids as in man, in whom, however, it may be found, rarely (Giacomini, 1881). When the lacrimal gland is well developed Harder's gland is poorly developed and vice versa (Wiedersheim, 1898).

Fishes and aquatic amphibians have no lacrimal organs, the eyes being bathed by the surrounding media.

The first rudiment of a gland appears in amphibia between the conjunctiva and the skin of the lower lid. In the tortoise there is one gland for the two eyes. In snakes the lacrimal gland is absent, but the Harderian gland is large and is at the medial angle or sometimes surrounds the globe. In certain snakes (Thyphlopidæ) it practically fills the orbit, being ten times bigger than the eye, which is rudimentary. In birds, also, the gland is very big.

THE LACRIMAL GLAND

The lacrimal and Harderian glands have a common origin in a single gland situated in the lower lid. The medial part produces the Harderian gland, which tends to remain in its original position, while the lacrimal gland tends to move towards the lateral canthus, then to the upper lid. Its origin from the lower lid is, however, seen by some of the ducts which always open under this.

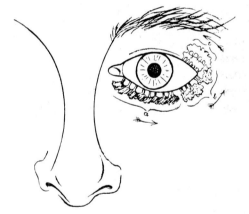

FIG. 458.—DIAGRAM TO ILLUSTRATE EVO-LUTIONARY MIGRATION OF THE LACRIMAL GLAND.

(From Whitnall, after Wiedersheim.)

Thus the rudiment in the lower lid of amphibia is really the rudiment of both lacrimal and Harderian glands.

In the newt (Triton), this rudiment is more developed towards the nasal side, and forms a rudimentary Harderian gland. Also in this animal a rudimentary lacrimal gland is developed on the temporal side.

In birds the lacrimal gland is placed at the lateral angle.

In the rabbit the lacrimal gland is partly in the upper lid, but mostly in the lower.

The tortoise, unlike other aquatic animals, has a large lacrimal gland situated posteriorly. This is due to the fact that the tortoise crosses dry sandy tracts when it wants to lay its eggs, and has to keep its eyes as moist as usual.

In the whale the secretion is fatty, like that of the tarsal glands.

In man the lacrimal ducts open on the conjunctiva.

In the tortoise, bird, rodent, and sheep the ducts unite to form one, and open in the lower lid.

In the primates there are several ducts which open mainly in the upper lid, but some always open under the lower.

The lacrimal organs are supplied by the second trigeminal division in all animals up to the mammal. In mammals the main supply comes from the first trigeminal division, indirectly also from the second.

The lacrimal secretion is watery or mucous, the Harderian secretion being oily. In some ungulates—pig, sheep, goat—and in the dog it is mucous. The Harderian gland is sebaceous (Wendt, 1877) in marine and "lower" land animals, becoming more like the lacrimal secretion in "higher" mammals.

The lacrimal gland is, in fact, a modified skin gland. In *Spelerpes*, a salamander, it is continuous with these.

In snakes, which have a large lacrimal gland, the ducts open into the mouth— hence the gland is salivary in function.

The Lacrimal Passages

Generally smaller than in man, they are absent in the turtle (Sardemann, 1884), seal, hippopotamus and elephant.

There is a single passage in the rabbit, pig and sheep, and double, as in man, in many other mammals.

Lacrimal papillæ are found only in man.

In the pig the canaliculi lie in bony canals in the lacrimal bone.

In the ophidia the lacrimal passages open into the mouth.

The Orbital Muscles

Poorly developed in the invertebrates, they are will marked in the vertebrates. In the invertebrates there are rudimentary muscles in relation to their ocelli.

Crustaceans and molluscs have mobile eyes on stalks.

Cophilia, a phyllopod crustacean, has a mobile retina.

Daphnia has a single median eye 0·1 mm in diameter formed by a number of ommatidia. This eye is provided with four muscles resembling our recti, which keep it in a constant state of vibration and move it in various directions.

In vertebrates there are 4 recti, 2 obliques, and usually a retractor.

The muscles are relatively small in birds, and the eye relatively little mobile, for the animal moves its head instead.

Thus also there is little mobility in fishes, reptiles, and amphibia, except aquatic turtles, sharks, and a teleost, *Periophthalmus*, the mud-skipper.

In fishes and birds they may be very oblique and often almost at right angles to the optic nerve.

In the bony fishes the muscles a short distance from their origin are placed in a canal.

The two oblique muscles form an almost complete girdle round the globe. In man they are inserted behind the equator. In other animals the insertion tends to be in front of this.

In most vertebrates, too, they have their origin close together near the front of the orbit. The reflected portion of the superior oblique is thus the original muscle, and is fleshy in many mammals. The trochlea is developed, as the origin comes to be placed farther back, to retain the direction of pull. In mammals there is a posterior attachment and a trochlea.

The two obliques cross the recti, sometimes between them and the globe, sometimes outside them.

In man the superior passes inside, the inferior outside, the corresponding rectus. In fishes both obliques are outside, In birds, and in the elephant and chimpanzee, the inferior oblique is outside; but in other mammals usually inside.

In the tiger the obliques split to enclose the corresponding rectus. In the lion only the superior does this.

The retractor bulbi (choanoid muscle) is well developed in the large Herbivora, but is also found in the tortoise, lizard, and amphibians. It is absent in birds and snakes, man, and the higher apes.

This muscle, which has the form of a cone, arises at the apex of the orbit and surrounds the back of the globe to the equator. It has a tendency to be divided into several portions; thus in the whale there are two, and in the amphibians three portions. It is supplied by the abducent nerve.

The main function is to retract the globe. It may support the globe in those animals which hang their heads for hours, and prevent the congestion which would otherwise result. In man, Grimsdale (1921) ascribed this function to the tonic action of the recti. In man, also, this muscle is missing, but Nussbaum (1902) found a trace.

THE ORBITAL VESSELS

In mammals, the general tendency is for the eye to be supplied by the external carotid; but as we ascend the animal scale, more and more comes from the internal carotid.

In the dog there are two ophthalmic arteries, one from each source, with an anastomotic branch between them.

In man the ocular and orbital vessels come from the internal carotid. We must not, however, forget the recurrent lacrimal artery, which is an anastomosis between the lacrimal derived from the internal carotid and the middle meningeal, which comes from the external. This branch may enlarge and take the place of the ophthalmic, thus reproducing the condition in the lower mammals.

A Hyaloid Artery is constant in mammals, but tends to disappear later than in man, and remnants are more commonly found. In the cat, for instance, it remains until one month after birth, and in the mole the hyaloid artery is permanent (Ciaccio, 1881).

The Retinal Vessels.—The central vessels usually pierce the sheaths of the optic nerve nearer the globe than in man.

The Ciliary Vessels are usually more important in the supply of the retina than in man, and often the central vessels are so small as to be negligible. Indeed, it is disputed whether the dog, cat and fox have an arteria centralis. Occasionally, while at the nerve head no arteria centralis was seen, a very small vessel was found farther back in the centre of the nerve (Wolff and Davies, 1931.)

In the dog, we found the retina supplied by cilioretinal vessels only. These pierce the *sclera* (not the nerve sheaths), and enter the nerve at the level of a ridge of retinochoroidal pigment, i.e. necessarily in the globe.

A central retinal vein, on the other hand, may be present for a very short distance only, but it also leaves the nerve inside the globe. In no case did we see the main retinal vessels cross the subarachnoid space, as they do in man.

The depth to which the retinal vessels penetrate into the retina varies. In man they reach the periphery of the outer nuclear layer, i.e. just into the outer plexiform layer. In the lower animals they penetrate less deeply. In the cat, for instance, only to the ganglion layer; in the horse and rabbit they are confined to the nerve fibre layer.

Mann (1928) found that rodent embryonic retinal vessels form a membrana vasculosa retinæ. Later the vessels sink in to become partially embedded in the nerve fibre layer.

Regarding the amount of retina which is vascularised, Leber (1903) makes the following classification:

1. *Holangiotic* (ὅλτς = entire).—Entirely supplied by vessels, as in the primates, some insectivores, carnivores, ungulates, pig, some rodents, marsupials, pinnipeds (seals and walruses).

2. *Merangiotic* (μέρος = partly).—Partly supplied with vessels, as in the rabbit and hare. The vessels are limited to the areas of the medullated nerve fibres (Fig. 445).

3. *Paurangiotic* (παῦρος = small). Slightly supplied with vessels, as in the bat, horse (Fig. 444), elephant, guinea-pig. The vessels are very small, and extend only a small distance from the disc.

4. *Anangiotic.*—The retina contains no vessels, as in the rhinoceros, porcupine, *Echidna*, a monotreme.

In the agouti, a rodent which has a retina almost anangiotic, and in some marsupials there is a cone which is characteristic of the reptiles. In the other anangiotic animals, one often finds a capillary vascularisation of the disc which may be visible ophthalmoscopically, and which is analogous to the cone of reptiles or the pecten of birds (Johnson, 1901; Mann, 1928).

THE RETINAL VESSELS

True retinal vessels are found only in mammals.

In the lower vertebrates, except the eel and a few others, the retina is avascular. It is the fate of the hyaloid system which determines the final method by which the retina gets its nourishment.

The retina may, in fact, be nourished in four ways (Mann, 1964):

1. A completely avascular retina, the blood-supply being entirely from the choroid (avascular type).

2. An avascular retina associated with a pecten projecting from the optic disc (pecten type).

3. An avascular retina supplied by vessels lying on its inner surface (membrana vasculosa retinæ type).

4. A vascular retina supplied by vessels ramifying in its substance.

1. *The Avascular Type* (without a pecten or its homologue) is found in many species; for instance, in certain fishes, reptiles, and mammals.

In the reptiles of this group there is, however, often a trace of a rudimentary pecten. Thus in the crocodile there are a few capillaries and some pigment in the nerve head.

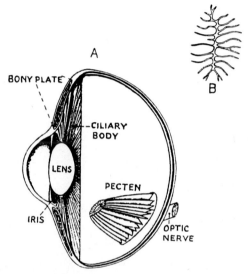

Fig. 459.—A = Vertical Section of the Temporal Half of the Eye of the Ostrich (Struthio camelus). B = Transverse Section of the Pecten.

(*From Butschli.*)

Among mammals the avascular retina is seen in the monotreme (*Echidna*); edentates (hairy armadillo); rodents (Brazilian porcupine, common guinea-pig, and chinchilla). Sometimes in ungulates and Chiroptera (rhinoceros and Australian fruit bat) (Johnson, 1901).

Most of these animals have a capillary vascularisation of the nerve head, which is visible ophthalmoscopically, and a visual acuity which does not reach a high standard.

2. *The Pecten Type* is seen in animals of a high degree of visual acuity.

The pecten is best developed in birds, but it has homologues in the cone of reptiles and the processus falciformis of certain fishes.

The Pecten of Birds (Figs. 459, 460) is a triangular pleated membrane, which extends from the optic disc (and cauda), which it covers, forwards for a variable distance into the vitreous. It is composed of a loose and folded connective tissue richly supplied with vessels and completely covered with pigment. It is this that gives it a velvety appearance.

In some birds, such as the swan and duck, it touches the lens; in others, especially in some nocturnal species, it is often rudimentary.

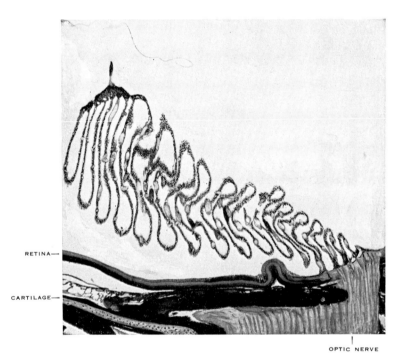

RETINA—

CARTILAGE—

OPTIC NERVE

FIG. 460.—THE PECTEN OF THE FOWL.

It has much the structure of ciliary process—vessels covered by epithelium and pigment.

(*McDonagh and Wolff, 1939.*)

The pecten is an ectodermal structure which is secondarily vascularised.

The *function* is essentially nutritive, taking the place of the retinal arteries which are absent in birds. Some hold that it has erectile properties, and thus offers a defensive mechanism against too strong light.

Kajikawa (1923) held that the pecten regulates the tension (thus a capillary venous reservoir), the secretion, and the temperature of the eye, especially at high altitudes (thus a heat radiator).

The pecten is always attached to the lens, although this may in some cases be by very fine fibrils only.

The Cone of Reptiles is analogous to the pecten of birds, but instead of being triangular, it is a cone-shaped projection from the disc. It is well developed in the lizard and chameleon, and rudimentary in the tortoise and serpent. It is also ectodermal in origin, being formed by a vascularisation of Bergmeister's papilla, which has grown forward into the vitreous.

The Processus Falciformis of fishes is a filamentary process which is probably homologous with the pecten. It passes from the disc to the back of lens, where it spreads out to form an enlargement called the *campanula of Haller*. This contains muscle fibres which form an ectodermal retractor lentis muscle.

It is also a vascular organ, but covered by epithelium. It is derived from the lips of the optic fissure, thus ectodermal, and is secondarily vascularised.

3. *The Membrana Vasculosa Retinæ Type.*—Here, branches of the hyaloid artery spread out over the *surface* of the retina without actually entering its substance. Ophthalmoscopically, they appear to be retinal vessels, but their true nature is found on microscopic section (Hirschberg, 1882).

This type is best seen in snakes, but is also found in amphibians (frog) and ganoid fishes (*Amia calva*).

In the embryos of certain rodents a similar condition obtains, while in the adult white rat the vessels sink to some extent into the nerve fibre layer, and thus form a link between this and the following type (Mann, 1929).

4. *The Arteria Centralis Retinæ Type* is typical of the primates. It will be remembered that this form of blood-supply develops in the first place like the pecten, i.e. by a vascularisation of Bergmeister's papilla. But instead of being confined to this, vascular buds grow out into the retina (see p. 454).

THE UVEAL VESSELS

The choroidal vessels are much the same throughout the vertebrates, except that in the bony fishes a great thickening of the choriocapillaris posteriorly forms the choroidal "gland".

The iris vessels, however, show many variations (see Mann, 1929 and 1931).

IN FISHES the iris is usually supplied by two anterior ciliary arteries, which run in the horizontal meridian towards the pupil, round which they form an arterial circle. The venous drainage lies deep, obscured by the silvery membrane (argentea).

IN AMPHIBIANS, also, the arteries are superficial. They enter the iris at irregular points, and run circumferentially. The veins are deep. Both arteries and veins are often obscured by pigment.

IN REPTILES the arteries, inferior and temporal, constantly enter the iris at six and eight o'clock, and then run circularly at the periphery of the iris. Often a superficial set of radial veins is also found.

In snakes, however, there is an irregular network of vessels.

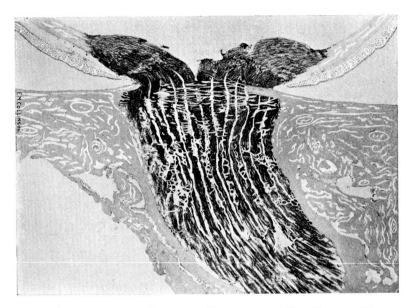

FIG. 461.—ANTEROPOSTERIOR SECTION OF NERVE-HEAD OF DOG (STAINED WEIGERT).

Note.—Normal medullation of nerve-head. Unlike when this occurs in the human as an abnormality, the fibres are medullated in region of lamina cribrosa.

BIRDS have deep circular arteries with superficial radial veins, and often a dense capillary plexus.

IN MAMMALS only is there a superficial system formed by the pupillary membrane. Hence only in mammals are there direct arteriovenous anastomoses in the

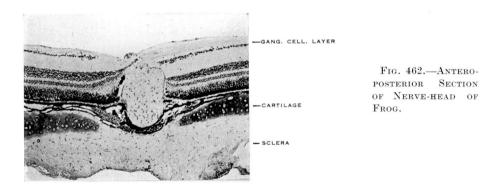

FIG. 462.—ANTEROPOSTERIOR SECTION OF NERVE-HEAD OF FROG.

region of the lesser circle. The greater circle often lies at the base of the iris, not, as in man, in the ciliary body. Also the ciliary processes tend to be in contact with the back of the iris.

In mammals generally (as opposed to man) the vorticose veins have their exit in front of the equator. Anterior to the vorticose veins, and not far from the corneo-scleral margin, the ciliary veins form an intrascleral circular anastomosis known as the circle of Hovius (Leber, 1903), well developed in the seal and porpoise. It drains into the vorticose veins, and may replace partly the anterior ciliary veins and the sinus venosus scleræ.

THE OPTIC NERVE

There is no optic ganglion in the vertebrates, such as is present in the invertebrates (Fig. 435).

In the vertebrates the nerve fibre layer of the retina is directly continuous with the optic nerve.

The form and structure of the optic nerve vary much, depending essentially on the number of fibrous partitions. In some the septa are absent, and then the nerve may be in the form of a ribbon; for instance, in the sword-fish and cartilaginous fishes.

In the eel a single partition divides the nerve into two.

According to Deyl, 1895, the higher the species of animal the more developed the framework. But Greeff (1900) recorded many exceptions to this.

THE CHIASMA

The chiasmal crossing is characteristic of the vertebrates; in *Myxine*, a cyclostome, it is actually in the brain substance. Below the mammals the crossing is complete. In the bony fishes there is a simple crossing, one nerve, usually the right, passing dorsal to the other.

In the herring one nerve passes through the other. In the parrot-fish each nerve divides into two, the halves crossing like two fingers of one hand with two of the other (Fig. 463).

In most reptiles and amphibians the nerves divide into many bundles, which, however, cross completely, likewise in birds.

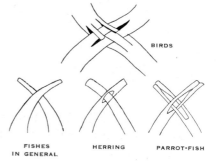

FIG. 463.—THE CHIASMAL CROSSING.
(*L.W., after Ovio.*)

In all mammals, except monotremes, a variable fraction of the optic fibres do not cross. Approximately, the less lateral the eyes are directed, and the more nearly they approach a completely forward gaze, as in man and other primates, the greater the proportion of fibres which do not cross—50% in man. About 15% are ipsilateral in Equidæ, whose laterally directed eyes permit a degree of panoramic vision. In Carnivora 25–30% are ipsilateral, permitting a considerable degree of binocular vision. (See Walls, 1963.)

A.E.—33

THE LATERAL GENICULATE BODY

The beginning of a lateral geniculate body is seen in the cyclostomes. It is small in most fishes, but shows better development in the teleosteans (Kappers, Huber and Crosly, 1936). In the amphibians, reptiles, and birds, it is still small, and does not send any fibres to the cortex (Smith, 1919).

In mammals it reaches its full development. It consists essentially of two nuclei which are dorsal and ventral in the primitive animals. It represents, in fact, the whole of the lateral geniculate body of the lower animals. As we pass up the scale the dorsal nucleus becomes more important, and the lateral geniculate body rotates so that what was dorsal becomes lateral or sometimes anterior. In the primates the ventral nucleus is practically non-existent (Clark, 1932), and only the dorsal nucleus is known to be cortically represented.

The ventral nucleus usually receives crossed fibres only, gives off the superior brachium, and is connected with the reflex centres of the midbrain (see Woollard, 1926). The retinal projection to the ventral, or pregeniculate, nucleus is in mankind said to be bilateral, but some observers deny that any optic nerve fibres reach it.

Minkowski showed that enucleation of the eye in man, cats, and monkeys (all having a partial crossing in the chiasma) results in the degeneration of certain layers or zones of both lateral geniculate bodies. He concluded that the crossed and uncrossed fibres go to alternate layers. (See Minkowski, 1913, 1920, and p. 358.)

In the human lateral geniculate body, as in that of monkeys, six laminæ are found. The two superficial ones are formed of large, deeply staining pyriform cells, from the deep aspect of which long branching processes arise, while the four deeper laminæ are composed of medium-sized cells, triangular and fusiform in shape, and fairly closely packed together (Clark, 1932). A great volume of work on the lateral geniculate nucleus has been recorded, chiefly in primates and common experimental animals. For some introductory references see p. 358.

PARIETAL AND PINEAL EYES (Figs. 464 *et seq.*)

Parietal and Pineal Eyes are very similar and closely associated.

In cyclostomes two diverticula, associated topographically with the epiphysis or pineal, grow from the most caudal limit of the diencephalon, at its junction with the mesencephalon. They are the sole survivors of paired visual organs which are considered to have been present near the dorsal midline of the head in pro-vertebrate forms. They reach the surface in cyclostomes, but are not arranged as a pair, being both in the midline. They are:

(*a*) The epiphysis or pineal body, connected with the posterior commissure.

(*b*) The parietal or parapineal body, placed anterior to the above and connected with the habenular commissure.

Now, while these outgrowths are usually glandular, they may develop into eyes which show variable differentiation.

The Parietal Eye is found in certain saurians (reptiles and birds). It lies under the skin in the parietal foramen, which is analogous to our anterior fontanelle. It is a closed vesicle, which is connected to the habenular commissure by a band known as the parietal nerve.

The eye structure is best seen in the primitive reptiles. In the lizard, *Lacerta ocellata*, for instance, there is a lens and behind it a cavity filled with a liquid like the vitreous, also a retina in which the rods and cones can be distinguished and a trace of a choroid. The pigment it contains has been noticed to move under the influence of light.

This eye is poorly developed in the ordinary lizards, it is absent in gecko, and is only seen during embryonic life in other saurians. In these latter, in fact, the parietal eye disappears more or less completely; it degenerates, alters; and is penetrated by fibrous partitions and vessels, which mask its primitive structure, and it is in the latter condition that we find the pineal body in all other vertebrates.

The considerable size of the parietal foramen in many fossil reptiles makes it probable that in them the parietal eye was of great functional importance; the pineal or parietal eye of living species, however, plays a very small role in vision.

The Pineal Eye is much like the parietal. The lamprey, a cyclostome, has both a parietal and a pineal eye.

The pineal eye, too, is placed under the skin, through the transparency of which it is visible. It develops from the extremity of the pineal gland, and is connected to the posterior commissure by the pineal nerve. In it there is a kind of retina, with sensory cells and calcareous nodules in place of pigment.

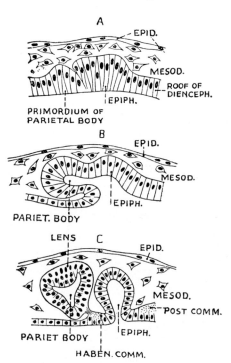

FIG. 464.—THE DEVELOPMENT OF THE PARIETAL EYE AND EPIPHYSIS (PINEAL) OF THE EMBRYO LIZARD (LACERTA).

A = embryo of 3-mm section through the roof of the diencephalon, showing primordium of epiphysis and parietal organ. B = somewhat later. C = the parietal organ and epiphysis have separated and the nervus parietalis has formed.

(*From Bütschli, after Novikoff.*)

In elasmobranch fishes the glandular pineal body itself has a bony stalk, and is placed in the parietal foramen under the skin. In the young frog, only, a pineal eye is found which degenerates later.

It is probable that the pineal gland of vertebrates is derived from paired symmetrical organs which have fused and which correspond to the distal eyes of the *Salpa* (Todaro, 1875). This is a swimming member of the sessile tunicates, which include the ascidians or sea-squirts, forms probably close to the origin of chordates.

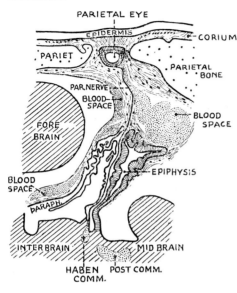

FIG. 465.—MEDIAN SECTION THROUGH THE HEAD AND PARIETAL EYE OF THE ADULT LIZARD (LACERTA AGILIS).

(From Bütschli, after Novikoff.)

In *Petromyzon* the pineal apparatus is at first paired and symmetrical, and later one of these develops into the pineal organ, while the other becomes the parapineal or parietal organ, which is placed in front of the other.

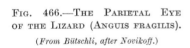

FIG. 466.—THE PARIETAL EYE OF THE LIZARD (ANGUIS FRAGILIS).

(From Bütschli, after Novikoff.)

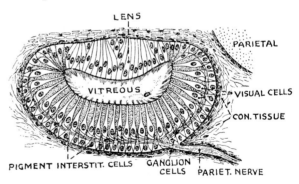

In no species possessing such median eyes in a functional state have any traces of ocular muscles, or indeed any accessory ocular structures, been observed. It is probable, therefore, that the mode of visual information provided by pineal and parietal eyes has always differed from that mediated by the lateral pair of eyes.

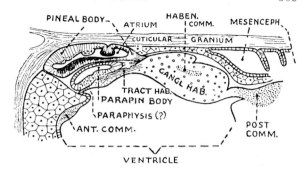

FIG. 467. — SAGITTAL SECTION THROUGH THE ROOF OF THE FORE-, INTER-, AND MIDBRAINS OF THE LARVA OF PETROMYZON PLANERI TO SHOW THE PINEAL AND PARA-PINEAL ORGANS.

(*From Bütschli, after Studnitzka.*)

THE OCULOMOTOR NUCLEUS

It is a general truism that as the vertebrate animal has evolved to more and more complex forms, in some groups the eyes, which at first lie laterally, come more and more to the front of the head. The same changes occur ontogenetically in man. In the embryo the eyes are first lateral, then later swing round to the front.

Associated with these changes there are some changes in the appearance of the oculomotor complex of nuclei. It has been claimed (Brouwer, 1918 and others) that as eyes move more and more to the front in phylogenetic history, and as binocular vision is correspondingly more developed and convergence becomes more important, the median nucleus of Perlia is formed, and joins together the originally separate lateral nuclei. On the other hand, the nucleus of Edinger-Westphal, originally single and median, was regarded as showing a tendency to divide into two.

The Edinger-Westphal nucleus, which appears earlier in phylogenetic history than that of Perlia, is single in the cetacea, rodents, pinnipedia, and carnivora, and paired in the higher apes and in man. However, these facile arguments can easily be demolished by other, more extensive but less frequently quoted observations. Tsuchida (1906) found the central nucleus of Perlia absent in 20% of human midbrains, and Clark (1926), Crosby *et al* (1943), and Warwick (1954) have all found this nuclear entity most variably and in general ill-developed or absent in primates. Its association with convergence is untenable, and attempts to equate the phylogeny and ontogeny of the oculomotor complex with this function fail on topographical, comparative and experimental grounds.

THE DORSAL CROSSING OF THE TROCHLEAR NERVE (see p. 291)

The trochlear nerve arises from a nucleus directly continuous with the oculomotor. It shows, like other cranial motor nerves, a central decussation, in this case complete. It differs, however, in the position of this decussation, which is dorsal to the aqueduct, and in the dorsal emergence of the nerve, just beyond this decussation.

It supplies the superior oblique, which in gnathostomes forms the most dorsal muscle (Fürbringer, 1875).

The ontogenetic history shows that the dorsal position of the nervus trochlearis and superior oblique muscle is acquired very early in embryonic life. The superior oblique arises from the dorsal portion of the mandibular myotome. (See Pearson, 1943.) Several theories have been advanced to account for this dorsal decussation. Fürbringer (1875) considered the trochlear nerve originally the motor supply of the pineal eye.

According to Gaskell (1908), migration of certain dorsal muscles to supply the lateral eyes can be seen in certain fossil animals. Neal (1914) held that the muscle fibres of the myotome of the second somite, which is supplied by the trochlear nerve, wandered over to the opposite side, and with the formation of the head fold acquired a ventral position. All the dorsal portion of the myotome degenerated except the superior oblique. The most convincing explanation is due to Cooper (1947). By observations in human embryonic and fetal material she was able to explain the decussation by the growth mechanics of the region.

THE CILIARY GANGLION

The ciliary ganglion is essentially a relay station for the parasympathetic fibres of the oculomotor nerve.

Sensory ganglion cells (which have wandered from the trigeminal ganglion) have also been described, but must be of little importance. A highly polemical literature on the ganglion's neuronal population has been reviewed by Warwick (1954). He observed no sensory cells, but a very small number of cells which might be sympathetic were seen. As in birds (see below) the human ganglion cells are much larger than usual autonomic neurons (sympathetic or parasympathetic). They compare with somatic multipolar neurons in size (Warwick, 1954). In birds this may be associated with the striated nature of the ciliary muscle, an explanation which cannot be applied in man.

Schwalbe (1874) found that in teleosts, amphibians and reptiles, the ganglion is connected with the oculomotor, and in many species no fibres come from the trigeminal or sympathetic. Also in ganoid fishes, in selachians, and chelonians (Pitzorno, 1913), the ciliary ganglion is associated with the oculomotor. In mammals the connection with the oculomotor is constant, although the sensory and sympathetic may be absent, as is sometimes the case even in man.

Structure.—In birds (Lenhossek, 1911, and Carpenter, 1906) the cells are cerebrospinal in type and the fibres do not divide in a T-shaped manner. Pitzorno also could find no sympathetic cells in the ganglion. In the equidæ the ganglion is microscopic. In the artiodactyls, pig, boar, buffalo, goat, and in the rabbit, the ganglion is double. In birds there is only a motor and no sensory or sympathetic roots. These join the ciliary nerves.

Experimentally in the dog, cat, and monkey, the ciliary muscle was found, long ago, to contract either on stimulating the oculomotor or the short ciliaries (Hensen and Völckers, 1868). Destruction of the iris and ciliary body causes degeneration of the cells of the ciliary ganglion (see Warwick, 1954, for original studies). If the ciliary ganglion is painted with nicotine, the motor path is blocked while the cornea is not affected. This shows that it is an autonomic cell station. This experiment could not be repeated in birds, in which the ciliary muscle is striated (Langendorf, 1894; Lodato, 1910).

Embryologically.—Cells are frequently found migrating along the oculomotor to the ganglion, and some have also been described coming from the trigeminal ganglion (Carpenter, 1906; Ganfini, 1911, 1917).

The Brain

With successively more complex evolution of vertebrate types, coupled with a general increase in body size, there has been a general tendency, among the mammals especially, towards an increasing size and complexity of the central nervous system. This is particularly true of the cranial end of the neuraxis, the brain, which also becomes *relatively* large again, especially in the mammals. This text is not a suitable place to deal with the details of this process, except in a most superficial manner, but a synopsis of the larger changes, particularly in regard to vision, may be helpful.

In all vertebrates the cerebral cavity or vesicle forms, by differential growth three primary divisions, the fore-, mid- and hindbrain vesicles. The three major regions thus formed, the *prosencephalon, mesencephalon,* and *rhombencephalon,* may be associated with the three great sensory inputs: olfactory, optic and vestibulocochlear. They may be further subdivided:

1. Telencephalon—the cerebral hemispheres.
2. Diencephalon—the thalamus and hypothalamus.
3. Mesencephalon—the midbrain.
4. Metencephalon—the pons.
5. Myelencephalon—the medulla oblongata.

The Prosencephalon, by a thickening of its roof, forms the pallium, which later develops into the cerebral hemispheres, while a thickening in the floor forms a basal nucleus which will form the corpus striatum.

In the Diencephalon a thickening at the sides forms the thalamus and hypothalamus, while the roof remains thin, and is often infolded as the tela choroidea, with its choroid plexuses.

In the Mesencephalon the roof forms the two optic lobes, and in mammals the four colliculi (corpora quadrigemina), while the floor forms the cerebral peduncles.

In the metencephalon the cerebellum is developed in the roof, while the pons develops in the floor.

In the Myelencephalon the floor forms the medulla oblongata, while the roof remains thin and is often folded in its cranial half, where the choroid plexuses of the fourth ventricle develop. Thus we see that the roof of the diencephalon and that of the myelencephalon remain thin, and the vessels with which they are richly provided form the choroid plexuses. Thickenings in the roof of the former, however, form the ganglion habenulæ and the parietal and pineal organs (q.v.).

Briefly, the main differences in the major classes of vertebrates are as follows.

In Fishes.—In the central nervous system of *Amphioxus* there is a simple enlargement of the neuraxis at its anterior end. Some authors hold that one can differentiate the olfactory, trigeminal and facial nerves, but this is doubtful. In the selachians the whole of the anterior region of the brain is olfactory, which is more developed than the visual portion. The optic lobes are, however, quite large, and the optic nerve terminates in them. The pallium, the future cerebral cortex, is poorly developed. The prosencephalon is thus largely olfactory in its connections, but there are unconfirmed suggestions that other sensory pathways, perhaps including visual projections, may reach the posterior end of the large but primitive cerebral hemispheres.

In the teleosts, on the other hand, the optic lobes are larger than the olfactory part of the brain and receive many sensory paths.

The diencephalon is poorly developed in fishes, although there is a small thalamus and rudimentary geniculate bodies. The hypothalamus is relatively well formed.

The cerebellum is very small in cyclostomes, large in selachians, and very large in the teleosts. The medulla oblongata is large, owing to the great development of the nerve nuclei, especially in the trigeminal, facial, and vestibulocochlear.

From the midbrain passes the tectospinal tract, which runs to the medial longitudinal fasciculus. The midbrain is often the largest part of the brain in teleosts and has most complex connections, receiving pathways, from not only the visual organs but also almost all other sensory systems, except olfactory.

In Amphibians the olfactory region is reduced; the pallium is further developed and there is a well-established tactile projection to the forebrain. Optic connections are invading the diencephalon. There is a rudimentary thalamus. The optic lobes are fairly well developed, especially in the anura, and the optic nerve goes to them. The medulla oblongata is small, and so is the cerebellum.

In Reptiles the pallium is still further developed, and, in fact, shows the first indication of a cortex, which is olfactory. There is a rudiment of the corona radiata passing from the basal ganglion to the cortex. The cerebral hemispheres are consequently larger than in amphibians; the thalamus is also increased in relative size.

The optic lobes are large, and in the crocodile there is an indication of an inferior colliculus (posterior quadrigeminal body).

From the roof of the diencephalon the parietal eye is developed.

In Birds there is a further development of the non-olfactory areas of pallium in the cerebral hemispheres. The optic lobes are large and the thalamus small. The geniculate nuclei are well developed. The cerebral hemispheres extend back over the optic lobes. The tractus occipito-mesencephalicus unites the occipital cortex with the optic lobes, and is perhaps the first clear connection between eye and cortex. The optic fibres mostly terminate in the optic lobes, but many pass to the geniculate bodies and thalamus.

Up to this level of vertebrate evolution the optic tracts are, of course, complete in their decussation.

In Mammals the striking feature is the great development of the cerebral hemispheres. They cover the diencephalon, the midbrain, and part of the cerebellum. But the midbrain is reduced and the quadrigeminal bodies (colliculi) are smaller than the optic lobes of the lower vertebrates. It is of interest to note here that the laminar pattern of the superior colliculi, well-marked in birds, shows a progressive simplification in mammals. The precursors of the colliculi, the "optic" lobes of non-mammalian forms, function as learning regions in, for example, teleosts. In mammals, with the increasing predominance of forebrain connections, the processes of learning move into it from the midbrain level.

The diencephalon is well developed, and so are the thalamus, geniculate bodies and peduncles. The thalamus becomes a great co-ordinating and relay centre for sensory impulses.

The olfactory region varies. It is very large in edentates, still well developed in the carnivora, but much reduced in aquatic mammals.

The geniculate bodies receive few optic fibres in the lower vertebrates. Even in the lower mammals, for instance the rabbit, more go to the superior colliculi. In the primates the geniculate bodies receive more and more visual fibres (in man, at least 90%).

Up to the sauropsida (bird and reptiles) the tectum of the midbrain is not divided into two pairs of colliculi. This change from a bigeminal to quadrigeminal arrangement may be linked with increasing cochlear development.

One of the most obvious generalizations in connection with brain evolution is the progressive invasion of a largely, if not exclusively, olfactory forebrain by projections of other modalities of sensation, or rather by their connections. This process, often spoken of as telencephalization, does not imply that the sensory and accompanying motor circuits, which become established at "higher" levels, completely supplant brainstem and particularly midbrain systems of sensorimotor interaction. As has been alluded to earlier (p. 353), it is a dangerous oversimplification to think of mesencephalic visual mechanisms as purely reflex, or to consider the geniculocortical pathway of mammals as the only true "visual" system. Much current research is blurring these earlier concepts.

It is impossible to over-emphasize the importance of vertebrate emancipation from olfactory domination and the accompanying development of highly dis-criminative binocular vision. Without this, and the retention of a primitive pentadactyl fore-limb, refined by the development of opposition in the hand and supination-pronation in the forearm, the evolution of primates would have been impossible. Grafton Elliot Smith, who was Eugene Wolff's chief during his demonstratorship at University College (a period during which this book was conceived), was an outstanding proponent of the significance of vision in the evolution of mankind. For this reason the author concluded this volume with an extensive quotation from a Bowman lecture, delivered by Elliot Smith in 1928. Although some of the details of this quotation have been superseded or modified during the subsequent decades, the majority of it is here appended, for its his-torical import and in the hope that it will stimulate the reader of this, necessarily morphological text, to extend this reading to more recent observations of the complex events occurring in the structural arena of the visual system.

"In all vertebrates the nerve-fibres proceeding from the retina cross (wholly or only in part in most mammals) to the other side of the brain, where they end in two masses of grey matter—the lateral geniculate body, which is part of the thalamus, and the superior quadrigeminal body, which is part of the midbrain. The former connection is concerned with the awareness of vision, the phenomena of consciousness, and the latter (midbrain) with such unconscious functions as the reflex actions of the eye-muscles and the general musculature of the whole body.

"In mammals the lateral geniculate body, for the first time in the vertebrate series, emits a large strand of fibres (optic radiation) to provide a path for visual impulses to the cerebral cortex. But the neopallium also begins to assume some of the motor control, which hitherto has been a function of the quadrigeminal bodies.

"With the acquisition of binocular vision (in mammals such as the cat or, better, monkeys) the fibres of the optic tracts become rearranged. The fibres from the lateral part of each retina no longer cross to the other side of the brain, but become connected with the same side, so as to bring into connection the terminations of the fibres coming from the medial side of one retina and the lateral side of the other, which, in binocular vision, necessarily act together so as to merge in consciousness the two images of one object.

"But this rearrangement of the optic tracts necessarily affects the endings of these tracts in the geniculate and quadrigeminal bodies. Instead of modification of the retinal localisation in the quadrigeminal body to adapt it to the new conditions, the cerebral cortex seems more fully to usurp its motor-controlling functions. With the loss of such functions the quadrigeminal body also loses most of the direct connections with the optic tracts, and the cerebral cortex acquires a correspondingly enhanced control of the quadrigeminal body.

"In monkeys and man further profound changes occur in the whole of the visual system. A definite macula lutea develops in the retina, and each of the percipient cells in the area of acute vision transmits its impulse (indirectly) to a separate fibre of the optic nerve. In the rest of the retina and in the retinas of other mammals groups of sensory cells (rods) transmit their impulses into one granule and ganglion cell, so that there are far more percipient elements than nerve-fibres in the optic nerve. Hence, when the macula develops in monkeys and man, this small area adds a contribution to the optic nerve and tract that is out of all proportion to its size. The macular fibres form more than a third of the optic nerve, and there is added to the geniculate body a new formation as a macular receptive mechanism.

"The development of macular vision confers upon man the ability to see the world and appreciate its meaning in a way that no other living creature is able to do. His new vision depends upon powers of visual perception as distinctive as the use of articulate speech to give expression to what he sees and thinks."

BIBLIOGRAPHY

ABBIE, A. A. (1933) *J. Anat.*, **67**, 491.
—— (1933) *Brain*, **56**, 233.
—— (1934) *J. Anat.*, **68**, 433.
—— (1938) *Med. J. Aust.*, **2**, 199.
ABD-EL-MALEK, S. (1938) *J. Anat.*, **72**, 518.
ABELSDORFF, G. (1898) *Arch. Anat. Physiol. (Abt. Physiol.)*, 115.
—— (1905) *Arch. Augenheilk.*, **53**, 185.
ADACHI, B. and HASEBE, K. (1928) *Das Arteriensystem der Japaner.* Kyoto.
ADLER, F. H. (1959) *Physiology of the Eye*, 3rd ed. St. Louis: Mosby.
—— (1965) *Physology of the Eye*, 4th ed. St. Louis: Mosby.
AIZAWA, K. (1958) *Acta Soc. Ophthal., Jap.*, **62**, 2283.
ALEZAIS, M. M. and D'ASTROS, L. (1892) *J. Anat. Physiol., Paris*, **28**, 519.
ALLEN, L., BURIAN, H. M. and BRALEY, A. E. (1955) *Archs Ophthal., Chicago.*, **53**, 783.
ALPERN, M. (1969) *The Eye*, vol. 3, Ed. H. Davson, London: Churchill.
ALPERS, J. B., BERRY, R. G. and PADDISON, R. M. (1959) *Archs Neurol. Psychiat., Chicago.*, **81**, 409.
ANDERSON, D. R. (1969) *Archs Ophthal.*, **82**, 800.
ANDERSON, D. R. and HOYT, W. F. (1969) *Archs Ophthal.*, **82**, 506.
AREY, L. B. (1932) *Cytology and Cellular Pathology of the Nervous System*, vol. 2. Ed. W. Penfield. New York.
ARLT, F. (1863) *Albrecht v. Graefes Arch. Ophthal.*, **9**, 64.
ARNOLD, F. (1851) *Handbuch der Anatomie des Menschen.*, vol. 2. Freiburg.
ASCHER, K. W. (1942) *Am. J. Ophthal.*, **25**, 31.
—— (1949) *Archs Ophthal.*, **42**, 66.
ASHTON, N. (1952) *Br. J. Ophthal.*, **26**, 465.
—— (1969) *Trans. ophthal. Soc. U.K.*, **89**, 526.
ASHWORTH, B. (1973) *Clinical Neuro-ophthalmology*, Oxford University Press.
ASK, F. (1907) *Anat. Anz.*, **30**, 107.
AUBARET, E. (1908) *Archs Ophthal., Paris.* **28**, 211. (Abstr. in *Ophthalmoscope*, 1908, **6**, 900.)
AXENFELDT, T. (1907) *Berl. Versamm. ophthal. Ges.*, **34**, 300.
BACH, L. and SEEFELDER, R. (1911–12) *Atlas zur Entwicklungsgeschichte des Menschlichen Auges.* Leipzig.
BACH-Y-RITA, P., COLLINS, C. C. and HYDE, J. E. (1971) *The Control of Eye Movements.* New York: Academic Press.
BACH-Y-RITA, P. and MURATA, K. (1964) *Q. J. exp. Physiol.*, **49**, 408.
BAIRATI, A. and ORZALESI, N. (1966) *Z. Zellforsch. microsk. Anat.*, **69**, 635.
BALAZS, E. A. (1961) *Structure of the Eye.* Ed. G. K. Smelser. New York: Academic Press.
BALBUENA, B. (1930) *Bull. Soc. Ophtal. Paris*, 286.

BALLANTYNE, A. J. and MICHAELSON, I. C. (1962) *Textbook of the Fundus of the Eye.* London: Churchill.

BARBER, A. N. (1955) *Embryology of the Human Eye.* London: Kimpton.

BATINI, C. and BUISSERET, B. (1974) *Archs ital. Biol.,* **112**, 18.

BAURMANN, M. (1923;–24) *Albrecht v. Graefes Arch. Ophthal.,* **111**, 352; **114**, 276.

BEAUVIEUX, J. and RISTITCH, K. (1924) *Archs Ophthal., Paris,* **41**, 352.

BEEVOR, C. E. (1907) *Brain,* **30**, 403.

—— (1908) *Phil. Trans. R. Soc.,* **200**, 1.

BEHR, C. (1935) *Albrecht v. Graefes Arch. Ophthal.,* **134**, 227.

BELL, C. (1822–3) *Phil. Trans. R. Soc.,* Pt. 1, 289.

BENDER, M. B. and WEINSTEIN, E. A. (1943) *Archs Neurol. Psychiat.,* **49**, 98.

BERGER, E. (1882) *Albrecht v. Graefes Arch. Ophthal.,* **28** (2), 28.

—— (1887) *Beiträge zur Anatomie des Auges im normalen und Pathologischen Zustande.* Wiesbaden.

BERGSTROM, B. (1973) *Acta oto-lar.,* **76**, 162, 173, 331.

BERNHEIMER, S. (1897) *Albrecht v. Graefes Arch. Ophthal.,* **44**, 481.

BILLINGS-GAGLIARDI, S. M., CHAN-PALAY, V. and PALAY, S. L. (1974) *J. Neurocytol.,* **3**, 619.

BJÖRKMAN, A. and WOHLFART, G. (1936) *Z. mikrosk.-anat. Forsch.,* **39**, 631.

BLAND-SUTTON, J. (1920) *Selected Essays and Lectures,* 4th ed. London: Heinemann.

BOEKE, J. (1927) *Z. mikrosk.-anat. Forsch.,* **4**, 448.

BOWMAN, W. (1849) *Lectures.* London: Longman.

BOYCOTT, B. B. and DOWLING, J. E. (1969) *Phil. Trans. R. Soc.,* **225**, 109.

BRODAL, A. (1969) *Neurological Anatomy,* 2nd ed, Oxford University Press.

BRODAL, A., POMPEIANO, O. and WALBERG, F. (1962) *The Vestibular Nuclei and their Connections, Anatomy and Functional Correlations.* Edinburgh: Oliver and Boyd.

BRODMANN, K. (1900) *Vergleichende Localisationlehre der Grosshirnvinde.* Leipzig.

—— (1909) *J. Physiol. Neurol. Lpz.,* **2**, 137.

BROUWER, B. (1918) *Z. ges. Neurol. Psychiat.,* **40**, 152.

—— (1925) *J. Neurol. Psychopath.,* **6**, 1.

BROUWER, B. and ZEEMAN, W. P. C. (1926) *Dt. Z. NervHeilk.,* **89**, 9.

—— (1926) *Brain,* **49**, 1.

BRÜCKE, E. (1846) *Arch. Anat. Physiol., wiss. Med.,* 370.

BRUESCH, S. R. and AREY, L. B. (1942) *J. comp. Neurol.,* **77**, 631.

BUDGE, J. and WALLER, A. (1851) *C. r. hebd. Séanc. Acad. Sci., Paris,* **33**, 370.

BUMKE, O. and TRENDELENBURG, W. (1911) *Klin. Mbl. Augenheilk.,* **49**, 145.

BURKARD, O. (1902) *Arch. Anat. Physiol. (Anat. Abt.) Suppl.,* **79**.

BUSACCA, A. (1943) *Elements de Gonioscopia,* São Paulo.

BUSACCA, A., GOLDMANN, H. and SCHIFF-WERTHEIMER, P. (1957) *Biomicroscopie du Corps Vitré et du Fond de l'Oeil,* Paris.

BÜTSCHLI, O. (1921) *Vorlesungen über vergliechende Anatomie,* Berlin.

BUTLER, T. H. (1923) *Trans. ophthal. Soc. U.K.,* **43**, 579,627.

BUZZARD, F. (1908) *Proc. R. Soc. Med., Neurol. Sect.,* **1**, 83.

CAJAL, S. R. (1893) *Cellule,* **9**, 17.

—— (1894) *Die Retina der Wirlbeltiere,* Trans. R. Greef. Wiesbaden.

—— (1909–11) *Histologie du Système Nerveux de l'Homme et des Vertébrés.* Paris.

CALSANS, O. M. (1953) *Annls Fac. Med. Univ. São Paulo*, **27**, 3.

CAMERON, M. E. (1959) *Br. J. Ophthal.*, **43**, 471.

CAMPBELL, A. N. (1905) *Histological Studies on the Localization of Cebebral Function.* Cambridge.

CARPENTER, F. W. (1906) *Bull. Mus. comp. Zool. Harv.*, **47**, 2.

CARPENTER, M. B., NOBACK, C. R. and MOSS, M. L. (1954) *Archs. Neurol. Psychiat., Chicago*, **71**, 714.

CARPENTER, M. B. and PETER, P. (1971) *J. Hirnforsch.*, **12**, 405.

CARRIÈRE, J. (1885) *Die Sehorgane der Tiere vergliechend-anatomisch dargestellt.* München.

CASSIDY, J. V. (1952) *Archs Ophthal., Chicago*, **47**, 141.

CHACKO, L. W. (1948) *Br. J. Ophthal.*, **32**, 457.

—— (1955) *J. anat. Soc. India*, **4**, 201.

CHAN-PALAY, V., PALAY, S. L. and BILLINGS-GAGLIARDI, S. M. (1974) *J. Neurocytol.*, **3**, 631.

CIACCIO, G. V. (1873) *Memorie R. Accad. Sci. Ist. Bologna*, 3.s., **4**, 460.

—— (1874) *Moleschott's Untersuch. zur Naturlehre des Menschen u.d. Thieren.*, **11**, 420.

—— (1875;–81) *Memorie R. Accad. Sci. Ist. Bologna*, 3.s., **5**, 74; 4.s., **11**, 577.

CIBA (1965) *Symposium on Colour Vision.* London: Churchill.

CLARK, W. E. LeGROS (1926) *J. Anat.*, **60**, 426.

—— (1932) *Br. J. Ophthal.*, **16**, 264.

—— (1941) *J. Anat.*, **75**, 419.

—— (1942) *Trans. ophthal. Soc. U.K.*, **52**, 241.

CLARK, W. E. LeGROS and PENMAN, G. G. (1934) *Proc. R. Soc.*, B, **114**, 291.

COGAN, D. G. (1956) *Neurology of the Ocular Muscles*, 2nd ed. Springfield, Illinois: C. C. Thomas.

COGAN, D. G. and KUWABARA, T. (1967) *Archs Ophthal.*, **78**, 133.

COHEN, A. I. (1965;–67) *Invest. Ophthalmol.*, **4**, 433; **6**, 694.

COLONNIER, M. (1967) *J. Anat.*, **98**, 327.

COMBERG, W. (1922) *Ber. Versamm. dt. ophthal. Ges.*, **43**, 259.

—— (1924) *Klin. Mbl Augenheilk.*, **72**, 692.

CONEL, J. L. (1939–59) *Post-natal Development of the Human Cerebral Cortex.* Cambridge, Mass.: Harvard University Press.

CONTINO, A. (1907;–09) *Albrecht v. Greafes Arch. Ophthal.*, **66**, 505; **71**, 1.

COOPER, E. R. A. (1945) *Brain*, **68**, 222.

—— (1947) *Br. J. Ophthal.*, **31**, 257.

—— (1951) *J. Physiol.*, **113**, 463.

COOPER, S. and DANIEL, P. M. (1949) *Brain*, **72**, 1.

COOPER, S., DANIEL, P. M. and WHITTERIDGE, D. (1955) *Brain*, **78**, 564.

COOPER, S. and FILLENZ, M. (1955) *J. Physiol.*, **127**, 400.

COPE, V. Z. (1916–17) *Br. J. Surg.*, **4**, 107.

CORDS, E. (1922) *Z. ges. Anat. Abt. 2. Anat. Entwicklungsgesch.*, **65**, 277.

CORNEA WORLD CONGRESS (1965) London: Butterworth.

CREVATIN, F. (1903) *Anat. Anz.*, **23**, 151.

CROSBY, E. C. (1953) *J. comp. Neurol.*, **99**, 437.

CROSBY, E. C., HENDERSON, J. W. and WOODBURNE, R. T. (1943) *J. comp. Neurol.*, **78**, 441.

CROSBY, E. C., HUMPHREY, T. and LAVER, E. W. (1962) *Correlative Anatomy of the Nervous System*. New York: Macmillan.

CROSBY, E. C. and WOODBURNE, R. T. (1943) *J. comp. Neurol.*, **78**, 441.

CUNEO, B. (1904;–11) in *Traité d'Anatomie Humaine*, Ed. Poirier and Charpy, 2nd ed, vol. V; 3rd ed, vol. V, Paris.

DANIEL, P. M. (1946) *J. Anat.*, **80**, 189.

DANIEL, P. M. and PRITCHARD, M. M. L. (1957) *Q. Jl exp. Physiol.*, **42**, 237.

DANIS, P. C. (1948) *Am. J. Ophthal.*, **31**, 1122.

DARTNALL, A. T. A. and LYTHGOE, J. N. (1965) in *Ciba Symposium on Colour Vision*. London: Churchill.

DAVSON, H. (1963;–72) *Physiology of the Eye*, 2nd ed; 3rd ed, London: Churchill.

—— (1969;–74) Ed. *The Eye*, vols. I and III; vol. VI, London: Academic Press.

DEJEAN, C., HERVOUËT, F. and LEPLAT, G. (1958) *L'Embryologie de l'Oeil et sa Tératologie*. Paris.

DEWULF, A. (1971) *Anatomy of the Normal Human Thalamus*. Amsterdam: Elsevier.

DEXLER, H. (1893) *Z. vergl. Augenheilk.*, **7**, 147.

DEYL, J. (1895) *Bull. int. Acad. Sci. Prague*, **12**, 120.

—— (1896) *Anat. Anz.*, **11**, 687.

DIMMER, F. (1907) *Albrecht v. Graefes Arch. Ophthal.*, **65**, 486.

DOGIEL, A. S. (1890) *Anat. Anz.*, **5**, 483.

—— (1891) *Arch. microsk. Anat. Entwmech.*, **37**, 602.

DOWLING, J. E. and BOYCOTT, B. B. (1966) *Proc. R. Soc.*, **166**, 80.

DRAULT, A. (1912) *Traité d'Anatomie Humaine*. 3rd ed. Ed Poirier, Paris.

DUBREUIL, L. (1907) *Les Glandes Lacrymales des Mammifères et de l'Homme*. Lyon: Thèse Méd.

DUCHENNE, G. B. A. (1883) *Selections from the Clinical Works of Dr. Duchenne*. Trans. and Ed. A. V. Poore, London: New Sydenham Society.

DUCKWORTH, W. (1904) *Morphology and Anthropology*. Cambridge.

DUKE-ELDER, J. S. (1927) *The Nature of Intra-Ocular Fluids*, London: Putman.

—— (1930) *The Nature of the Vitreous Body*. London: Putman.

—— (1932) *Textbook of Ophthalmology*, vol. 1. London: Kimpton.

DUKE-ELDER, J. S. and COOK, C. (1963) *System of Ophthalmology*. Vol. III. London: Kimpton.

DUKE-ELDER, J. S. and WYBAR, K. C. (1962) *System of Ophthalmology*, Vol. II. London: Kimpton.

DUVERNEY, D. (1749) *L'Art de Disséquer Méthodiquement les Muscles, etc.* Paris.

DUVERNOY, H. (1975) *The Superficial Veins of the Human Brain*. Berlin.

DUVERNOY, H. and KORITKE, J. G. (1964) *C. r. hebd. Séanc. Acad. Sci., Paris*, **258**, 6533

—— (1968) *J. Hirnforsch*, **10**, 227.

ECCLES, J. C., ITO, M. and SZENTÁGOTHAI, J. (1967) *The Cerebellum as a Neuronal Machine*. Berlin.

ECONOMO, C. VON and KOSKINAS, G. N. (1925) *Die Cytoarchitecktonik der Hirnrinde*, Berlin: Springer-Verlag.

EHLERS, N. (1965) *Acta ophthal,*. Suppl. 81, 9.

EICHNER, D. (1958) *Z. Zellforsch. mikrosk. Anat.*, **48**, 137.

EISLER, P. (1930) *Kurzes Handbuch der Ophthalmologie*, vol. 1. Ed. Schiek and Brückner.

ELIŠKOVÁ, M. (1969) *Br. J. Ophthal.*, **53**, 326.

—— (1973) *Br. J. Ophthal.*, **57**, 766.

ELSCHNIG, A. and LAUBER, H. (1907) *Albrecht v. Graefes Arch. Ophthal.*, **65**, 428.

FAWCETT, E. and BLACHFORD, J. V. (1906) *J. Anat.*, **40**, 63.

FAZAKAS, S. (1933) *Zentbl. ges. Ophthal.*, **28**, 494.

FEENEY, M. L., GRIESHABER, J. and HOGAN, M. L. (1965) In *The Structure of the Eye.* Ed. J. Rohen, Stuttgart.

FINCHAM, E. J. (1925) *Trans. ophthal. Soc. U.K.*, **26**, 39.

—— (1929) *Trans. ophthal. Soc. U.K.*, **30**, 101.

—— (1937) *Br. J. Ophthal.*, mon. Suppl. VIII.

FINE, B. S. (1963) *Archs Ophthal.*, **69**, 83.

FISCHEL, A. (1929) *Lehrbuch der Entwicklung des Menschen.* Berlin.

FISHER, J. H. (1904) *Ophthalmological Anatomy.* London: Frowde & Hodder.

FITZGERALD, M. J. J. (1956) *J. Anat.*, **90**, 520.

FLECHSIG, P. (1927) *Meine myelogenetische Hirnlehre.* Berlin.

FORTIN, E. P. (1938) *Rétine Humaine.* Buenos Aires.

FOSTER, G. E. (1973) *Liverpool University Thesis*, Liverpool University Press.

FRANÇOIS, J. (1948) *Bull. Soc. belge Ophthal.*, **3**, 55.

FRANÇOIS, J. and NEETENS, A. (1974) *The Eye*, vol. 5, Ed. H. Davson and L. T. Graham. London: Academic Press.

FRANÇOIS, J., NEETENS, A. and COLLETTE, J. M. (1955) *Am. J. Ophthal.*, **40**, 491.

—— (1955;–56;–59) *Br. J. Ophthal.*, **39**, 220; **40**, 730; **43**, 394.

FUCHS, E. (1855;–78;–84) *Albrecht v. Graefes Arch. Ophthal.*, **2** (3), 39; **24** (3) 1; **30**, 1.

—— (1907) *Arb. neurol. Inst. wien. Univ.*, **15**, 1.

—— (1917) *Textbook of Ophthalmology.* Trans Duane, 5th English ed., Philadelphia.

FUKUDA, M. (1970) *Jap. J. Ophthal.*, **14**, 91.

FÜRBRINGER, A. (1875) *Jena. Z. Naturw.*, **9**, 11.

FUSZ, S. (1906) *Virchows Arch. path. Anat. Physiol.*, **183**, 465.

GANFINI, C. (1911;–17) *Archs ital. Anat. Embriol.*, **10**, 574; **16**, 43.

GARZINO, A. (1953) *Rass. ital. Oftal.*, **22**, 3.

GASKELL, W. (1899) *Brain*, **22**, 329.

GASKELL, W. H. (1908) *The Origin of Vertebrates.* London.

GÉNIS-GÁLVEZ, J. M. (1957) *Anat. Rec.*, **127**, 219.

GERLACH, J. (1880) *Anatomie des Auges.* Leipzig.

GIACOMINI, C. (1887) *Archs. ital. Anat. Embriol.*, **9**, 119.

GILBERT, P. W. (1957) *Contr. Embryol.*, **36**, 59.

GILLILAN, L. A. (1941) *J. comp. Neurol.*, **74**, 367.

—— (1955) *Anat. Rec.*, **121**, 466.

—— (1959) *J. comp. Neurol.*, **112**, 55.

—— (1962) *Correlative Anatomy of the Nervous System.* Ed. Crosby et al., New York, Macmillan.

GIVNER, I. (1939) *Arch. Ophthal.*, **22**, 82.

GLEES, P. (1941) *J. Anat.*, 75, 434.

—— (1961) *The Visual System*, ed. Jung, R. and Körnmuller, H., Berlin.

GLOSTER, J., PERKINS, E. and POMMIER, M. (1957) *Br. J. Ophthal.*, **41**, 103.

GOLDBERG, J. M. and WURTZ, R. H. (1972) *J. Neurophysiol.*, **35**, 542.

A.E.—34

GOLDMANN, H. (1954) *Opthalmologica, Basel*, **127**, 334.

GREEFF, R. (1900) *Handbuch der gesamten Augenheilkunde*, 2nd ed, vol. 1., Graefe and Saemisch, Leipzig.

GREEN, L. (1894) *Albrecht v. Graefes Arch. Ophthal.*, **40** (1), 1.

GRIMES, P. and SALLMANN, L. VON (1960) *A. M. A. Archs Ophthal.*, **64**, 81.

GRIMSDALE, H. (1921) *Trans. ophthal. Soc. U.K.*, **41**, 357.

GROSS, C. G., ROCHA-MIRANDA, C. E. and BENDER, M. B. (1972) *J. Neurophysiol.*, **35**, 96.

GROYER, F. (1903) *Sber. Akad. Wiss. Wien*, **112**, 51.

—— (1903) *Wien. klin Wschr.*, **16**, 959.

GRYNFELLT, E. (1899) *Annls Oculist*, **121**, 331.

GUILLERY, R. W. (1971) *Exp. Brain Res.*, **12**, 184.

—— (1974) *Essays on the Nervous System.* Ed. Bellairs, R. and Gray, E. G., Oxford University Press.

GUILLERY, R. W. and COLONNIER, M. (1970) *Z. Zellforsch. mikrosk. Anat.*, **103**, 90.

HAGEDOORN, A. (1928) *Br. J. Ophthal.*, **12**, 479.

HAMBURG, A. (1959) *Ophthalmologica, Basel*, **138**, 81.

HAMILTON, W. J., BOYD, J. D. and MOSSMAN, H. W. (1972) *Human Embryology*, 4th ed. Cambridge: Heffer.

HANNA, C., BICKNELL, D. S. and O'BRIEN, J. E. (1961) *Archs Ophthal.*, **65**, 695.

HARMAN, N. B. (1899) *J. Anat. Physiol., Lond.*, **34**, 1.

HASSLER, O. (1966) *Neurology, Minneap.*, **16**, 505.

HASSLER, R. (1955) *Sixth Latin-American Congress on Neurosurgery.* Montevideo, p. 254.

HAYREH, S. S. (1969) *Br. J. Ophthal.*, **53**, 721.

HAYREH, S. S. and VRABEC, F. (1966) *Am. J. Ophthal.*, **61**, 136.

HEESH, K. (1926) *Breithefte Dres. u. Leipz.*, **23**, 78.

HENLE, J. (1853) *Handbuch der topographischen Anatomie*, Wien.

—— (1866) *Handbuch der systematischen Anatomie des Menschen*, vol. 2, Braunschweig.

HENKIND, V. (1967) *Br. J. Ophthal.*, **51**, 115.

—— (1969) *Trans. Am. Acad. Ophthal. Oto-lar.*, **73**, 890.

HENSCHEN, S. E. (1898) *Neurol. Zentbl.*, **17**, 194.

HENSEN, V. and VÖLCKERS, C. (1868) *Experimental-untersuchungen über de Mechanismus der Accomodation*, Kiel: Schwers.

HERMAN, L. H. (1966) *Anat. Rec.*, **154**.

HESS, C. VON (1898) *Albrecht v. Graefes Arch. Ophthal.*, **35** (1), 1.

—— (1907;–08;–10) *Arch. Augenheilk.*, **58**, 182; **60**, 327; **67**, 341.

—— (1913) *Handbuch der Vergleichenden Physiologie*, vol. 4. Jena.

—— (1922) *Medsche Klin.*, **18**, 1214.

HESSE, R. (1895;–96;–97;–98; 1900;–03;–05;–07) *Z. wiss. Zool.*, **61**, 393; **62**, 527; **62**, 671; **63**, 456; **65**, 446; **68**, 379; **70**, 347; **72**, 565.

HESSER, C. (1913) *Anat. Hefte.*, **49**, 1.

HINES, M. (1931) *Am. J. Anat.*, **47**, 1.

HIPPEL, A. VON (1898) *Albrecht v. Graefes Arch. Ophthal.*, **45**, 286.

—— (1899) *Beiträge zur Augenheilkunde*, Halle.

HIRSCHBERG, J. (1882) *Arch. Anat. Physiol.*, **81**, 493.

HIS, W. (1880) *Arch. Anat. Entwicklungs*, **5**, 224.

HOGAN, M. J. (1961) *Trans. Pacif. Cst oto-ophthal. Soc.*, **42**, 61.

—— (1963) *Invest. Ophthalmol.*, **2**, 418.

HOGAN, M. J., ALVARADO, J. A. and WEDDELL, J. E. (1971) *Histology of the Human Eye*, Philadelphia.

HOGAN, M. J. and FEENEY, L. (1963) *J. Ultrastruct. Res.*, **9**, 10, 29, 47.

HOLMBERG, A. S. (1959) *Archs Ophthal.*, **62**, 6, 956.

HOLMES, G. (1918) *Br. J. Ophthal.*, **2**, 353, 449, 508.

HOLMES, G. and LISTER, W. T. (1915) *Brain*, **39**, 34.

HONRUBIA, F. M. and ELLIOTT, J. H. (1968) *Invest. Ophthalmol.*, **2**, 418.

HORNER, W. (1824) *Philad. J. med. phys. Sci.*, **8**, 70.

HORRIDGE, C. A. (1968) *Interneurons*, Reading: W. H. Freeman.

HOVELACQUE, A. (1927) *L'Anatomie des Nerfs Craniens et Rachidiens*, Paris.

HOVELACQUE, A. and REINHOLD, P. (1917) *Revue anthrop.*, **27**, 277.

HOWE, L. (1907) *The Muscles of the Eye*, New York.

HUBEL, D. H. and WIESEL, T. N. (1961;–62;–68) *J. Physiol., Lond.*, **155**, 385; **160**, 106; **195**, 215.

—— (1965) *J. Neurophysiol.*, **28**, 229.

—— (1969) *Nature, Lond.*, **221**, 747.

—— (1972) *J. comp. Neurol.*, **146**, 421.

HUECK, A. F. (1841) *Bewegung der Krystallinse*, Leipzig.

ICHIKAWA, A. and NAKAJIMA, Y. (1962) *Tohoku J. exp. Med.*, **77**, 136.

INGLE, D. and SCHNEIDER, G. F. (1969) *Science, N.Y.*, **168**, 1493.

INGVAR, S. (1923) *Brain*, **46**, 301.

ISHIKAWA, T. (1962) *Invest. Ophthalmol.*, **1**, 587..

IWANOFF, A. (1865;–69) *Albrecht v. Graefes Arch. Ophthal.*, **11** (1), 135; **15** (3), 284.

—— (1874) *Handbuch der gesamten Augenheilkunde*, Vol. 1, 8.

JAKUS, M. A. (1964) *Ocular Fine Structure*, Boston: Little, Brown.

JAYATILAKA, A. D. P. (1965) *J. Anat.*, **99**, 635.

JAYLE, G. E. (1939) *Appareil Lacrymal*, in *Traité d'Ophtalmologie*, Paris, **1**, 331.

JOHNSON, G. L. (1901) *Phil. Trans. R. Soc.*, **194**, 1.

JOHNSTON, J. B. (1909) *J. comp. Neurol.*, **19**, 593.

JONES, E. G. (1974) *The Neurosciences*, Ed. F. O. Schmitt and F. G. Worden, M.I.T. Press.

JONES, E. G. and POWELL, T. P. S. (1969;–70) *Brain*, **92**, 477; **93**, 793.

JONES, F. W. (1939) *J. Anat.*, **73**, 583.

KAJIKAWA, J. (1923) *Albrecht v. Graefes Arch. Ophthal.*, **112** (2), 260.

KAPLAN, H. A. (1956) *Acta radiol.*, **46**, 364.

KAPLAN, H. A. and FORD, P. M. (1966) *The Brain Vascular System*, Amsterdam.

KAPPERS, C. U. A., HUBER, G. C. and CROSBY, E. C. (1936) *The Comparative Anatomy of the Nervous System of Vertebrates Including Man*, New York.

KARPLUS, J. P. and KREIDL, A. (1909;–10;–13) *Pflügers Arch. ges. Physiol.*, **129**, 401; **135**, 138; **145**, 115.

KEENEY, A. H. (1972) *Modern Ophthalmology*, vol. 1, 2nd ed. Ed. A. Sorsby, London: Butterworth.

KEITH, A. (1913) *Human Embryology and Morphology*, London.

KERR, E. W. L. and LYSAK, W. R. (1964) *Archs Neurol., Chicago*, **11**, 593.

A.E.—34*

KESSING, S. V. (1966) *Acta ophthal.*, **44**, 439.

KEY, A. and RETZIUS, G. (1875) *Studien in der Anatomie des Nervensystems*, Stockholm.

KHAN, N. M. (1969) *Blood Supply of the Midbrain*, Thesis, London University.

KIER, E. L. (1966) *Invest. Radiol.*, **1**, 346.

KOKOTT, W. (1934) *Klin. Mbl. Augenheilk.*, **92**, 117.

KÖLLIKER, A. VON (1861) *Entwicklungsgeschichte des Menschen*, Leipzig.

KOLMER, W. (1936) in *Handbuch der mikroskopischen Anatomie des Menschen*, Ed. von Möllendorff, vol. 3, Berlin.

KOLMER, W. and LAUBER, H. (1936) in *Handbuch der mikroskopischen Anatomie des Menschen*, Ed. von Möllendorff, vol. 3 (2), Berlin.

KONIGSMARK, B. W., KALYANARAMAN, U. P., CORY, P. and MURPHY, E. A. (1969) *Bull. Johns Hopkins Hosp.*, **125**, 146.

KOSAKA, K. and HIRAIWA, K. (1915) *Folia neuro-biol.*, **9**, 367.

KRAUSE, C. (1842) In *Handbuch der menschlichen Anatomie*, **2**, Hanover.

—— (1879) In *Handbuch der menschlichen Anatomie*, 3rd ed, W. Krause, **2**, 29.

KRAUSE, W. (1854) *Z. rationelle Med.*, **4**, 337.

—— (1867) *J. Anat. Physiol., Lond.*, **1**, 346.

—— (1886) *Int. Mschr. Anat. Histol.*, **3**, 218.

KRÜCKMANN, E. (1905) *Albrecht v. Graefes Arch. Ophthal.*, **60**, 350, 452.

KUHN, R. A. (1961) *Am. J. Roentg.*, **86**, 1040.

KUHNE, W. and SEWALL, H. (1880) *Unters. physiol. Inst. Univ. Heidelberg.*, **3**, 221.

KUHNT, H. (1877) *Zentbl. med. Wiss.*, **15**, 337.

—— (1890) *Jena. Z. Med. Naturw.*, **24**, 177.

KUNTZ, A. (1953) *The Autonomic Nervous System*, 4th ed. London: Baillière Tindall.

KUPFER, C., CHUMBLEY, L. and DONNER, J. (1967) *J. Anat.*, **101**, 393.

KUZETSOVA, L. V. (1963) *Trudy šestoj naučnoj konterencii po vozrastnoj morfologii, fysiologii i biochimii*, Moskva.

LAGRANGE, F. (1920) *Archs Ophthal., Paris*, **37**, 641.

LANDOLT, E. (1870) *Arch. mikrosk. Anat., Berlin*, **7**, 81.

LANGENDORFF, O. (1894) *Pflügers Arch. ges. Physiol.*, **56**, 525.

LANKESTER, E. R. (1890) *Q. Jl. microsc. Sci.*, **31**, 124.

LANKESTER, E. R. and BOURNE, A. G. (1883) *Q. Jl. microsc. Sci.*, **23**, 177.

LATIES, A. M. (1967) *Archs Ophthal.*, **77**, 405.

LAWSON, G. (1895) *Trans. ophthal. Soc. U.K.*, **15**, 185.

LAZORTHES, G. (1961) *Vascularisation et Circulation Cérébrales*, Paris.

LAZORTHES, G., POULHES, J., BASTIDES, G. and ROULLEAU, J. (1958) *Revue neurol.*, **99**, 617.

LEBER, T. (1872) *Albrecht v. Graefes Arch. Ophthal.*, **18** (2), 25.

—— (1903) in *Handbuch der gesamten Augenheilkunde*, Ed Graefe and Saemisch, 2nd ed, vol. 2, Leipzig.

LE DOUBLE, F. (1897) *Traités des Variétés du Système Musculaire de l'Homme*, Paris.

LEESON, T. S. (1970) *Can. J. Ophthalmol.*, **15**, 609.

—— (1971) *J. Anat.*, **108**, 135.

LELE, P. P. and WEDDELL, G. (1956) *Brain*, **79**, 119.

LENDE, R. A. and POULOS, D. A. (1970) *J. Neurosurg.*, **32**, 336.

LENHOSSEK, M. (1911) *Anat. Anz.*, **37**, 137.

—— (1911) *Arch. mikrosk. Anat., Berlin*, **76**, 745.

LENZ, G. (1924) *Klin. Mbl. Augenheilk.*, **72**, 769.

LEPLAT, G. and DE JEAN, C. (1939) in *Traité d'Ophthalomologie*, Ed P. Baillart, C.. Couteau, E. Redslob and E. Velter, Paris.

LERCHE, W. (1965) in *The Structure of the Eye*, Ed. J. W. Rohen, Stuttgart.

LEWIS, P. R. and SHUTE, C. C. D. (1959) *Nature*, **183**, 1743.

LEWIS, W. H. (1912) in *Manual of Human Embryology*, vol. II, Ed. F. Keibel and F. P. Hall, Philadelphia and London.

LINDAHL, C. (1912) *Arch. Augenheilk.*, **72**, 213.

LOCKWOOD, C. (1886) *J. Anat. Physiol.*, **20**, 1.

LODATO, O. (1910) *Archs ottalm. Palermo*, **8**, 165.

LODDONI, G. (1930) *Ann. ottalm.*, **58**, 468.

LOWENFELD, I. E. (1966) *Natn. Acad. Sci. N.R.C. Publ.*, **1272**, 17.

LOWENSTEIN, O. and LOWENFELD, I. E. (1969) in *The Eye*, 3rd ed, vol. 3, Ed H. Davson, New York and London: Academic Press.

LYLE, T. K. (1958) *Applied Physiology of the Eye*, London: Baillière, Tindall & Cox.

MACMASTERS, R. E., WEISS, A. H. and CARPENTER, M. B. (1966) *Am. J. Anat.*, **118**, 163.

MAEDA, J. (1959) *Jap. J. Ophthal.*, **3**, 37.

MAGGIORE, L. (1917;–24) *Ann. ottalm.*, **40**, 317; **52**, 625.

MAGITOT, A. (1908) *Contribution à l'Étude de la Circulation Artérielle et Lymphatique du Nerf Optique et du Chiasma*, Paris.

—— (1946) *Physiologie Oculaire Clinique*, Paris.

MANN, I. C. (1927) *Trans. ophthal. Soc. U.K.*, **47**, 142.

—— (1928;–57;–64) *The Development of the Human Eye*, 1st, 2nd and 3rd ed, London: B.M.A.

—— (1929;–31) *Trans. ophthal. Soc. U.K.*, **49**, 202; **51**, 63.

———— (1931) *Trans. zool. Soc. Lond.*, **21**, 355.

—— (1933) *Br. J. Ophthal.*, **17**, 449.

—— (1957) *Developmental Abnormalities of the Eye*, London: B.M.A.

MANNHARDT, F. (1871) *Albrecht v. Graefes Arch. Ophthal.*, **17** (11).

MANNI, E. (1967) *Expl. Neurol.*, **22**, 1.

MANNI, E., BERTOLAMI, R. and DE SOLE, C. (1966) *Expl. Neurol.*, **16**, 226.

—— (1967) *Bull. Soc. ital. Biol. sper.*, **43**, Comm. 66.

MANZ, W. (1859) *Z. rationelle Med.*, 3.s., **5**, 122.

MARINA, A. (1898; 1901) *Dt. Z. NervHeilk.*, **14**, 356; **20**, 369.

MARQUARDT, R. (1966) *Klin. Mbl. Augenheilk.*, **148**, 50.

MARSHALL, J. and ANSELL, P. L. (1971) *J. Anat.*, **110**, 91.

MAURICE, D. M. (1969) in *Physiology of the Eye*, 2nd ed, Ed M. Davson, London: Churchill.

MAWAS, J. (1910) *Region Ciliare de la Rétine*, Thése de Lyon.

MAWAS, J. and MAGITOT, A. (1912) *Archs Anat. microsc.*, **14**, 41.

MECKEL, J. F. (1748) *De Quinto Pare Nervorum Cerebri*, Göttingen.

MEIBOMIUS, H. (1666) *De Vasis palpebrarum*, Helmstadi.

MEIKLE, T. H. and SPRAGUE, J. M. (1964) *Int. Rev. Neurobiol.*, **6**, 150.

MENSHER, J. H. (1974) *Surv. Ophthal.*, **10**, 1.

MERKEL, F. (1885) *Handbuch der topographischen Anatomie*, 2nd ed, Braunschweig.

—— (1887) *Anat. Anz.*, **2**, 17.

MERKE and KALLIUS (1901) Makroskopische Anatomie des Auges, in *Graefe-Saemisch, Handbuch der gesamten Augenheilkunde*, 2nd ed, **1**, chap. 1.

MEYER, F. (1887) *Morph. Jb.*, **12**, 414.

MICHAELSON, I. C. and CAMPBELL, A. C. P. (1940) *Trans. ophthal. Soc. U.K.*, **66**, 71.

MEISCHER, G. (1923) *Arch. mikrosk. Anat., Berlin*, **97**, 326.

MINKOWSKI, M. (1913) *Arb. hirnanat. Inst. Zürich*, **7**, 255.

—— (1920) *Schweizer Arch. Neurol. Psychiat.*, **6**, 201; **7**, 268.

MISHIMA, S. (1965) *Archs Ophthal., Chicago*, **73**, 233.

MISSOTTEN, L. (1965) *The Ultrastructure of the Human Retina*, Brussels.

—— (1965) in *The Structure of the Eye*, Ed J. W. Roben, Stuttgart.

MISSOTTEN, L. and VAN DEN DOOREN, E. (1966) *Bull. Soc. belge Ophtal.*, **144**, 800.

MITCHELL, G. A. G. (1953) *Anatomy of the Autonomic Nervous System*, Edinburgh, Churchill Livingstone.

MOLL, J. (1857) *Albercht v. Graefes Arch. Ophthal.*, **3** (2), 258.

MONTAGNA, W. (1967) *Advances in the Biology of the Skin*, New York.

MONTAGNA, W. and HU, F. (1967) *Advances in Biology of the Skin*, Vol. 8, The Pigmentary System, Oxford: Pergamon Press.

MOODY, M. F. (1964) *Biol. Rev.*, **39**, 43.

MORGAN, M. W. and HARRIGAN, R. F. (1951) *Am. J. Optom.*, **28**, 242.

MOSES, R. A. (1965) *Invest. Ophthalmol.*, **4**, 935.

MOTAIS, E. (1887) *L'Appareil moteur de l'Oeil*, Paris.

MOUNTCASTLE, V. B. and HENNEMAN, E. (1952) *J. comp. Neurol.*, **97**, 409.

MÜLLER, H. (1855;–57) *Albrecht v. Graefes Arch. Ophthal.*, **2** (2), 1; **3** (1), 1.

—— (1858) *Z. wiss. Zool.*, **9**, 541.

—— (1859) *Verh. phys.-med. Ges. Würzb.*, **19**, 244.

—— (1872) *Gesammelte und unterlassene Schriften*, Leipzig.

—— (1875) *Z. wiss. Zool.*, **8**, 1.

—— (1875) *Verh. phys.-med. Ges. Würzb.*, **10**, 179.

NATHAN, H. and GOLDHAMMER, Y. (1973) *Acta anat.*, **84**, 590.

NATHAN, H., OUAKNINE, M. D. and KOSARY, I. Z. (1974) *J. Neurosurg.*, **41**, 561.

NATHAN, H. and TURNER J. W. A. (1942) *Brain*, **65**, 343.

NEAL, H. V. (1914) *J. Morph.*, **25**, 1.

NEGUS, V. F. (1958) *Comparative Anatomy and Physiology of the Nose and Paranasal Sinuses*, London: Livingstone.

NIPPERT, O. (1931) *Z. Morph. Anthrop.*, **29**, 1.

NORDMAN, J., MACK, G. and MACK, G. (1974) *Ophthal. Res.*, **6**, 216.

NUEL, I. P. (1892) *Archs Ophtal., Paris*, **12**, 70.

NUSSBAUM, M. (1893) *Anat. Anz.*, **8**, 208.

—— (1902) *Verh. anat. Ges., Halle*, 137.

NUTT, A. B. (1955) *Ann. R. Coll. Surg.*, **16**, 30.

OPPEL, O. (1963) *Albrecht v. Graefes Arch. Ophthal.*, **166**, 19.

OPPENHEIMER, O. R., PALMER, E. and WEDDELL, G. (1958) *J. Anat.*, **92**, 321.

O'RAHILLY, R. (1966) *Contr. Embryol. (Carnegie Inst.)*, **38**, 1.

O'RAHILLY, R. and MEYER, D. B. (1960) *Z. Entw. Ges.*, **121**, 351.

ØSTERBERG, G. (1935) *Acta ophthal.*, Suppl. 6, 1.

OVIO, J. (1927) *Anatomie et Physiologie de l'Oeil dans la Série Animale*, Trans. C. de Jean, Paris.

PAGET, D. M. (1945) The Circle of Willis, in *Intra-Cranial Arterial Aneurysms*, Ed. W. E. Dandy, New York.

PAPPAS, G. D. and SMELSER, G. K. (1958) *Am. J. Ophthal.*, **46**, 299.

PARSONS, J. H. (1902) *R. Lond. ophthal. Hosp. Rep.*, **15**, 81.

—— (1904–5) *The Pathology of the Eye*, vols 1–2, London.

PASIK, T. and PASIK, P. (1971) *Vision Res.*, Suppl. 3, 419.

PATON, L. and MANN, I. C. (1925) *Trans. ophthal. Soc. U.K.*, **45**, 610.

PAU, H. (1957) *Ophthalmologica*, **134**, 320.

PEARSON, A. A. (1943;–44) *J. comp. Neurol.*, **78**, 29; **81**, 47.

PEDLER, C. (1961) *Br. J. Ophthal.*, **45**, 425.

PEI, Y.-F. and SMELSER, G. K. (1968) *Invest. Ophthalmol.*, **7**, 672.

PERLIA, R. (1889) *Albrecht v. Graefes Arch. Ophthal.*, **35**, 287.

PETERS, A. and PALAY, S. L. (1966) *J. Anat.*, **100**, 451.

PETIT, F. P. du (1926) *Mém. Acad. Sci. Inst. Fr.*, 69–96.

PFEIFER, R. A. (1925) *Monogrn Gesamt-geb. Neurol. Psychiat.*, **43**, 1.

PFISTER, J. (1890) *Albrecht v. Graefes Arch. Ophthal.*, **36**, 83.

PHILLIPS, A. J. (1972) *Br. J. physiol., Optics*, **27**, 141.

PICK, J. (1970) *The Autonomic Nervous System*, Philadelphia: Lippincott.

PIERSON, R. J. and CARPENTER, M. B. (1974) *J. comp. Neurol.*, **158**, 121.

PIRENNE, M. A. (1967) *Vision and the Eye*, 2nd ed, London: Chapman & Hall.

PIRIE, N. W. (1949) *Br. J. Ophthal.*, **33**, 271.

PITZORNO, N. (1913) *Archs ital. Anat. Embriol.*, **11**, 527.

POCKLEY, F. (1919) *Med. J. Aust.*, **1**, 509.

POIRIER, P. (1911) *Traité d'Anatomie Humaine*, 3rd ed, **5**; fasc 2 (Les Organes du Sens).

POLYAK, S. L. (1941) *The Retina*, Chicago.

—— (1957) *The Vertebrate Visual System*, Chicago.

PRINCE, J. H. (1949) *Visual Development*, Edinburgh: Livingstone.

PURPURA, D. P. and YAHR, M. D. (1966) *The Thalamus*. New York: Columbia University Press.

QUAIN, R. (1894) *Elements of Anatomy*, Ed E. A. Schäfer and G. D. Thane, vol. III, part III, London.

—— (1898) *Elements of Anatomy*, Ed E. A. Schäfer and G. D. Thane, vol. I, part I, new ed, London.

—— (1900) *Elements of Anatomy*, Ed E. A. Schäfer and G. D. Thane, vol. III, London.

RABL, C. (1903) *Über den Bau und Entwicklung der Linse*, Leipzig.

RANSON, S. W. and MAGOUN, H. W. (1933) *Archs Neurol. Psychiat., Chicago*, **30**, 1193.

RASMUSSEN, L. and WINDLE, W. F. (1960) Ed, *Neural Mechanisms of the Auditory and Vestibular Systems*, Springfield: C. C. Thomas.

REDSLOB, E. (1927) *Annls Oculist.*, **164**, 107, 721.

—— (1932) *Le Corps Vitré*, Paris.

—— (1939) in *Traité d'Ophthalmologie*, vol. 1, Paris.

RHOTON, A. L., KOBAYASHI, S. and HOLLINSHEAD, W. A. H. (1968) *J. Neurosurg.*, **29**, 609.

RICHIARDI, S. (1887) *Atti Accad. naz. Lineci Rc.*, **1**, 193.

RIEHL, H. A. (1908) *Int. Mschr. Anat. Physiol.*, **25**, 181.

ROBERTSON, A. (1869) *Edinb. med. J.*, **14**, 696; **15**, 491.

ROCHON-DUVIGNEAUD, A. (1903) *Encycl. franc. d'Ophtal.*, **1**, 369.

—— (1933) *Recherches sur l'Oeil et la Vision chez les Vertébrés*, Paris.

—— (1943) *Les Yeux et la Vision des Vertébrés*, Paris.

RODIECK, R. W. (1973) *The Vertebrate Retina*, San Francisco.

ROHEN, H. (1964) in *Möllendorf's Handbuch der Mikroskopischen Anatomie des Menschen*, vol. III, part, 4, p. 239, Berlin.

ROSEN, E. S. (1969) *Fluorescence Photography of the Eye*, London: Butterworths.

ROSSIGNOL, S. and COLONNIER, M. (1971) *Vision Res.*, Suppl., 3.

RUSHTON, W. A. H. (1962) *Visual Pigments in Man*, Liverpool University Press.

RUSKELL, G. L. (1968;–71a;–74) *J. Anat.*, **103**, 65; **109**, 374; **118**, 195.

—— (1969) *Z. Zellforsch. mikrosk. Anat.*, **94**, 261.

—— (1970;–71b;–73) *Expl Eye Res.*, **10**, 319; **12**, 166; **16**, 183.

SALZMANN, M. (1912) *Anatomy and Histology of the Human Eyeball*, Trans E. V. L. Brown, Chicago.

SANDERS, O. (1974) *Br. J. Ophthal.*, **58**, 468.

SARDEMANN, E. (1884) *Zool. Anz.*, **7**, 569.

SÄTTLER, C. (1876) *Albrecht v. Graefes Arch. Ophthal.*, **22** (2), 1.

SCHALY, G. A. (1926) Thesis, Gröningen.

SCHIEFFERDECKER, P. (1905) *Z. Augenheilk.*, **14**, 186.

SCHIRMER, O. (1894; 1903) *Albrecht v. Graefes Arch. Ophthal.*, **56**, 468; **58**, 197.

SCHLOSSMAN, A. and PRIESTLEY, B. S. (1966) *Strabismis*, Boston.

SCHULTZE, M. (1873) in *Stricker's Manual of Human and Comparative Histology*, vol. 3, London.

SCHWALBE, G. (1874) in *Handbüch der gesamten Augenheilkunde*, Ed Graefe and Samisch, 1st ed, vol. 1, Leipzig.

—— (1887) *Lehrbuch der Anatomie der Sinnesorgane*, Erlangen.

SCHWARTZ, W. (1961) in *The Structure of the Eye*, Ed G. K. Smelser, New York: Academic Press.

SCHWARZ, J. (1925) *Z. Anat. Entw-Gesch.*, **75**, 361.

SCHWEINITZ, G. DE (1923) *Trans. ophthal. Soc. U.K.*, **43**, 12.

SCOTT, B. L. and PEASE, D. C. (1959) *Am. J. Anat.*, **104**.

SEEFELDER, R. (1930) in *Kurzes Handbüch der Ophthalmologie*, vol. 1, Ed F. Schieck and A. Brücker, Berlin.

SESEMANN, E. (1869) *Arch. Anat. Physiol. wiss. Med.*, p. 154.

SHELLSHEAR, J. E. (1920) *J. Anat.*, **55**, 25.

—— (1927) *Brain*, **50**, 236.

SHERRINGTON, C. S. (1905) *Proc. R. Soc.*, B., **76**, 160.

—— (1906) *The Integrative Action of the Nervous System*, London.

SILLITO, A. M. and ZBROZYNA, A. W. (1970) *J. Physiol.*, **211**, 461.

SINCLAIR, D. (1967) *Cutaneous Sensation*. Oxford University Press.

SINGH, S. and DASS, R. (1960) *Br. J. Ophthal.*, **44**, 193, 286.

SIVANANDASINGAM, P. (1973) *London University Thesis*, London.

SJÖSTRAND, F. S. (1948) *J. appl. Phys.*, **19**, 1188.

—— (1958) *J. Ultrastruct. Res.*, **2**, 122.

SMELSER, G. K. and ISHIKAWAS, T. (1966) *Acta XIX Cong. Ophthal. India*, **1**, 612.

SMITH, C. G. and RICHARDSON, W. F. G. (1966) *Am. J. Ophthal.*, **62**, 1391.

SMITH, G. E. (1907) *J. Anat. Physiol., Lond.*, **40**, 200.

—— (1919) *J. Anat.*, **53**, 271.

—— (1928) *Trans. ophthal. Soc. U.K.*, **47**, 64.

—— (1930) *J. Anat.*, **64**, 430.

SONDERMANN, R. (1933) *Acta ophthal.*, **11**, 280.

SORSBY, A. and SHERIDAN, M. (1960) *J. Anat.*, **94**, 192.

SPEMANN, H. (1938) *Embryonic Development and Induction*, New Haven, U.S.A.

SPITZNAS, M. (1970) *Albrecht v. Graefes Arch. Ophthal.*, **180**, 44.

STANFIELD, J. P. (1960) *J. Anat.*, **94**, 2, 251.

STANNIUS, H. (1839) *Handbuch der Anatomie der Wirbelthiere*, 2nd ed, Berlin.

STEELE, E. J. and BLUNT, M. J. (1956) *J. Anat.*, **90**, 486.

STEINER, L. (1923) *Annls Oculist.*, **160**, 137.

STEPHENS, R. B. and STILWELL, D. L. (1969) *Arteries and Veins of the Human Brain*, Springfield, Illinois: C. C. Thomas.

ST. HELEN, R. and MCEWEN, W. K. (1961) *Am. J. Ophthal.*, **52**, 539.

STIBBE, E. P. (1928) *J. Anat., Lond.*, **62**, 159.

STONE, J. and HANSEN, S. M. (1966) *J. comp. Neurol.*, **126**, 601.

STOPFORD, J. S. B. (1916;–17) *J. Anat. Physiol., Lond.*, **50**, 131; 255, **51**, 250.

STOTLER, W. A. (1937) *Proc. Soc. exp. Biol. Med.*, **36**, 576.

STREETEN, B. W. (1967) *Archs Ophthal.*, **81**, 383.

STUDNICKA, F. K. (1898) *Jena. Z. Naturw.*, **31**, 1.

SUMITA, R. (1961) *Acta Soc. ophthal. jap.*, **65**, 1188.

SUNDERLAND, S. and HUGHES, E. S. R. (1946) *Brain*, **69**, 301.

SZENTÁGOTHAI, J. (1942;–43) *Arch. Psychiat. NervKrankh.*, **115**, 127; **116**, 721.

—— (1970) in *The Neurosciences*, Ed F. O. Smith and F. G. Worden, New York.

—— (1973) in *Handbook of Sensory Physiology*, VIII, Ed R. Jung, Berlin.

SZILY, A. VON (1903) *Anat. Hefte*, **34**, 417.

—— (1908) *Anat. Hefte*, **35**, 649.

—— (1921) *Albrecht v. Graefes Arch. Ophthal.*, **101**, 195.

TARLOV, E. and TARLOV, S. R. (1971) *Brain Res.*, **34**, 37.

TENON, J. R.. (1806) *Mémoires et Observations sur l'Anatomie*, Paris.

THEOBALD, G. D. (1934) *Trans Am. ophthal. Soc.*, **32**, 574.

THOMSON, A. (1912) *Anatomy of the Human Eye*, Oxford.

THUMA, B. D. (1928) *J. comp. Neurol.*, **46**, 173.

TODARO, F. (1875) *Atti R. Accad. Lincei*, **2**, 55.

TOMINIAGA, Y. L. and IKUI, H. (1964) *Acta Soc. ophthal. jap.*, **48**, 397.

TORMEY, J. M. (1966) *Trans. Am. Acad. Ophthal. Oto-lar.*, 761.

TOUSIMIS, A. J. and FINE, B. S. (1959) *Am. J. Ophthal.*, **48**, 397.

TOUSSAINT, D. (1947) *A Treatise of Gonioscopy*, Philadelphia.

—— (1958) *Bull. Soc. belg. Ophtal.*, **120**, 589.

TOUSSAINT, D., KUWABARA, T. and COGAN, D. G. (1961) *Archs Ophthal.*, **65**, 575

TOZER, F. M. and SHERRINGTON, C. S. (1910) *Proc. R. Soc.*, B, **82**, 450.

—— (1910) *Am. J. Ophthal.*, **58**, 408.

TRAQUAIR, H. M. (1948) *An Introduction to Clinical Perimetry*, London: Kimpton.

—— (1957) *Clinical Perimetry*, 7th ed, Ed G. I. Scott, London: Kimpton.

TRIPATHI, R. C. (1971) *Expl. Eye Res.*, **11**, 116.

—— (1972) *Br. J. Ophthal.*, **56**, 157.

—— (1973) *Lancet*, **2**, 8.

TSAI, C. (1925) *J. comp. Neurol.*, **39**, 173.

TSCHERNING, M. H. A. (1898) *Optique Physiologique*, Paris.

TSUCHIDA, U, (1906) *Arb. hirnanat. Inst Zürich*, **2**, 1.

TURNER, A. L. (1901) *The Accessory Sinuses of the Nose*, London.

—— (1908) *Lancet*, ii, 396.

—— (1908) *Br. med. J.*, ii, 730.

URIBE-TRONCOSO, M. (1909) *Annls Oculist.*, **142**, 237.

—— (1921;–25) *Am. J. Ophthal.*, **55**, 321; **8**, 433.

VAN DER STRICHT, O. (1922) *Arch. d. Biol.*, **32**, 346.

VIDIĆ, B. (1968) *Anat. Rec.*, **162**, 511.

VILLARD, H. (1896) *Montpell. méd.*, **5**, 651, 672, 693.

VIRCHOW, H. (1881) *Z. wiss. Zool.*, **35**, 247.

—— (1882) *Beiträge zur vergleicherden Anatomie des Auges*, Berlin.

—— (1902) *Über Tenon'schen Raum und Teno'schen Kapsel*, Berlin.

—— (1906) in *Handbuch der gesamten Augenheilkunde*, Ed Graefe and Saemisch, 2nd ed, part 1, Leipzig.

—— (1910) in *Handbuch der gesamten Augenheilkunde*, Ed Graefe and Saemisch, 2nd ed, vol. 1, Leipzig.

VOGT, A. (1921) *Klin. Mbl. Augenheilk.*, **66**, 321, 718, 838.

VRABEC, F. (1952) *Ophthalmologia*, **123**, 210.

—— (1955) *Čslká Oftal.*, **11**, 213.

—— (1966) *Am. J. Ophthal.*, **62**, 926.

WALKER, A. E. (1938) *The Primate Thalamus*, Chicago.

WALLS, G. L. (1942) *The Vertebrate Eye*, New York: Cranbrook.

—— (1963) *The Vertebrate Eye* (reprint), New York: Haffner.

WALSH, F. B. and HOYT, W. F. (1969) *Neuro-Ophthalmology*, Baltimore.

WARD, F. O. (1858) *Outlines of Human Osteology*, 2nd ed, London.

WARWICK, R. (1953) *J. comp. Neurol.*, **98**, 449.

—— (1954) *J. Anat.*, **88**, 71, 555.

—— (1955) *Brain*, **78**, 92.

—— (1956) *Ann. R. Coll. Surg.*, **19**, 36.

—— (1964) in *The Oculomotor System*, Ed M. B. Mercer, New York.

WARWICK, R. and WILLIAMS, P. L. (1973) *Gray's Anatomy*. 35th ed. London and Edinburgh: Churchill Livingstone.

WATTS, J. W. (1934) J. Anat., **68**, 534.

WEDDELL, G. (1941) *J. Anat.*, **75**, 346.

WEDDELL, G., PALMER, E. and PALLIE, W. (1955) *Biol. Rev.*, **30**, 159.

WEEKERS, R., GRIETEN, J. and LAVERGNE, G. (1961) *Ophthalmologica*, **142**, 650.

—— (1961) *Bull. Soc. belge. Ophthal.*, **129**, 361.

WEEKERS, R., GRIETEN, J., LAVERGNE, G. and LEKEUX, M. (1963) *Ophthalmologica*, **146**, 57.

WEISKRANTZ, L. (1972) *Proc. R. Soc.*, B, **182**, 427.

WEISS, L. (1887) *Anat. Hefte*, **8**, 191.

WENDT, E. C. (1877) *Über die Harder'sche Drüse der Säugethiere*, Strassburg.

WHITE, J. C., SMITHWICK, R. M. and SIMEONE, F. A. (1952) *The Autonomic Nervous System*, 3rd ed. London: Kimpton.

WHITFIELD, I. C. (1967) *The Auditory Pathway*, London: Edward Arnold.

WHITNALL, S. E. (1911) *J. Anat. Physiol., Lond.*, **46**, 36.

—— (1932) *Anatomy of the Human Orbit*, 2nd ed, Oxford: Blackwell Scientific.

WHITTERIDGE, D. (1937) *J. Physiol.*, **89**, 99.

WIEDERSHEIM, R. (1898) *Grundriss der vergleichenden Anatomie der Wirbelthiere*, 4th ed, Jena.

WIESEL, T. N. and HUBEL, D. H. (1966) *J. Neurophysiol.*, **29**, 1115.

WILLBRAND, H. (1929) *Der Faserverlauf durch das Chiasma*, Berlin.

WILLIAMS, P. L. and WARWICK, R. (1975) *Functional Neuroanatomy of Man*, Edinburgh: Churchill Livingstone.

WILLIS, T. (1664) *Cerebri Anatome*, Amsterdam.

WINCKLER, C. (1927) *Manuel de Neurologie*, Haarlem.

WINCKLER, G. (1937) *Archs Anat. Histol. Embryol.*, **23**, 219.

—— (1956) *C. r. Ass. Anat.*, **43**, 848.

WISE, G. N., DOLLERY, C. T. and HENKIND, P. (1971) *The Retinal Circulation*, New York: Harper Row.

WOLFF, E. (1946) *Trans. ophthal. Soc. U.K.*, **66**, 291.

—— (1951) *Lancet*, **260** (1), 888.

—— (1953) *Brain*, **76**, 455.

WOLFF, E. and DAVIES, F. (1931) *Br. J. Ophthal.*, **15**, 609.

—— (1938) *Proc. R. Soc. Med.*, **31**, 1104.

WOLFF, E. and PENMAN, C. G. (1950) *Proc. int. Congr. Ophthal., London*, **2**, 625.

WOLFRING, E. (1872) *Anatomy of the Human Orbit*, 2nd ed, Oxford.

WOLFRUM, M. (1907;–08;–08) *Albrecht v. Graefes Arch. Ophthal.*, **65**, 220; **67**, 307, 670; **69**, 145.

WOLTER, J. R. (1955) *A.M.A. Archs Ophthal.*, **53**, 201.

—— (1959) *Am. J. Ophthal.*, **48**, 370.

—— (1961) in *The Structure of the Eye*, Ed G. H. Smelser, New York: Academic Press.

WOOD, C. A. (1917) *The Fundus Oculi of Birds*, Chicago.

WOOLLARD, H. H. (1925) *Proc. zool. Soc. Lond.*, **127**, 1071.

—— (1926) *Brain*, **49**, 77.

—— (1927) *Recent Advances in Anatomy*, London.

—— (1931) *J. Anat.*, **65**, 225.

WOOLLARD, H. H. and BEATTIE, J. (1927) *J. Anat.*, **61**, 414.

WOOLSEY, C. N. (1964) in *Cerebral Localization and Organization*, Ed G. Shalterbrand and C. N. Woolsey, Madison, U.S.A.

WYBAR, K. C. (1954) *J. Anat.*, **88**, 94.

XUEREB, G. P., PRICHARD, M. M. L. and DANIEL, P. M. (1954) *Q. Jl exp. Physiol.*, **39**, 119, 219.

YAMAMOTO, T. (1966) *Jap. J. Ophthal.*, **10**, 1, 40.

ZAKI, W. (1960) *Archs Anat. Histol. Embryol.*, **45**, 105.

Zander, E. and Weddell, G. (1951) *J. Anat.*, **84**, 397.
Zeis, E. (1835) *Z. ophthal.*, **4**, 231.
Zeitzschmann, O. (1904) *Albrecht v. Graefes Arch. Ophthal.*, **58**, 61.

INDEX